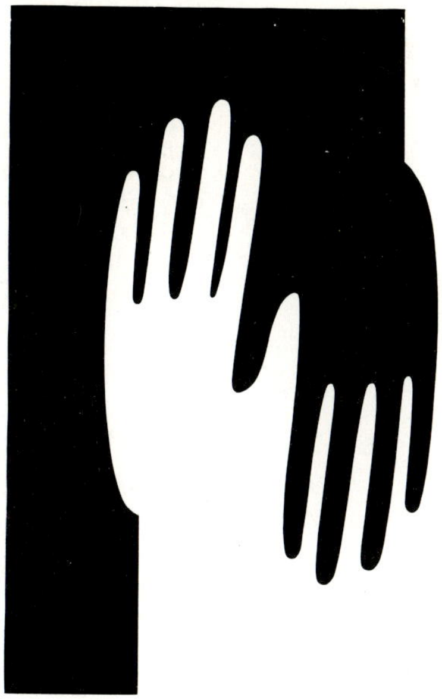

The Hand

Surgical and Non-surgical Management

EDITED BY

EUGENE S. KILGORE, JR., M.D.

Clinical Professor of Surgery, Director of the Hand Services, Department of Surgery, University of California Medical School, San Francisco, California

WILLIAM P. GRAHAM, III, M.D.

Professor of Surgery, Chief, Division of Plastic and Reconstructive Surgery, Pennsylvania State University College of Medicine, Hershey, Pennsylvania

LEA & FEBIGER · PHILADELPHIA

1977

The decorative device used appears through the courtesy and with the permission of Abbey Press, Saint Meinrad, Indiana.

Library of Congress Cataloging in Publication Data

Main entry under title:

The Hand.

Includes index.
1. Hand—Surgery. 2. Hand—Wounds and injuries.
3. Hand—Diseases. I. Kilgore, Eugene S. II. Graham,
William P. [DNLM: 1. Hand. 2. Hand—Surgery.
3. Hand injuries—Therapy. WE830 H234]
RD559.H36 1977 617′.575 76-40478
ISBN 0-8121-0534-6

Published in Great Britain by Henry Kimpton Publishers, London

PRINTED IN THE UNITED STATES OF AMERICA

Print Number: 4 3 2 1

To our many teachers, and with great appreciation to our families who have provided so much encouragement: our wives Mimi Kilgore and Susan A. Graham and our children Eugene and Bee Kilgore and Elizabeth and Susan P. Graham.

When amulets and talismans are lost, the mouth dry, the bladder empty, and time too short for prayers and incantations, the hand is quickly available.

(Gifford, Ed., Jr., M.D., *The Evil Eye,*
Macmillan Press, 1958)

Preface

Many texts dealing with the hand exist, some of which are superb. However, all have limitations in covering and making readily accessible the information needed for diagnosis and management of all common clinical problems. Perhaps it is impossible to do so, but this text is an effort in that direction. It is born out of frustration in searching for opinions and the answers to reach a solution to existing cases. Hopefully, it will fill such voids as a reference for most students and clinicians dealing with the hand, regardless of the extent of their experience or existing library source.

There is no claim to originality, for, indeed, today, such a claim is usually but a reflection of inadequate knowledge of the experience of others, whether published or not. On the contrary, credit is given, even if not specified, to all who have shared in furthering knowledge and experience of treatment of the hand. It is particularly extended to the masters of the past, most of whom are founder members of the American Society for Surgery of the Hand.

An effort has been made to emphasize a method rather than all methods of management, and, thus, for the sake of practicality and simplicity, avoid an encyclopedic approach. The methods cited have stood the test of experience and proven as effective and predictable as any others. There has been extensive collaboration between the distinguished contributors and the editors in order that the format of the text be consistent. Information of purely historical or academic and limited clinical value has not been included.

Chapters have been included on subjects not generally covered in other texts but, nevertheless, germane to the care of patients with hand problems. These include functional anatomy, anesthesia, common skin disorders of the hand, stiffness, pain, pitfalls of treatment and psychological aspects of hand injury. Photographs and illustrations have been discreetly chosen. Particular attention has been paid to indexing so as to facilitate the reader's search for information.

We are deeply indebted to the many hand surgeons who have contributed to and cooperated dedicatedly on this endeavor, as well as to the non-contributors (including medical students and patients) who have stimulated and supported us. To one mentor, J. William Littler, we are particularly grateful, for his stimulus, enthusiasm, dedicated teaching and innumerable ingenious designs of effective and worthy surgical techniques served to initiate our interest in the hand and, now, this text. His influence has embodied much more than technique. It has reached the core of medicine and surgery: Mastery of the patient's needs, awareness of the practicalities of any treatment, practice of the art of medicine, execution of esthetic surgery with precision and humility about any outcome.

Most of all we are thankful to our families, our colleagues Dr. William L. Newmeyer, III, Dr. Stephen H. Miller, and Dr. Thomas S. Davis, our secretaries Donna Morris, Helen Caldwell, Virginia Osborne, and Nancy Ebersole, our artist, Kelly Alsedek, and the executive editor of Lea & Febiger, Mr. Edward H. Wickland, Jr., for their great help and patience throughout these seven years.

Finally, no effort of this sort is ever without room for improvement. We always welcome criticism and advice.

San Francisco, California
Hershey, Pennsylvania

EUGENE S. KILGORE, JR., M.D.
WILLIAM P. GRAHAM, III, M.D.

Contributors

HAROLD W. BALES, M.D. (deceased)
Associate Professor of Plastic Surgery
University of Rochester Medical School
New York

JOHN L. BELL, M.D.
Professor of Clinical Surgery
Northwestern University Medical School
Chicago

F. WILLIAM BORA, JR., M.D.
Associate Professor of Orthopedic Surgery
University of Pennsylvania School of Medicine
Philadelphia

JOHN A. BOSWICK, M.D.
Professor of Surgery
University of Colorado
Chairman of Hand Surgery and Rehabilitation Services
Denver

RICHARD I. BURTON, M.D.
Chairman of Section for Surgery of the Hand,
Department of Orthopaedics
Associate Professor of Orthopaedics
University of Rochester Medical School
New York

SYLVESTER CARTER, M.D.
Clinical Professor of Surgery
New York Medical College
Director of Hand Surgery
Flower & 5th Avenue Hospital; Metropolitan Hospital Center; Sydenham Hospital; and West Chester Medical Center.

W. BRUCE CONOLLY, F.R.C.S. (Eng.), F.R.A.C.S., F.A.C.S.
Honorary Surgeon
Sydney Hospital, Paramatta Hospital, St. Luke's Hospital
Surgeon in Charge
Sydney Hospital Hand Clinic, NSW, Australia

THOMAS E. DRAKE, M.D.
Assistant Clinical Professor of Dermatology
University of California Medical School
San Francisco

RICHARD G. EATON, M.D.
Co-Director, Hand Surgery Service
Department of Surgery
The Roosevelt Hospital
Associate Clinical Professor of Surgery
Columbia University
New York

WILLIAM P. GRAHAM, III, M.D.
Professor of Surgery
Chief, Division of Plastic and Reconstructive Surgery
Pennsylvania State University College of Medicine
Hershey

MICHAEL HARTY, M.A., M. Ch., F.R.C.S.
Professor of Anatomy and Orthopedic Surgery
School of Medicine
University of Pennsylvania
Philadelphia

EUGENE S. KILGORE, JR., M.D.
Clinical Professor of Surgery
University of California Medical School
Co-Director of the Hand Service
San Francisco General Hospital
San Francisco

HOWARD MAIBACH, M.D.
Professor of Dermatology
University of California Medical School
San Francisco

STEPHEN H. MILLER, M.D.
Associate Professor of Surgery
Division of Plastic and Reconstructive Surgery
Pennsylvania State University College of Medicine
Hershey

WILLIAM L. NEWMEYER, III, M.D.
Associate Clinical Professor of Surgery
University of California Medical School
Co-Director of the Hand Service
San Francisco General Hospital
San Francisco

KARL ROSENFELD, M.D.
Orthopedic Surgeon
Paoli Memorial Hospital
Paoli

RONALD H. ROSILLO, M.D.
Assistant Professor of Psychiatry and of Physical Medicine and Rehabilitation
University of Pennsylvania School of Medicine
Philadelphia

JAMES W. SMITH, M.D.
Associate Professor of Clinical Surgery
Cornell University Medical College
Associate Attending Surgeon, The New York Hospital—Cornell Medical Center
New York

LINTON A. WHITAKER, M.D.
Associate Professor of Surgery (Plastic)
University of Pennsylvania School of Medicine
Philadelphia

Contents

1 Historical Aspects of Modern Hand Surgery

Since the early part of this century surgery of the hand has evolved from a consideration of hand infections into a broad field of regional specialization, including the entire upper extremity. If all important contributions were to be mentioned, the story of the development of hand surgery would be a book in itself.

The first major advance in modern surgery of the hand was the publication of Allen B. Kanavel's book, *Infections of the Hand,* in 1912. It was the culmination of nearly ten years of systematic studies of the applied anatomy of the fascial spaces of the hand. These studies, as they were applied to clinical practice, revolutionized the treatment of hand infections. The book was widely accepted throughout the world and its popularity was attested to by the publication of seven editions up to 1939. It was the only practical textbook on the hand during World War I; the second and third editions appeared in 1914 and 1916.

Although other special fields such as plastic, orthopedic and thoracic surgery benefited by the war experiences of 1917–1918, no important progress was made in hand surgery as a result of World War I. The fear of infection deterred most surgeons from attempting either primary or secondary procedures. Generally, hand injuries were treated in a random manner: many were left open to drain, and initial treatment consisted mainly of pouring antiseptic solutions into the wounds. Toward the end of the war, however, the principle of primary wound excision followed by delayed closure began to be applied by military surgeons. Unfortunately, that method was not uniformly carried over to civilian practice. Reconstructive procedures were seldom attempted and crippled hands usually remained functionless.

During World War I, Sterling Bunnell developed a deep interest in surgery of the hand. In 1918, his first article on the hand dealt with tendon repairs of the fingers and appeared in *Surgery, Gynecology and Obstetrics,* a leading surgical journal with Allen B. Kanavel as its associate editor. Bunnell, Sumner L. Koch, Henry Marble and Michael L. Mason, all destined to become notable figures in the fields of trauma and hand surgery, served with the U. S. Army Medical Corps in France from 1917 to 1919.

Hand Surgery from World War I to World War II

In the interval between World War I and World War II, hand surgery developed steadily but slowly. During that time the significant advances could be attributed only to the repeated efforts of a relatively few surgeons in North America and overseas. After infections were better understood, the basic principles of treatment of open hand injuries remained to be established. Halsted's precepts regarding tissue handling in relation to wound healing were quickly adopted by certain surgeons who eventually became noted in the field of hand surgery. In 1921 Bunnell introduced the term *atraumatic technique,* which was to become the byword of hand surgery throughout the world.

The pioneers of hand surgery in the years before World War II would not be called hand surgeons in the sense of the term as it is understood today. These men had a broad background and experience in general surgery, and for the most part did not limit their endeavors to any particular region. Kanavel was considered a master surgeon and was noted for major contributions in the fields of neurological and abdominal surgery as well as for an intense interest in subjects pertaining to the hand. Bunnell, Koch, Marble, Mason and other recognized contributors to hand surgery maintained a wide interest in many other surgical areas throughout their careers.

After World War I, in Chicago, Kanavel was joined in the practice of surgery by Sumner L. Koch, who became interested in the treatment of burns and open wounds with particular reference to the hand. Michael Mason entered practice with them in 1928, and after Kanavel's retirement in 1935 Harvey S. Allen joined the internationally known group. In addition to their teachings and many articles about the management of acute injuries of the hand, the Chicago group made many of the early outstanding contributions on such subjects as Dupuytren's contracture, tuberculous tenosynovitis and congenital anomalies of the hand. The experimental studies on the process and rate of tendon healing by Mason, Shearon and Allen established a basis for successful tendon repair and have withstood the test of time for more than thirty years.

For many years Kanavel's book on infections was the only practical text available to those undertaking treatment of surgical disorders of the hand. There were no books concerning topics other than infections until Iselin's monograph appeared in 1933. The next textbook on the hand was published in England in 1940. The author, R. M. Handfield-Jones, dedicated the book to Dr. Kanavel whose tragic death occurred in an automobile accident in 1938. It was not until 1942 that a textbook on hand surgery was published in the United States. The book was written by Condict W. Cutler, Jr., of New York, and entitled *The Hand: Its Disabilities and Diseases.*

In addition to Bunnell and his colleague, Joseph H. Boyes of California and the Chicago group, other names appeared in the surgical literature pertaining to infections and other disorders of the hand. Among them were: Hugh Auchincloss, Condict Cutler, Jr., and Leo Mayer of New York City; Marc Iselin of Paris; Deryl Hart of Duke University; and Henry Marble of Boston. All of these surgeons strove to upgrade the quality of care for hand injuries and infections, which unfortunately was often carried out by untrained practitioners or inexperienced house officers. Furthermore, most of the surgical world considered the treatment of injuries and infections of the hand in the realm of minor surgery until after World War II.

Hand Surgery in World War II

Surgery of the hand as an area of regional specialization began, for the most part, in the United States Army during the last two years of World War II. Until that time no special consideration had been given to the treatment of soldiers with hand injuries or other wounds affecting hand function. In 1944, Major General Norman T. Kirk, the Surgeon General, sought to alleviate the haphazard situation which existed regarding military hand casualties. He requested that Sterling Bunnell of San Francisco be appointed as a special civilian consultant to the Secretary of War in order to develop hand surgery in the Army. This appointment was implemented by the designation of nine hand services within the Zone of Interior to receive serious hand injury cases.

In November, 1944, many soldiers with disabling hand deformities were scattered in military hospitals throughout the United States. There was no comprehensive plan for managing hand casualties, and few surgeons were sufficiently experienced to treat and follow a complex hand case to a point of optimal functional return. The overall result was a high incidence of functionless hands.

By early 1945, military casualties with severe hand injuries were referred to hand surgery services at the nine general hospitals in the Army's Zone of Interior. Although those hospitals were functioning then as plastic surgery centers, the hand surgery services were designated as autonomous units. The hospitals selected for hand services were: Newton D. Baker, William Beaumont, Crile, Cushing, Dibble, Northington, Valley Forge and Wakeman General Hospitals.

The first edition of Bunnell's comprehensive textbook *Surgery of the Hand* was published in 1944. It was adopted immediately as an official text by the Army and was widely distributed throughout military medical installations.

On November 29, 1944, Dr. Bunnell began the first of eight extensive teaching tours which continued for the next two years. Comprehensive courses, each lasting three to four days, were given in large general hospitals. The programs included operative clinics conducted by Dr. Bunnell, patient presentations, conferences and lectures. As many as sixty patients were examined during the course of each session. The courses were popular, and were attended by many officers throughout each service command. Some 1945 photographs showed as many as thirty persons crowded around Dr. Bunnell as he operated on a soldier's hand.

During the tours made by the special consultant, twenty-three courses were given in twenty different hospitals and forty-nine additional visits made to twenty-seven other hospitals.

It was Dr. Bunnell's conviction that a hand surgeon be a master of the entire region and not merely a tissue specialist. A chief of a hand service required a good general surgery background but also experience in orthopedic, plastic, and neurosurgery. In addition, he had to be able to teach to provide for future hand surgical teams. The overall results obtained at the special hand centers far surpassed anything heretofore known in the annals of military surgery. Many of the participating surgeons had to be retained on active service long after other military surgeons had been discharged because there were no adequate replacements to handle the extensive load of patients needing reconstructive surgery of the hand.

Many of the officers stationed at hand centers during World War II continued an active interest in hand surgery after they were discharged from military duty. A roster of chiefs of service of their hospitals during the peak period, June to October, 1945, included: Major S. B. Fowler at Baker; Lt. William H. Frackelton at Beaumont; Major Gilbert Hyroop at Crile; Captain J. W. Littler at Cushing; Major Donald R. Pratt at Dibble; Major Arthur J. Barsky at Northington; Major George S. Phalen at O'Reilly; Major Walter C. Graham at Valley Forge; and Major Lot D. Howard, Jr., at Wakeman General Hospital.

Following one of the wartime tours by Dr. Bunnell, the idea of forming a postwar group for continuing education in hand surgery was conceived. Darrel T. Shaw consulted with Joseph H. Boyes, a former resident and associate of Dr. Bunnell. One night during the fall of 1945, five military surgeons with a common interest in surgery of the hand met informally and the basic plan for the American Society for Surgery of the Hand was formulated. The surgeons who participated at that meeting were J. H. Boyes, S. B. Fowler, R. L. Payne, Jr., D. T. Shaw, and George Webster.

The concept of such an association was embraced immediately by Dr. Bunnell, who was asked to submit names of prospective members. Dr. Boyes was selected chairman of an organizational meeting to be held in Chicago in January of 1946. Twenty-six of the thirty-five founding members were present at that meeting. Sterling Bunnell was elected president of the new society and in his 1947 presidential address accurately predicted a forthcoming worldwide interest in the development of the field.

Hand Surgery Following World War II

The early activities of the American Society for Surgery of the Hand had an outstanding influence upon the development of hand surgery in the United States. At the first scientific meeting in 1947, more than two hundred fifty doctors registered for the program. By the end of its third year the Society's membership doubled in number. Open discussions of common problems and the interchange of new ideas and techniques attracted the attention of many enthusiastic surgeons and residents from the fields of general, orthopedic and plastic surgery.

Immediately following the war there was an almost explosive demand for all kinds of specialty training by returning medical officers and postwar intern classes. For a considerable period not enough places were available to meet the ever-increasing demand for training in hand surgery. At that time preceptor training was the usual method for continuing education in the field. Because of the lack of programs and postgraduate courses, many early aspirants had to be content to visit the relatively few hand centers as observers.

Gradually, more preceptor and residency training programs were established in the United States. Practically all the directors of the hand surgery programs were members of the American Society for Surgery of the Hand. By 1970, fifty-six centers in North America and three overseas were available for advanced training. At present, however, there is no formal standardization of hand training programs, and minimum training requirements in hand surgery by specialty boards are not well defined.

The spread of the American Society's activities stimulated development of hand associations in many countries. In 1951, the Scandinavian Society for Surgery of the Hand was formed and continued to develop under such men as Moberg, Önne, Carstam and Bang-Rasmussen. In Great Britain two associations for hand surgery were started: the Hand Club of Great Britain in 1952 and the Second Hand Club in 1956. Those two groups soon combined to form the British Society for Surgery of the Hand under the leadership of such men as Pulvertaft, Seddon, Kilner, Capener, Clarkson, Graham Stack, Furlong, Molem and others. In 1957, Joseph H. Boyes was influential in organizing the Japanese Society for Surgery of the Hand.

Other hand organizations have continued to develop overseas and regionally in the United States and Canada. There are now associations for France and Switzerland, Italy, Brazil and Portugal. The Spanish-speaking countries of South America have a hand society and an association of hand surgeons has developed in the German-language countries of Europe.

Liaison among ten international hand organizations was established in 1968 with formation of an International Federation of Societies for Surgery of the Hand. Moberg of Sweden and Pulvertaft of England have served as presidents, and Barsky of New York serves as secretary-general. Committees composed of international representatives have been established for such subjects as standardization of nomenclature, accident prevention, disability and functional evaluation, bibliography and congenital malformations.

The world medical literature now abounds with material about the upper extremity. Since 1967, the American Society for Surgery of the Hand has sponsored a computerized listing of all publications pertinent to the field of hand surgery. The 1970 volume of the *Bibliography of Surgery of the Hand* contained over four hundred pages with separate listings of articles and authors.

Following the introduction of Bunnell's textbook on hand surgery in 1944, numerous other books have been published on the subject through the ensuing years. Some have weathered through several editions. Boyes was responsible for the major revision of Bunnell's book in 1964 and again for the fifth and sixth editions. Rank and Wakefield, now joined by Hueston, are considered the leaders of hand surgery in Australia. Their book, *Surgery of Repair as Applied to Hand Injuries,* now in its third edition, remains the most outstanding primer on the acutely injured hand. Flatt's book on acute hand injuries can well be considered a complementary text to the work of the Australian authors. Kaplan's text, *Functional and Surgical Anatomy of the Hand,* continues as a practical reference for surgeons. The limitation of space prevents acknowledgment of other notable books in the field of hand surgery.

It would be difficult to undertake a critical review of all outstanding advances in surgery of the hand since World War II. Various names have appeared repeatedly in the world literature and on postgraduate programs pertaining to hand surgery. Many of them are known internationally for their particular skills, interests, contributions or teaching abilities.

Bunnell, Boyes, Mason, Pulvertaft, Littler, Riordan, Verdan, Brand, Goldner, White and a host of others are considered highly in the areas of tendon repair, tendon grafts and transfers. Skoog, McIndoe, Larsen and Posch, Luck, L. D. Howard, Hueston and many others are noted for introducing changing concepts and techniques in Dupuytren's disease. Moberg's critical evaluation of the importance of sensibility in relation to hand function has stimulated a continuing search for improved methods of nerve repair.

The surgical treatment of rheumatoid disease has developed steadily over the past fifteen years. In any discussion of the subject the names of Flatt, Lipscomb, Marmor, Niebauer, Phalen, Straub, Swanson and Vainio constantly appear. A consideration of reconstruction of the thumb would bring forth the work of Hilgenfeldt, Gosset, Moberg, Littler, Peacock and many others. Buncke, Davis, Jacobson, Kleinert and J. W. Smith have made outstanding contributions in the development of microsurgical techniques for hand surgery.

The problem of attaining uniformly satisfactory results following primary or secondary tendon procedures continues as a major challenge. Peacock and Cameron have experimented with the use of homologous composite grafts of the entire digital flexor tendon mechanism. Hunter, Carroll and others have approached the problem by clinical use of artificial tendon implants. Investigations by Peacock, Madden and others on the biological control of scar tissue represent a major breakthrough toward solving the complex problems of wound healing in relation to gliding function.

There is an expanding interest in the social and economic significance of hand injuries. Approximately one of every three industrial or home accidents involves the hand. The surgeon who undertakes the care of the injured or disabled hand will be challenged by the increasing demand for higher standards of both care and result.

References

1. Boyes, J.H.: *Bunnell's Surgery of the Hand,* 5th ed. J.B. Lippincott, Philadelphia, 1970.
2. Bunnell, S., Ed.: *Hand Surgery in World War II.* Office of the Surgeon General, Department of the Army, Washington, 1955.
3. Bunnell, S.: *Surgery of the Hand.* J.B. Lippincott, Philadelphia, 1944.
4. Cutler, C.W., Jr.: *The Hand: Its Disabilities and Diseases.* W.B. Saunders, Philadelphia, 1942.
5. Flatt, A.E.: *The Care of Minor Hand Injuries,* 2nd ed. C.V. Mosby, St. Louis, 1963.
6. Handfield-Jones, R.M.: *Surgery of the Hand.* Williams and Wilkins, Baltimore, 1940.
7. Iselin, M.: *Chirurgie de la Main.* Masson et Cie, Paris, 1933.
8. Kanavel, A.B.: *Infections of the Hand.* Lea & Febiger, Philadelphia, 1912.
9. Kaplan, E.B.: *Functional and Surgical Anatomy of the Hand,* 2nd ed. J.B. Lippincott, Philadelphia, 1965.
10. Mason, M.L.: Fifty year's progress in surgery of the hand. Int. Abstr. Surg., 101:541, 1955.
11. Rank, B.K., Wakefield, A.R. and Hueston, J.T.: *Surgery of Repair as Applied to Hand Injuries,* 3rd ed. Williams and Wilkins, Baltimore, 1968.

2 Anatomy

Man has been compared and contrasted with many animal species, both favorably and unfavorably, since the dawn of time. Nowhere has his dominance been more commonly expounded than in the structural and functional adaptions encountered in the hand. This organ has been recognized as the symbol of man's power, the outward reflection of his inner mind, the precise instrument of his perception, in fact the indispensable tool of his inheritance and independent livelihood. The human foot is specifically adapted for weight bearing, balance, stability and locomotion. The conversion from pronograde to bipedal orthograde position has liberated the hand for man's technological and cultural advances, constructive or destructive as they may be.

The prime functions of the hand are feeling (sensibility) and motion. These modalities have become highly refined and adaptive and, together with the evolution of the thumb, have endowed man's hand with superior aptitudes that have fostered his intellectual advance. The thumb is the prime digit responsible for this achievement. It is natural, therefore, that it dominates the representation of the extremity in the sensory and motor cortex.

To accomplish its function, the hand is powered by an intricate system of synergistic and antagonistic muscles acting on a long cantilevered skeletal frame. The major part of this frame is designed primarily to position the hand. Musculotendinous units running from it to the hand provide power while the small intrinsic muscles of the hand itself position the thumb and provide dexterity.

In correcting disorders of the hand, the focus is always on the maintenance and restoration of basic function: pinch and grasp. Therefore, all physical management is oriented toward maintaining the "position of function" (Fig. 2-1). It is varied to meet individual needs but, in the main, is defined as the position that permits the most basic requirements of hand function. This position should facilitate feeding and toilet requirements and comfortable, forceful, non-fatiguing effort.

Generally speaking, the elbow should be held to a right angle, the forearm neutral, the wrist extended 30° and the fingers furled to within meeting distance of the pronated thumb. This ensures the independence of the patient in daily survival in spite of the most overwhelming afflictions of the hand.

Sound diagnosis and treatment of hand disorders are predicated on the understanding of functional

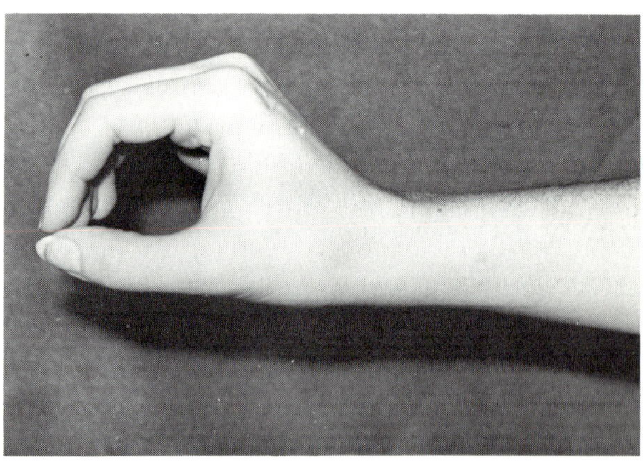

Figure 2-1. *The "position of function" maintains the longitudinal and transverse arches of the hand while positioning the digits for grasp or pinch.*

anatomy. Without this, it is impossible to foresee the functional consequence of any problem and to avoid the creation of disability by iatrogenic misadventure.

Nomenclature

All references to the forearm and hand should be made to the volar (palmar) or dorsal (extensor) surfaces and to the radial and ulnar sides (not lateral and medial). The digits are identified as the thumb—ray I, index finger—ray II, long (middle) finger—ray III, ring finger—ray IV, and little finger—ray V (Fig. 2-2).

Surface Anatomy

The surface anatomy of the hand presents a number of landmarks and characteristics which are of clinical importance.

Joints

The radiocarpal joint is found immediately beneath the proximal skin creases of the volar and dorsal aspect of the wrist. The distal radioulnar joint lies off the center of the wrist and immediately subcutaneous to the proximal dorsal wrist crease. The basal joint of the thumb (carpometacarpal joint) is at the distal limit of the anatomical snuffbox. The metacarpophalangeal joints of the fingers lie beneath the distal fourth of the palm.

Bony Prominences

The tip of the radial styloid is at the proximal margin of the anatomical snuffbox. Here the abductor pollicis longus and flexor pollicis brevis emerge from their fibro-osseous sheath and form the radial border of the snuffbox. Lister's tubercle, the pulley for the extensor pollicis longus, can be felt on the dorsal radius. Distally, the extensor pollicis longus forms the ulnar boundary of the snuffbox (Fig. 2-3).

The base of the index and long metacarpals can be readily palpated at the level of the distal extensor crease. When the fist is clenched, the tensed tendons of the extensor carpi radialis longus and brevis can be felt just proximal to these metacarpals. The prominence of the base of the thumb metacarpal lies radially and receives the abductor pollicis longus, primarily a radial wrist deviator.

Four bony prominences can be felt in the heel of the hand. These prominences are the points of

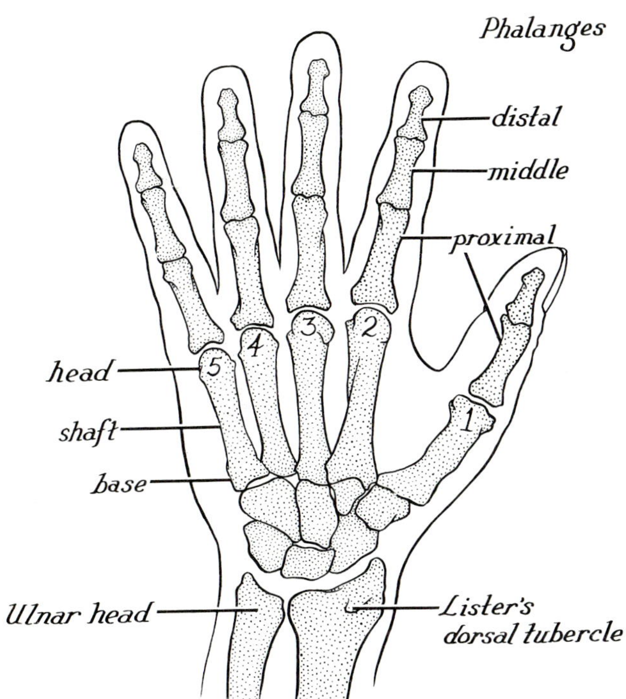

Figure 2-2. *Proper nomenclature for the hand.*

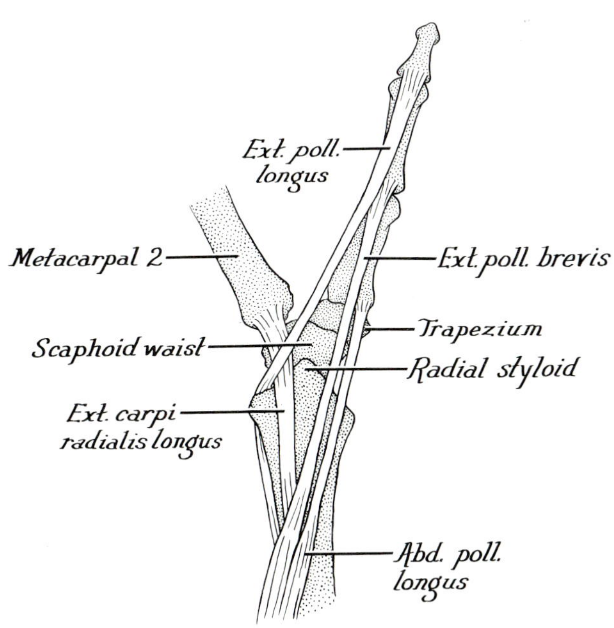

Figure 2-3. *Schematic representation of the "anatomical snuffbox."*

attachment of the flexor retinaculum.* On the extreme ulnar side, at the distal flexion crease, is the slightly mobile pisiform bone, the sesamoid of the flexor carpi ulnaris. Just distal to this is the hook of hamate, about which lie the two important distal branches of the ulnar nerve, the deep motor branch and the superficial sensory branch.

The tubercle of the scaphoid at the distal flexor crease of the wrist and the slightly more distal ridge of the trapezium are the two radial bony prominences. The distal edge of the flexor retinaculum is felt with deep pressure in the center of the heel of the palm. The tendon of the flexor carpi radialis disappears into the hand after passing over the scaphoid tuberosity. The palmar carpal ligament bridges the flexor carpi radialis radially and the loge de Guyon on the ulnar side of the heel of the hand.

On the volar aspect of the metacarpophalangeal joint of the thumb, sesamoid bones lie on either side of the floor of the flexor sheath.

Tendons

The snuffbox on the dorsal radial aspect of the wrist can be demonstrated only with active extension—abduction of the thumb (Fig. 2-3). The radial boundary of the snuffbox is formed by the extensor pollicis brevis superficial to the deeper lying abductor pollicis longus. The ulnar border of the snuffbox is the extensor pollicis longus. Further ulnarward are the powerful radial wrist extensors previously described. On the ulnar side of the wrist just distal to the styloid of the ulna, the extensor carpi ulnaris may be palpated when the patient makes a tight fist.

Centrally on the dorsum, the long extensors of the fingers become prominent with simultaneous extension of the wrist and fingers as they emerge from under the extensor retinaculum.

Volar to the wrist joint are three wrist flexors which are easily demonstrated by flexing the wrist against resistance as the thumb and little finger are pinched together. These are the flexor carpi radialis passing over the tubercle of the scaphoid, the centrally located palmaris longus joining the palmar fascia, and the flexor carpi ulnaris. The latter is more easily palpated when the hand is spread. In the distal palm the prominence of the proximal pulleys of the fingers can generally be palpated over the center of axis of the different metacarpals.

*This is the combined term for the palmar carpal ligament and the deeper, thicker and more distal transverse carpal ligament (the roof of the carpal canal).

Fascia

The distal edge of the extensor retinaculum lies under the proximal extensor crease of the wrist. All the extensors of the digits and wrist pass under it on their way from the forearm. On the flexor side, the leading edge of the flexor retinaculum can be palpated. The only other fasciae that are normally palpable are the natatory ligaments across the apices of the webs. The fascia most commonly affected and palpable in disease is the palmar fascia which thickens with Dupuytren's fasciitis.

Nerves and Vessels

On the dorsum are the prominent veins. On the volar aspect of the radial and ulnar styloids are the palpable radial and ulnar arteries respectively. The former can be traced in the floor of the anatomical snuffbox, and the latter can sometimes be felt in the heel of the hand just distal to the hook of the hamate.

The radial nerve can be rolled under the palpating finger just proximal to the radial styloid and the much smaller dorsal branch of the ulnar nerve just distal to the ulnar styloid. The median nerve is either subcutaneous or just deep to the palmaris longus on the midvolar aspect of the wrist. Proximal to the flexion creases it is quite vulnerable and usually will give a slightly positive Tinel's sign upon percussion. At the elbow, proximal to the antecubital flexion crease, the median nerve can be rolled under the examiner's finger along the medial border of the biceps tendon.

The superficial sensory branch of the ulnar nerve can be rolled on the hook of the hamate in the palm. The main ulnar nerve is vulnerable to pressure in the groove behind the medial humeral epicondyle.

The volar digital nerves and the arteries deep to them can be easily compressed against the phalanges anywhere along their course.

Skin

The dorsal skin is loose and pliable, whereas the volar skin is thick and tethered by the underlying fascia. The palmar creases are points of fixation by fascia to the underlying bone. It must be remembered that the point of maximum concentration of critical functional structures in the hand (nine flexor tendons, the median nerve, the motor branch of the ulnar nerve and two arterial arches) lies in an area in the center of the heel of the hand which can be covered by a 1.5-cm circle. The center of this hub is at the intersection of the central axis of the long finger ray and the volar border of the fully extended thumb.

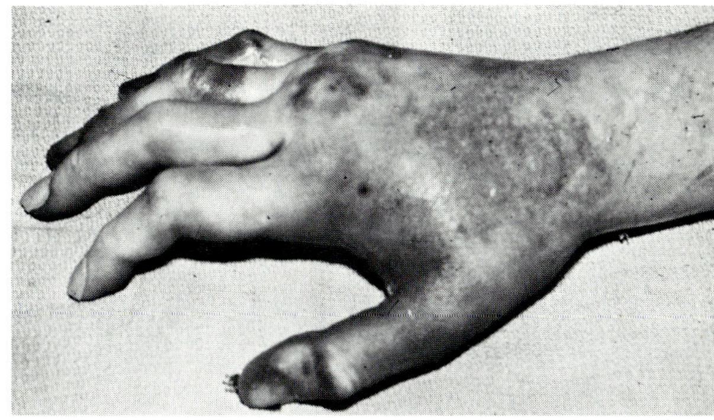

Figure 2-4. *"Claw hand in disguise." A deep dermal burn of the dorsum is initiating metacarpophalangeal joint extension due to the tight dorsal skin and underlying edema.*

Anatomy of the Skin

The skin of the forearm and hand is, for the most part, untethered except in the palm and the palmar side of the digits. Although it is elastic, it can become a venous tourniquet in the presence of excessive swelling. Functionally it varies in the hand from the dorsal to the volar aspect.

Volar skin is tethered by an extensive network of fascial strands to stabilize it for efficiency of grasp and pinch. The concentration of these strands is greatest at the level of the palmar and digital creases and the lateral borders of the digits and palm. These become a problem when they restrict expansion and stretching of skin to accommodate congestion. Thus the tourniquet effect of the skin over the palmar fat pads is easily aggravated by injury or infection.

The palmar skin is also thick and has a rich concentration of sweat glands. This complements the skin lines in providing needed friction. Although thick, it is not particularly tough, but has the propensity for relatively rapid hypertrophy and the development of protective calluses. The sensory innervation gives the fingertips some of the most exquisite epicritic sensibility of any skin of the body. The disadvantage of this is appreciated when wounds give rise to sensitive scars or neuromata.

The dorsal skin is untethered and subject to much more excursion and stretching than the palmar skin. This is functionally necessary in order to allow the fist to close without restricting the transverse and longitudinal arches. In going from a flat hand to a tightly closed fist, the adult stretches the dorsal skin at least 2 to 3 cm in the longitudinal and transverse planes.

Under the dorsal skin lies the predominant venous and lymphatic drainage of the hand, so that tightness here serves to compress and choke the circulation. The looseness of the skin favors the sequestration of edema fluid beneath it, and with distension of the subcutaneous space the tense skin forces the metacarpophalangeal joints into extension and the thumb ray into adduction ("a claw hand in disguise") (Fig. 2-4). The looseness of the skin also favors skin avulsions from tangential forces (e.g. wringer injury).

In contrast to volar skin, two specialized appendages of the dorsal epidermis—the hairs and nails—can give rise to problems of infection.

Functionally, the skin may be thought of as a protective cloth, covering the forearm and the hand. It is seldom appreciated by the novice that the long finger of the average adult male needs 56 cm^2 of skin for coverage and that the body of the hand exclusive of the fingers requires 250 cm^2 of skin to cover it.

Anatomy of Fat

The fat of the hand is specialized and does not regenerate. Therefore it must be respected and protected. Its prime function is to cushion the palm. It is maintained in position throughout the volar aspect by fascial strands. There are not true septae, so isolated "compartments of fat" as such do not exist.

Palmar fat remains constant in amount and does not fluctuate in response to changes in body weight. However, it does atrophy with sensory denervation. The fat of the forearm and dorsum of the hand is similar to body fat elsewhere, and varies with the obesity of the patient.

Clinically, the importance of fat is twofold in surgery of the hand: (1) It is invaluable as a medium for vascularizing tendons and establishing favorable adhesions for excursion of the tendons. (2) It is at times indispensable as a cushion around nerves, tendons, and bony prominences.

Fascia

The functions of fascia are the stabilization of structures, the maintenance of form and the restriction of motion. It accomplishes these by its composition of collagen and connective tissue with limited elasticity. It is identified by its white and relatively avascular appearance and is recognized at surgery by the fact that it can easily be placed under tension for orderly dissection.

It exists in many different forms—from relatively thin, even delicate strands or sheets to highly developed, tough structures such as collateral ligaments and pulleys. The dictum of atraumatic surgery is to cut only the tissue that can be tightened with the retractors and flicked with a probe, namely, the fascia.

The inelasticity of fascial tissue and its propensity for swelling, thickening, and shrinking are the bases for a host of pathological states. Often it proves dispensable in treating these. The fascial sleeves of the forearm, hand, and digits, tight pulleys of tendons and ligaments of joints, and strands that tether the palmar skin must often be split, sectioned, or removed to relieve congestion, constriction, and stiffness.

Fascia of the Forearm

The clinical importance of the fascia at this level is its definition of three compartments: (1) the passage for the ulnar nerve at the elbow (ulnar groove and cubital tunnel), (2) the flexor wad including a sling, the lacertus fibrosus, and (3) the extensor wad. The tunnel for the ulnar nerve is dispensable when it causes constriction. The fascia forming this tunnel bridges from the medial epicondyle to the olecranon.

The fascia of the extensor and flexor wads is the deep fascia of the forearm and has numerous septae to the long bones. These septae have to be divided in mobilizing musculotendinous units and achieving access to vessels and nerves. Once divided, the anatomy of these structures becomes quite clear. The greatest cause for clinical concern about this deep fascia is its ability to deceptively choke the circulation to these separate muscle wads, leading to ischemic necrosis and fibrosis (Volkmann's contracture). Too often, the tightness of one compartment or the other has been masked by the overlying padded skin or the surgical release of one compartment has obscured the need for releasing the other. Slitting this fascia does not impose any functional handicap at all and should be done routinely as a prophylatic measure in the conduct of reparative surgery of musculotendinous and neurovascular structures of the forearm.

Fascial Structures About the Wrist

The deep fascia of the forearm condenses on the dorsum of the wrist to form the six compartments that house the extensor tendons. This is a rather broad structure approximately 2.5 to 3.5 cm wide. It blends with the deep fascia of the volar side at the radial and ulnar borders of the wrist. It has relatively little functional significance but clinically has to be respected in the conduct of tenorrhaphies and the relief of stenotic changes (de Quervain's tenosynovitis). In acting as a pulley system of the extensors it necessitates the coexistence of the extensor synovial bursae which secrete the lubricating fluid. These bursae extend well distal and proximal to the limits of the retinaculum and, like their counterparts on the flexor surface, are avenues for the rapid spread of infection. They are also the site of other common pathological states, namely, non-infectious tenosynovitis and extensor sheath ganglia.

On the volar aspect of the wrist, the deep fascia of the forearm merges with the palmar carpal ligament, the superficial and proximal portion of the flexor retinaculum. The stouter component of this retinaculum is the transverse carpal ligament which is deeper and slightly more distal. The fibers of the palmar carpal ligament are transverse. The palmaris longus tendon which is longitudinally oriented interdigitates with the ligament as it passes into the palmar aponeurosis to form the pretendinous bands.

The palmar carpal ligament is a condensation of the deep fascia of the forearm as the fascia passes over the wrist. To stabilize the volar skin, the fascia attaches to the pisiform and the fifth metacarpal on the ulnar side, where it blends with the flexor carpi ulnaris to form a roof over the ulnar nerve and artery (loge de Guyon). On the radial side, it blends with the tubercle of the scaphoid and covers the flexor carpi radialis from which it extends into the fascia of the thenar wad and becomes fixed to the first metacarpal. A network of vertical strands anchors the palmar skin to this ligament over the heel of the hand.

Blending loosely to the deep side of this ligament is the transverse carpal ligament, the roof of the carpal canal. It is one of the toughest ligaments of the body. It is approximately 2.5 cm wide and at times is 5 to 7 mm thick. It is anchored on the radial side to the tubercle (ridge) of the greater multiangular (trapezium) and on the ulnar side to the hook of the hamate (Fig. 2-5). The median nerve is immediately beneath this ligament on the radial side of the carpal canal. The tiny thenar motor branch of this nerve usually hooks around the distal margin of the ligament. Its many variations must be known (Fig. 15-17). Competing for space in this narrow tunnel are the nine long flexor tendons to the digits and their synovial bursae. Occasionally there is a large median artery as well.

The clinical significance of the flexor retinaculum lies in the fact that its transverse carpal ligament binds the median nerve and flexor tendons. This produces either a carpal tunnel syndrome or permits restrictive adhesions to form when there has been any injury of the tendons passing through the carpal canal. In these instances, this relatively dispensable ligament is sectioned.

The synovial bursae are avenues for the spread of infection and the target of non-infectious tenosynovitis (rheumatoid) (Fig. 2-6). The radial and ulnar bursae may communicate with one another. The ulnar bursa of the little finger encompasses all

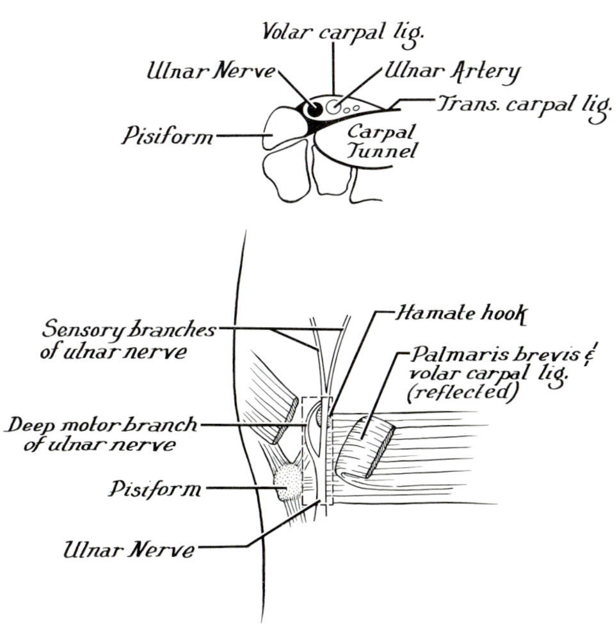

Figure 2-5. *Anatomy and relationships of the flexor retinaculum.*

of the long flexors of the wrist and passes through the carpal tunnel into the distal forearm. The bursae around the tendons of the index, long, and ring fingers extend to the midpoint of the palm. The radial bursa runs from the thumb into the distal forearm. Parona's space is deep to the radial and ulnar bursae and superficial to the pronator quadratus. This space becomes infected by extension from the radial or ulnar bursa.

Fascia of the Body of the Hand

In the dorsum of the hand, the fascia blends with the extensor retinaculum but is considerably thinner. It creates two spaces in the dorsum of the hand, the dorsal subcutaneous and subaponeurotic spaces. The plane between these two contains the digital extensors. Laterally this fascia fuses with the palmar fascia and fixes to the marginal metacarpals, especially at the level of the metacarpophalangeal joints. Over the web spaces where this fascia thins, edema fluid and pus from the palm can gain access to the dorsum of the hand. The dorsal nerves and veins are superficial to this fascia. A deeper fascia covers the intrinsic muscles (interossei and adductor of the thumb).

Clinically this fascia forms three spatial levels. The two superficial spaces (subcutaneous and subaponeurotic) are frequent reservoirs for abscess formation which may require separate drainage. The fascia investing the intrinsic muscles must be split in the presence of congestion if ischemic fibrosis and secondary contractures are to be avoided.

The palmar aponeurosis is an extensive system of longitudinal, transverse and vertical components. These compartmentalize the tendons, lumbricals, and neurovascular structures, running longitudinally to the fingers. The palmar skin is tethered by innumerable fascial strands stretching from the aponeurosis and its anchorage to the marginal metacarpals where it blends with the dorsal fascia.

The longitudinal components (pretendinous bands) are the extensions of the palmaris longus and run over the flexor tendons to the metacarpal heads. A separate, but lesser, band is sometimes found over the thumb ray. The configuration of this sheet of fascia is that of a ribbed fan, with transverse fibers between the pretendinous bands (ribs) forming the superficial transverse ligament in the midpalm. The pretendinous bands, although volar to this transverse ligament, are intimately interwoven with it. All fibers regardless of direction

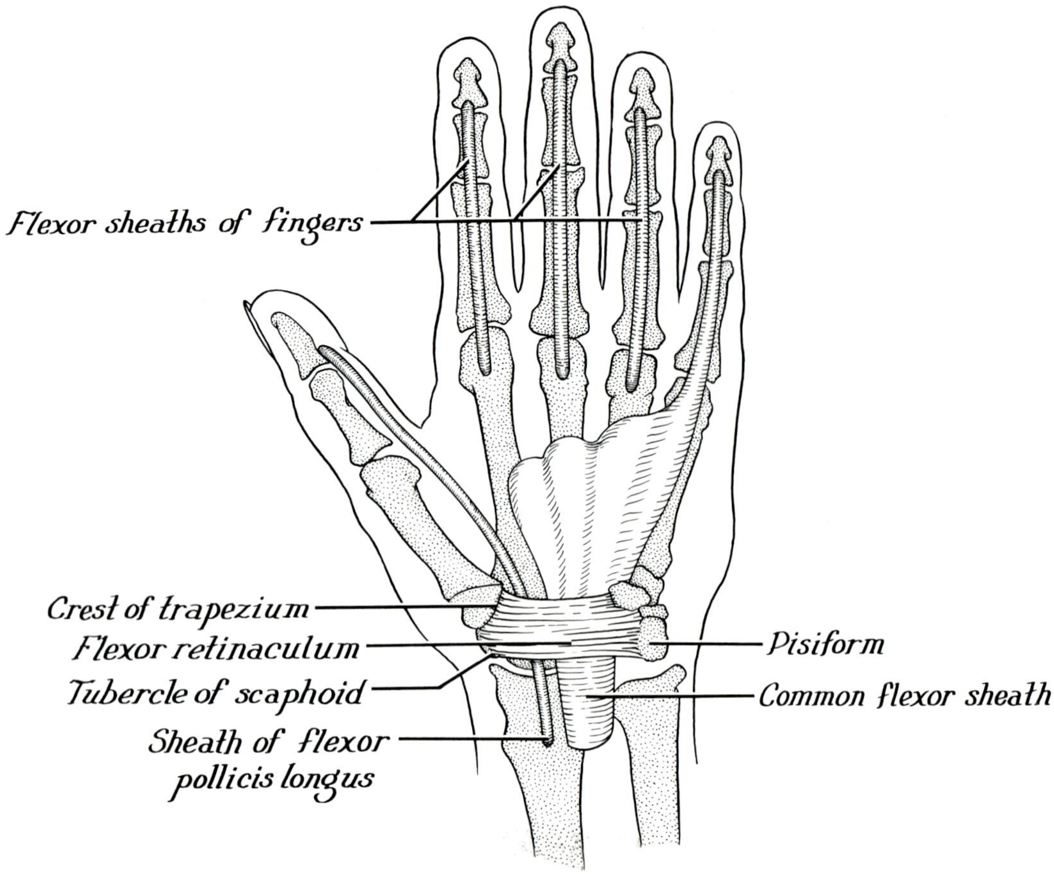

Figure 2-6. *Flexor synovial bursae.* (*Redrawn from Cunningham.*[3])

(longitudinal, vertical, or transverse) fuse without predictable anatomical planes at the margins of the seven tunnels (four tendinous and three neurovascular and lumbrical spaces) formed by the vertical septae.

Except in the midpalm, the long flexor tendons of the fingers are surrounded by the synovial sheaths. The proximal flexor pulleys of the flexor sheaths are found in the distal palm. These are totally distinct from the juxtaposed palmar fascia and can easily be spared in any dissection of the latter.

The web spaces contain additional fascia sheets, the natatory (interdigital) ligaments. These ligaments also have transverse fibers which fuse with the flexor sheaths and with the yoked lateral extensions of the pretendinous bands and lateral fascial sheets of the proximal phalanges. Between the superficial transverse ligament and the natatory ligaments of Grapow are windows which are devoid of fascia and through which the distal palmar fat pads bulge. The neurovascular bundles bifurcate deep in these windows.

The deep fascia of the palm is that which overlies the volar interossei and the adductor of the thumb. Deeper than the palmar aponeurosis is the fascia investing the hypothenar and thenar musculature.

The clinical significance of the fascia of the palm resides in its capability to restrict expansion in accommodating edema, its separation of the palm into spaces and its capacity of undergoing the changes of Dupuytren's fasciitis with the development of nodules and contractures. Unlike dissections on the forearm and dorsum of the hand, the ramifications of the palmar fascia are one of the principal factors contributing to the intricacy, complexity, and prognostic dilemmas of hand surgery.

Fascia of the Digits

The fascia of the digits is composed of an encircling membrane and specific restraining ligaments of the skin and extensor hood mechanisms symmetrically arranged on the radial and ulnar sides of the digits. In addition, it forms the specialized retinacular system of the flexor tendon sheaths and bursae. The encircling membrane is not unlike the fascia of the forearm. However, it is often barely definable on the volar hemisphere. On the sides of the digit it can be identified as the lateral fascial sheet closely allied to the skin, and dorsally as a membrane immediately over the extensor band.

There are specific subdivisions (septae and bands) of this system which have important functions in stabilizing the skin against tangential motion. The volar fat pads are tethered to the underlying bone or flexor sheath with a myriad of fine vertical strands erroneously referred to as septae. At the flexion creases the fat pads are reduced and the fascia acts as a drawstring to pull in the skin so flexion can occur. In so doing, it also creates what is referred to as the "anterior closed spaces" by almost interrupting the continuity of the fat pads.

Dorsally, the skin of the distal phalanx, from the distal joint to the crest of the eponychium, is markedly tethered. Laterally in the proximal and middle phalanges, the skin is tethered and the volar neurovascular bundles are straddled by two sheets of fascia. The volar one is Grayson's ligament, the transverse fibers of which join the flexor sheath (Fig. 2-7). The dorsal one is Cleland's ligament, with oblique fibers securing the skin to the phalanges. Both of these ligaments attach to the lateral fascial sheet. The natatory ligament of the web joins the proximal limit of this sheet. The pretendinous band of the palmar aponeurosis normally phases out as a distinct structure when it reaches the proximal digital fat pad and encircling membrane of the digit. However, it may form recognizable "spiral bands" as yoke-like connections with the lateral sheet (Fig. 2-8).

The extensor hood mechanism of the digit is held in place and its action complemented by the static forces of three retinacular bands—the oblique retinacular ligament of Landsmeer distally, the transverse retinacular ligament centrally, and the sagittal bands (transverse) proximally. These are discussed under extensor tendons (Chap. 14).

The flexor sheath system holds the tendons snugly in position during flexion. Condensations act as pulleys to counteract the forces of bowstringing. The synovial bursae described previously begin at the insertion of the long flexors on the distal phalanges. Those of the index, long, and ring fingers terminate in the distal palm.

The clinical importance of the fascia of the digit

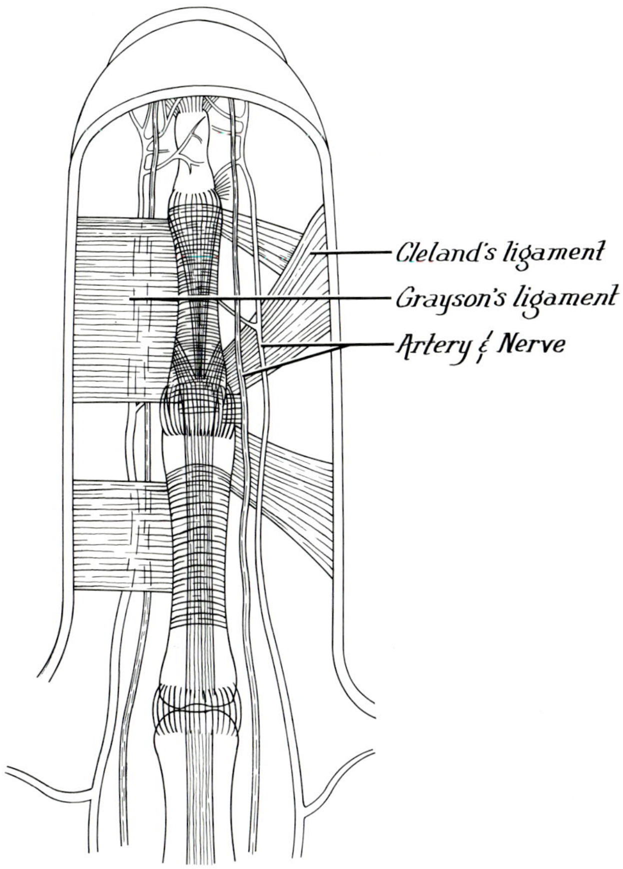

Figure 2-7. *Grayson's ligament (transverse) and Cleland's ligament (oblique). (Redrawn from Milford, L.*[8])

parallels that of the fascia in the palm. In addition, there are some special problems related to the extensor retinacular system which are discussed in Chapter 14.

Anatomy of the Bones and Joints

The basis for architectural excellence and functional supremacy of the hand can be appreciated in part by focusing attention on the skeletal properties before adding the contributions of the soft tissues.

The positioning of the cantilevered system of the upper extremity and the execution of acts of dexterity are dependent upon a wide range of motion of many joints. Fortunately, there is an overlap of the functional range of one joint or many joints to another not only in the extremity but in the trunk as well, so that an impairment in one area can be well compensated for and, in fact, escape notice. Thus, the shoulder serves well to compensate for function of the loss of forearm and wrist motion,

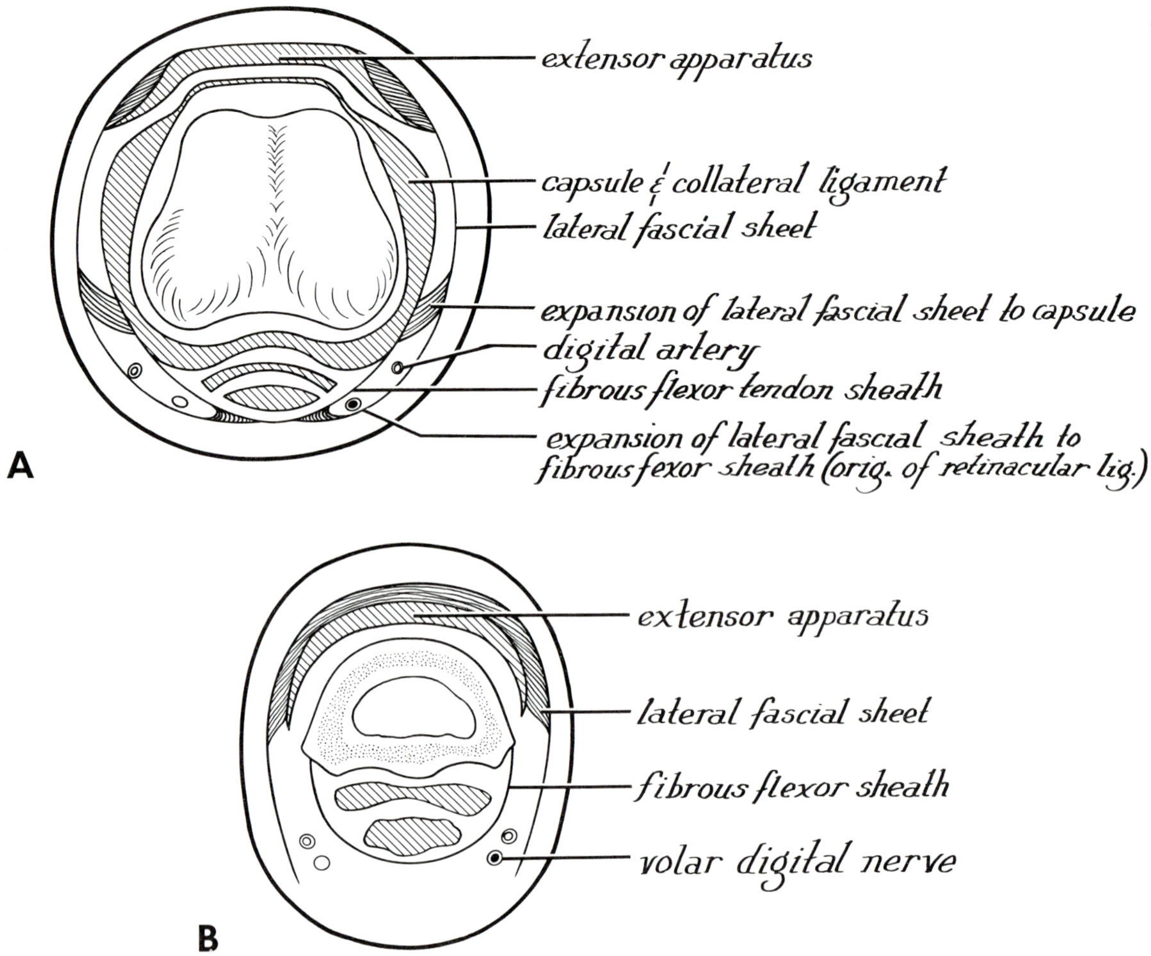

Figure 2-8. *Diagrammatic representation of the terminations of the pretendinous bands in the lateral fascial sheet of the digit.* (*Redrawn from Hueston, J.T. and Tubiana, R.*[6])

while the back, neck, and wrist will compensate for the elbow. In the thumb any two joints usually compensate for the loss of one. In the case of the fingers, any two joints may compensate for the loss of any one of the other joints of the ray.

The forearm rotates about an axis that runs through the radial head to the tip of the long finger. In pivoting around this axis, the radius rotates around the distal ulna through a range of 140° from full pronation to full supination. The hand can be circumducted about this axis by the wrist (the key joint of the hand) which moves at two levels of the carpus. Maximal extension (±50°) is at the level of the intercarpal joint and maximal flexion (±50°) is at the level of the radiocarpal joint. This is in contrast to extension of ±35° at the radiocarpal joint and flexion of ±35° at the intercarpal joint. All of the lateral motion is at the radiocarpal joint (±35° ulnar deviation, ±20° radial deviation). Thus, there is an aggregated range of wrist extension of ±85° for a total range of 170° and a total lateral excursion of 55°.

The prime weight-bearing surfaces at the wrist are between the concavity of the radius and the lunate and scaphoid. The centripetal stress along the forearm is transferred from the radius to the ulna by the interosseous membrane. This is attested to by the obliquity of the fibers of membrane which are directed distally from the radius to the ulna. Any derangement of the articulations of the radius and the interosseous membrane in relation to the ulna threatens forearm rotation. The dominance of the radius in transmitting force from the hand renders its distal and proximal extremes common targets for trauma (Colles' fracture distally and radial head fracture-dislocation proximally).

At the metacarpophalangeal joints there is similar circumduction; in the case of the thumb, this is greatly augmented by the saddle configuration of the carpometacarpal joint which is specifically adapted to this function.

Basic hand function requires that the fingers extend to a straight line at their three joints and in flexion that the tips meet the proximal, middle, and distal palm. The aggregate range of joint motion to accomplish this is $\pm 250°$. For the fingertip to meet the proximal palm flexion at the proximal and middle joints is required. To meet the middle palm flexion of all three joints is necessitated. Flexion of the middle and distal joints enables the tip to approximate the distal palm.

The interphalangeal joints are hinge joints with a plane of motion from extension to flexion without any deviation. Such deviation, abduction, adduction, occurs only at the metacarpophalangeal joint. Here the relationship of the cupped base of the proximal phalanx through the asymmetrical convexity of the metacarpal head together with collateral ligaments of fixed length allows for the additional excursion in the lateral plane ($\pm 45°$) including circumduction.

The metacarpophalangeal joint has a cam-like action. The axis of rotation in the anterior-posterior plane is dorsal. Thus, the effective distance (radius) of the phalanx from this axis is short in flexion and long in extension. In addition, there is a lateral flare (similar to a pear) in the head of the metacarpal in going dorsal to volar. Thus, the collateral ligaments are forced to accommodate this lateral flare and increased anterior-posterior radius when the joint is flexed. This tightens the ligaments drastically and brings the proximal phalanges into side-by-side adduction. When this happens, they cannot be spread apart. Hence, to spread the fingers, which requires ligamentous laxity, the metacarpophalangeal joints have to be in extension. The clinical significance of this is the stiffness in extension that occurs as a result of any condition that causes swelling and shortening of these ligaments (the swollen hand or injured metacarpophalangeal joint). The long, ring, and little fingers are the fingers that hold contraction without fatigue at the proximal interphalangeal joints* for extended periods of time. This function is, to a large extent, dependent on the integrity of the metacarpophalangeal joint.

The versatility and adaptability of the thumb in executing its functions of pinch and grasp result from its wide range of motion. The directions of motion are in three planes: flexion-extension, adduction-abduction, and pronation-supination (Fig. 2-9). In circumduction, the thumb passes through each of these planes of motion. The greatest versatility of motion is at the carpometacarpal joint, a universal joint fashioned as a double saddle. This

*Monkeys and apes always hang on a flexed proximal interphalangeal joint because the superficialis can tolerate prolonged contraction but the profundus cannot.

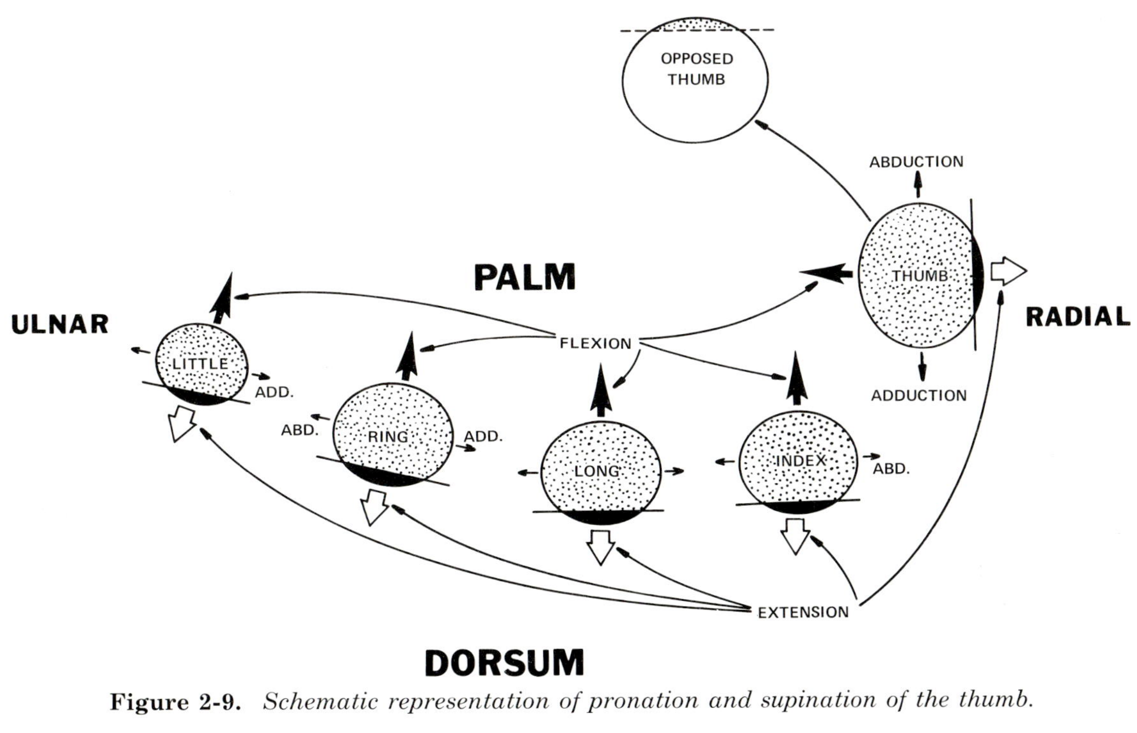

Figure 2-9. *Schematic representation of pronation and supination of the thumb.*

joint moves ±35° in the abduction-adduction plane and ±50° in the flexion-extension plane.

Although the metacarpophalangeal joint of the thumb does not have the saddle configuration, it nonetheless has quite an extensive range of motion in the same planes indicated for the carpometacarpal joint. The interphalangeal joint has a simple hinge action in the flexion-extension plane. All the joints of the thumb have variable degrees of motion. However, a lack at one joint is often compensated for by the other two joints.

The thumb is recessed to the level of the proximal interphalangeal joint of the index finger. This, together with its excursion, makes possible its prime functional movements: (1) spreading the thumb web, which should be possible to about 90°, and (2) rotation (pronation) of the thumb so it will fall in the path of the opposing tips of the index, long, and ring fingers as they furl toward the tubercle of the scaphoid. This act is called opposition.

The essential transverse and longitudinal arches of the hand cannot be assumed without proper mobility. These arches are necessary to cup the palm and oppose the thumb to the fingertips. The most critical motion for the assumption of the transverse arch is pronation of the thumb and of the ring and little finger rays around the central fixed unit (the immobile index and long metacarpals anchored to the distal carpal row). The carpometacarpal joint of the ring finger moves about 15° and that of the little finger about 30° in establishing this arch. The most important joints for the establishment of the longitudinal arch are the metacarpophalangeal joints of the fingers.

Anatomy of the Ligaments

The anatomy of the collateral ligaments of the digits must be understood to appreciate the basis for certain problems of stiffness. They pass from their dorsal proximal origin as fan-shaped structures to their insertion distally and slightly volar. The volar half is somewhat thinner and more membranous than the stout dorsal half and is often referred to as the accessary collateral ligament.

The configuration of the head of the proximal articulating bone varies in respect to the articular arc it creates. This in turn governs the anatomy of the ligaments. The origin of those about the interphalangeal joints corresponds to the center of rotation. Since the arc of flexion has an equal radius, the change in tension on the ligament is minimal from extension to flexion.

The changes in tension that do occur are different in the dorsal and volar halves of the ligament depending upon the position of the joint. In extension the dorsal half is loose and the volar half is tight; on flexion the reverse pertains.

The eccentricity of the metacarpophalangeal joint causes a lengthening of the radius of the arc in passing from full extension to full flexion. Therefore, the ligament is very lax in extension and is tightened by flexion. Thus, any shortening of the ligaments of a metacarpophalangeal joint results in stiffness in extension.

The carpometacarpal joint of the thumb has a stabilizing anterior oblique ligament which anchors the metacarpal to the intercarpal ligaments and is a substitute for a volar plate. This ligament has to resist the subluxating force of the abductor pollicis longus at the base of the metacarpal in its action as a powerful radial wrist deviator.

Each interphalangeal and metacarpophalangeal joint is protected on its palmar aspect by a volar plate which passes from distal to proximal and acts as a trapdoor keeping the flexor tendons from buckling into the joint. The leading edge of this small, tough structure is always proximal and is quite thin centrally with two marginal extensions (checkrein ligaments) which attach to the volar periosteum. Dislocation ruptures the proximal or distal portion of the volar plate and sometimes tears a variable portion of one or both collateral ligaments. At times, the volar plate folds into the joint, locking it in extension.

The volar plates of the metacarpophalangeal joints of the fingers and thumb give rise to the sagittal bands (sling ligaments) of the extensor hood mechanism. The intermetacarpal ligaments between the finger metacarpals also insert on the volar plates, and for this reason are more appropriately called the intervolar plate ligaments. These attachments to the volar plate are the principal factors which hold it dorsally in dislocations of the metacarpal head into the palm. Encircling the neck of the "buttonholed" (dislocated) metacarpal head of the finger are: (1) the superficial transverse ligament of the palmar fascia, (2) the lumbrical, (3) the flexor tendons and the pretendinous bands, and distally and dorsally (4) the natatory ligament and the volar plate. The constraint on the volar plate by its retinacular attachments is the principal factor in preventing reduction. This restriction is readily relieved through a dorsal approach by simply splitting the volar plate down the center.[1] The separation of the two halves of the volar plate relaxes the constricting ring, permitting reduction. There is a great variation in laxity of the digital joints which is governed by the length of the collateral ligaments and the checkreins of the volar plates. The degree of laxity is the key to the vicissitudes of habitus of the digits after injuries to nerves and tendons. When the ligaments of the metacarpophalangeal joints are tight and hyperextension impossible, digital clawing does not develop after median and ulnar nerve palsies. Similarly, loss of superficialis muscle function does not result in hypertension (recurvatum) of the proximal interphalangeal joint if these periarticular structures are tight.

On the dorsum of the digital joints the capsule has no equivalent of the volar plate and is simply a synovial membrane subject to considerable inflammatory and post-traumatic changes.

The wrist has a myriad of crisscrossing ligamentous structures overlying the synovial capsule (Figs. 2-10 and 2-11). When there is sufficient separation of ligamentous fibers, the synovium can herniate, creating a ganglion. The ulnar and radial collateral ligaments are at times like the digital ligaments, the focus of a desmitis. The volar radiocarpal ligament is incriminated in the development of non-union of fractures of the waist of the scaphoid which it crosses and presses upon in the course of pronation and supination.

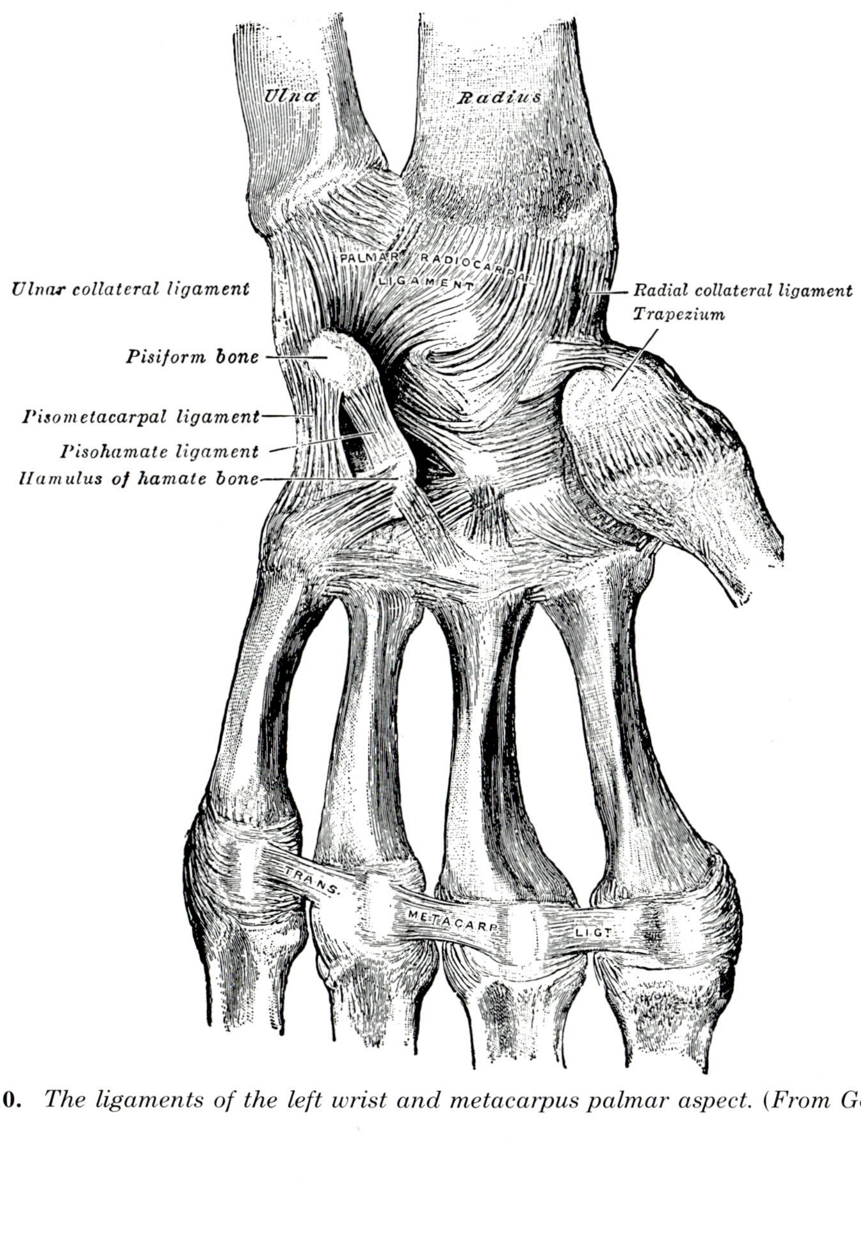

Figure 2-10. *The ligaments of the left wrist and metacarpus palmar aspect.* (*From Goss, C.M.*[5])

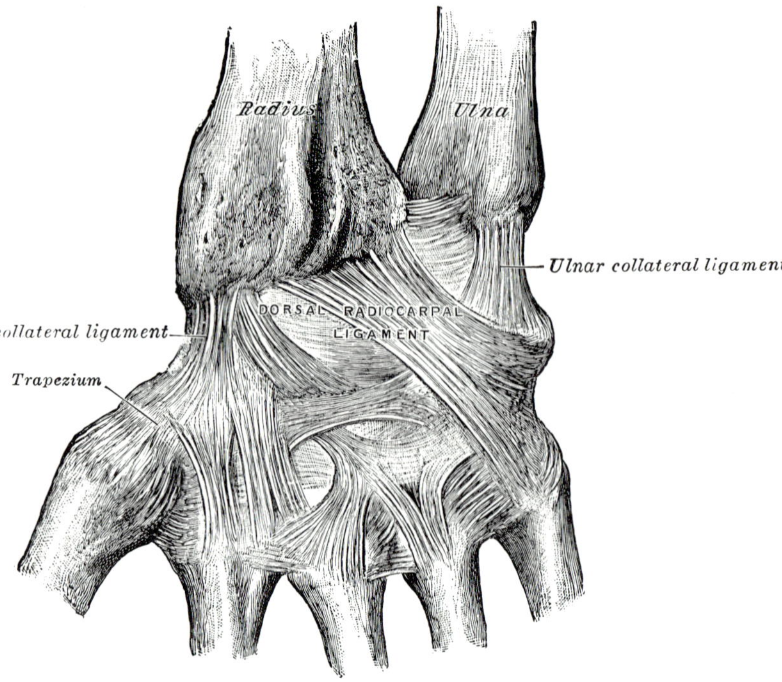

Figure 2-11. *The ligaments of the left wrist, dorsal aspect.* (*From Goss, C.M.*[5])

The Anatomy of the Musculotendinous Units

The extrinsic and intrinsic muscles are the two categories governing hand function. The massive extrinsic group provides the power and endurance needed by the hand. Each is the prime mover of just one joint, although in transit the digital extrinsics may move more than one joint. In contrast, each intrinsic muscle does not have such a clear-cut prime joint to move and instead, by specific design, spreads its action to more than one joint. The intrinsic muscles function as positioners of the digits and as such render the essential function of dexterity. This is not to say that they are lacking in power, for paralysis of the ulnar nerve often diminishes power grip by as much as 50 per cent. Furthermore, the adductor pollicis (prime flexor of the metacarpophalangeal joint of the thumb), has power equal to or in excess of the flexor pollicis longus.

The Anatomy of the Extrinsic Muscles

The extrinsic muscles consist of the forearm flexor-pronator wad (14 muscles) and the forearm extensor-supinator wad (14 muscles). The excursion of the extensor and flexor tendons is variable (maximum of 85 mm to a minimum of 18 mm). The median nerve innervates all the flexor-pronator wad except the flexor carpi ulnaris and the flexor profundus to the ring and little fingers which are innervated by the ulnar nerve. The radial nerve innervates the extensor-supinator wad.

The primary wrist movers are on the collateral borders of the forearm. The intervening space is occupied by the long digital flexors and extensors (Figs. 2-12 to 2-15). The primary wrist flexors are the flexor carpi radialis, inserting on the base of the second and third metacarpal, and the flexor carpi ulnaris, which incorporates the pisiform as it passes on to insert on the hamate and fifth metacarpal. These are synergistic to the long finger extensors which they stretch. The extensor carpi radialis longus, brevis, and ulnaris are the primary wrist extensors and are synergistic to the long digital flexors which they stretch. These wrist extensor muscles insert on the bases of metacarpals II, III and V respectively.

Ulnar deviation of the wrist is brought about by the integrated action of the antagonistic flexor and extensor carpi ulnaris. Radial deviation of the wrist is primarily a function of the abductor pollicis longus which inserts on the base of the thumb metacarpal. Assisting in radial deviation are the extensor pollicis brevis and the protagonistic flexor and extensor carpi radialis muscles.

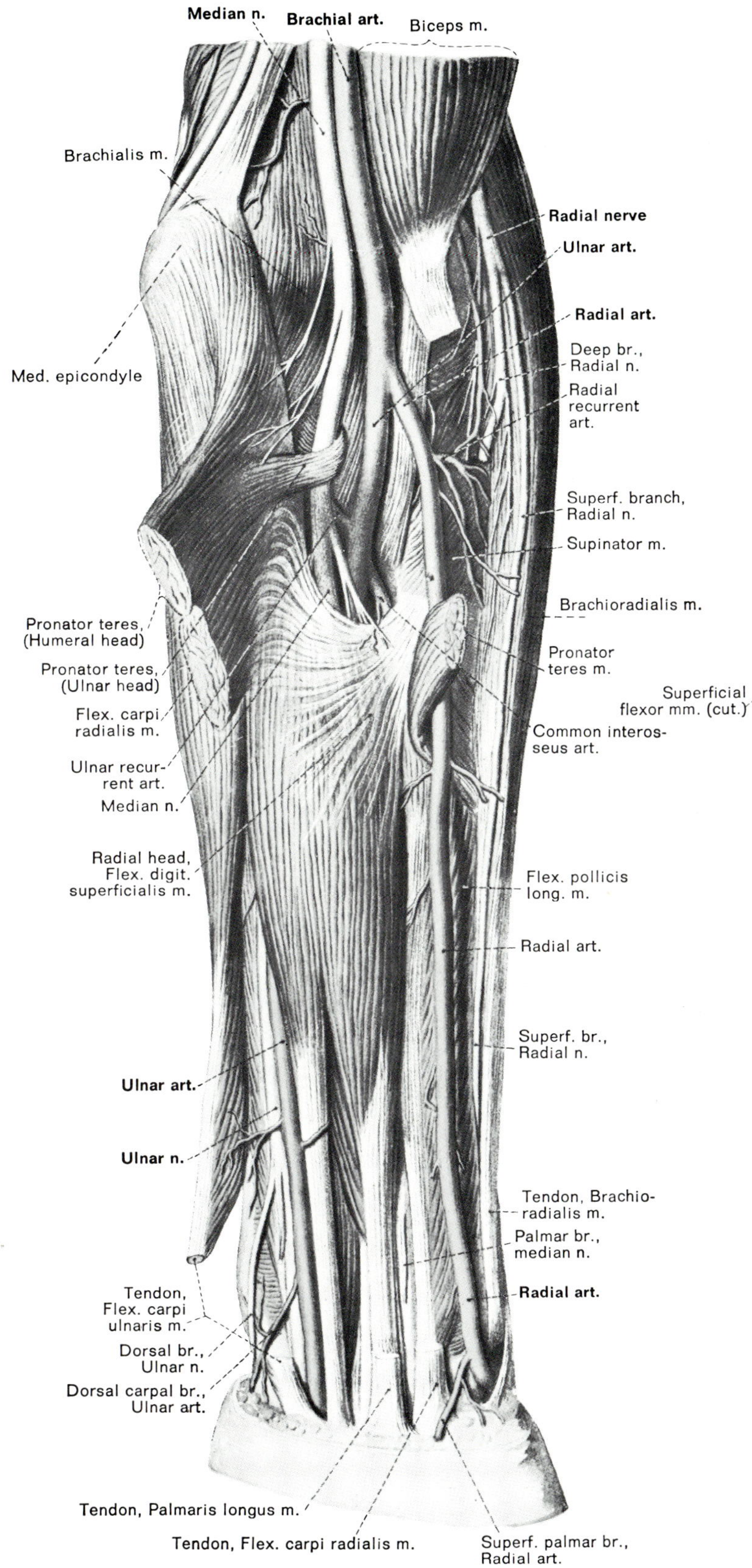

Figure 2-12. *Nerves and arteries, left volar aspect forearm (superficial dissection). (From Clemente, C.D.*[2]*)*

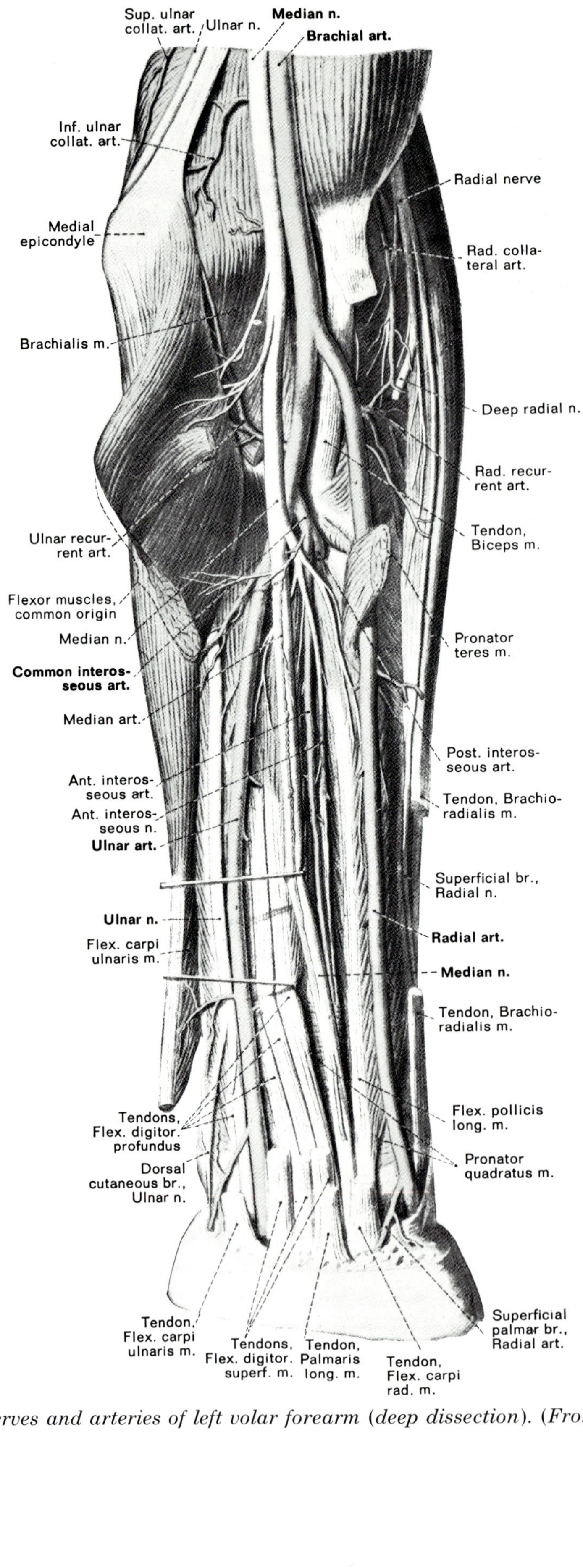

Figure 2-13. *Nerves and arteries of left volar forearm (deep dissection).* (*From Clemente, C.D.*[2])

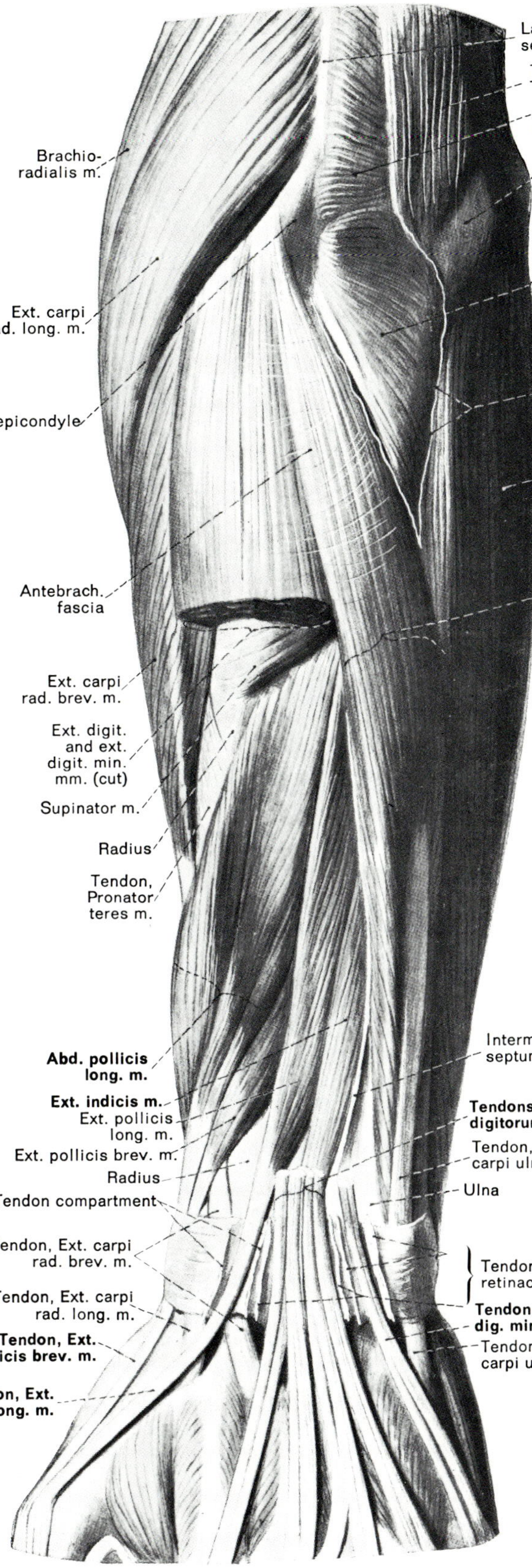

Figure 2-14. *The muscles of the left dorsal forearm.* (*From Clemente, C.D.*[2])

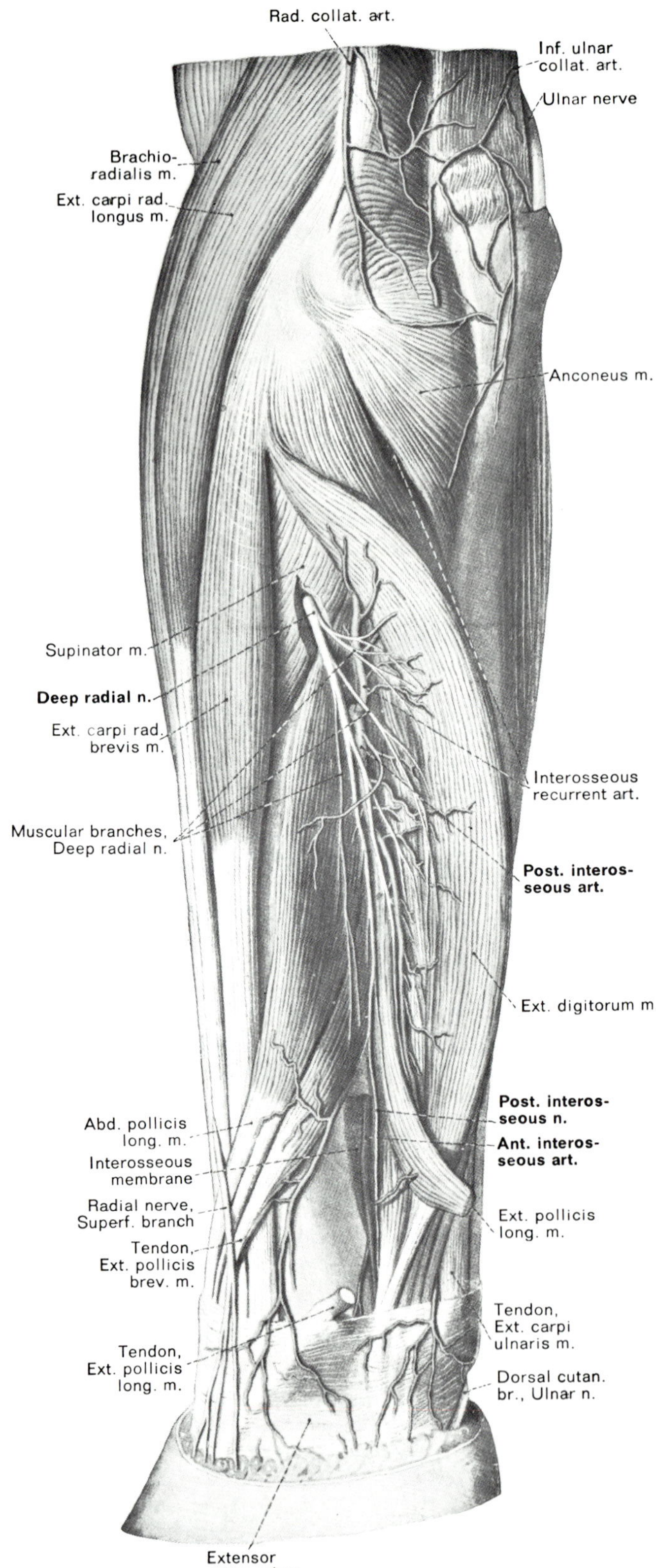

Figure 2-15. *Nerves and arteries of the left dorsal forearm (deep dissection). (From Clemente, C.D.*[2]*)*

Most of the flexor pronator group of muscles arise from the area of the medial humeral epicondyle. The anterior and medial aspects of the ulnar shaft are covered by the large belly of the flexor digitorum profundus, which can be palpated on the volar aspects of the subcutaneous border of the ulna. The ulnar and median nerves on either side of the ulnar artery lie on its volar surface. Distally, the tendons in the palm give rise to the lumbrical muscles and thereafter pierce the tendons of the flexor superficialis to insert broadly over the proximal and palmar surfaces of the distal phalanges. The distal interphalangeal joints are the prime joints that the profundus muscles move. Inasmuch as the profundus tendons came from a common muscle, they must all act together to be effective. The profundus muscle to the index, at times, is totally independent. The profundus muscles have a split innervation which usually has some overlap. In terms of reconstruction it should be noted that the innervation of the digital skin generally corresponds to the motor innervation of this muscle.

The flexor digitorum superficialis originates from the humerus and the ulna with a thin aponeurotic slip from the radius. The aponeurotic ring between these two heads forms a window which allows passage of the median nerve and ulnar artery. The flexor digitorum superficialis forms a superficial belly which sends tendons to the sides of the middle phalanges of the long and ring fingers and a deeper belly which sends similar tendons to the index and little finger.

In accommodating the passage of the profundus tendon, a superficialis tendon splits and the two halves spiral behind the profundus to decussate before terminating laterally in their insertions on the shaft of the middle phalanx (Fig. 2-16).

The superficialis function is generally independent for each finger. However, the tendons to the ring and little finger are frequently joined and act together. The prime joints flexed are the proximal interphalangeal joints.

The flexor pollicis longus is the deepest long extrinsic on the radial side of the forearm where it arises from the radius and has totally independent action. It inserts broadly on the shaft of the distal phalanx of the thumb and is the prime flexor of its interphalangeal joint.

The excursion of the long digital tendons has its maximal range at the wrist level where the amplitude may reach 4 to 5 cm. At the metacarpophalangeal joints this range is reduced by 1 to 1.5 cm.

At the insertion of each long flexor in the digit is a substantial condensation of the mesotendon in the form of the vincula brevia (the vascular stalk). This may tether a divided tendon and keep it from retracting. More proximally the vincula longa, which are more friable, may do the same. Sensory awareness of motion and of tension along the musculotendinous unit depends on the integrity of nerve endings about other tissues, e.g. skin, subcutaneous tissue and joints, which are secondarily stimulated.

All of the digits have retinacular flexor sheaths

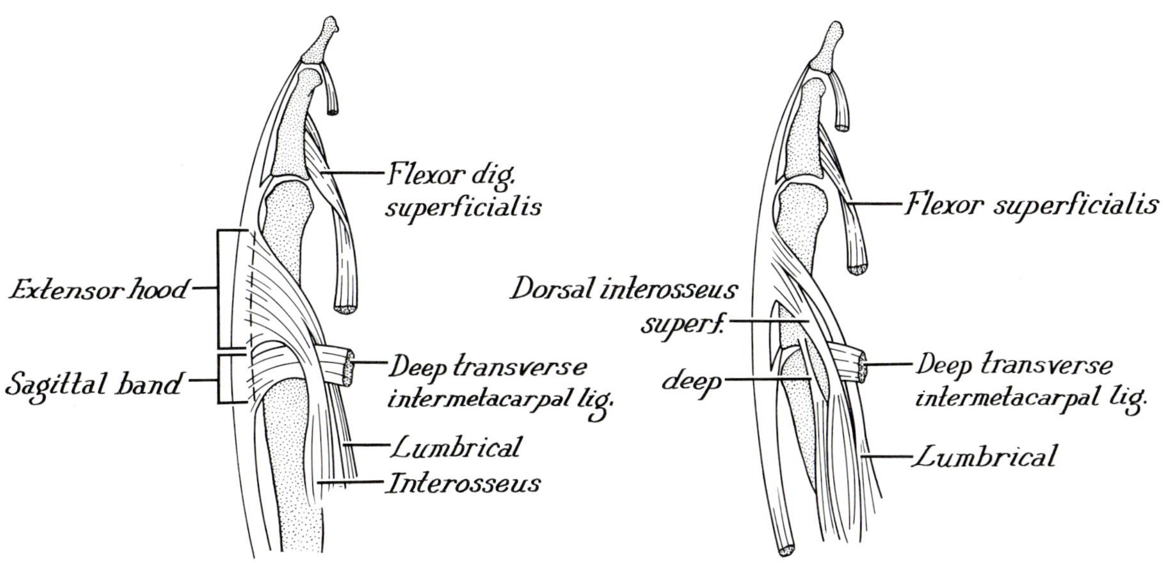

Figure 2-16. *Diagrammatic representation of the spiraling of the flexor superficialis near its insertion and the intrinsic muscle insertions about the metacarpophalangeal joint.*

housing the long flexor tendons and the synovial bursae that lubricate them. These sheaths begin at the point where the tendons are prone to start bowstringing, namely, at the head of the metacarpals. The adaptation to resist bowstringing where its tendency is maximal has resulted in thickenings of the sheath which are called pulleys. The minimum functional requirement for such pulleys is one for each phalanx beyond the proximal. Hence, for the thumb one is needed and for the fingers, two. The most proximal of these is to be found in the distal palm and is a distinctly separate structure from any other tissue. It is fixed to the volar plate of the proximal phalanx and, in the case of the fingers, the subjacent intervolar plate ligaments blend with it. Distal to this are three more stout bands, one over the shaft of the proximal phalanx, one over the volar plate of the proximal interphalangeal joint and the last at the midportion of the middle phalanx. Between the three terminal ones are cruciate rings. Between these pulleys the flexor sheath is thin and at times transparent. The ideal finger pulleys to save in reconstruction so that the tip of the finger will meet the middle palm in flexion are the most proximal and most distal (Fig. 2-17).

The biceps (innervated by the musculocutaneous nerve) enters the forearm to insert on the radial tubercle deep in the antecubital fossa. A stout aponeurotic bridge (lacertus fibrosis) runs medially from its musculotentinous junction to the antebrachial fascia over the flexor wad. The prime function of the distal biceps is to supinate the forearm. A lesser function is to complement the brachialis as the flexor of the elbow. Underneath the lacertus fibrosis are the median nerve and the brachial artery. Beneath it is also found the proximal limit of the flexor wad, the pronator teres, which usually has two heads, one from the medial epicondyle and one from the ulna. This muscle traverses the forearm obliquely and inserts on a broad aponeurotic plane on the middle third of the radius over the flexor superficialis muscles and under the extensor carpi radialis longus. The

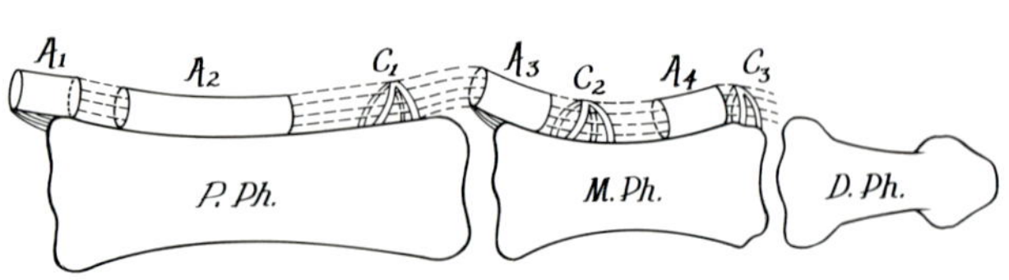

Figure 2-17. *Schematic representation of the reticular flexor tendon sheath. (From Doyle, J.R. and Blythe, W.*[4]*)*

median nerve passes under or through it and may be constricted here by a fibrous ring.

Distally, the pronator quadratus lies as a transversely oriented quandrangular muscle in the floor of the forearm under all the long flexor muscles.

Most of the extensor-supinator group of muscles arise from the lateral epicondyle. The extensor carpi ulnaris forms the posterior-lateral border and the brachioradialis the anteriomedial border, with the small anconeus triangulated between the olecranon and the lateral epicondyle. The brachioradialis originates from the humerus and inserts on the radial styloid with the radial nerve running out on the dorsal aspect distally from beneath it. The prime function of the brachioradialis is flexion of the elbow. However, depending upon the position of the forearm, it may act as a pronator or supinator.

The supinator is the deepest muscle arising from the posterior aspect of the lateral epicondyle and along a line on the radial side of the olecranon and proximal ulna. Its fibers run obliquely across the radial border of forearm and are inserted into the lateral edge of the radial tuberosity and the radius as far as the pronator teres. The proximal fibers form an aponeurotic window, the arcade of Frohse (Fig. 15-21), through which the radial nerve enters after it passes from between the brachialis and brachioradialis. The nerve continues through the planes of the muscle and emerges distally deep to the extensor communis and on the surface of the abductor pollicis longus and extensor pollicis brevis. The supinator's prime function is forearm supination.

The anconeus aids in extending the elbow. Running to the ulnar styloid along the distal border of the anconeus is the extensor carpi ulnaris which inserts on the base of the fifth metacarpal. On the radiodorsal margin of the extensor wad but just deep and parallel to the brachioradialis is the extensor carpi radialis longus arising from the humerus and inserting on the base of the index metacarpal. Adjacent to it is the companion extensor carpi radialis brevis arising around the lateral epicondyle and inserting centrally at the base of the third metacarpal. The latter two tendons pass deep to the abductor pollicis longus and the extensor pollicis longus and brevis. The more centrally located extensor carpi radialis brevis is the most important of the carpal extensors. It preserves the transverse arch and acting alone does not cause lateral deviation of the wrist.

In the center of the extensor wad between the carpal extensors lie the extensor digitorum communis and extensor digiti minimi, which also arise primarily from the lateral epicondyle. Deep to these muscles over the interosseous membrane lie the abductor pollicis longus, the extensor pollicis brevis, the extensor pollicis longus, and the extensor indicis from the radial to the ulnar aspect in the forearm.

The abductor pollicis longus and the extensor pollicis brevis have an oblique course up to the extensor retinaculum. The abductor pollicis longus is often composed of multiple tendons which may occasionally pass in separate sheaths and insert about the thumb metacarpal and the trapezium. Its prime function is radial deviation of the wrist; however, it also has an obligatory function in abducting the thumb. The extensor pollicis brevis running on the surface of the abductor pollicis longus joins the extensor mechanism of the thumb and immediately inserts centrally on the base of the proximal phalanx. The prime joint it moves is the metacarpophalangeal joint. The extensor pollicis longus has an oblique course after traversing its fibrous sheath and passing around Lister's tubercle. It joins the extensor hood to the ulnar side of the extensor brevis and passes on to insert on the base of the distal phalanx. It has a stout insertion as compared to that of the extensor insertion of the fingers. The prime function is forceful extension, including hypertension, of the interphalangeal joint. All three of these tendons to the thumb pass under the major terminal sensory branches of the superficial radial nerve.

The extensor digiti quinti and the extensor indicis propius have entirely independent functions from the extensor communi. After traversing the wrist (where the extensor digiti minimi has its own sheath) they run deep to the extensor communi and join their respective digital extensor hoods on the ulnar side of the extensor communis tendons with which they blend. The extensor communi lack independence. They pass through a common sheath across the wrist and are tethered together over the body of the hand by highly variable oblique interconnections, the conexus intertendineus (Fig. 2-18). They join the extensor hood centrally over the apex of the metacarpal heads and

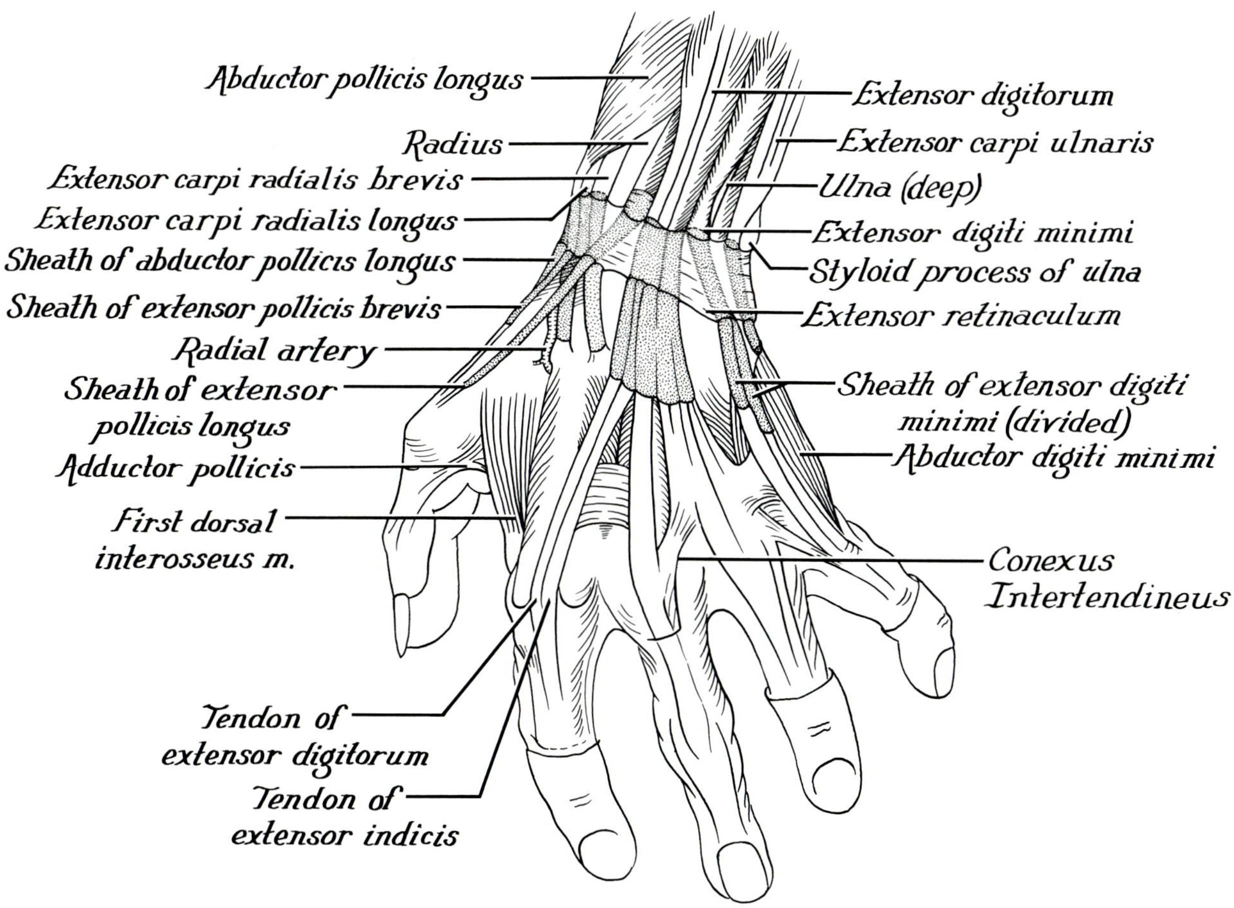

Figure 2-18. *The extensor tendons and the juncturae tendinae (conexus intertendinous) on the dorsum of the hand. (Redrawn from Cunningham.[3])*

become the middle extensor tendon (central slip) of that structure. On either side lie the radial and ulnar sagittal bands (sling ligaments) which hold the extensor over the apex of the metacarpal head. These bands are anchored to the volar plate and intermetacarpal ligament. Although the middle extensor tendon goes to the base of the middle phalanx where it terminates as a relatively thin insertion, it also, in most instances, has a slip inserting into the base of the proximal phalanx.

The prime joint extended is the metacarpophalangeal joint. However, with progressive flexion of this joint, the long extensor becomes a strong extensor not only of the proximal interphalangeal joint but, by virtue of the interconnections in the extensor hood, also the distal interphalangeal joint.

Anatomy of the Extensor Hood

The extensor hood is an aponeurotic sheet of intricate design which, spread out on the dissecting table, resembles an impressionistic Christmas tree. It consists of an interweaving of tendinous and fascial elements which allow the forces of pull from the extrinsic extensors and the intrinsic muscles to act in concert (Fig. 2-19). The integrated action extends the interphalangeal joints. Simultaneously, the hood allows antagonistic activity of flexion by the intrinsics and extension by the extrinsic extensors at the metacarpophalangeal joint. In addition to these dynamic stresses by the muscles acting on the extensor hood, there are ligaments which at one point in the course of active motion become static agents of motion by the tension that develops on them.

The middle extensor tendon is the central tendon of the hood and the lateral extensor tendons are the intrinsic tendons. The three separate along the distal half of the proximal phalanx just before the middle extensor tendon inserts on the base of the middle phalanx. Just beyond this the lateral extensor tendons fuse into a common terminal extensor tendon which inserts as a very thin sinew on the terminal phalanx. There is no window in this sheet of tissue but there are bilaterally symmetrical expansions in the form of fascial retinacular bands. These act to secure the tendinous portions against displacement which compromises their function. Depending on the existing degree of extension, the tension directed along the axis of their fibers makes them contribute to the movement and stabilization of the metacarpophalangeal and distal interphalangeal joint. Proximally are the previously described sagittal bands at the beginning of the extensor hood. With extension of the joint to a straight line, they become sufficiently taut to direct the pull of the long extensor over the waist of the proximal phalanx, facilitating hyperextension.

From the lateral margins of the terminal extensor tendon is a fascial veil which narrows into the oblique retinacular ligament, passing close to the phalanx in an oblique direction to terminate in the flexor sheath of the proximal phalanx. This lies volar to the axis of movement of the proximal interphalangeal joint and is tightened with extension of this joint. Therefore, in extension of the proximal interphalangeal joint, it complements the muscle forces which are tightening the terminal extensor tendon and extending the distal joint. In fact, should the continuity of the terminal extensor tendon be broken proximally without compromising the oblique retinacular ligament, this ligament is capable of executing full extension of the distal joint, providing it is stretched by extension of the proximal interphalangeal joint.

The sling that holds the middle extensor tendon, the lateral extensor tendon, and the oblique retinacular ligaments in place over the dorsum of the proximal interphalangeal joint and prevents lateral and volar shift of these structures is the transverse retinacular ligament. It is the counterpart of the sagittal bands proximally and is anchored on either side of the volar plate and flexor sheath of the middle joint.

Anatomy of the Intrinsic Muscles

The intrinsics are the muscles which originate entirely distal to the wrist. There are 20 of them, 15 of which are innervated by the ulnar nerve. They consist of three muscles each for the thenar and hypothenar wads, four dorsal interossei, three volar interossei, four lumbricals, the adductor of the thumb (largest and most powerful intrinsic), the deep, short flexor of the thumb and the palmaris brevis. There are no muscles, only tendons, distal to the metacarpophalangeal joint. The five muscles innervated by the median nerve are the three thenar muscles and the radial two lumbricals.

The overall function of the intrinsics is understood best by thinking of them as cupping the palm and spreading the hand. The former action they execute by flexing the metacarpophalangeal joints

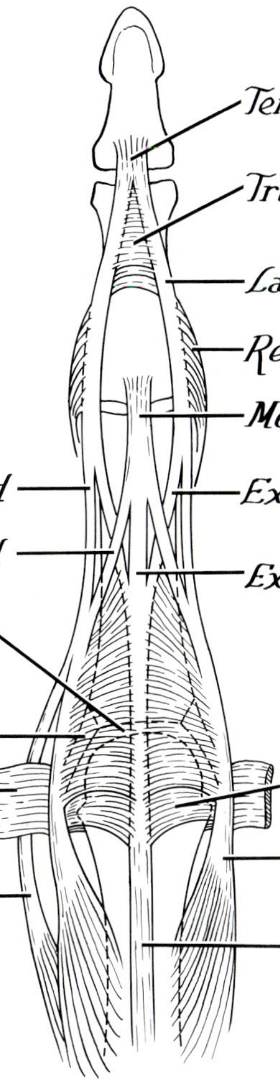

Figure 2-19. *Schematic representation of the digital extensor mechanism.* (*Redrawn from Tubiana, R. and Valentin, P.*[10])

and extending the interphalangeal joints and by adducting the digits and by pronating the radial and supinating the ulnar borders of the hand. When exaggerated, this becomes the "intrinsic plus" hand (Fig. 2-20). Spreading the hand requires abduction of the digits. An analysis of the configuration of the cupped hand shows that the intrinsic muscles are indispensable to both the transverse and longitudinal arches of the hand. When paralyzed, the palm is totally flat, the metacarpophalangeal joints are extended, the interphalangeal joints are flexed, and the webs are open midway between full adduction and abduction. This is the claw deformity of the "intrinsic minus" hand (Fig. 2-21).

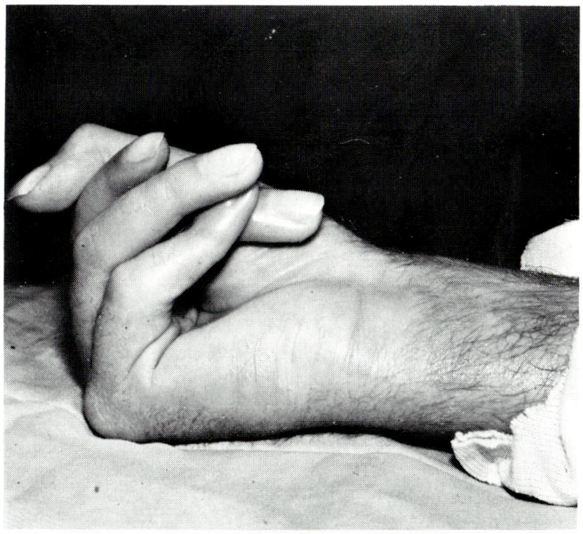

Figure 2-20. *"Intrinsic plus" deformity. The metacarpophalangeal joints are flexed and the interphalangeal joints extended. Pronounced cupping of the hand occurs with adduction of the digits.*

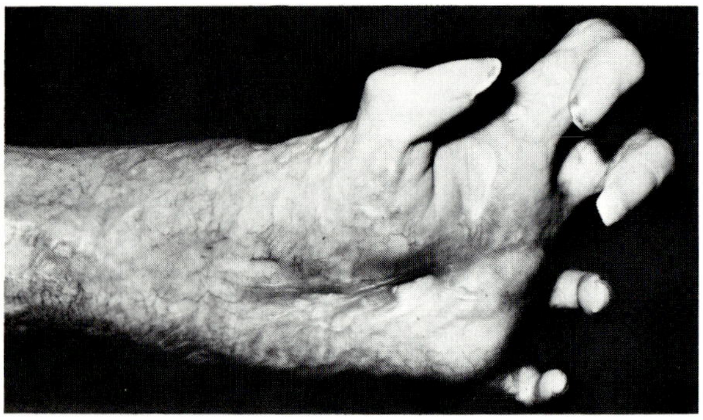

Figure 2-21. *"Intrinsic minus" deformity. Laxity of the intrinsic muscles with the extrinsic extensors and flexors acting as synergists.*

THE ORIGIN, INSERTION AND ACTION OF THE INTRINSIC MUSCLES

The interosseus muscles, four dorsal and three volar, are situated between the metacarpal shafts. The tendons pass distally beside the metacarpophalangeal joints and on the dorsal side of the deep transverse intervolar plate ligament when present. The larger dorsal group have a bipennate origin from the contiguous sides of the adjacent metacarpal shafts and, distally, a bifid insertion. The deeper connection is to the bases of the proximal phalanges with loose attachments to the collateral ligaments. The more superficial portion blends with and helps to form the lateral extensor tendon of the hood. The smaller unipennate palmar interossei arise from a metacarpal shaft, insert on the margins of the proximal phalanges and contribute to the lateral extensor tendons of the extensor hood. A wide variation is encountered not only in the number and attachments of the interossei but also in their innervation and even in their nomenclature. Current opinion holds that these variations have no effect on manual power, skills or dexterity.

Thus, at the metacarpophalangeal joints of all five digits, a radial and ulnar deviator is found attached to the base of the corresponding proximal phalanx, to the extensor hood, or to both. All except the abductor pollicis brevis are commonly innervated by the ulnar nerve. This simple functional and practical concept avoids the problems of adduction and abduction to and from an axial digit.

The four lumbricals arise from the flexor profundus tendon in the palm. They pass on the volar side of the deep intermetacarpal ligament (transverse metacarpal ligament) and, crossing on the radial side of the proximal phalanx, give rise to the lateral extensor tendon of the extensor hood (intrinsic band, lateral band). These are the only muscles of the hand that have a mobile attachment at both ends, allowing them to constantly adjust their contractile efficiency (stretch tone) with respect to flexion of the metacarpophalangeal joints. They are considered the prime flexors of these joints. The interossei, not having a mobile base, can only increase their contractile efficiency by the stretch incurred in association with metacarpophalangeal joint extension by the extrinsic extensor muscles. The maximum efficiency of the interossei is reached with full extension of these joints.

By the design of the extensor hood, all three musculotendinous groups are integrated. The tension (position of the metacarpophalangeal joint) placed on any one group will modify its efficiency. Thus, maximum efficiency of the interossei is allowed with progressive extension of the metacarpophalangeal joint, while the extrinsic extensors reach their maximal efficiency with progressive flexion of that joint.

THE INTRINSIC MUSCULOTENDINOUS UNITS OF THE HAND

The thenar wad of muscles on the radial side of the thumb are balanced by muscles of the web space on the ulnar side so that the thumb "post" is

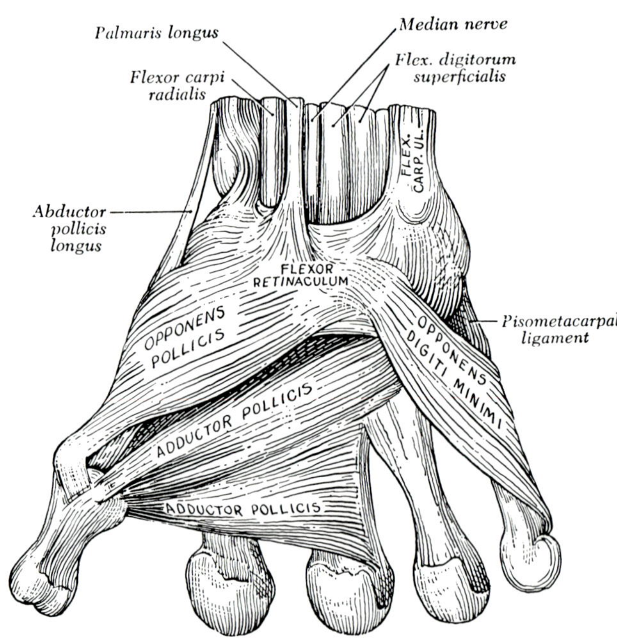

Figure 2-22. *The muscles of the thumb.* (*From Goss, C.M.*[5])

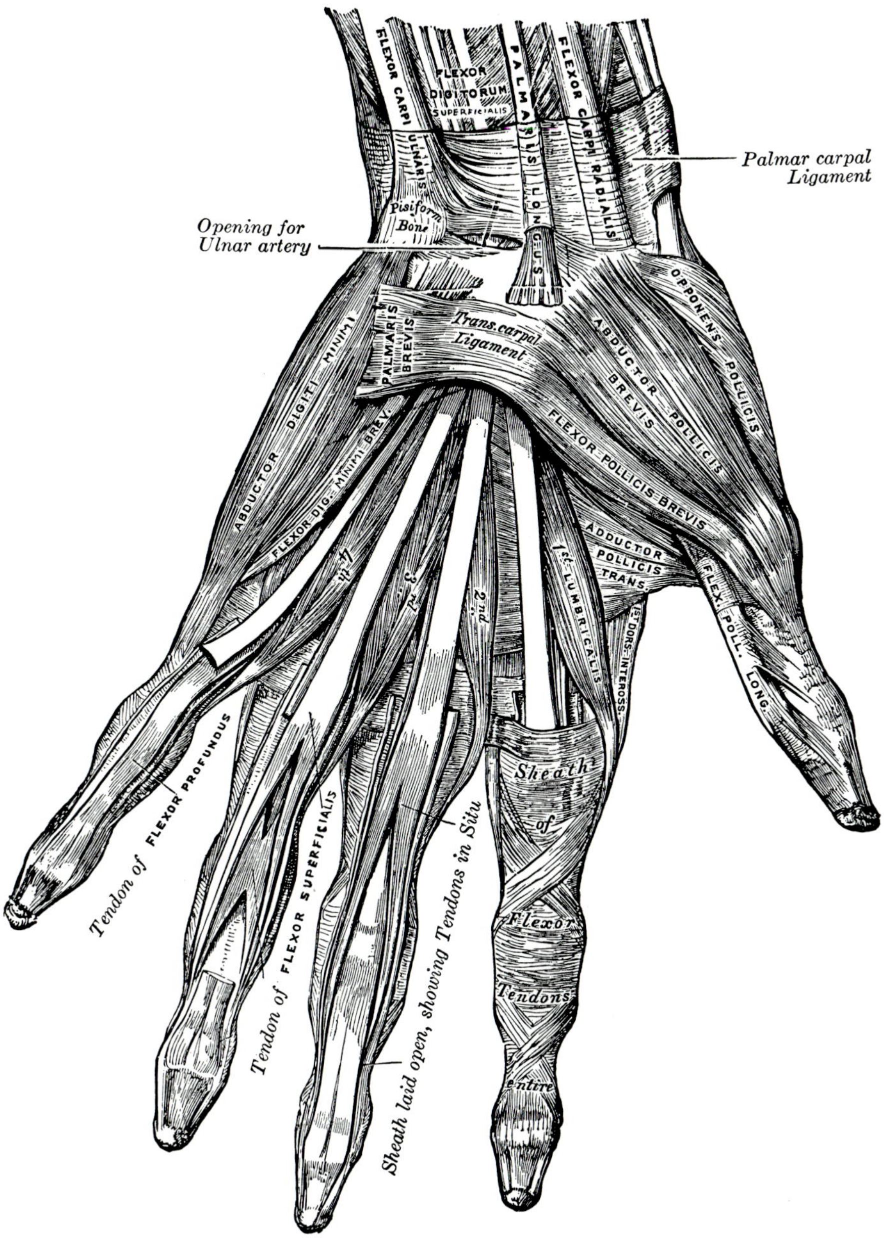

Figure 2-23. *The muscles of the left hand, palmar surface.* (*From Goss, C.M.*[5])

harmoniously stabilized or moved at any point in the arc of pronation-supination or abduction-adduction (Figs. 2-22 and 2-23). There are three muscles in the thenar wad which act synergistically to abduct, pronate and oppose the thumb (Fig. 2-9). They may all be innervated by the recurrent motor branch of the median nerve. However, in up to 50 per cent of cases, there is overlap of innervation by the ulnar nerve. The abductor pollicis brevis, which hugs the radial border of the metacarpal, is the one most rarely innervated by the ulnar nerve. Accordingly, assessment of its function is a good reflection of function of the median nerve.

The other muscles, the opponens pollicis and, further volar, the superficial head of the flexor pollicis brevis originate, together with the abductor brevis, from the transverse carpal ligament and the radial carpal bones. The insertion of these muscles is akin to that of the intrinsics to the fingers. A dorsal extensor hood is formed but is somewhat less distinct than that of the fingers.

The thumb web muscles are three in number: the small, deep head of the flexor pollicis brevis, the huge triangulated adductor pollicis which serves primarily as powerful flexor of the metacarpophalangeal joint, and the first dorsal interosseus. The radial deviator (abductor) of the index finger is an accessory adductor of the thumb by virtue of the fact that part of its origin is on the ulnar side of the thumb metacarpal. The adductor arises by two heads, a distal transverse and proximal oblique, from the metacarpal of the long finger. The short flexor arises from the ulnar side of the thumb metacarpal.

The insertions of these intrinsic muscles are variable, but the overall functional effect is consistent. That is one of forceful flexion of the metacarpophalangeal joint, extension of the interphalangeal joint (but not hyperextension nor extension with force), and abduction-pronation versus adduction-supination. The insertions on the radial side are on the metacarpal (by the opponens), the volar aspect of the base of the proximal phalanx and the equivalent of the lateral extensor tendon of the extensor hood. The insertions on the ulnar side are similar. However, the adductor has the most extensive insertion about the volar base, usually incorporating a sesamoid bone. In addition it has a long slip deep to the flexor pollicis longus which inserts with the flexor brevis and abductor pollicis brevis on the radial side.

THE HYPOTHENAR MUSCULATURE

These muscles are analagous to those of the thenar group. However, all are innervated by the superficial palmar branch of the ulnar nerve. Their functions are abduction and flexion of the proximal phalanx of the little finger and supination of its metacarpal. The origin of the opponens digiti quinti is from the hamate and the palmar carpal ligament, and its insertion is broadly over the ulnar aspect of the metacarpal shaft. The flexor digiti quinti (sometimes absent) has the same origins but inserts on the volar-ulnar aspect of the proximal phalanx. The superficial abductor digiti quinti is the largest and of clinical importance as a choice of motor for opponensplasty. Its origin is from the pisiform and the tendon of the flexor carpi ulnaris. Its inserts like the flexor brevis and its function is similar.

The least important intrinsic muscle is the twentieth, the palmaris brevis, which is innervated by the ulnar nerve and passes across the heel of the hand from the transverse carpal ligament and palmar aponeurosis to be inserted into the skin on the ulnar side of the hand. It aids in cupping the palm.

Anatomy of Nerves

The major motor and sensory nerves of the upper extremity originate from the cervical thoracic roots C-5 to T-1. These roots interweave in the brachial plexus (Fig. 2-24) and are joined by the sympathetics. The latter arise from the stellate ganglion, which is a fusion of the inferior cervical and upper thoracic sympathetic ganglion, lying behind the vertebral artery between the seventh cervical vertebral transverse process and the neck of the first rib. The sympathetic system has a much greater impact on the extremity in relationship to disease and pain than is often appreciated. It controls all autonomic functions of the limb, including those identified with the parasympathetic system.

The mixed motor and sensory fibers in peripheral nerves are an important limitation in orienting axons at the time of neurorrhaphy. The location of axons within a funiculus is constantly shifting millimeter for millimeter (Fig. 15-5). This further complicates the difficulty of axonal matching in neurorrhaphy when there is any loss of substance. The longitudinal epineurial vessels which distinguish a nerve from a tendon are a guide to orientation in nerve repair. Vessels within a nerve may give problems from bleeding.

Nerves are ensheathed by tough connective tissue sleeves, externally the epineurium and internally the perineurium, around each individual funiculus. Up to 50 per cent of the cross-sectional area of a nerve may be comprised of these connective tissue sleeves. Neurorrhaphy attempts to match the funiculi by size and position by suturing their perineurium. The nerve receives its blood supply segmentally from its adjacent vascular plexus through a mesoneurium.

The musculocutaneous nerve arises from C-5, C-6, C-7 and the lateral cord giving off motor branches to the brachialis and biceps terminating as the lateral antebrachial cutaneous nerve of the forearm. It exits between the brachialis laterally and the distal biceps innervating the volar-radial skin of the forearm.

The radial nerve arises from C-5, C-6, C-7, C-8, and T-1 and is the prime contribution of the posterior cord. It lies deep to the axillary artery and

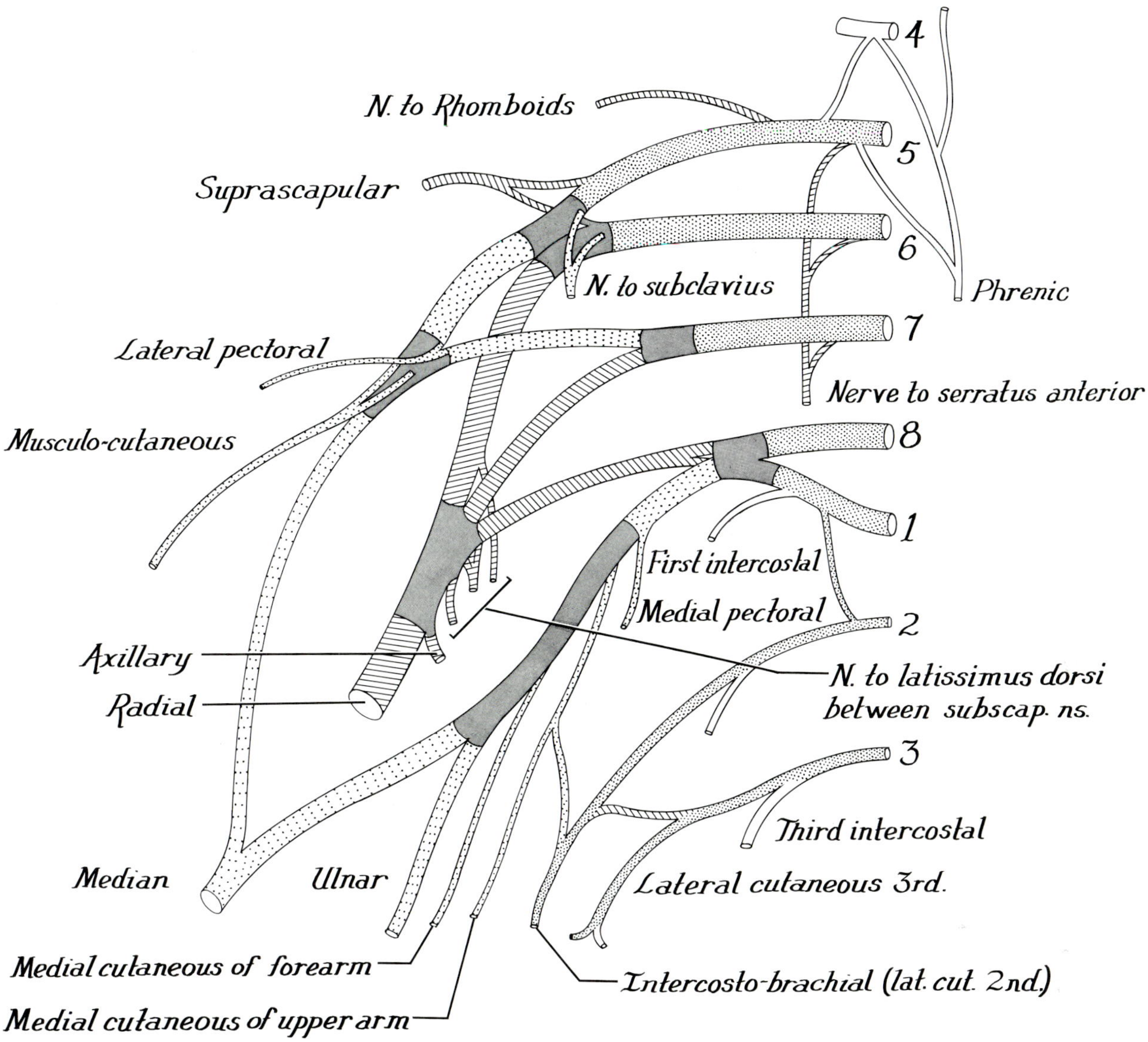

Figure 2-24. *Brachial plexus.* (*Redrawn from* Cunningham's Manual of Practical Anatomy.[3])

spirals about the posterior aspect of the humerus in spiral groove to supply the triceps and anconeus in the arm, emerging between the brachialis and brachioradialis. It divides under cover of the brachioradialis into a deep and superficial branch. The latter runs under the cover of this muscle to emerge dorsally in the distal third of the forearm. The sensory function is not crucial but injury to the sensory nerve in the distal forearm can produce disabling neuromas. The deep motor branch (dorsal interosseous) traverses the substance of the supinator through the arcade of Frohse (Fig. 2-25) to innervate the extensors and long abductor of the thumb. The radial nerve thus innervates all the extrinsic extensors of the wrist and digits. Its most

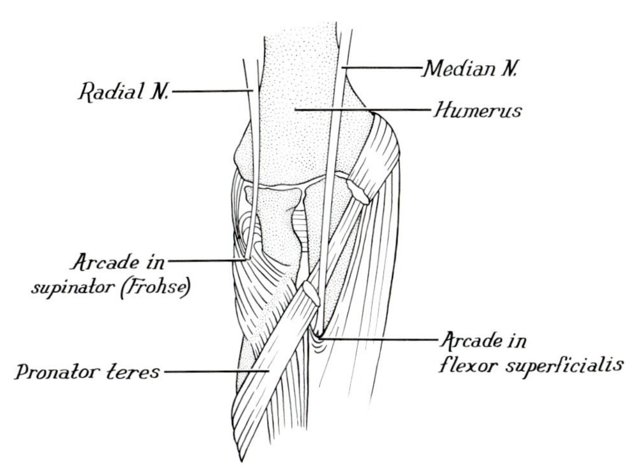

Figure 2-25. *Schematic anatomy of the anterior relationships of the median and ulnar nerves at the elbow.*

important function is innervation of wrist extensors, which are indispensable for grip.

This nerve is vulnerable to injury in several areas:

1. Through compression (usually external) of the middle and distal thirds of the arm (spiral groove).
2. By compression within the fascial sleeve of the extensor wad of muscles of the forearm.
3. By isolated entrapment at the arcade of Frohse.
4. By direct injury in its subcutaneous course in the arm and forearm.
5. By direct injury over the bare area of the proximal radius.

The median nerve arises from C-6, C-7, C-8 and T-1 plus the lateral and medial cords of the brachial plexus. It is the most important nerve to the hand, because its injury renders the radial half of the palm and the prime digits of the hand "blind" or hypersensitive. These digits are the thumb, index, long and radial half of the ring finger. All the volar aspects of these digits, and in the case of the fingers additionally the dorsal aspects of the distal two phalanges, are supplied by the median nerve. It innervates the forearm pronators, all the extrinsic flexors except the flexor carpi ulnaris and the ulnar two profundi segments. In addition, it innervates the thenar muscles and the radial two lumbricals. Thus, 11 of the 14 extrinsic flexor pronator group muscles and 5 of the 20 intrinsic muscles of the hand are innervated by this nerve. It lies anterior to the brachial artery in the upper arm and assumes a medial relationship to it as it enters the forearm alongside the biceps. It passes through or under the substance of the pronator teres and shortly thereafter deep to the superficialis muscle through an aponeurotic window (Fig. 2-25). After entering the superficialis muscle, it gives off the volar (anterior) interosseous nerve to the flexor pollicis longus, pronator quadratus, and profundus to the index and long fingers.

The main body of the median nerve emerges on the radial border of the superficialis muscle protected by the palmaris longus (if present) in the midline of the forearm at the wrist. Here it gives off an important sensory branch to the palmar area (palmar cutaneous branch of the median nerve), which when injured may cause a painful neuroma or a numb palm. The nerve then passes through the carpal tunnel volar to the nine flexor tendons and immediately under the stout transverse carpal ligament.

The recurrent motor branch varies in its size and origin and must be meticulously protected and identified during dissection. Although usually arising on the radial side and entering the thenar muscles distal to the transverse carpal ligament, it may arise on the ulnar side of the nerve or penetrate the ligament to reach the thenar muscles (Fig. 15-17). The nerves to the two radial lumbricals arise from their respective common volar nerves. Beyond the ligament are the common volar digital nerves which lie deep to the superficial arterial arch and divide in the midpalm into the proper digital nerves. As they reach the web they become superficial (volar) to the digital arteries and shortly thereafter give off dorsal branches to the middle and distal phalanges of the fingers and the distal phalanx of the thumb.

Areas of entrapment of the median nerve are:

1. Under the ligament of Struthers, the uncommon oblique ligament from the medial epicondyle to the supracondylar process.
2. Within the flexor-pronator muscle mass of the forearm.
   a. Isolated compression by the pronator teres.
   b. Isolated compression by the aponeurosis of the superficialis.
   c. Within the flexor wad secondary to massive congestion or fibrosis.
3. In the carpal tunnel.

The ulnar nerve arises from C-8 and T-1 through the lower trunk and medial cord to pass along the medial aspect of the brachial artery. It enters the cubital tunnel after passing around the medial epicondyle in the ulnar groove. This superficial position is readily accessible for regional anesthesia. The nerve enters the forearm through a window in the flexor carpi ulnaris (cubital tunnel) and comes to lie on the forearm deep to the flexor carpi ulnaris and to the ulnar side of the profundus muscles of the ring and little fingers which it also innervates. In the distal third of the forearm it gives off its dorsal sensory branch and then proceeds with the ulnar artery into the fibrous canal (loge de Guyon) at the base of the hypothenar musculature. Here, it gives off the muscular branches to the hypothenar muscles, as well as the deep motor branch (Fig. 2-26). The latter passes around the hook of the hamate into the depths of the palm but superficial to the deep arterial arch to supply all the interossei, the adductor of the thumb, the deep head of the flexor pollicis brevis and the two ulnar lumbricals. The termination of the motor portion of the ulnar nerve is in the first dorsal interosseous.

The superficial sensory nerve in the palm sup-

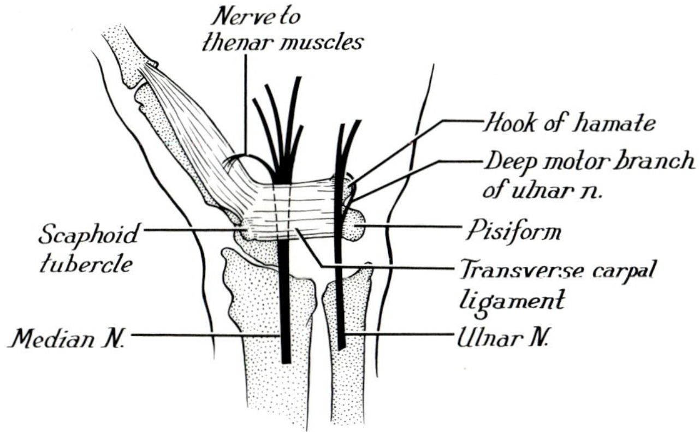

Figure 2-26. *Anatomy of the median and ulnar nerves at the wrist.*

plies the little finger and the ulnar half of the ring finger with dorsal branches to the middle and distal phalanges of each. Thus the prime importance of this nerve is the innervation of 15 of the 20 intrinsic muscles and sensibility on the ulnar aspect of the hand.

The sites of potential entrapment of the ulnar nerve are:

1. The ulnar groove.
2. The cubital tunnel.
3. Loge de Guyon.

Anatomy of Circulation

The major veins and lymphatics are predominantly on the dorsum of the digits and the body of the hand where they cannot be compressed with gripping. However, there is a deep network of fine veins on the volar aspect and with each artery are companion venae comitantes. The major superficial veins of the forearm and dorsum of the hand are the cephalic vein on the radial side, the basilic vein on the dorsal ulnar side and the median antebrachial vein on the volar ulnar side (Fig. 2-27).

The lymphatic drainage of the hand and forearm is through a superficial and deep system. The superficial network is in two layers, a fine subcutaneous system and a deeper system over the deep fascia. There are intercommunications between these components of the superficial system and at the elbow with the deep system accompanying the arteries. The superficial system aggregates into trunks on the collateral margins of the digits and the body of the hand. The network is extremely fine and diffuse on the volar side as compared to the dorsum, where the main large vessels drain into the forearm. The lymphatic drainage follows the distribution of the major venous trunks. Thus, the radial half of the hand drains by the cephalic veins and in the antecubital fossa splits to follow the course of both the cephalic and basilic veins lead-

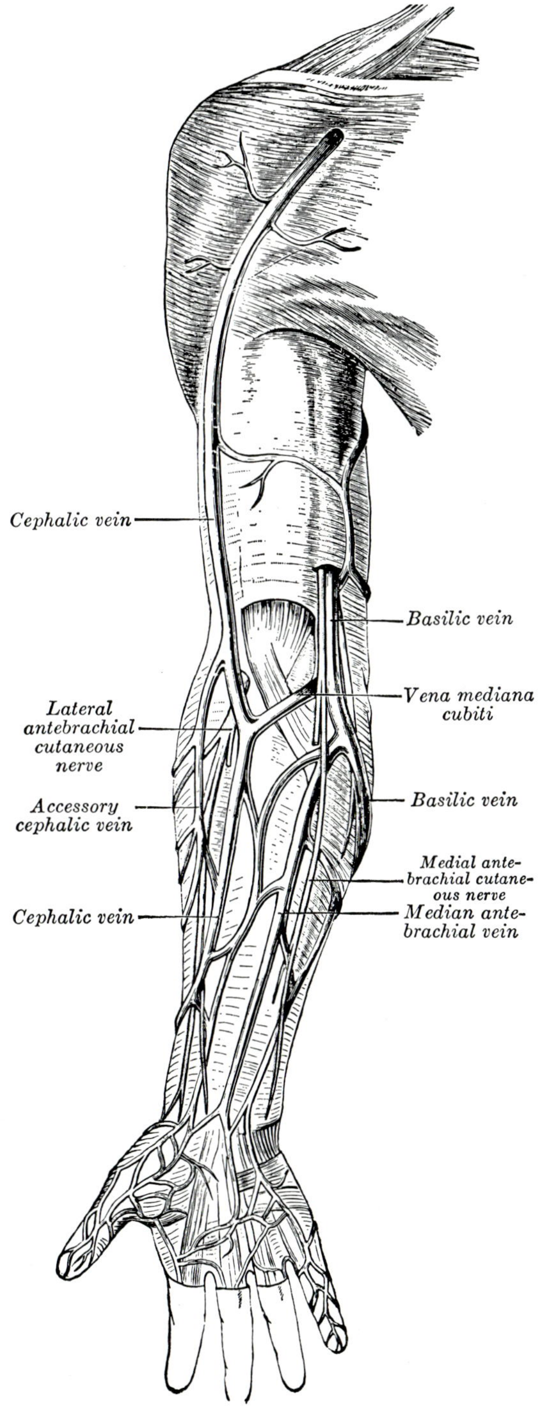

Figure 2-27. *The superficial veins of the upper limb. (From Goss, C.M.*[5]*)*

ing to the axillary and deltopectoral nodes. In contrast, the ulnar side of the hand drains primarily near the basilic vein and the median antebrachial vein volarly to the supratrochlear (epitrochlear) nodes and subsequently to the axillary nodes. Thus, supratrochlear nodes are less likely to be affected by lymphatic drainage from the radial side of the hand.

It is apparent, therefore, that a predominant part of the major venous and lymphatic trunks of the forearm and hand is subcutaneous, where the vessels are easily compressed by tight skin, clothing, and jewelry. Similarly, the deep venous and lymphatic systems that accompany the arteries are within the fascial compartments and are easily compromised by any congestion therein.

The most important features of the arterial circulation are: (1) the richness of the collateral circulation, (2) the considerable anatomical variability, and (3) relationships of surgical importance.

The axillary artery becomes the brachial artery at the level of the teres major where it is surrounded by the major nerves of the arm as well as the basilic vein. It runs on the medial aspect of the biceps with the median nerve crossing it anteriorly to subsequently lie lateral to the nerve under the lacertus fibrosus. Just distal to the antecubital flexion crease and at the proximal edge of the pronator teres it splits into the radial and ulnar arteries. About the elbow is a rich anastomotic complex joining the bifurcation of the radial and ulnar arteries (radial recurrent and anterior and posterior ulnar recurrent) with the brachial artery in the arm.

The radial artery leaves the flexor muscle wad to run under the cover of the brachioradialis and superficial to the flexor pollicis longus. At the radial styloid it splits into the superficial palmar branch and the larger dorsal branch. The former crosses at right angles through the substance of the thenar muscles to anastomose with the terminus of the ulnar artery (the superficial palmar arch) (Fig. 2-28). The deep branch runs in the floor of the anatomical snuffbox (on occasions superficially). It gains access to the palm through the apex of the thumb web and becomes the deep palmar arch which is joined on the ulnar side by the deep branch of the ulnar artery. This arch is proximal to the superficial arch and volar to the deep motor branch of the ulnar nerve but dorsal to the flexor tendons and the lumbricals. This deep arch is often the principal and sometimes the only parent artery of the princeps pollicis and the arterial circulation of the index finger. Therefore, the surgeon must be

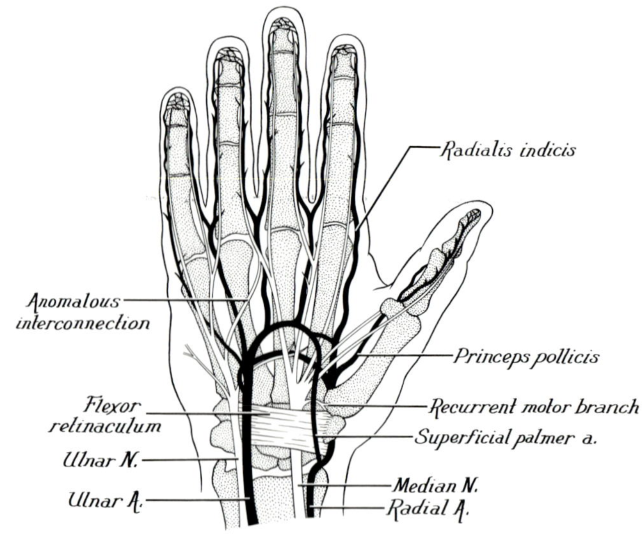

Figure 2-28. *Arterial arches of the palm.* (*Redrawn from* Cunningham's Manual of Practical Anatomy.[3])

wary of this in elective surgery about the wrist, especially for the common ganglion. It is the easiest artery to palpate because of its superficial position proximal to the wrist flexion crease.

The ulnar artery enters the flexor muscle compartment of the forearm through the aponeurotic window formed by the radial and ulnar heads of the superficialis muscle. It crosses behind the median nerve and gives off the common interosseous artery as the nerve gives off its volar interosseous branch. The common interosseous artery immediately branches into two or three major arteries: the constant anterior (volar) interosseous and posterior (dorsal) interosseous arteries and the infrequent median artery. The latter may also arise from the anterior interosseous.

The median artery normally disappears in later fetal development but may persist as the dominant artery of the hand. This fact must be recognized in the conduct of any surgery involving the carpal canal, when the median artery lies adjacent to the median nerve.

The anterior interosseous artery runs down the center of the forearm on the interosseous septum between the profundus and the flexor pollicis longus beside the anterior interosseous nerve. It dissipates in its dorsal and palmar branches over the pronator quadratus, contributing to the collateral circulation of the wrist.

The smaller posterior interosseous artery at the level of the pronator teres passes proximal to the interosseous membrane and joins the posterior interosseous nerve on the deep side of the extensor digitorum communis and on the surface of the abductor pollicis longus. It will be found emerging through the supinator. Distally, like its volar counterpart, it contributes to the collateral circulation of the wrist.

The larger ulnar artery crosses deep to the flexor pronators and median nerve to lie on the body of the flexor digitorum profundus. In the distal half of the forearm it parallels the radial side of the ulnar nerve. It enters the hand through Guyon's canal where it gives rise to the superficial palmar arch. This arcade is found immediately under the palmar aponeurosis and just distal to the transverse carpal ligament. The nerves and tendons are deep to it.

Generally, the ulnar artery provides the major arterial circulation to the hand, but upon occasion the thumb and index finger receive most, if not all, of their circulation from the radial artery via the deep palmar arch. Whenever arterial ligation is necessary, an Allen's test (Chap. 10) should be done to assure satisfactory collateral circulation from the remaining vessel.

References

1. Becton, J.L., Christian, J.D., Goodwin, H.N. and Jackson, J.G.: A simplified technique for treating the complex dislocation of the index metacarpophalangeal joint. J. Bone Joint Surg., 57A:698, 1975.
2. Clemente, C.D.: *Anatomy: A Regional Atlas of the Human Body.* Lea & Febiger, Philadelphia, 1975. Illustrations taken from Fernes and Staubesand, Eds.: *Sobotta Bechur, Atlas der Anatomie des Menschen,* 17th ed. Urban and Schwarzenberg, Munich.
3. *Cunningham's Manual of Practical Anatomy,* Vol. I, 11th ed. Oxford University Press, London, 1948.
4. Doyle, J.R. and Blythe, W.: Macroscopic and functional anatomy of the flexor tendon sheath. Presented at the 29th Annual Meeting of the American Society for Surgery of the Hand, Dallas, January 15–17, 1974.
5. Goss, C.M., Ed.: Gray's *Anatomy of the Human Body,* 29th American Edition. Philadelphia, Lea & Febiger, 1973.
6. Heuston, J.T. and Tubiana, R.: *Dupuytren's Disease.* Grune and Stratton, New York, 1974.
7. Kilgore, E.S., Graham, W.P., Newmeyer, W.L. and Brown, L.G.: The extensor plus finger. Hand, 7:159, 1975.
8. Milford, L.: *Retaining Ligaments of the Digits of the Hand.* Philadelphia, W.B. Saunders, 1968.
9. Spinner, M.: *Injuries to the Major Branches of Peripheral Nerves of the Forearm.* Philadelphia, W.B. Saunders, 1972.
10. Tubiana, R. and Valentin, P.: The anatomy of the extensor apparatus of the fingers. Surg. Clin. North Am., 897, 1964.

3 Examination of the Hand

Disorders of the hand are manifested as either acute or elective problems. The approach varies somewhat for the two categories. In the acute case, most often an injury, treatment must be rendered relatively promptly and there is little opportunity to assess the psychological makeup of the patient. Often considerable anxiety is present which substantially influences the patient's attitude and the course of his recovery.

In contrast, an elective problem generally allows the surgeon to thoroughly orient himself and the patient to the disorder of the hand and the risks and prognosis of treatment. This is important because much of the success of any hand surgery is dependent upon a favorable and responsible attitude by the patient during the convalescence, which may be extended.

Although priorities will vary depending upon the type of case, acute or chronic, certain principles must be kept in mind during any evaluation.

The record must be detailed and accurate. Notes and diagrams must be made during the course of the examination.

The environment of the evaluation should be one that will not generate anxiety on the part of the patient and will serve the purposes of confidentiality. If necessary for the patient's comfort, he should be supine.

Every source should be exploited for an accurate history. The diagnosis may hinge entirely upon the precise details of the mechanism of an injury or the chronology of the natural history of the disorder and its treatment. A system of evaluation should always include the following information:

Age
Sex
Occupation and working status
Hand dominance
General health
Allergies
Preexisting hand problems
Chief complaint and date of onset
History of disorder and mechanism of injury
Precipitating, aggravating and relieving factors
Present status:
  Subjective factors
  Objective factors
Diagram (where indicated)

Recognition of the patient's age is important. The physical and economic magnitude of the problem and the psychological and physical capacity to respond to treatment, especially surgery, will vary greatly depending upon whether the patient is a child, adolescent, adult, or elderly person.

Certain elective procedures are often postponed in the very young to await their maturity and potential to understand and cooperate. Adolescents often hide the magnitude of their ego-generated concern over relatively insignificant problems. Failure to recognize this and give adequate reassurance may vastly magnify the problem for the patient. In middle life, the economics of family support may be in peril if a course of treatment generates prolonged disability. Failure to recognize this may produce an unsatisfactory psychological and physical result. The elderly hand is more prone to stiffness and its limited tolerance to surgery and immobilization must be recognized in choosing proper treatment.

Certain problems are more frequent in one sex than the other. Males are more likely to have thick heavy hands that easily stiffen, whereas women more often present cosmetic problems and some specific disorders such as carpal tunnel syndrome.

The functional requirements of the hand are to a large extent governed by the patient's occupation. This, in turn, influences the surgeon's choice of treatment. A musician may be inordinately handicapped by loss of digital length or mobility, while this would be an insignificant disability for someone else. A stiff, anesthetic, reimplanted little finger might be required for cosmetic reasons in a receptionist. In someone else the same finger would be in the way and very disabling.

The knowledge of the working status of the patient gives insight into the magnitude of the disability as well as his motivation. In considering treatment the prognosis is always more favorable in the patient who insists upon working in spite of the handicap of his disability.

Hand dominance plays an important role in any hand disability. Grip strength and dexterity are generally greater in the dominant hand, and greater surgical efforts to restore these are usually justified.

Coexisting health problems may influence disorders of the hand and its repair and recovery. Awareness of these will guide the clinician in his program of treatment.

Psychological aberrations of the patient are some of the most common problems encountered. Indeed, all too often the hand problem is a reflection of the basic psychological one. Patients with substantial basic anxieties are subject to hand injuries and are prone to the formation of thick scar and stiffness regardless of the original pliability of the tissues.

Patients with psychoses, mental retardation, epilepsy, and spastic disorders are usually unable to cooperate in a complex treatment program. Alcoholics and other drug addicts present similar handicaps to treatment. A patient with claustrophobia may not be able to tolerate the confinement of a pedicle flap or immobilization in a cast.

Some patients by their low pain threshold make it impossible to inject any medication because of their apprehension toward the needle.

Hypertension and bleeding tendencies will aggravate the bleeding and swelling from an injury or surgery. In elective cases this may be controlled (antihypertensive treatment, reduction of aspirin ingestion, etc.).

The coexistence of systemic infection or infection within the involved extremity is a matter of concern in dealing with a hand problem. The same concern exists in the face of peripheral vascular insufficiency, and with any systemic state of metabolic depletion or anemia.

A knowledge of the patient's allergies is essential. The common categories which are germane to the treatment of the hand are: (1) antibiotics, e.g. penicillin; (2) anti-inflammatory agents, e.g. phenylbutazone; (3) analgesics, e.g. aspirin or codeine; (4) contact irritants, e.g. adhesive tape; (5) certain suture materials, e.g. catgut.

The failure to recognize preexisting hand problems can lead to improper diagnosis and assignment of liability for injury, and improper selection of treatment and erroneous prognosis. There can be problems of appearance and form or function brought about by previous injury, disease or congenital malformation. Clues to the existence of previous problems are often gained only through suspicious attention to details of the history, examination and roentgenograms. An example is the bipartate scaphoid mistaken for a fractured scaphoid, or a non-union with sclerotic edges mistaken for a fresh fracture.

For diagnostic reasons, and for proper treatment planning, it is essential to learn the time of onset of the patient's problem and the details of his chief complaints (subjective and objective factors).

With wounds, the interval from wounding to treatment dictates the need for antibiotics for the risk of infection. It also indicates the extent of the healing process that has already taken place. After three to four weeks it may be impossible to reduce a fracture and after two to four months to retrieve a divided flexor tendon. At this stage it is necessary to go into the details of the history of the development of the disorder and the mechanism of the injury. In evaluating the risk of infection it is important to know where, how, and when a wound occurred. If it occurred in soapy dishwater the risk is small compared to its having occurred in a barnyard.

In considering a fracture there must be some history of violence. Hence we should know the forces involved and their direction. The history must reflect the physical findings. An abrasion with a crust and dry gangrene of a fingertip are not acute injuries. The location and amount of injury created by broken glass puncture wounds are far less predictable than are those created by local incision with a knife. The innocuous wound of entrance of a high-pressure injection injury of the hand may belie the severity of the problem initiated. The importance of these details is obvious when comparing the location of the stumps of the flexor tendon injured in a fall on the outstretched palm to their location when the injury is sustained in grabbing a knife.

Essential to a thorough history and important in planning treatment is a list of precipitating and aggravating factors. It does little good to advise the patient to use his hand at work if that circumstance is an aggravating one. Examples of this are: (1) the identification of cervical nerve root compression by the history of extremity pain consistently produced by certain positions of the neck, (2) the recognition of Raynaud's phenomenon by its initiation when the hand is exposed to cold or the patient is extremely tense, (3) the relationship of highly repetitive activity (e.g. clipping the lawn) and myositis crepitans of the abductor pollicis longus and (4) the relationship of skin exposure to detergents and the eruption of dermatitis.

The existence and character of previous treatment are of utmost importance. In acute cases such knowledge avoids unnecessary duplication and helps materially in planning future treatment. Were tetanus toxoid and antibiotics administered at the onset of injury? Was an effort already made to reduce this difficult dislocation? What was the previous response of this de Quervain's tenosynovitis to steroid injection? Has the patient already had an adequate program of physiotherapy?

With all of this available past information about the patient, it is equally important to establish the present status and compare it with the past. Progressive subjective and objective improvement, no improvement or deterioration must be noted and related to the extent and duration of previous treatment.

In an acute injury showing progressive neurological impairment, some form of decompression may be urgent. In contrast to this, the stiffness of the digit that has had every modality of treatment without any change in a period of 2 to 3 months is permanent.

A diagram is indispensable to good recording of certain hand problems, and is often far more succinct and definitive than the written word. It shows the topography of subjective and objective problems. The examination of the patient should begin by focusing attention on the total patient, the neck, both upper extremities and finally the involved part of the hand. This pertains to both acute and chronic cases and should be modified only in the presence of hemorrhage, marked pain, circumstances of severe mangling and the like. The surgeon should allow ample time within the limits of good treatment to become aware of coexisting psychological and physical problems and their magnitude. Good light and a well-ventilated room with proper help and equipment are needed for an adequate efficient examination.

With acute problems, the need of facilities for comfort is often more pressing than in the case of chronic disorders. Having the patient supine will generally accomplish this, and will obviate syncope and its hazards. Clothing and jewelry should be completely removed from the upper extremity.

The usual acute problems consist of injuries and pain initiated by infection and occasionally nontraumatic vascular disorders. The priorities in evaluating the acutely injured hand are: (1) the control of hemorrhage, (2) the extent of viability (vascular integrity), (3) the appreciation of motor and sensory nerve function, (4) the maintenance of skeletal alignment and joint function, (5) the control of pain by suitable systemic, regional, or local analgesia and (6) the evaluation of the wound and the injuries within it.

The initial control of bleeding should be attempted by direct pressure by sterile dressings against the bleeding point. More definitive control can then follow with a sphygmomanometer as an arterial tourniquet. This should be padded with cast padding and secured with more cast padding or adhesive tape. The tubing should be directed toward the shoulder, the extremity elevated and the tourniquet inflated rapidly to 250 to 300 mm Hg. The tubing should then be clamped at the cuff by a large hemostat and the inflation valve released. Tolerance of the tourniquet under these circumstances is excellent in the average patient for at least 20 to 30 minutes. The use of the tourniquet serves as an effective psychological distraction. If not done previously, the wound should now be rendered anesthetic by suitable field or nerve block with 1 per cent lidocaine without epinephrine. The skin can now be suitably cleansed and the extremity draped. The final control of the bleeding point can then be discretely done by precise identification and ligation. This often requires the use of a magnifying loupe, extension of the wound, and removal of clots. Ligatures should be non-reactive, e.g. nylon. This technique avoids iatrogenic injury to uninjured nerves and other structures.

At this point it is possible to survey the extent of injury and to determine the best facilities for treatment. Complex injuries, flexor tendon, nerve and difficult bone and joint problems, as well as some extensor tendon injuries, should generally be referred to the operating room.

Acute pain exclusive of that caused by direct trauma and wounds is most commonly caused by infectious and non-infectious inflammatory states. The criteria for their diagnosis are given in Chapter 8. Another, rare, cause of pain is acute vascular insufficiency secondary to vascular accident, e.g. embolus or intra-arterial drug injection.

The evaluation of chronic problems comprises two categories: the initial examination and the follow-up examination. The initial examination differs from that for acute injury primarily because bleeding, a fresh wound and the attendant anxiety and pain are lacking. Accordingly, more detailed attention can be directed at the total patient, the comparison of the upper extremities, a systematic approach to the musculoskeletal and neurological function, and the state of other soft tissues.

A routine should be followed. The whole upper extremity and neck should be bared. The patient should be watched as he disrobes. This is an ideal opportunity to observe his function and the consistency of any deficit.

The patient should be asked to sit or stand squarely and to elevate both extremities simultaneously to the ceiling. At a glance the range of motion of the shoulders and elbows and the existence of abnormalities of form (e.g. atrophy, tumors) can be seen.

Even more important, however, is the fact that the hands are brought into prominence without the distracting background of patterned clothing and jewelry. By pronation and supination the dorsal and volar aspects of the hands can be compared, the fists made to close and open rapidly, the digits made to spread and meet, and the thumbs made to approximate the fingertips in succession. Eliciting these maneuvers with the hands overhead reduces the likelihood of deliberate restriction of function by the patient and highlights any abnormalities.

The patient is then asked to bring both elbows tightly to his waist and to move his forearms through full pronation and supination. The integrity of wrist function is then compared by the palm-to-palm pray position while the shoulders are abducted, after which the hands are placed dorsum to dorsum.

Digital lengths are compared by matching digits palm to palm (crease by crease). Digital motion is compared by moving the fingertips from a straight line to meet the proximal, middle and distal palm and the thumb from full abduction-extension to flexion to meet the ulnar side of the hand. Any abnormal configurations of form and alignment are noted.

Specific attention is then directed to the skin, its color, temperature and perspiration. Scars, contractures, wounds and other lesions are noted, as is the character of the fingernails. The radial and ulnar pulses are palpated, and where appropriate an Allen's test is done (Chap. 10). Abnormal pulsations or bruits are recorded.

The neuromuscular evaluation must specifically identify the integrity of the three major nerves and of the individual musculotendinous units. The integrity of the radial nerve is tested by forceful wrist extension and extension of the metacarpophalangeal joints and by pinprick within the dorsum of the thumb web. The ulnar nerve is tested by forceful spreading of the fingers and flexion of distal joint of the ring and little fingers and by pinprick over the eponychium of the little finger. The median nerve is tested by forceful flexion of the wrist and of the interphalangeal joints of the thumb and index finger and by pinprick over the eponychium of the index and long fingers. A test should be made of the distal phalangeal flexors and of the independence of action of the superficialis tendons, the independent extensors of the thumb, index and little fingers and of the wrist flexors and extensors.

A critical test of sensory function of the median nerve is the blindfold coin-discrimination test in which the patient is asked to identify coins while blindfolded.

Where appropriate, points of tenderness must be elicited and the mechanism of pain reproduced. The instability of ligaments and the existence of crepitation and trigger phenomena must be established by appropriate testing. Circumferential measurements of the biceps, forearm and digits will verify atrophy or swelling and goniometer readings of extension and flexion will demonstrate deficits in range of motion. Pinch and grip meter readings are necessary to evaluate the power of these functions objectively.

Adjuncts to the history and physical examination consist of roentgenographic studies and laboratory tests. Musculoskeletal injury generally requires initial and follow-up roentgenograms to aid in diagnosis and treatment. Where results are inconclusive it is often helpful to have comparable views of the opposite extremity and to obtain views in multiple planes. Many scaphoid fractures have been missed because of failure to get a plane of exposure that passes exactly parallel to the plane of the fracture. Roentgenograms are also helpful in cases of tumefaction and inflammation of bone and with some soft tissue tumors and foreign bodies. Special examinations—tomography, magnification views, cineroentgenography and arthrography—can aid in the diagnosis of certain difficult problems.

The principal laboratory studies for evaluating problems in the hand are: complete blood count, sedimentation rate, uric acid, latex fixation tests, histological examination, culture of pathogenic organisms, and the conduction velocities and latencies of nerves.

The usual pitfalls in the evaluation of the hand lie in an inadequate history and incomplete initial and subsequent examinations. An accurate diagnosis requires consistency on the part of the patient in his subjective and objective complaints and their correlation with consistent physical and laboratory findings. It also requires a knowledge of the manifestations of disorders and of compensatory mechanisms which can mask the problem in whole or in part. A typical example is the failure to recognize a divided extensor pollicis longus tendon since the distal phalanx of the thumb still extends to a straight line (a function of the intrinsics of the thumb). Similarly, a carpal tunnel syndrome may not be recognized because the patient gives a history of pain radiating from the forearm to the shoulder and chest. A trigger thumb in an infant may not be recognized because it is assumed that the limited extension is a fault of the extensor mechanism. In addition, pitfalls of omission and commission exist, such as the failure to detect a foreign body in a wound because the examination was not carried out with a proximal tourniquet, or the failure to recognize the presence of gout because of a normal uric acid determination.

The development and maintenance of a practice in hand surgery depend upon the extent of effective communication between the treating physician and interested parties. These include referring physicians, insurance companies and employers. The latter two are administratively responsible for the great volume of industrial injuries and must be informed to meet their obligations in supporting the patient during his disability and in maintaining effective replacement during his absence. Reports, particularly the initial report, are psychologically and administratively urgent. The initial report should give succinct details of the history, physical status, diagnosis and proposed treatment, an estimate of the treatment period and time to be lost from work. The physician must guard against underestimating the latter two issues and in making any initial commitment regarding permanent disability.

4 Facilities

In the locations where treatment is rendered to the hand, the office, the emergency room and the operating room, certain specially trained personnel and specific equipment are needed. The least appreciated and attended factor about the patient with a hand problem is its psychological impact upon him. Loss of hand function through pain, disease or injury may not only be frightening but threatens economic security and ego, constituting a crisis. Hence the environment of treatment can have a lasting effect in preparing the patient to deal with the problem and conditioning him to a smooth or difficult convalescence. The patient is suggestible, with blunted discrimination between favorable and unfavorable influences. He has a predilection to absorb pessimistic rather than optimistic suggestion. Looks, behavior, remarks, noises, silence, odors and the activity around him all play on his senses and his imagination. Thus a sympathetic, prompt, orderly approach, flavored with encouragement and sparing him details of the adverse experiences of others and unusual hazards, will go far to relieve his anxiety and to conserve the energy which it consumes.

Office and Emergency Room Facilities

Ideally, the requirements for the care of the hand in the emergency room and the office are parallel. Twenty-five to thirty per cent of all emergency room cases involve hand problems and any office specializing in the hand will treat a sizable number of patients daily. Hence, the flow of patient traffic with priority for special problems must be constantly monitored. Tidy, esthetic waiting rooms and examination facilities, with congenial, compassionate and efficient personnel, will go far to implement this.

Patients suffering acute injuries with pain and bleeding must be seen immediately for comfort and prompt attention. Patients who are to be seen very briefly in follow-up should be taken care of in advance of those requiring a time-consuming evaluation and treatment. Receptionists, nurses and surgeons must be mindful of the exigencies of individual patients. The maintenance of the ideal atmosphere of the waiting and treatment area can be enhanced by the speedy processing of the disruptive patient, e.g. abusive, non-hygienic adult or wailing child. Some waiting is unavoidable, but the sting of this can be reduced by facilities for distraction, e.g. background music, reading material, etc., and, even more important, by a genuine reception and careful attention to the treatment of the problem.

At the initial visit the individual identifying data for each patient must be accurately recorded so that his needs for the execution of insurance reports and disability papers, as well as the bookkeeping needs of the office and hospital, can be promptly and efficiently processed.

The treatment area should be quiet, well lighted, and, where necessary, appeal to the privacy needed for a given patient. The floor space should be sufficiently liberal to avoid congestion. The frequently used dressings and instruments should be immediately available to any given treatment table. An autoclave is essential but the delays incurred by dependence on it can be reduced by the use of disposable syringes and needles.

The common materials and instruments which should be available at each treatment area are as follows:

Materials Available on the Treatment Table for Hand Care

- Tabletop contains:
  - Sponge forceps
  - Sponge forceps container
  - Solution for soaking instruments
  - Container of sterile 4 x 4 gauze pads
  - Container of sterile 2 x 2 gauze pads
  - Container of alcohol sponges
  - Container of sterile cotton-tipped applicators
  - Container of sterile tongue blades
  - Container of Xeroform* gauze strips
  - Airtight bottles, 8 oz
    - Ether
    - Benzene
    - Alcohol
    - Hydrogen peroxide
  - Bottle, 4 oz, tr. benzoin
  - Jar, 16 oz, zinc oxide
  - Baby powder
  - Tube gauze applicators (2 sizes)
  - Aromatic ammonia ampules
- Top drawer contains:
  - Band-Aids (assorted)
  - Kling (assorted)—elastic gauze bandage
  - Kerlix (assorted)
- Second drawer contains:
  - Ace bandages (assorted)
  - Digital splints (assorted)
  - Slings
- Third drawer contains
  - Reston (½″ and ¼″ sheets)—adhesive-backed foam sponge
- Fourth drawer contains:
  - Micropore tape (assorted)—non-allergic paper tape
  - Miscellaneous
- Wall-mounted tape dispenser

Instruments Available on the Treatment Table for Hand Care

- Scalpels (sterile)—#15 and #11 blades
- Forceps (sterile)
  - Large smooth
  - Fixation (fine multitoothed)
  - Fine smooth tying
- Hemostats (sterile)
  - Fine curved mosquito
  - Standard straight Crile
- Scissors
  - Bandage (sterile and unsterile)
  - Fine short-bladed curved pointed iris (sterile)
- Magnifying loupe, 2 power

Additional Instruments and Supplies for Surgery and Special Procedures

- Bottle, 8 oz, 1 per cent iodine
- Paint brush in alcohol
- Sphygmomanometer with heavy clamp for tubing
- Boat of antiseptic solution containing:
  - Scissors
    - Large curved Mayo
    - Small iris
    - Littler type
  - Forceps
    - Large smooth
    - Fixation
    - Fine smooth tying
    - Jeweler's
  - Hemostats—curved mosquito
  - Retractors
    - Small right-angle double-ended (Ragnell)
    - Vein
    - Strong heavy single hooks
    - Double fine hooks
    - Self-retaining, spring
  - Needle holder, smooth-jawed—Webster
  - "Dental probe" (dural dissector)
  - Nail clipper
  - Rongeur (double action)—Hibbs small
  - Razor blades or Goulian knife
- Bunnell hand drill (sterile)
- Kirschner wires (sterile)—.035, .045, .062
- Wire cutters (sterile)
- Blunt-nosed pliers to remove K wires (sterile)
- Ring cutter
- Sutures—3-0, 4-0, 5-0, 6-0 monofilament nylon with fine cutting needle
- Gloves (sterile)
- Sheets and towels (sterile)
- Hyfrecator
- Tin snips and pliers

Special Materials

- Injectables
  - Lidocaine 1 per cent
  - Triamcinolone, 10 mg and 40 mg/ml
    - Tetanus toxoid } Refrigerated
    - Antibiotics, injectable } Refrigerated
    - Bacitracin } Refrigerated
- Syringes (disposable)—assorted
- Needles (disposable)—gauge 18 to 30
- Resuscitation kit
- Wheelchair

The instruments listed are a composite of those used in plastic and ophthalmologic surgery. The

*Xeroform: 3% bismuth tribromophenate impregnated gauze. Chesebrough-Ponds, Greenwich, Connecticut.

heavier instruments used in general and orthopedic surgery are not acceptable for the treatment of the hand. Disposable and discarded instruments are likewise unsatisfactory.

Figure 4-1 shows a typical examination table for treating an extremity with the patient sitting. This is ideal for the evaluation and treatment of painless problems, e.g. dressing changes, application of splints and removal of some sutures. When privacy is not important there may be several of these in one room.

Figure 4-2 is an example of an examination and treatment table with a Mayo stand on which to place the extremity during treatment. The patient can lie either way on this flat table by merely shifting the Mayo stand and the pillow. Figure 4-3 shows the operating table in the emergency room, which can be raised or lowered to serve the preference of the surgeon. For all areas a good light is essential. These facilities must be complemented by good adjustable lighting, magnifying loupes, and a tourniquet (sphygmomanometer) for adequate care of the hand.

The equipment and supplies needed for the application and removal of casts are listed below:

Cast cutter with vacuum
Plastic bucket
Cast padding, assorted
Plaster, fast-setting, assorted
  3- and 4-inch wide strips 15″ long
  3- and 4-inch wide rolls
Cotton stockinette

The equipment needed for measuring function, motion and atrophy is as noted:

Cloth tape measure (metric)
Ruler (metric)
Goniometer for digits
Goniometer for wrist and elbow
Grip dynamometer, Jamar
Pinch dynamometer
Compass (2-point tester)
Coins—assorted
Sandpaper—assorted
Percussion hammer

The emergency evaluation and treatment of the hand have traditionally been relegated to the novice, intern and resident. Not until every physician who makes the initial evaluation of a hand injury has been indoctrinated with the fundamentals of diagnosis and treatment will the proper emergency care of the hand begin. There still is a real void in the adequate training of nurses to assist properly in this specialty.

For the physician adequately trained in the care of the hand, the treatments which can be routinely rendered in the office and emergency room are outlined below.

INJECTIONS AND ASPIRATIONS

The patient should be supine and the hand supported on an arm board. The skin is cleansed with alcohol. The needles must be sharp and introduced

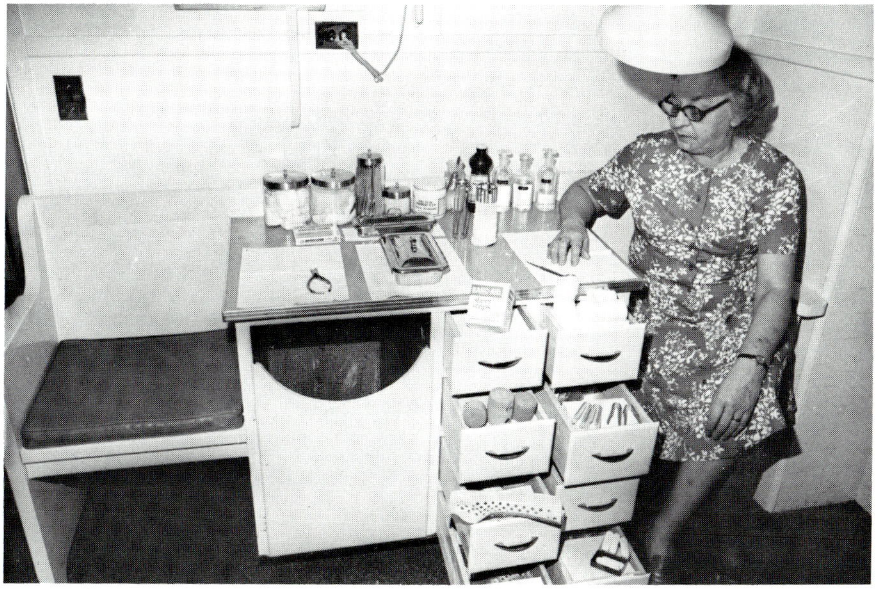

Figure 4-1. *Examination table suitable for a patient who is seated.*

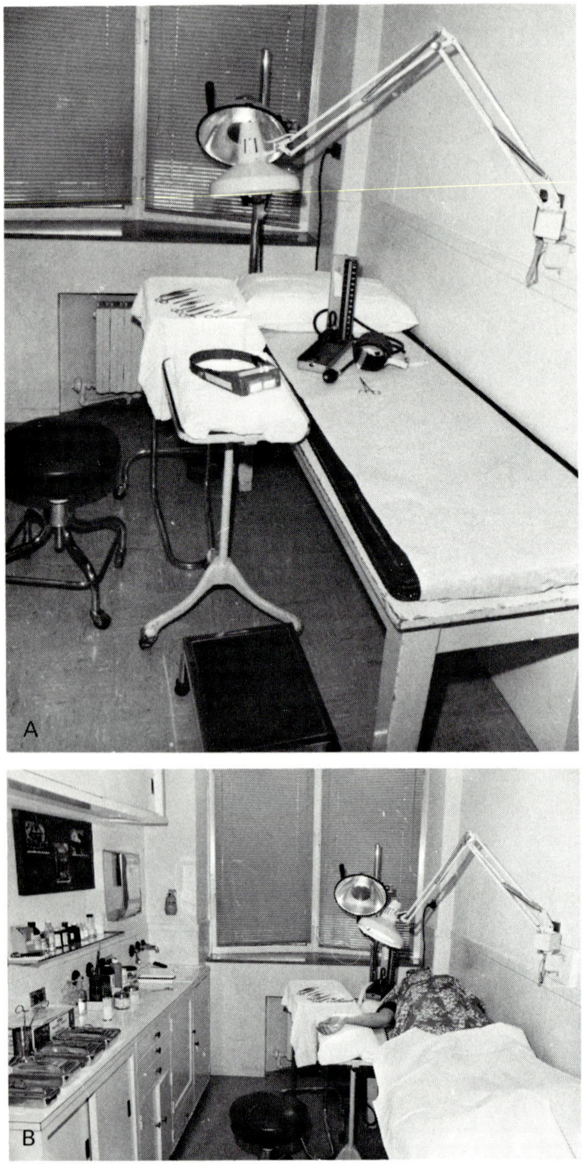

Figure 4-2. *An examination table for the recumbent patient which can be used with the patient lying in either direction by reversing the position of the pillow and the Mayo stand.*

perpendicular to the skin. The injection should always be slow and never in such volume as to cause tissue tension. With the exception of tetanus toxoid and antibiotics, most injections in the upper extremity should be combined with lidocaine to avoid pain. Nerves and vessels should not be injured. Short 26- to 30-gauge needles should be used for injections close to the surface. For deeper injections (e.g. the carpal canal) a $1\frac{1}{2}$-inch, 25-gauge needle may be used. If a steroid has been administered, its diffusion will be facilitated by gentle massage combined with active opening and closing of the fist. Aspirations of synovial spaces and cysts may require an 18- or 19-gauge needle after the area has been anesthetized.

FRACTURES, DISLOCATIONS, AND SPRAINS

The patient should be supine if reduction is necessary or if pain is bothersome. Reduction requires suitable regional or local anesthesia. Difficult reductions must be referred to the hospital for operating room care by possible open treatment. Simple intermedullary fixation may be undertaken, as may any external fixation (Chaps. 11 and 12).

CONTUSIONS AND SUBUNGUAL HEMATOMAS

Barring extreme pain, the patient may be sitting for evaluation of contusions. If there is any suspicion of bony injury, roentgenograms should be obtained. All constrictive clothing and jewelry should be removed and, depending upon the amount of swelling and pain, consideration should be given to the use of a forearm cast to immobilize the wrist for several days. No effort should be made to aspirate a hematoma nor to inject it with enzymes. Patients with serious injuries should be hospitalized and, where indicated, fasciotomies performed.

The subungual hematoma should be decompressed if it is painful. To do this, the patient must be supine. If the lake of blood is extensive no anesthesia is necessary. The nail is most easily perforated by twirling a #11 scalpel or 19-gauge needle attached to a syringe at an oblique angle to the

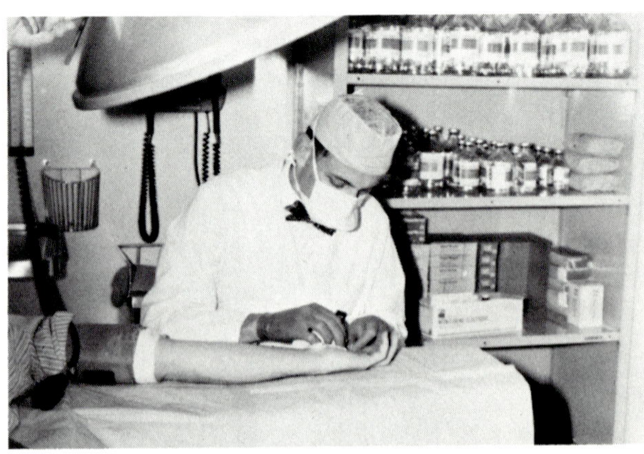

Figure 4-3. *Adjustable arm board and operating table for emergency room use. Note tourniquet and adequate illumination.*

surface of the nail. A wet dressing or zinc oxide compress is applied for 24 hours. A roentgenogram is needed in all of these injuries to rule out the presence of a fracture.

LIMITED BURNS AND ABRASIONS

Suitable cleansing and debridement are done, usually with the patient recumbent (Chap. 18).

PUNCTURE WOUNDS AND FOREIGN BODIES

The prime obligation in the office or emergency room is to assay the extent of contamination and complexity of the injury, thus determining the need for hospitalization. Simple puncture wounds may require no more than advice to the patient regarding control of swelling and activity, augmented by the administration of tetanus prophylaxis and antibiotics. Many foreign bodies can be retrieved under tourniquet ischemia and adequate anesthesia in the office and emergency room. Magnification must be available. However, the physician must be selective in the technique and timing of the removal (Chap. 9).

SKIN WOUNDS (UNCOMPLICATED)

Most wounds of skin and fat are amenable to removal of clots, irrigation, closure, drainage and splinting in the office or emergency room, providing the procedures are not so time consuming as to disrupt the expedient care of other patients. When that is the case, the wound should be dressed, the part immobilized, antibiotics administered and the patient hospitalized for definitive care.

AVULSION INJURIES

The major consideration with respect to such an injury is whether it will prove to be too extensive or time consuming to treat without hospital admission. Most fingertip amputations and loss of substance injuries of less than 2.5 cm^2 can be treated with an onlay split-thickness skin graft in the office or emergency room (Chaps. 9 and 16).

EXTENSOR TENDONS

If the separation of extensor tendon lacerations is 0.5 cm or less, the injury can be suitably repaired in the office or emergency room. When the separation is greater than 0.5 cm, the retrieval of the proximal stump and its approximation to the distal stump may be difficult, and such repairs should be done in the operating room. In treating these problems the surgeon must be mindful of the potential for the development of mallet and buttonhole deformities (Chap. 14). Division of extensor tendons in the wrist and forearm should be repaired in the operating room.

INCISION AND DRAINAGE OF INFECTIONS

When regional or local anesthesia is feasible, a great many abscesses may be incised and drained in the office or emergency room. However, extensive infections of subcutaneous spaces, and infections of bones, joints, and tendon sheaths, must generally be treated in the hospital (Chap. 20).

MISCELLANEOUS

These procedures include: biopsies, limited excisions of cutaneous and some subcutaneous lesions, certain cases of subcutaneous fasciotomy for Dupuytren's fasciitis, removal of internal fixation, etc.

PREPARATION OF THE PATIENT FOR REFERRAL TO THE HOSPITAL

The patient with a freshly injured hand should be made comfortable with proper splinting and positioning of the hand. Wounds may be temporarily sutured or dressed after standard surgical preparation of the skin. Contaminating injuries may require the immediate institution of local and systemic antibiotic coverage as well as drainage. The reason for hospitalization should be explained but the details of definitive care and orientation about its consequences should be left to the discretion of the surgeon to whom the patient is referred. The physician should send as much historical information as possible to the hospital with the patient; he should include details of allergy, specific requests made by the patient and his family, and details of any treatment rendered (including medications and the time given). When general anesthesia is anticipated within 6 to 8 hours, the patient should be instructed to avoid oral intake. Conditions which are referred to the hospital and not treated in the office or emergency room are listed below. Specific details of management are given in the appropriate chapters.

Time-consuming simple surgical procedures
Complex procedures
Surgical procedures requiring a general anesthetic
Flexor tenorrhaphy
Extensor tenorrhaphy (widely separated tendon stumps)
Neurorrhaphy
Vascular anastomosis
Major grafts and flaps
Complex fracture reductions and fixation
Mangling and complex injuries
Extensive infections
Amputations and loss of substance injuries not amenable to limited and simple grafting
Extensive burns

Preoperative Care

Before reconstructive procedures are undertaken, the surgeon must take the time to study the physical abnormalities and to understand the psychological makeup of the patient, his needs, and the reasons for the contemplated operation. The success of surgery is largely governed by the patient's ability to assume his full responsibility in implementing the treatment program and accepting, without apprehension, the length of convalescence. Irreversible stiffness and scar formation are generated by fear and anxiety as well as by indifference and reluctance to mobilize the extremity actively postoperatively. This must be recognized by the surgeon in planning the treatment, which must be adapted to the patient's idiosyncrasies of age, occupation and physical and mental health. The surgeon must develop, from his pool of experience, the simplest treatment to meet the needs of the patient. When there is little to gain and much to risk in terms of function, time and expense, the plan should be simplified or the condition accepted as it is. When the functional loss is overwhelming, a little improvement may justify considerable reconstructive effort.

It is a mistake to generate apprehension for treatment that has good promise, but it is just as much a mistake to hide from the patient the realities of significant uncertainties, drawbacks or hazards of treatment. To aid the patient in understanding his problem and to hold his confidence over the course of treatment, consultation by a qualified hand expert may be very helpful. A patient should never be coerced into acquiescence to an operation.

After the initial evaluation of the injury, further observation of the patient over a period of time may be crucial to the proper selection of the operation to be done and its timing. This period will help to recognize the inception of an infection, impairment of circulation or the existence of other more serious injuries. It also gives a chance to assay the patient's attitude toward the planned treatment.

Except when the problem is urgent, operations should be scheduled when the patient and the surgical team are at their best. A good night's sleep on the part of the patient and his physicians may be invaluable to meet the psychological and physical demands of a challenging operation. Urgent problems requiring prompt care are hemorrhage, impaired circulation with cyanosis or pallor and associated cooling of all or part of the extremity, severe pain, mangling or marked disruption of alignment, systemic toxicity and rapidly progressive swelling and paralysis.

Certain prerequisites with respect to the condition of the tissues must be met if reconstructive surgery is contemplated. There must be good circulation and pliable skin and fat in the operative area. If tenorrhaphies and tendon transfers are contemplated, there must be good passive mobility of the involved joints and intact muscles with adequate power. The tissues should have good sensibility whenever possible.

A helpful set of routine preoperative orders for hand surgery is given below.

Note and record any allergies
Give nothing by mouth
Keep the trunk flat and extremity comfortably elevated on pillows so that hand is above the heart
Infuse in the normal arm 1000 cc 5 per cent dextrose in water with antibiotics over 3 hours
Give tetanus toxoid 0.5 cc i.m. in thigh if not already administered*
Conduct routine laboratory tests
Order morphine sulfate, 10 mg i.m. on call
Order scopolamine, 0.4 mg i.m. on call
Sign operative consent for: ____________

This must be modified to meet the individual needs of the patient.

*To be ordered specifically depending on the adequacy of previous immunization.

Operating Room Procedure

Regardless of whether the patient is asleep or not, any discussions within earshot must be disciplined to avoid increasing his anxiety. He should be kept warm and comfortable and transported from his room to the operating table with dispatch.

Preparation of the Skin

A properly padded tourniquet is placed about the upper arm. It is not to be inflated until preparations prior to incision are complete unless hemorrhage is a problem. Blind clamping of bleeding points should not be done to avoid injury to nerves. Tourniquet time must be conserved and should rarely exceed 2 to $2\frac{1}{2}$ hours. The gauge should be tested for accuracy before each use and set at 100 mm Hg above the patient's systolic blood pressure.

Shaving is not necessary except where an incision will be made or adhesive tape applied. When there is a fresh wound with blood and dirt on the skin, hydrogen peroxide or soap and water may be needed to remove it. Otherwise a simple coating of the skin with 1 per cent iodine and alcohol suffices. This is most easily applied with an ordinary paint brush. The "prep" solution should not enter an open wound. Care is directed toward washing the iodine from the skin with alcohol and preventing the iodine from saturating the tourniquet padding. Vigorous scrubbing of the skin is not necessary.

Method of Draping

The arm is positioned with comfort on an arm board which may consist of two operating table arm boards, side by side, or a specially made board with a leg. The former facilitates raising and lowering the operating table to meet the preferences of the surgeon to stand or sit at work. Drapes are applied to the arm in the following manner: A single stockinette is placed on the hand and rolled up over the tourniquet like a sleeve. This should be fastened proximally or should be snug enough to hold its position. If possible, this is done with the patient's cooperation while he is still awake, thus avoiding the difficulty of putting the sleeve on a flaccid, anesthetized extremity.

A sterile waterproof layer of either plastic or paper drape is placed over the arm board and covered with towels. Next, a long drape is placed directly under the arm, folding the edge nearest the body into a 6- or 8-inch cuff. The arm is placed on this drape so that the edge of the cuff lies just distal to the limit of the prepared skin. The top drape is then placed over the body and upper arm so that its edge coincides with the edge of the cuff below. The margins of the two drapes are secured with towel clips. The clips adjacent to the arm secure both sheets and the stockinette but not the skin. This allows the arm to be easily moved about in all directions without opening up undraped and unsterile areas (Fig. 4-4A–D).

Surgical Procedure

At this point the patient is anesthetized. Anesthesia precedes the skin preparation and draping only when (1) the patient is in pain or excessively anxious, or the tourniquet is applied to control bleeding, (2) a regional anesthesia is preferred. Care is then taken to control the anesthetized extremity and prevent its contamination.

Skin incisions are always planned with a marking dye with crosshatches for proper alignment at closure; this may be done with methylene blue applied with a long sharpened applicator or with commercially available skin-marking pens. To obtain the most bloodless field, a large roll of soft gauze is placed in the palm; the stockinette is brought over the hand and an elastic roll is carefully wrapped centripetally up to the tourniquet, which is then inflated. In the absence of an Esmarch bandage, adequate emptying of blood is achieved by the highest elevation of the arm without constricting it. If local anesthesia is to be used, the tourniquet is first inflated. This precludes venous congestion of the wound by the block. When a digital block is complete, a wide Penrose drain may be applied completely flat as a finger tourniquet and the upper-arm tourniquet released.

There are certain contraindications to the use of an Esmarch bandage prior to tourniquet inflation: infection, extensive hemorrhage, divided tendons, fractures, significant soft tissue injury, thin-walled cysts, and certain foreign bodies, e.g. glass. Basically, the bandage should not be used if it is prone to create further damage by spreading extravasated blood or pus, or by displacing divided tendons.

A tourniquet must be applied to the upper arm for all operations unless the proximal limits of the

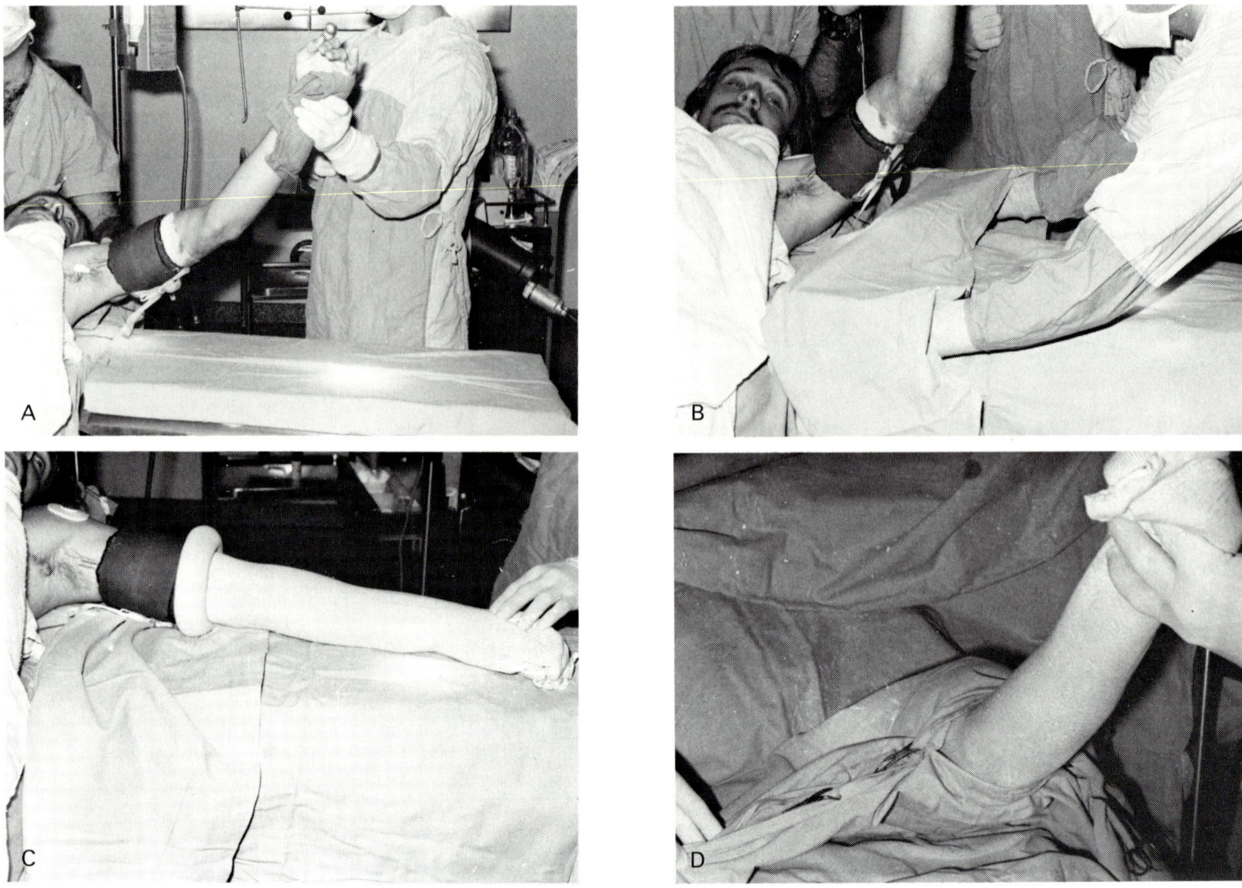

Figure 4-4. *Proper method of draping the upper extremity to permit easy movement of the arm and free positioning of the hand. (See text.)*

operative field negate it. Inflation may be withheld during debridement of ischemic tissue until the exact limits of viability can be determined. When a critical dissection has been completed in a long procedure, the definitive repair (replantation or neurorrhaphy) may be undertaken after deflation of the tourniquet and the subsidence of reactive hyperemia.

Tourniquet tolerance has been known to exist without detriment in certain instances for more than 3 hours. In anticipation of a period of surgery exceeding $2\frac{1}{2}$ hours the tourniquet is released after applying a compressive dressing, saturated with lactated Ringer's solution, to the wound. The extremity is elevated, the wound compressed by the surgeon and all constrictive factors of the drape relieved. Ten minutes later, after simple suspension (occasionally after pressure exsanguination), the tourniquet may be reinflated. A magnifying loupe must always be available to provide at least 2.5 magnification at a focal length of not less than 20 cm. If greater detail is needed higher magnification should be used.

The preferred scalpel has a #15 blade which should be mounted on a broad handle for control. The knife is held like a pencil, using fine digital rather than wrist control. The cutting is done with the tip and not the body of the blade; for the most part the blade is used only to incise the skin. The deeper dissection is performed with short, curved-bladed, pointed and sharp-edged scissors. By rapid, repetitive and minimal spreading of the blades, coupled with tension on the tissues by appropriate vertical retraction, the fat and neurovascular structures will fall away from the fascia. The points of the blades are always in view as the strands of fascia are divided to open the wound. A blunt "dental probe" (biology dissecting probe or dural dissector) is indispensable in putting fascial structures and scar under tension during dissection.

Small vessels are electrocoagulated with the needle point as they are encountered during the course of dissection. Vessels much larger than 1 mm should be individually ligated with 6-0 nylon. To identify a previously bleeding vessel, the adjacent soft tissue may be slightly compressed; this usually makes the vessel bleed again.

The skin is not compressed with forceps. Retraction is accomplished either by fine skin hooks or by nylon stay sutures placed through the dermis and held by mosquito clamps shod with plastic or rubber tubing.

Since padding of the hand is indispensable, its fat must not be traumatized during dissection. Its protection is particularly critical in developing flaps, and the surgeon must protect the small vessels supplying it and the skin. Whether in elective or emergency surgery, the direction of dissection must always be from healthy tissues into abnormal tissues; the only exception to this is drainage of an abscess.

The operative field must be kept moist by the use of wetted instruments and sponges moistened with lactated Ringer's solution. During microsurgical procedures the small cellulose sponges used in ophthalmologic surgery are helpful.

The operator changes his position around the arm board, or has the table raised or lowered as necessary, to allow comfortable, easy dissection with ideal vision.

In fresh injuries an adequate assay of the tissues requires adequate exposure (wound extension if necessary) and visualization. The latter is a function of removing clots and debris, generally referred to as debridement. It is essential that no viable tissue with functional importance be violated. The intent of debridement is not synonymous with making the skin margins and tissues "look good" to the surgeon. Too frequently this has resulted in unwarranted new hemorrhage and venous congestion when the skin is closed. Contrary to common belief, stained and tattooed tissues do not generally predispose to infection, whereas contaminated clots, foreign bodies and devitalized tissues do. These should be debrided. If this is not feasible the wound should be irrigated with antibiotics and either left open or closed loosely with adequate drainage.

Closure of the Wound

Clots are mechanically removed from the wound. They must be distinguished from blood in the interstitial spaces which usually does not glisten and cannot be removed. Where indicated, antibiotic solution (bacitracin, penicillin) or steroid (triamcinolone) is placed in the wound. No subcutaneous sutures are required in the digits or body of the hand. The skin is always closed with an everting technique. To effectively prevent blood clots from forming in the wound, the tourniquet is kept inflated until gentle compression of the completed dressing can be applied, unless an unrecognized major arterial leak is suspected and must be looked for prior to wound closure. The hand should immediately be observed for the return of circulation. A loose drain should be employed whenever a contaminating injury predisposes to infection of a dead space. To prevent dead space in elective cases (fasciectomy for Dupuytren's disease) a small suction drain is most useful (Fig. 6-2).

Dressings and Immobilization

Fine mesh gauze is smoothly applied over the wound. It should be trimmed and notched so it will lie wrinkle free. This is followed by a dressing which prevents dead space in the wound or congestion of the wound. Soppy wetness facilitates sequestration of blood and serum into the dressing. The right amount of compression is achieved by a flatly and loosely laid coarse-meshed gauze (Kling or Kerlix*) applied without constriction. Proper cushioning with foam sponge (Reston†) before any circumferential wrapping is done obviates the chance of constriction by shrinkage of the drying gauze. The wet dressing invariably dries before maceration occurs (Fig. 4-5A–E).

If the problem of sweating exists and maceration is anticipated, a thin membrane of gauze may be placed between the fingers. The greatest care must be taken to avoid bulky and tight dressings in the web spaces to prevent digital congestion and adduction contracture of the thumb. If it is desired to keep the dressing wet for a day or more, it is covered with a waterproof wrapping.

Immobilization is the key to successful repair. For this purpose, plaster of Paris is generally preferred. It must be adequately cushioned to prevent undue tightness. This is achieved by the use of loosely wrapped cast padding over plastic foam (Reston). Generally the position of function is preferred (Fig. 2-1). When this is not possible, extremes of joint extension or flexion must be avoided. In wrapping the forearm, the elbow

*Kling: Elastic gauze bandage, Johnson & Johnson, New Brunswick, New Jersey. Kerlix: Gauze bandage, Johnson & Johnson, New Brunswick, New Jersey.

†Reston: Adhesive-backed foam sponge, 3M Company, Minneapolis, Minnesota.

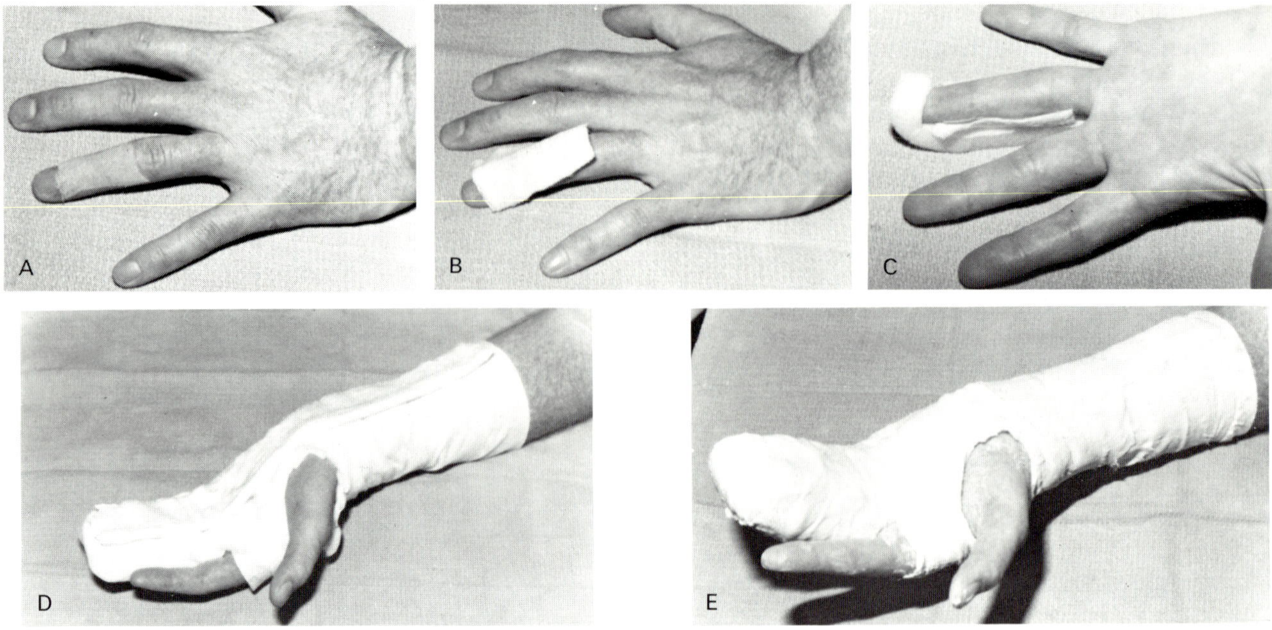

Figure 4-5. *The technique of dressing the hand after elective surgery.*
A: *Single layer of Xeroform gauze on wound.*
B: *Wet plain gauze pad cut to conform to basic wound.*
C: *Padding of wound with foam sponge (Reston).*
D: *Ample padding of extremity with cotton sheeting and placement of a keel to reinforce volar aspect.*
E: *Light plaster shell which can incorporate all fingers in boxing-glove fashion if desired.*

should be maintained at 90° of flexion, at which point the forearm circumference is maximal. If this is unheeded the cast will be too tight and the antecubital fossa will be encroached upon by the dressing and cast, choking the forearm when the patient flexes his elbow to elevate the hand.

The desired position of immobilization will be held most easily if fast-setting plaster and warm water are used. The maintenance of this position will be ensured by the use of circumferential plaster. It need not be thick and heavy; in fact, it may be eggshell thin as long as a 6-inch section of the volar aspect of the wrist is reinforced with a "keel."

Flexor tendon repairs, nerve repairs, many fractures and other procedures within the body of the hand are immobilized best with a boxing-glove type of cast. Covering one or more digits is no problem as long as the patient has sensibility and the padding is carefully applied. For youngsters and irresponsible adults, a long-arm boxing-glove cast is preferred. Children should keep the extremity against the chest inside a T-shirt at all times to avoid abusing the cast in play. The cast for an adult requires 2 rolls of padding, a 3 x 15-inch volar slab of plaster and a 3- or 4-inch roll of plaster.

Postoperative Care

Typical postoperative orders for hand care are:

Do not place tight sleeves or blood pressure cuffs on the operated arm.
Keep the operated arm above the heart at all times.
In bed, keep the patient supine and the arm comfortably elevated on one or more pillows with the hand above the heart.
Do not suspend the arm.
Have patient pass all unsplinted joints of the upper extremity through a full range of active motion hourly during the day.
Report throbbing pain not relieved by elevation immediately to the physician.
Give codeine 60 mg i.m. or p.o., q 4 hours p.r.n. pain; notify physician if inadequate.
Give regular diet.
Give diazepam 10 mg h.s. p.r.n.
Allow patient bathroom privileges.
Administer antibiotics: ______________________.

The two most important items in the postoperative treatment are (1) the preservation of ideal circulation by the prevention of congestion and

(2) the relaxation of repaired tissues in a comfortable position. Proper attention to these points requires the full-time cooperation of the patient and close supervision by the physician and nursing staff.

Throbbing pain is the telltale clue of failure of this regimen. If it is unrelieved by elevation and the release of any constricting and compressive forces, the surgeon must be promptly notified. Such pain is evidence of excessive pressure and must be relieved mechanically, not by mere analgesics. The surgeon may have to remove the cast, reposition the part, and even open the skin and fascia. Unless the patient is in a long arm cast with the elbow at 90°, suspension is contraindicated because the weight of the arm causes the forearm cast to shift, choking the hand at the wrist.

Having the patient move all the upper extremity joints that are not restricted by the dressing and cast promotes good circulation and prevents stiffness. This is no license to move these joints with force, as this may unconsciously and synergistically put enough tension on the healing tissues within the cast to disrupt them.

When the patient is out of bed he should be encouraged to keep his hand overhead. When he is fatigued he should either be supine in bed or sit in a chair beside the bed so that he can elevate his hand on pillows.

Prophylactic antibiotics are liberally used in non-elective operations to prevent infection. The antibiotic of choice should be one that empirically has good control over gram-positive organisms. The initial dose should be high and should be given as early as possible; subsequent doses are administered around the clock. The preferred route of administration is by mouth. Bacterial cultures are not necessary unless there is clinical evidence of infection. As a rule, the antibiotics are given for three days.

The average postoperative period of hospitalization is 12 to 24 hours. Therefore, it is important that the patient be informed of the need to continue the measures to control congestion and pain. During his transportation home, he may wear a sling. In most instances there should be a follow-up telephone call from the patient to the doctor or an office visit within 72 hours.

Upon discharge, the patient should be instructed as follows:

In order for your hand to heal, the two most important items requiring your constant attention are:

1. *The prevention of any congestion of the blood flow to your hand.*
   You must avoid clothing that feels the least bit tight when your elbow is bent. Furthermore, until you are instructed otherwise, you should avoid lying on your arm or placing your hand below your heart. Your sling should only be used when you are traveling. At home you should keep pillows under your forearm when sitting or lying so that your hand will be propped above your heart. This must be comfortable.
2. *The constant relaxation of all your muscles.*
   The healing in your hand is made possible by protecting it from strain. For this reason you have a protective splint, but this is not enough. Any forceful movement of the parts that are not covered up will automatically place strain on the healing area. However, without using force, and by being very gentle, you can improve the circulation to your hand by moving the joints of your shoulder and elbow, as well as those of your fingers that are not covered up, as far as they will go. This movement should be done several times a day to prevent stiffness. You must not use this arm or hand to lift or pull or twist anything.

If you have any questions or if you have any pain that pounds with your heart call the doctor. Be sure to follow his instructions about medications and see him as you have been directed.

Your next appointment to see Dr. ________ is:

Date ______________________________

Place ______________________________

Physician's telephone number: ______________.

When to change casts and dressings, or to obtain follow-up roentgenograms, depends upon the problem and the judgment of the surgeon. The specifics for postoperative care are cited in the appropriate chapters. Generally speaking, meddlesome cast and dressing changes are prone to disturb the tissues and hurt the patient with no benefit. There is no rush in removing nylon sutures. Placed without tension they cause no reaction and need not be removed for 3 to 4 weeks or longer. Zinc oxide can soften the old skin and facilitate the extraction of sutures which do not have to be removed the day they are cut.

Mobilization and Rehabilitation

A problem of the hand may or may not be disabling, depending not only upon the problem but upon the nature of the patient and his resourcefulness, or lack of it. Ideally, rehabilitation is initiated when the hand problem first manifests itself. The patient's initiative should lead him to suitable physical, intellectual and sociological activity to maintain a good input of sensory stimuli. This will reduce the forces of inactivity, anxiety, stiffness and pain that deter productivity. Patients lacking such initiative and independence need various degrees of supervision in rehabilitation and mobilization. Often this cannot be effectively begun until the need for immobilization has passed.

Once immobilization has been concluded, the uninhibited youthful patient will often require restraints to prevent him from doing too much too soon. The aging of tissues in the elderly patient increases the period of convalescence and the need for psychological and physical support.

Adults in the middle years of life often fall prey to impatience, resentment and frustration, becoming dependent upon the existing system of disability support. Confidence in their own productivity is easily lost and is transferred to confidence in the "crutch" of their dependence. To wean them from disability may require inordinate discipline and attendance at an extended daily program of physical and occupational therapy. When no progress is made under these circumstances in 4 to 6 weeks, the condition is probably static.

The most important aspect of mobilization and rehabilitation is education of the patient. In layman's terms, he must know what is wrong, what he can do about it, and what his goals should be. These points must be repeated frequently. It must be emphasized that physical and occupational therapy is merely a form of work, and that he should augment this institutional activity at home or on the job.

Progressive mobilization depends upon the "inevitability of gradualness" and the psychological support of the patient who is easily frustrated by the intolerance of his tissues to stress and activity. Pending the development of endurance, the schedule of hand effort should be four periods of the day (morning, noon, evening, and bedtime). The patient should be removed from all distraction and able to concentrate fully on active motion of the hand. His exercise should be one of mass action of his entire hand, applying maximal force through extremes of motion (opening and closing his fist, flexing and extending his wrist, pronating and supinating his forearm). When properly executed, there will be some discomfort as long as there is no sensory paralysis. Each moment of sustained mass effort of the hand should be followed by a period of total relaxation until full comfort has been reached. The development of sustained pain or swelling signifies excessive effort and requires temporary reduction in its duration. Initially endurance might be only 5 minutes q.i.d. This should be gradually built up to an hour or two q.i.d.

Total respites from the effort of mobilizing the hand are psychologically important. Hopefully, the patient can then find preoccupation with something entirely different. Certain devices psychologically helpful in gaining movement and strength are:

- Warm soapy water and a large sponge to squeeze
- Regular putty, Silly Putty, or Play Doh to squeeze
- Coarse sandpaper and a soft wooden dowel to sand down
- Surgeon's glove to pinch or grip and stretch with both hands
- Safety pins to open and close and cards to shuffle for dexterity
- Tennis ball to squeeze for power grip
- A 1- to 5-pound barbell for exercise for wrist motion
- A broom to hold by the handle during pronation and supination
- Weighted satchel to carry for elbow extension
- Finger walking up a wall for shoulder motion

Intractable pain and stiffness may be reduced or totally relieved by the injection of triamcinolone, with lidocaine analgesia, into the trigger point (Chaps. 21 and 27).

When active effort is not possible, dynamic splints may help but must be used cautiously. If applied with too much force and for too long they may aggravate rather than alleviate stiffness and pain. The surgeon must check the fitting of such a device before it is used (Fig. 4-6*A–X*).

As with active effort, the application should be consistent and periodic, with enough force to create pressure for brief periods of time (5 to 10 minutes) without a backlash of lingering pain and swelling. A period of complete relaxation and comfort must follow. The periodic reduction of the tension of the splint will allow active motion of joints to be maintained.

When active and passive effort fail to overcome stiffness in a period of 2 to 3 months, in selected cases surgery (arthrolysis, tenolysis and release of soft tissue contractures) may be beneficial (Chaps. 21 and 27).

For successful rehabilitation, the surgeon and his staff must show a high level of professional interest in the patient's progress. This should not only be demonstrated subjectively but also by objective measurements of motion and power at frequent

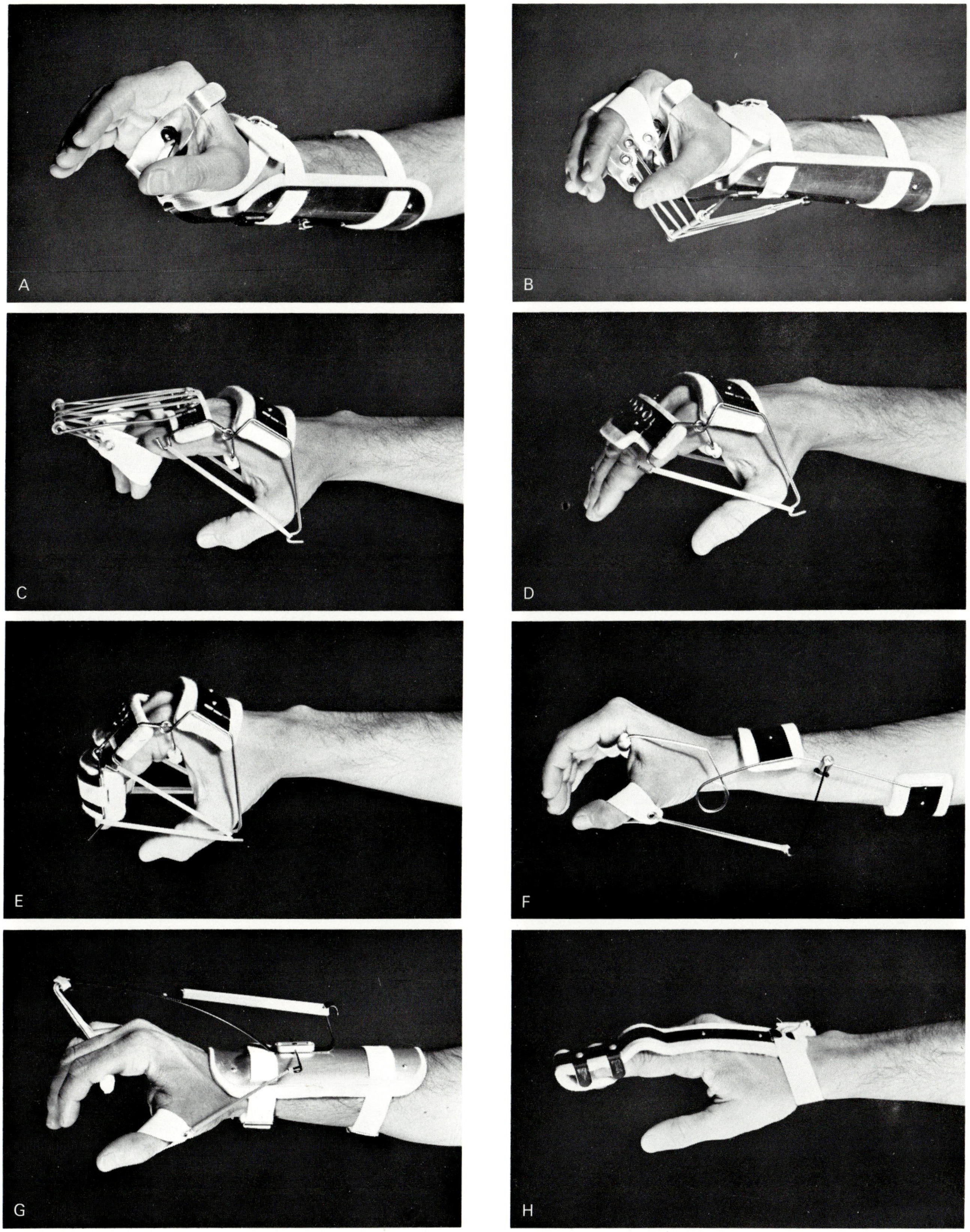

Figure 4-6. *Assorted dynamic splints for hand rehabilitation.* **A:** *Cock-up splint for dorsiflexion of the wrist.* **B:** *Spring cock-up splint with attachment to flex the metacarpophalangeal joints.* **C:** *Knuckle-bender splint to flex the metacarpophalangeal joints.* **D:** *Knuckle bender with outrigger to extend the distal finger joints.* **E:** *Knuckle bender with extra segment to flex the distal joints.* **F:** *Oppenheimer spring wire splint for radial palsy.* **G:** *Thomas suspension splint for radial palsy.* **H:** *Finger extension splint with clock spring to extend finger or thumb.*

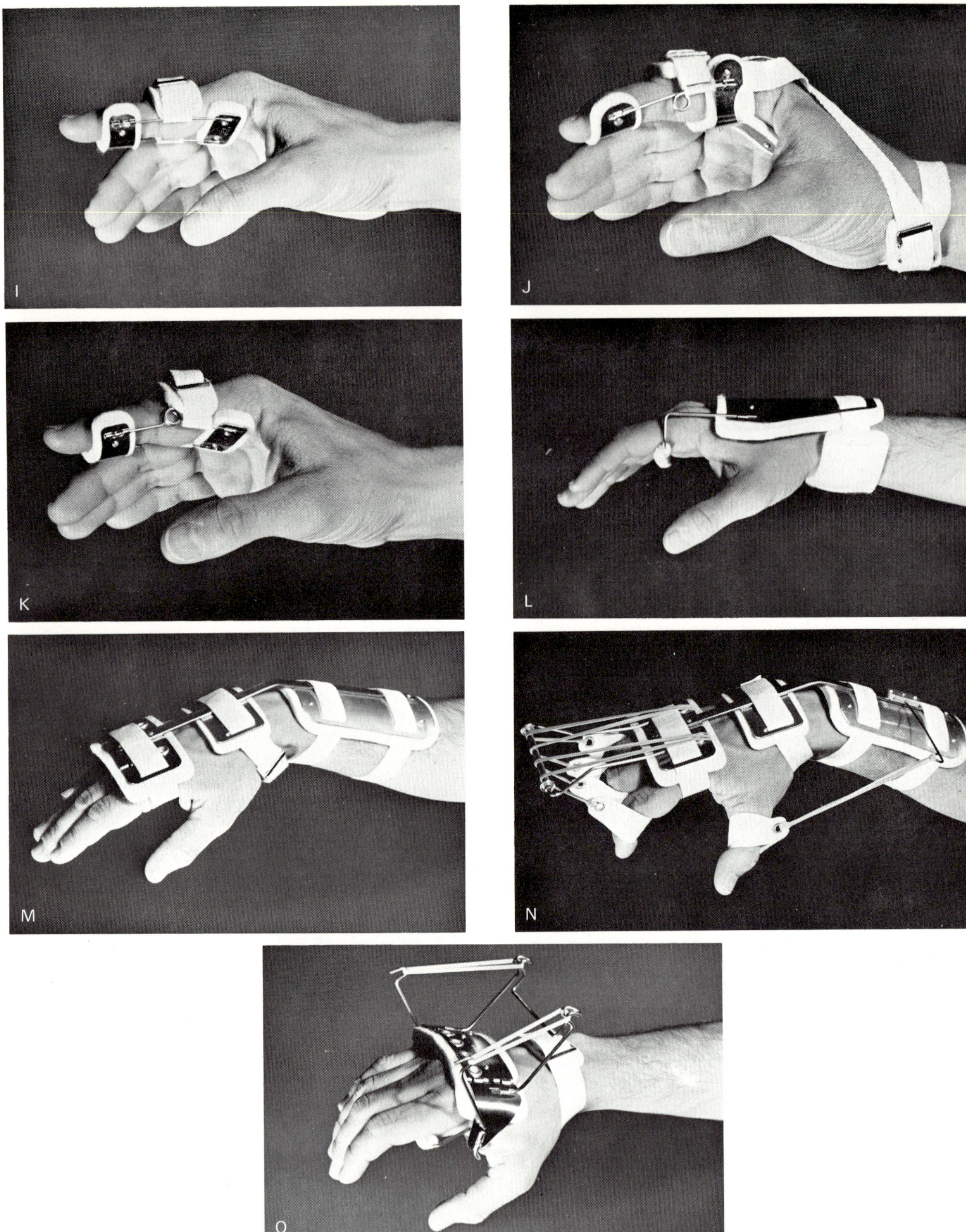

Figure 4-6 (cont'd). **I:** *Spring wire safety-pin splint to extend a finger.* **J:** *Finger extension splint with wrist support.* **K:** *Modified safety-pin splint to extend a finger.* **L:** *Palmar splint for use following Dupuytren's operation.* **M:** *Dorsal wrist splint.* **N:** *Dorsal wrist splint with outrigger attachment.* **O:** *Reverse knuckle-bender splint to extend the metacarpophalangeal joints.*

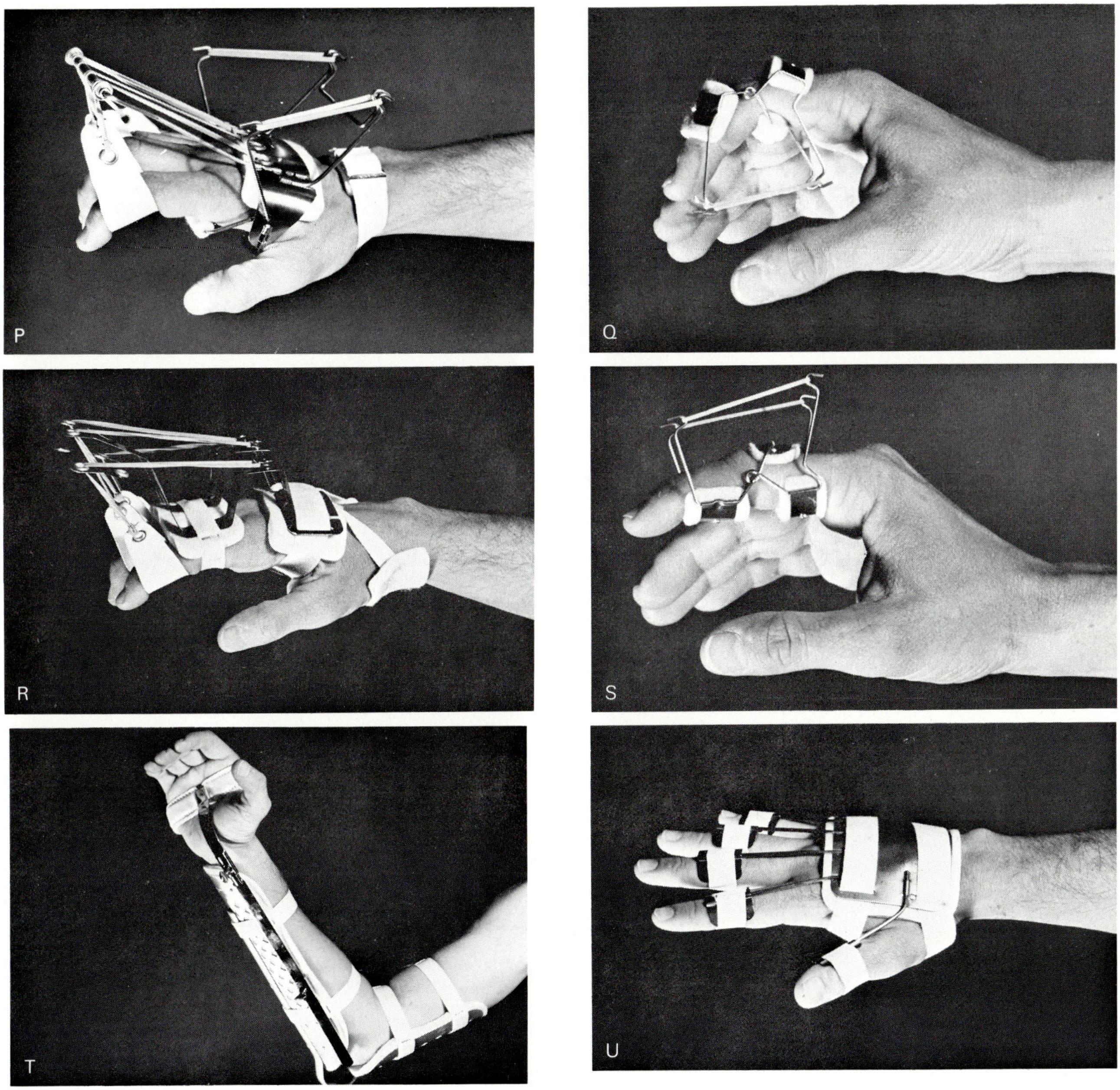

Figure 4-6 (cont'd). **P:** *Reverse knuckle bender with outrigger.* **Q:** *Finger knuckle bender to flex the middle finger joint.* **R:** *Composite spring and elastic splint to extend the fingers.* **S:** *Reverse finger knuckle bender to extend middle finger joint.* **T:** *Torsion bar to supinate or pronate the wrist unit to be clamped to a standard elbow splint.* **U:** *Spreading hand splint.*

intervals. Such observations help to encourage the patient toward further effort and improvement.

Every assistance should be given to enable the patient to return to modified work pending his maximal recovery. However, the existing fear of liability in our society has made many employers insist that the patient be 100 per cent, or maximally, recovered before accepting him back on the payroll. This fact tends to breed resentment and litigation. A small percentage of patients who are

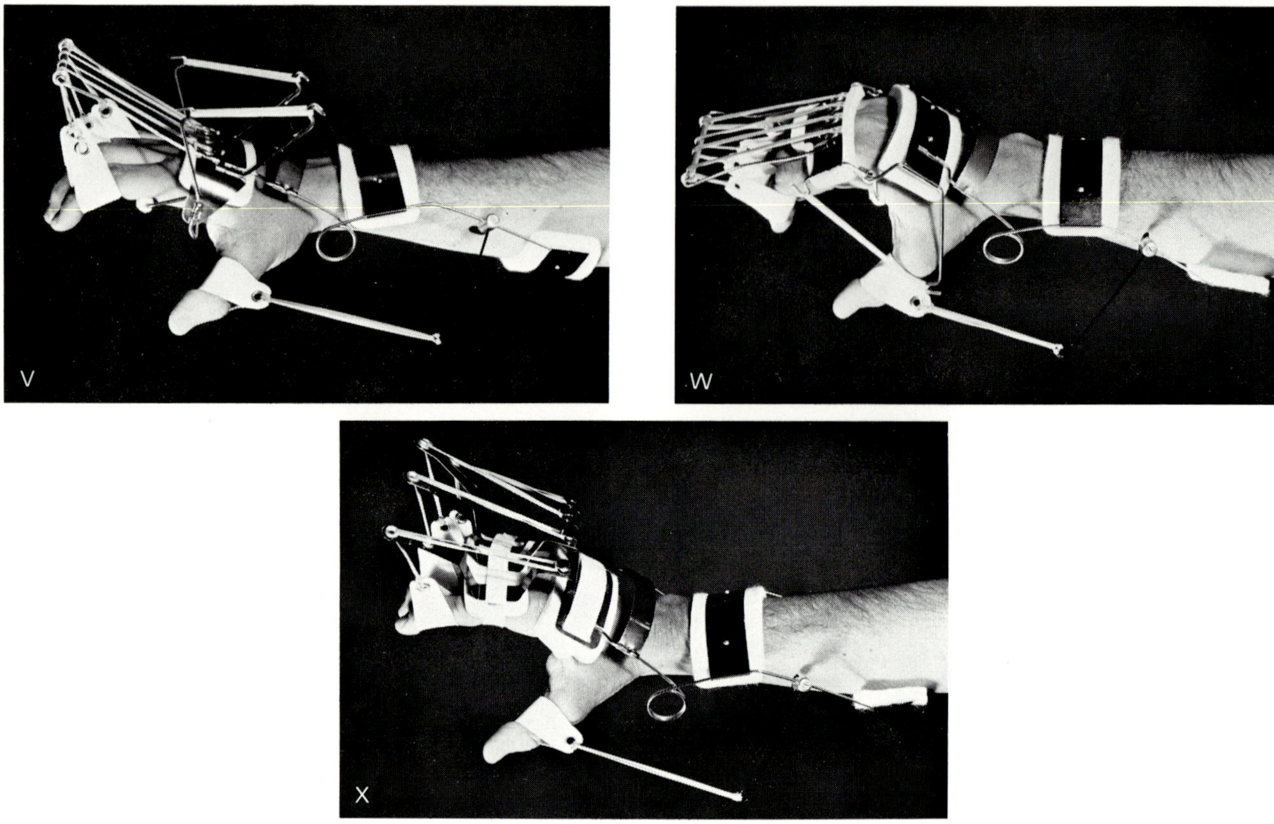

Figure 4-6 (cont'd). V: *Combination of spring Oppenheimer for wrist dorsiflexion. Knuckle bender to flex the metacarpophalangeal joints and outrigger to extend the distal finger joints.* **W:** *Combination of spring Oppenheimer for wrist dorsiflexion, reverse knuckle bender to extend the metacarpophalangeal joints and outrigger to extend the distal finger joints.* **X:** *Combination of spring Oppenheimer for wrist dorsiflexion with composite spring splint to prevent metacarpophalangeal hyperextension and outrigger to extend distal finger joints.* (*All figures in this series courtesy of Hittenberger's, San Francisco.*)

seeking rewards through litigation can usually be identified by the inconsistency of their objective findings, their haphazard attention to follow-up appointments and therapy schedules, and their complete failure to show the improvement which is reasonably expected. The sooner they are dismissed from treatment, rated for disability, and ordered to work, the better.

5 Pitfalls in Hand Surgery

In the spectrum of hand problems there are a host of pitfalls which are worthy of consideration. These result from ignorance, neglect, indifference or poor judgment. Awareness and avoidance of these traps in the course of treatment will markedly reduce complications as well as temporary and permanent disability.

Patient-generated Pitfalls

The patient has the prime responsibility for seeking care for his hand problem and executing the prescribed treatment plan. However, out of ignorance, fear or poor motivation, this responsibility is often not met. The patient's ignorance stems from inadequate education of the laity at large regarding the importance of early attention to certain hand problems. It also stems from the unfortunate fact that the physician and others participating in treatment often fail in their instruction of the patient.

The habit pattern of the patient is unintentionally prejudicial to some of the measures that must be invoked for proper treatment. These habits are difficult to modify. The patient may be asked to elevate his extremity and avoid lying on it at night. He may not be able to assimilate the importance of such measures when his daily habits involve activity and dependence on the extremity, the wearing of a wristwatch, and sleeping on the extremity which has become injured. Therefore, the change will be enforced only in relation to the patient's awareness of its importance and urgency. This may require repeated explanation and demonstration. In this regard, responsibility for the proper management of the hand problems of infants and children must be clearly detailed to and assumed by their guardians. Any limitation in motivation and indifference to responsibility impose a threat to the outcome of an incipient or established hand problem. This is particularly evident in patients whose life styles are characterized by such behavior (drug addicts, alcoholics, and patients needlessly on welfare).

A search for secondary gain on the part of the patient (compensation-mindedness) always thwarts the effectiveness of any treatment program. This may be difficult to recognize, and can be masked by the patient's demands for treatment and his flattery of the physician. The filing of an early final disability rating and report is the only way to arrest attempts at secondary gain.

The prolonged disability imposed by many hand problems easily leads to impatience and despondency unless the patient is programmed in his treatment and interval activity. It is fruitless, and often prejudicial, to involve him in active and passive exercises all day long when the signs of improvement are very limited. This can only lead to discouragement. Instead, the timing of physical effort should be limited to his tolerance and repeated at spaced intervals during the day. Between times his attention should be focused on other physical and intellectual challenges which will provide a positive psychological effect.

Children are prone to escape from the disciplines of physical rehabilitation of a hand as long as the other hand works perfectly well. To control this, appropriate measures must be instituted to curtail the use of the normal hand and force the use of the hand needing mobilization. An example of this is the restraint of the normal hand inside a mitten or T-shirt, with the abnormal, free, hand as the only agent of pinch and grip.

Anxiety, fear and pain vary tremendously in magnitude from one patient to another. During the initial treatment, substantial quantities of compassion and analgesia may be required. It is important to recognize factors in the patient's background which generate such patterns of response and direct efforts to developing confidence and motivation. This will enable the patient to be weaned from these supportive measures as soon as possible.

Physician-generated Pitfalls

The gamut of iatrogenic pitfalls includes: inadequate evaluation and diagnosis, lack of judgment regarding treatment, improper execution of primary and follow-up treatment, failure to adapt methods to the requirements of the patient, and failure to discard previous treatment plans the value of which has been disproven. Treatment of the hand is a discipline requiring specialized training. The lack of such training generates many of these pitfalls. A knowledge of functional anatomy and the fundamental mechanisms and dynamic effects of disorders of the hand is a prerequisite for any physician treating the hand.

History

The details of complaints, past and present history, mechanism of onset, and precipitating and aggravating factors are crucial to any accurate diagnosis. These must be integrated with an overall evaluation of the patient's social and economic background, his general state of health and, of course, his age, occupation, and the specific functional and/or cosmetic requirements for his hand. The accuracy of historical data is often critical for a correct diagnosis and may require repeated questioning of the patient and others who are knowledgeable about him, e.g. witnesses to an injury. The physician must be sensitive to the patient's requirement for confidence and privacy in exposing the history. Documentation of previous disorders of the extremity and prior treatment rendered the current problem is imperative for accurate diagnosis and the development of a therapeutic regimen.

Examination

The examination of both acute and chronic problems of the hand have certain similarities that should be attended to in avoiding misdiagnoses. In both instances, adequate facilities are needed, with proper instrumentation, good lighting and posturing of the patient that is comfortable and will forestall further injury should syncope occur. The opportunity to examine the entire head and neck area and both upper extremities must be provided. Repeated examinations are often necessary to ensure the accuracy of observations.

THE ACUTE INJURY

The patient is often apprehensive and may provide erroneous responses out of fear and pain. Analgesia may be needed, but no anesthetics should be instilled until sufficient initial examination has documented the amount of sensory and motor impairment. Blood may obscure the damaged tissues. Therefore, at the time of initial examination and any surgery, a tourniquet is usually essential for the accurate evaluation of injury and its repair. Likewise, the size or location of a wound should not lull the physician into complacency regarding the degree of injury, e.g. a small penetrating injury from glass may produce a functional loss far distant from the skin wound.

In the course of attending to the acutely injured hand, serious life-threatening injuries *cannot be overlooked.* Thus, a thorough examination of the whole patient is mandatory prior to the initiation of anesthesia and a potentially long surgical procedure on the hand.

THE CHRONIC INJURY

Less urgency attends the patient who is being evaluated for a chronic problem or elective surgery. The simple maneuver of asking the patient to raise both hands over his head and perform rapid repetitive motions (e.g. pinch and grip) avoids the distraction of clothing and frees the hands from the patient's watchful eye. To achieve an accurate diagnosis, repeated examinations will often be necessary to exclude inconsistencies.

Adequate clinical notes are necessary to provide a continuum of information about the progress of the patient. Drawings of the injured hand and serial measurements of strength and motion are helpful to document progress and avoid confusion in preparing reports.

Laboratory and Radiographic Evaluations

Basic roentgenograms are necessary in the complete evaluation of many hand problems. It is often necessary to compare roentgenograms of both hands, and at times only special views (e.g. carpal tunnel view to demonstrate a fracture of the hook of the hamate) are capable of demonstrating the problem. The radiologist must know what the physician seeks. By adequate communication between the two, the appropriate examinations can be obtained and the greatest information gained.

Certain laboratory evaluations must not be overlooked when problems of the hand elude diagnosis. Uric acid determinations and screening studies for rheumatoid disease may guide the physician to the diagnosis of inflammatory disorders of skin, joints and tendon sheaths. When a problem has become chronic and failed to respond as expected to therapy, suspicion must warrant further diagnostic procedures (e.g. biopsy or culture).

Judgment

Many of the pitfalls of caring for the hand can be avoided by recognizing the limits of the patient's needs and tolerances and avoiding overenthusiastic treatment. The trauma caused by a great deal of surgery with little hope of improvement may risk the impairment of existing function by further scarring. However, a considerable amount of surgery may be warranted to gain some essential function when very little, if any, is present. The performance of a procedure must not be based on the surgeon's ability to do it, but on the patient's need for it and the prognosis for improvement following it.

Roentgenograms are diagnostic aids, but should not be the prime basis of treatment. Perfect reduction is of no value if it is achieved only at the expense of such abnormal posturing that intractable stiffness and pain result (e.g. Cotton-Loder position for a Colles' fracture).

Treatment

No undertaking of hand treatment will succeed if pain is not controlled. Reconstructive and rehabilitative efforts will not be tolerated if the patient must deal with excessive misery.

Unlike other areas of the body, the hand does not compensate and hide surgical abuse. Two of the greatest aids in minimizing iatrogenic trauma to the hand during operation are a proximal arterial tourniquet and magnification. Each allows a more precise identification of tissues, better hemostasis and more effective conduct of the operation. During initial examination and subsequent surgery of a wound, gentleness is paramount in reducing scar and subsequent stiffness and pain.

Failure to gain adequate exposure is a prime cause of misdiagnosis and surgical complications. When the primary wound is inadequate to identify and repair the deeper damaged tissues, it is necessary to extend it, and to dissect from normal healthy tissues into the zone of injury. Incisions must be planned and drawn on the skin. They must be designed to give direct access to the pathological process and not compromise circulation or lead to iatrogenic loss of function by injury of critical structures or the formation of adverse adhesions or secondary contracture.

The basic tenets of careful surgical technique are nowhere more important than in the hand. Dead space must be eliminated by hemostasis (electrocoagulation and ligation) and appropriate drainage or excessive scarring will ensue and infection may occur. Tension and swelling are poorly tolerated by the hand. Both lead to stiffness. Surgical decompression must be instituted for relief of congestion if elevation and the reapplication of looser dressings are insufficient. The hallmark of tension, regardless of etiology, is throbbing pain which is caused by venous congestion. Ignoring this symptom threatens the development of ischemic fibrosis (Volkmann's contracture). Congestion follows injury, surgery, dependency, constrictive dressings, splints and the wearing of tight clothing or jewelry. It requires constant vigilance by all concerned, especially the patient, and must be treated mechanically and physically, not with analgesics. Localized burning pain at a bony prominence under a splint means that the pressure on the skin is causing localized congestion and ischemia which will lead to necrosis unless the pressure is promptly relieved.

Skeletal alignment must be achieved prior to wound closure or else the functional architecture may be destroyed and the circulation jeopardized (Fig. 5-1*A–C*). The primary repair and reconstruction of major structures will fail functionally unless the skin and subcutaneous covering are adequate. Many surgical procedures to tendons, nerves and blood vessels have failed because skin cover with satisfactory vascularity and fatty-areolar padding had not been provided.

Postoperative congestion and secondary fibrosis

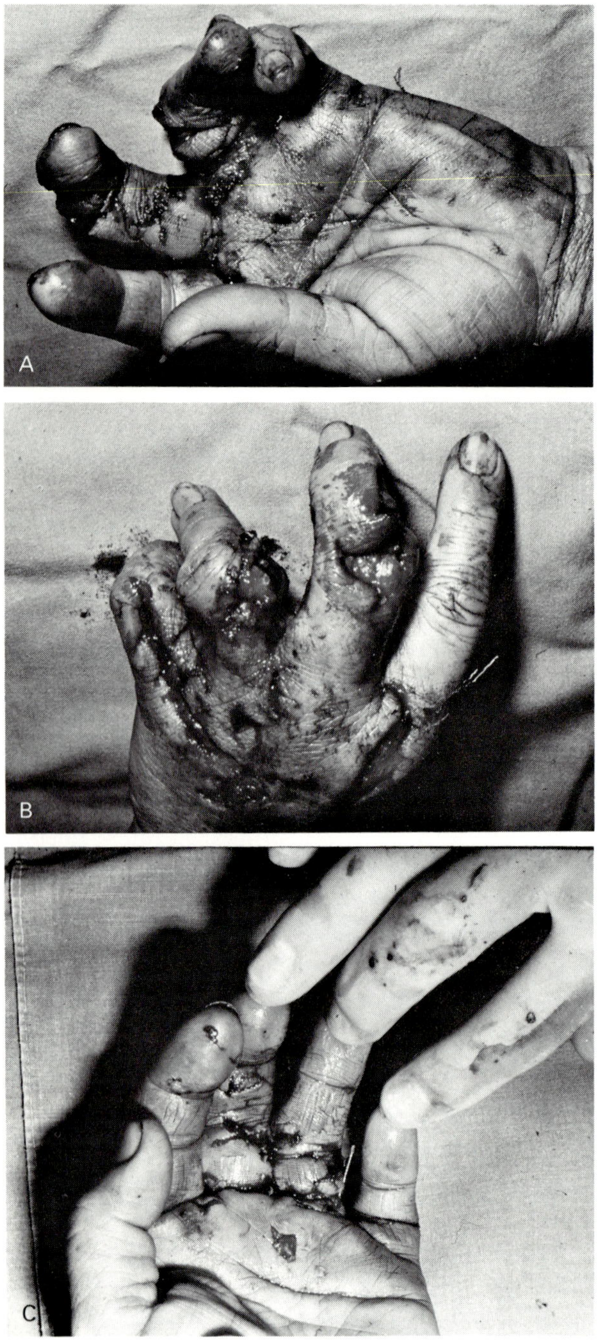

Figure 5-1. *Marked cyanosis of the ring finger was evident in this woman's crushed hand until reduction of the severely displaced fractures was done.*

vary proportionately to the volume and surface area of tissues injured and operated upon. Therefore, overall hand function may be worsened by an insistence on the surgical reapproximation of *all* damaged tissue, rather than simplification of function by the intentional resection of, or failure to reapproximate, some functionally dispensable structure. This is particularly true where multiple tendons are injured at one level of the hand or forearm.

It is essential that all joints acted upon by a musculotendinous unit have been fully mobilized prior to tenorrhaphy. Tenorrhaphy cannot be expected to improve any existing limitations in passive motion. Similarly, a tenolysis or arthrolysis and any procedure that requires prolonged splinting cannot be expected to succeed concomitantly. Tenolysis and arthrolysis procedures must be followed by active motion within 24 to 48 hours, which, of course, is incompatible with a procedure such as tenorrhaphy or bone grafting which requires several weeks of immobilization.

The misconception often exists that the essence of the hand procedure is the repair of the deep tissues and that skin closure, dressing and casting can be relegated to the less experienced assistant. The fact is that the success of the procedure depends equally on careful attention to every technical detail from preparation and draping to dressing and immobilization. Despite care with all details, violent emergence from anesthesia and lunging provoked by removal of an endotracheal tube can disrupt tissue repair, especially tenorrhaphy and the reduction of fractures.

Failure to employ antibiotics locally and systemically in adequate prophylactic doses has led to aggravation of many infections. If infection is likely, antibiotic therapy should be initiated without waiting for pus and the results of sensitivity tests. However, a history of any preexisting allergies must be established before the drug is selected.

The major pitfall in the use of anti-inflammatory agents is their threat to the exacerbation of preexisting peptic ulcer disease or systemic allergy. Local atrophy (skin and fat) and cutaneous depigmentation may occur at the site of steroid injections.

Pitfalls in Follow-up

It is a mistake to expect the patient to assimilate the features of his treatment and response thereto without adequate supervision. Similarly, it is impossible to assay the magnitude of his anxiety without close initial follow-up. Most postoperative cases and cases of infection must be seen in 24 to 72 hours, and even with suitable progress should, for a time, be seen once or twice a week if the original problem was a major one.

The evaluation on each visit should include a

survey of subjective and objective status, and should allow time to answer questions and to provide appropriate reassurances and instructions. This interest on the part of the physician is often reciprocated by better motivation and harder work by the patient.

Workmen's compensation injuries and other liability cases generally require initial and follow-up reports. The physician's timely attention to these is of great importance to ensure the rendering of appropriate administrative and fiscal matters which accompany any disability. Delay causes financial distress and, secondarily, impairment in motivation. However, the surgeon must be careful in making premature assertions about permanent disability, and in underestimating temporary disability. Except for certain injuries involving loss of substance, it is frequently impossible at the start of treatment to estimate accurately the existence and extent of eventual permanent disability.

Common Miscellaneous Pitfalls

Most acute hand problems are not urgent and, therefore, midnight surgery when the surgical staff is not at its best is seldom indicated. Ineffective immobilization and elevation are common pitfalls. Every postoperative case requires adequate immobilization. This invariably necessitates that the wrist be immobilized, inasmuch as it is the key joint of the hand. When it is free to move it invokes considerable tension on tendons so that peripheral joints and injured tissues are not relaxed. The extremity should never be tied up and suspended above the heart so that the weight of the arm (7 kg) drags against the point of suspension, for congestion, and even ischemia, will occur. Wherever possible, the hand is placed in the position of function and total rest of the involved digits is provided by covering them with a softly padded, lightweight boxing-glove cast. Ready-made splints are seldom without risk of congestion, stiffness, pain and deformity (Fig. 5-2). The webs of the fingers rarely need gauze padding. If applied, however, it should not be more than one or two thicknesses and never snug. Wet dressings over wounds help to draw out blood and prevent dead space. Prolonged immobilization that causes marked stiffness must be avoided. In this regard, clinical stability, not roentgenographic bone healing, should be the guiding factor in discontinuing immobilization.

Beware of surgical exuberance. Non-surgical measures should always take precedence over operative procedures if the chance of improvement is equal. All surgery is injury and, regardless of how carefully done, may give rise to disability. Contrariwise, reluctance on the part of the patient or physician to drain pus or to decompress a congested area of the hand or forearm (e.g. fasciotomy) easily leads to severe and permanent impairment of function.

Good circulation heals and prevents trouble, not closure of the wound. An open wound is not, per se, the reason for an infection, but the insistence on closing all wounds is the basis for the development of many infections. Closure of a wound with tension produces enough congestion and ischemia for infection to become established. The placement of reactive foreign material (catgut) further increases the congestion, the risk of infection and the likeli-

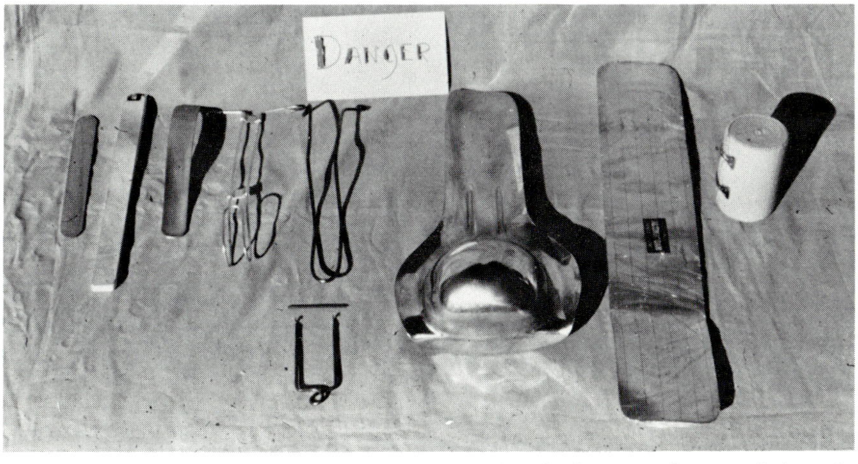

Figure 5-2. *Many ready-made splints and traction or compressive devices can do more injury than good to the hand. Splints and dressings for the hand must be custom fabricated.*

hood of excess scar. Dependency of the hand and premature motion aggravate these problems.

Beware of substituting a complex risky procedure for an effective simple one. In the primary treatment of wounds with loss of skin substance (e.g. fingertips), simplicity of grafting is the best means for achieving an uncomplicated and predictable success. In this regard, a thin, split-thickness skin graft is preferred in most instances. Such grafts will take on all viable dry wounds, including bone. Rarely do amputated fingertips truly survive. Therefore, reimplantation of such composite grafts is not advised.

Do not be reckless with fat about the hand. The palmar fat is indispensable as a cushion. Contrary to popular belief, this fat does not regenerate or hypertrophy as fat elsewhere does. Therefore, it should be meticulously preserved during any operative procedures on the hand.

In maintaining adequate immobilization, stiffness of unimmobilized joints must be prevented. During convalescence, all joints, including the shoulder, that are not specifically immobilized should pass through a complete range of motion several times a day. However, as long as there still is need for immobilization of a part of the extremity, the movements allowed must never be with force. Otherwise, the immobilized part may be synergistically moved unintentionally.

Work is the most effective method of mobilizing the hand. Its objective is to achieve full, forceful excursion of tendons and joints. Regardless of motivation, the power available for this is greatest in the finger flexors and weakest in the finger extensors. Accordingly, digits should not be immobilized for long in full digital flexion, but rather in moderate extension of the interphalangeal joints. The patient should not squeeze a ball to improve flexion but rather something that can be completely compressed, such as a soaking wet sponge. Physiotherapy is a means of supervising a program of work and it should be discontinued as soon as the patient is capable on his own.

Some Pathological States with Inherent Pitfalls

A diagnosis of *wrist sprain* should never be made without careful follow-up roentgenograms in 10 days to rule out the possibility of a fracture, especially of the scaphoid or lunate.

Extensor tendon injuries are frequently masked at first by the interconnecting and overlapping function of various components. A prime example of this is the insidious evolution of a buttonhole deformity.

The vincula frequently mask the *division of the long flexors of the digits.*

A *stenosing flexor tenosynovitis* (trigger finger) is often mistaken for an extensor tendon or skeletal problem.

Industrial injection injuries and electrical burns may be deceptively benign when first seen, but require constant watching and access to facilities for urgent treatment.

Injuries from teeth over the metacarpophalangeal joints also require urgent treatment to forestall a "human bite" infection.

Herpes simplex infection of the distal phalangeal area is commonly mistaken for a felon, and *Hutchinson's melanotic whitlow* for a chronic paronychia.

Gout is often mistaken for a bacterial cellulitis.

6 Incisions and Soft Tissue Repair

Incisions

Well-planned incisions are essential in hand surgery. A marking material such as methylene blue or vital green is necessary for designing incisions. Differences in the characteristics of the hairless, tightly adherent immobile volar skin and the loosely attached dorsal skin must be considered.[8] The capacity to compensate for scar contracture is less on the volar surface because of these characteristics. Volar incisions must therefore be planned more accurately than those on the dorsal surface.

Incisions must never compromise function and must not cross in a straight line surfaces that are normally subjected to repeated stretch (e.g. flexion creases). They must run longitudinally between the lateral limits of the flexion and extension creases of the digits (neutral zones), and should give ideal access and exposure while preserving the vascular integrity.[10] Whenever possible a skin-fat flap is raised over the zone of tendon or nerve suture so that the skin wound is removed from the underlying tenorrhaphy or neurorrhaphy.

Transverse incisions, or those paralleling skin creases, generally give the best functional and cosmetic result but, because they are often perpendicular to the underlying vessels, nerves and tendons, must be executed with extreme care (Fig. 6-1).

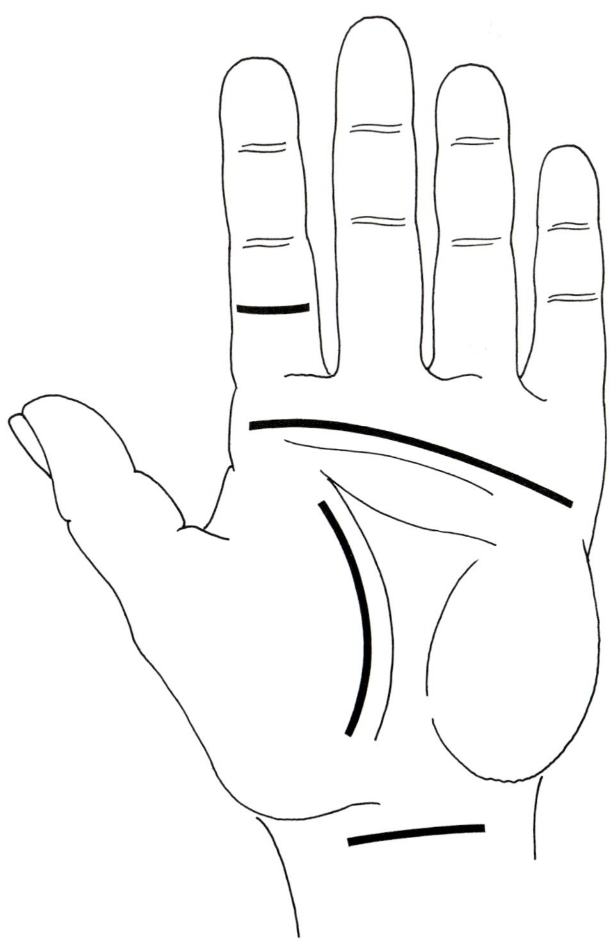

Figure 6-1. *Transverse incisions and incision parallel to creases commonly utilized in hand surgery.*

Magnification and hemostasis with a proximal tourniquet are used during dissection to avoid injury to important structures. Wound edges should be retracted in a near vertical direction with fine skin hooks, and only the strands and sheets of fascia placed under tension are cut. The incision is best made with a #15 blade, holding the knife handle as a pencil and cutting only through the epidermis and dermis. The remainder of the dissection is done with sharp-edged, curved, short-bladed (10- to 15-mm) pointed scissors, spreading the tissue minimally to tense the vertical fascial septae which are then cut.

Dissection should proceed from known to unknown or from normal to abnormal. A proximal pneumatic tourniquet should be used in all but the most superficial hand incisions. During the dissection small vessels can be electrocoagulated with a needle-point cautery and the larger ones identified and ligated. Drains should be used liberally, especially in contaminated wounds or in any wound where the adequacy of hemostasis is questionable. If there is a question about hemostasis the tourniquet should be deflated prior to wound closure and the major bleeding points either electrocoagulated or ligated. At times the finger or extremity may be gently squeezed to test hemostasis before closing the wound to identify any remaining open vessels. A drain should be used whenever there has been extensive dissection and if any suspicion about later oozing exists. If hemostasis is considered to be adequate, the tourniquet may be kept inflated until the wound is closed and the cast or bulky compressive dressing applied.

Drainage may be achieved through the use of Penrose drains or rubber catheters split longitudinally to form a trough. Our preference has been the use of a 19-gauge scalp vein apparatus and the 10-cc vacuum tubes used for blood collecting. The scalp vein hub attachment is removed and the tubing notched for additional draining. After the catheter has been placed in the wound the skin is closed and the dressing applied. The needle end of the apparatus is then inserted in a vacuum tube which is changed as necessary (Fig. 6-2).

In the hand and forearm, the skin should be closed as a single layer, usually with a non-absorbable, monofilament synthetic suture such as 4-0 or 5-0 nylon. Chromic catgut or polyglactin is used with young children, where removal of sutures may be a problem. Continuous sutures may be used except where flaps have to fit precisely.

Many traditionally used incisions designed to treat infections should be replaced by those with fewer complications. The classic fish-mouth incision for drainage of distal pulp-space infections (felons) and hockey-stick incisions should be replaced by direct incisions over the point of the abscess[6] on the volar surface and the underlying septae divided (Fig. 6-3). Bayonet incisions are sometimes useful, but more often other incisions are preferable which avoid dividing the vessels and lymphatics that are sectioned through the horizontal component of the bayonet. In the thumb transverse or zigzag wounds are preferable, especially on the volar surface of the distal phalanx.

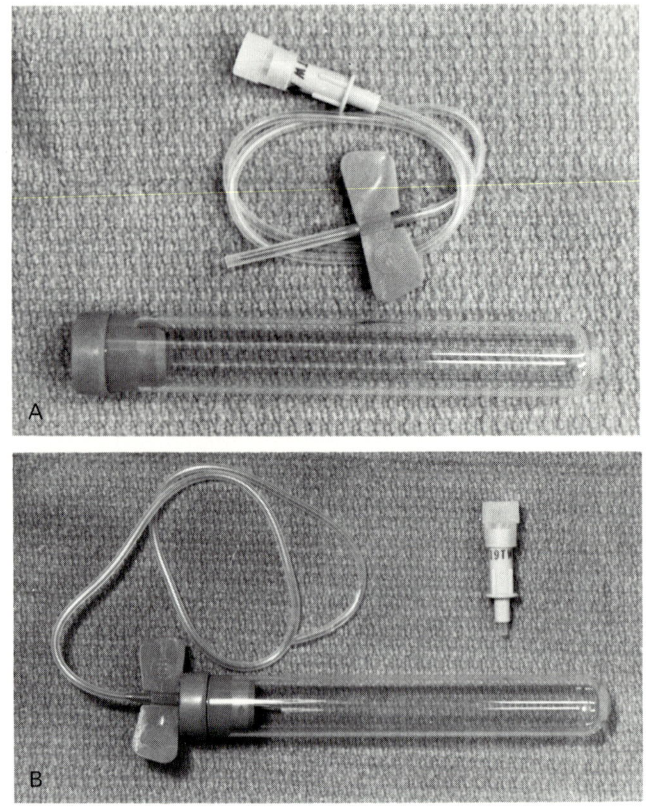

Figure 6-2. *A scalp vein apparatus and vacuum blood collecting tube make an excellent minisuction system for the hand.*

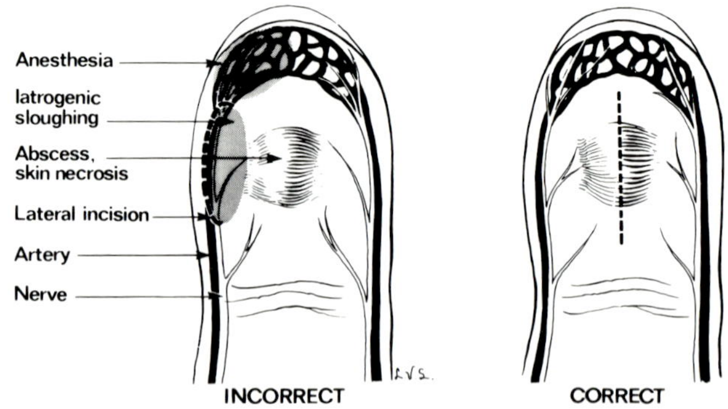

Figure 6-3. *Most felons can be drained by an incision over the point of maximum involvement. This avoids the risk of injury to the neurovascular structures and sloughing of skin. (From Kilgore, E.S., Brown, L.G., Newmeyer, W.L., Graham, W.P. and Davis, T.S.: Treatment of felons. Am. J. Surg., 130:194, 1975. Reprinted by permission of the American Journal of Surgery.)*

Midlateral or midaxial incisions are useful (Fig. 6-4) but may give less exposure than an oblique or zigzag incision on the volar side of the digit (Fig. 6-5).[5] Short longitudinal incisions directly over the proximal and distal ends of the involved sheath are usually best in treating infections of the tendon sheaths.[7]

In treating trigger finger the usual considerations for making volar incisions are followed. Vertical incisions extending from metacarpophalangeal joint crease to distal palmar crease are usually best, except at the thumb where a transverse or oblique incision should be used (Fig. 6-6).

Longitudinal incisions on the dorsum are preferred to protect venous and lymphatic drainage, while giving good exposure to the extensor mechanism for almost any procedure[8] (Fig. 6-7). The dominant force of the flexors will prevent the problems of contracture with this incision. A dorsal longitudinal incision with or without a transverse extension across the proximal edge of the nail fold (Fig. 6-7) is excellent for exposure and preservation of blood supply. Lateral incisions, when used, should be in the form of long flaps, preserving the digital veins and lymphatics as much as possible.[10] A transverse incision is used to expose the metacarpophalangeal joints, dorsally, directly over the distal ends of the metacarpals (Fig. 6-7). Undulation of this incision may reduce any tendency for limitation of motion at the metacarpophalangeal joints.[1] The large veins between the metacarpals should not be divided.

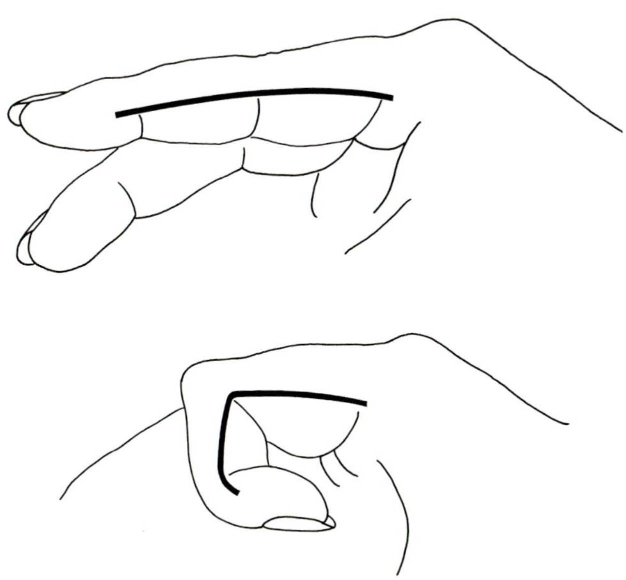

Figure 6-4. *The classical midaxial incision at the dorsal aspect of the flexion creases heals without contracture.*

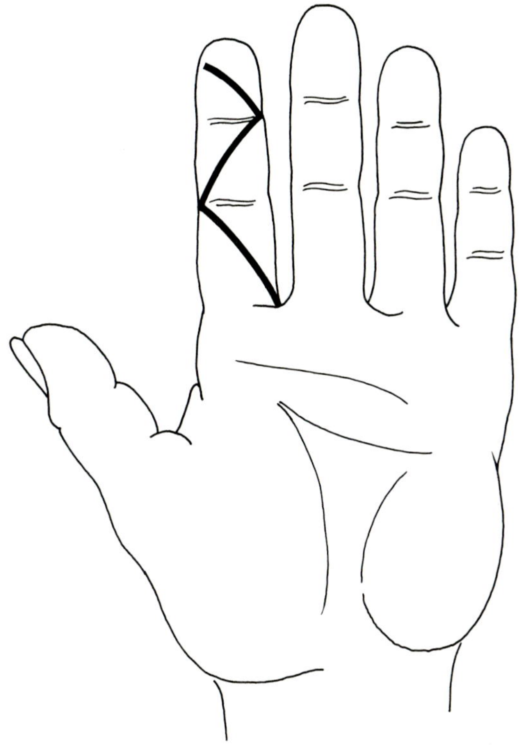

Figure 6-5. *The zigzag incision on the volar aspect of the finger provides excellent exposure.*

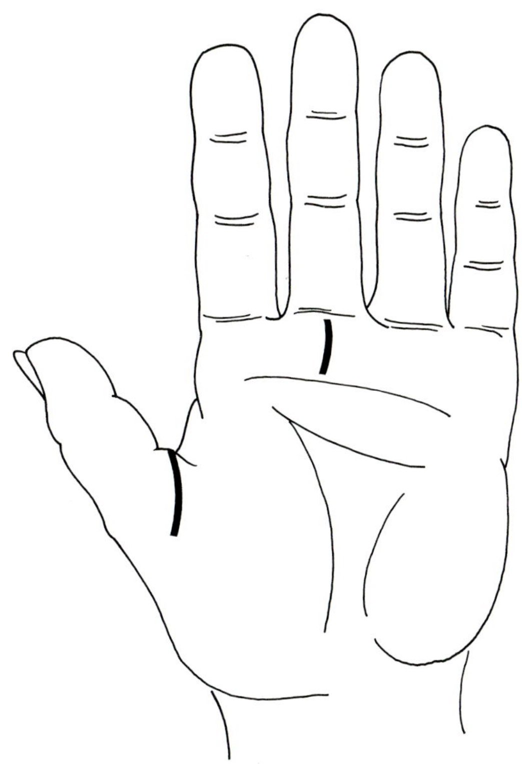

Figure 6-6. *For the release of the proximal pulley a vertical incision is adequate at the base of the fingers and a slight oblique incision is used for the thumb.*

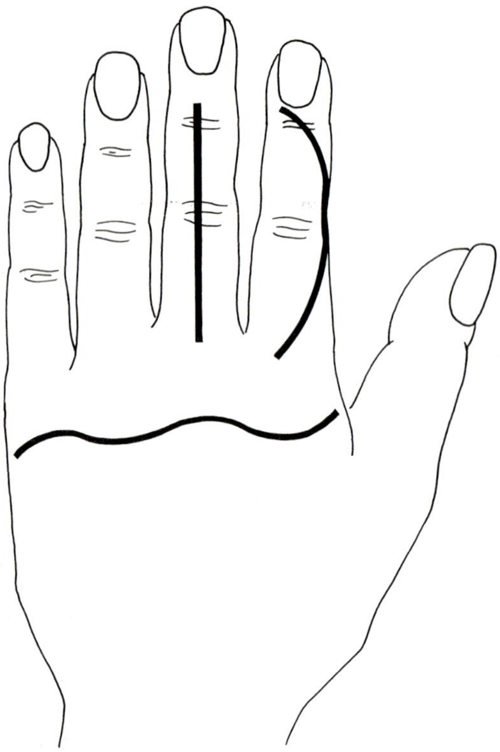

Figure 6-7. *A dorsal midline or lateral curved incision may be used for exposing the dorsal and lateral aspects of the finger. A gentle undulating incision is preferred over the metacarpals. The dorsal veins should not be injured in making these incisions.*

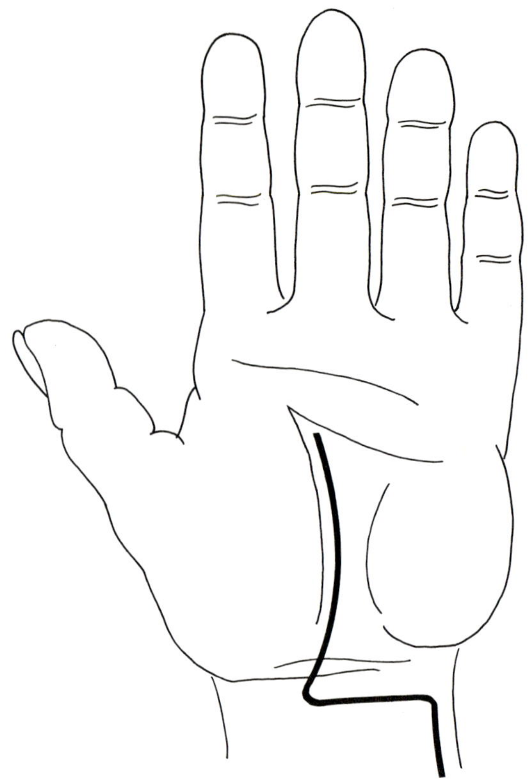

Figure 6-8. *Any incision across the wrist should not pass vertically but obliquely. The palmar cutaneous branch of the median nerve should not be injured.*

An incision extending from the proximal end of the transverse carpal ligament well into the palm allows exposure of the motor branch of the median nerve during operation on the carpal tunnel.[16] If more exposure is needed proximally, the incision is lengthened along the ulnar side of the wrist (Fig. 6-8). Injury to the palmar cutaneous branch of the median nerve can occur when this incision is placed too far toward the radial side of the wrist.

Incisions in the forearm are usually best made vertically along the radial or ulnar volar surfaces except in specific creases such as the wrist (Fig. 6-9)

Incisions are extended from the wrist into the palm or from palm to fingers by crossing flexion creases at an angle, thus avoiding straight-line contractures across the joint. Zigzag, undulating or right-angled incisions are the most common and useful methods of crossing joint creases (Fig. 6-10) on the volar surface of the hand (Fig. 6-11). On the dorsum joints may be crossed in a straight line, or the same types of incision used on the volar aspect may be utilized.

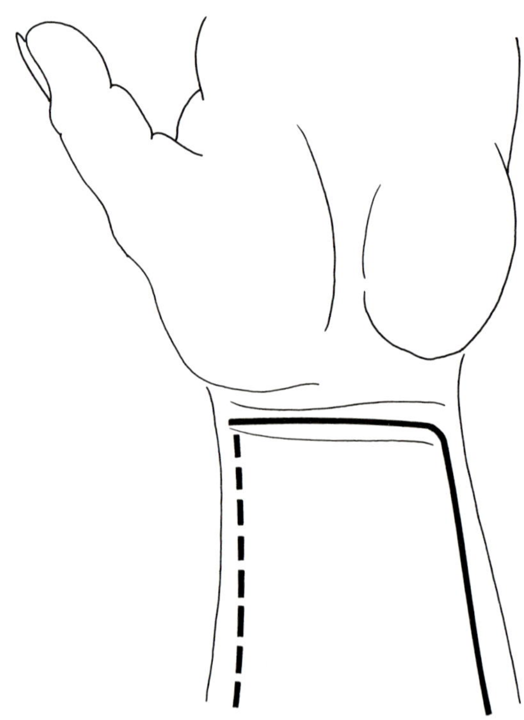

Figure 6-9. *Incisions in the arm are placed along the borders or alternatively as gentle S curves on the volar aspect.*

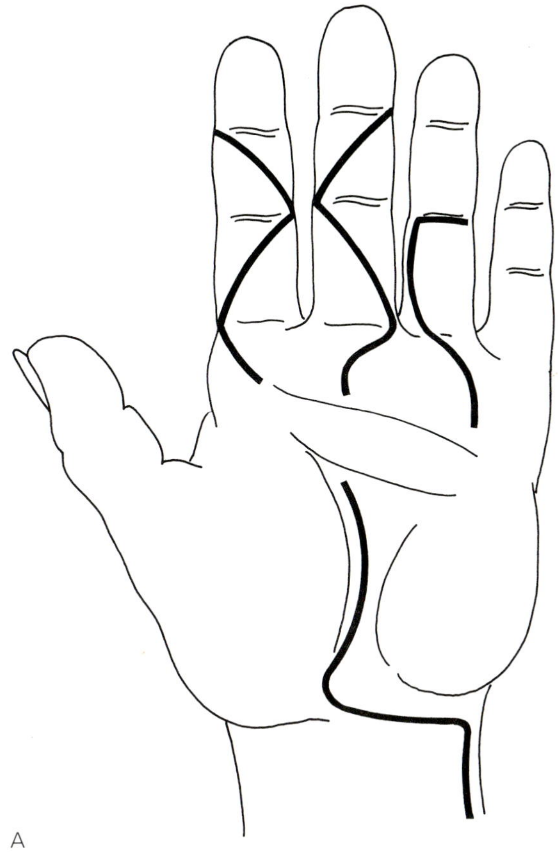

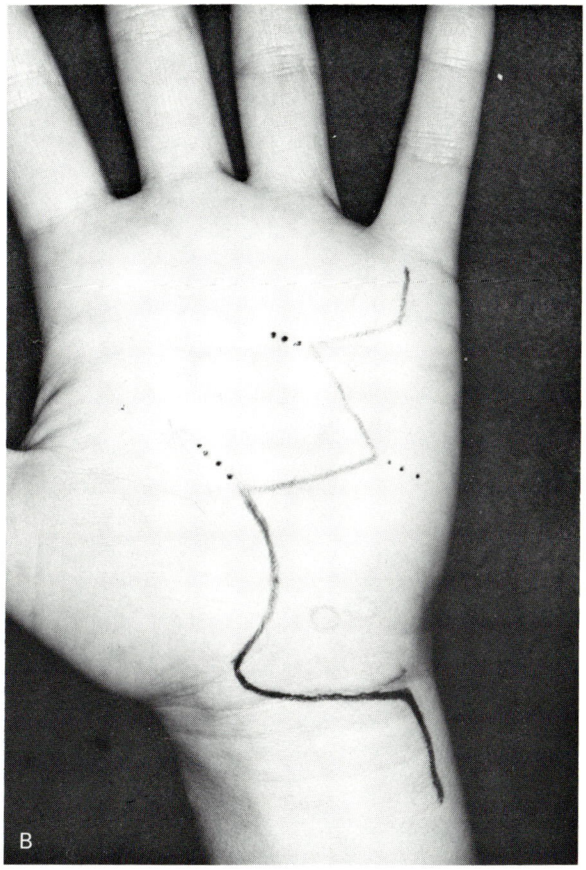

Figure 6-10. *Zigzag incisions are used to pass from one section of the hand to another* **(A).** *When length must be gained, a V-Y advancement technique can be used* **(B).**

Resurfacing

Hand wounds must be closed as expeditiously as possible to achieve early healing followed by early motion. Adequate soft tissue repair is the step of prime importance in the reconstructive process.[13] Other than direct wound closure, free grafts and pedicle flaps are the alternatives for soft tissue reconstruction. The types of free skin grafts available are split-thickness, full-thickness, and composite grafts. The types of pedicle flaps available are local, distant and island pedicle flaps. The final decision as to the fate of injured tissue may be delayed 3 to 4 days after injury without detriment to the wound, though all obviously devitalized tissue should be debrided and the tissue replaced immediately to achieve the earliest possible wound closure.[3]

The simplest method of closure is usually best. Flaps should be used when a wound is not suitable for a free graft, usually in cases of exposed bone or tendon denuded of periosteum or paratenon.

Free Grafts

Free grafts are preferable for the closure of most hand wounds because of their simplicity, relative certainty of success, and rapidity with which sensibility is achieved. Reinnervation of full-thickness skin grafts is usually better than that of split-thickness skin grafts, while flaps other than local rotation flaps or island pedicles rarely regain more than protective sensibility.[15]

Split-thickness skin grafts may be categorized into thin (.008 to .012 in), medium thickness (.012 to .016 in), and thick (.016 to .020 in). A full-thickness skin graft includes the full thickness of the epidermis and dermis and, depending on the area of the body, may vary considerably in thickness. Grafts including more than the full thickness of epidermis and dermis are composite grafts and have limited usefulness.

Donor sites in all cases should be selected with subsequent function and appearance of the donor area in mind.

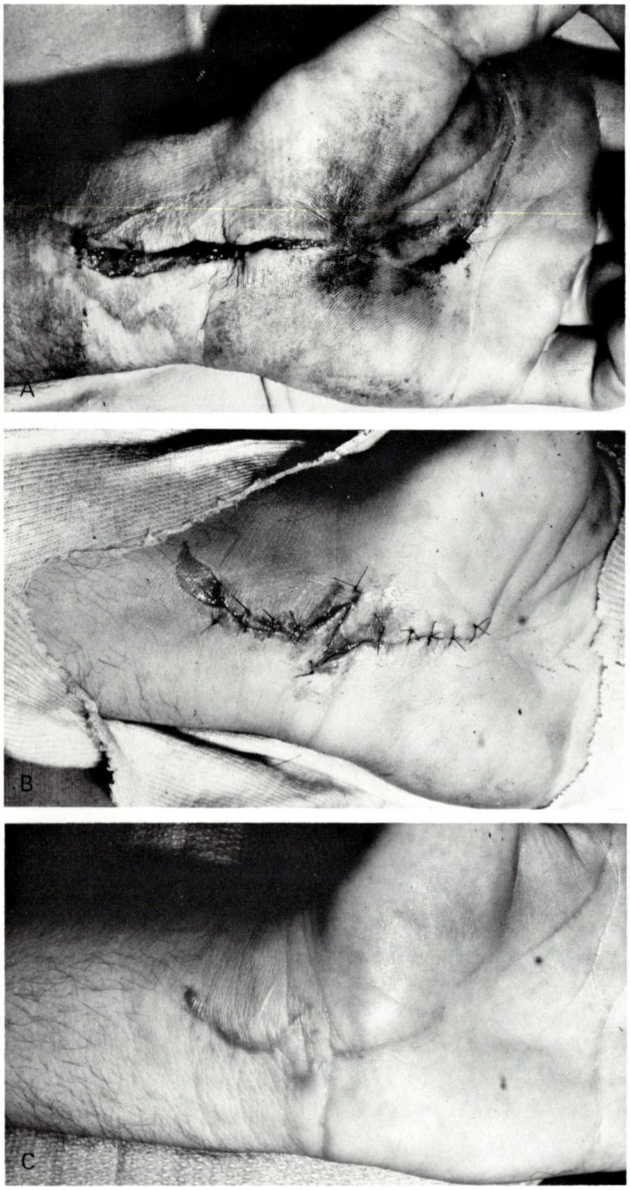

Figure 6-11. *A linear laceration across a joint crease can be broken up by a Z-plasty.*

FULL-THICKNESS SKIN GRAFTS

Full-thickness grafts are most useful in small wounds such as fingertip injuries where rugged coverage with maximum sensibility is desired. The successful use of full-thickness grafts requires ideal conditions encountered most often with limited elective surgery, as in the release of scar contracture or of a syndactyly.

The inguinal or groin fold is the donor site of choice for most full-thickness skin grafts. An ellipse of skin can be taken from this area about 2 to 3 cm in maximum width and 8 to 10 cm in maximum length in the average adult. Other possible donor sites include the wrist crease, the hypothenar eminence, the supraclavicular areas, and the antecubital fossa. The last is less commonly used today since an unpredictable degree of scarring can result from excisions in that area. This was the site of the classical Wolfe's graft for fingertip coverage.

The full thickness of skin is cut to the appropriate size after the area of the defect has been measured and transferred to the donor site. The wound can usually be converted to an ellipse or simply closed with a subcutaneous chromic catgut suture and a continuous dermal or skin suture of nylon. The graft is then trimmed of all extraneous fat so that only dermis and epidermis are left.

The graft is sutured in place with a continuous suture of nylon or occasionally with chromic catgut or polyglactin in small children. Several interrupted tie-over sutures of 4-0 silk are used for a bolus or tie-over dressing to hold the graft in place (Fig. 6-12). The part in question is immobilized with a bulky dressing or plaster cast and elevated. If there is any question about hemostasis, the wound should be inspected at 24 hours. If hemostasis is adequate, the dressing may be left for 4 to 5 days before the first inspection. At that time the bolus is removed and the sutures around the edges are left in place. A protective dressing is then placed on the graft. The sutures around the edge of the graft are removed at 10 to 14 days. If both ends of the silk sutures used for the tie-over dressing are left long, a second similar dressing may be utilized for continued immobilization.

SPLIT-THICKNESS SKIN GRAFTS

A partial thickness of the skin can be removed with a variety of instruments. These include the Ferris Smith knife using the freehand method, the Goulian or Humby knife which provides a guard to gauge the thickness of the graft, and various mechanical dermatomes. The Padgett-Hood and the Reese dermatomes employ the blade-and-drum principle for cutting grafts of specific thickness and give uniform depth and width but less rapid harvesting of grafts.

In general, thin grafts will provide the most certain "take" with the most rapid wound closure, but with the greatest subsequent contracture and the hazard of a less durable wound. As the thickness of the graft increases, the certainty of graft take decreases but durability and padding increase.

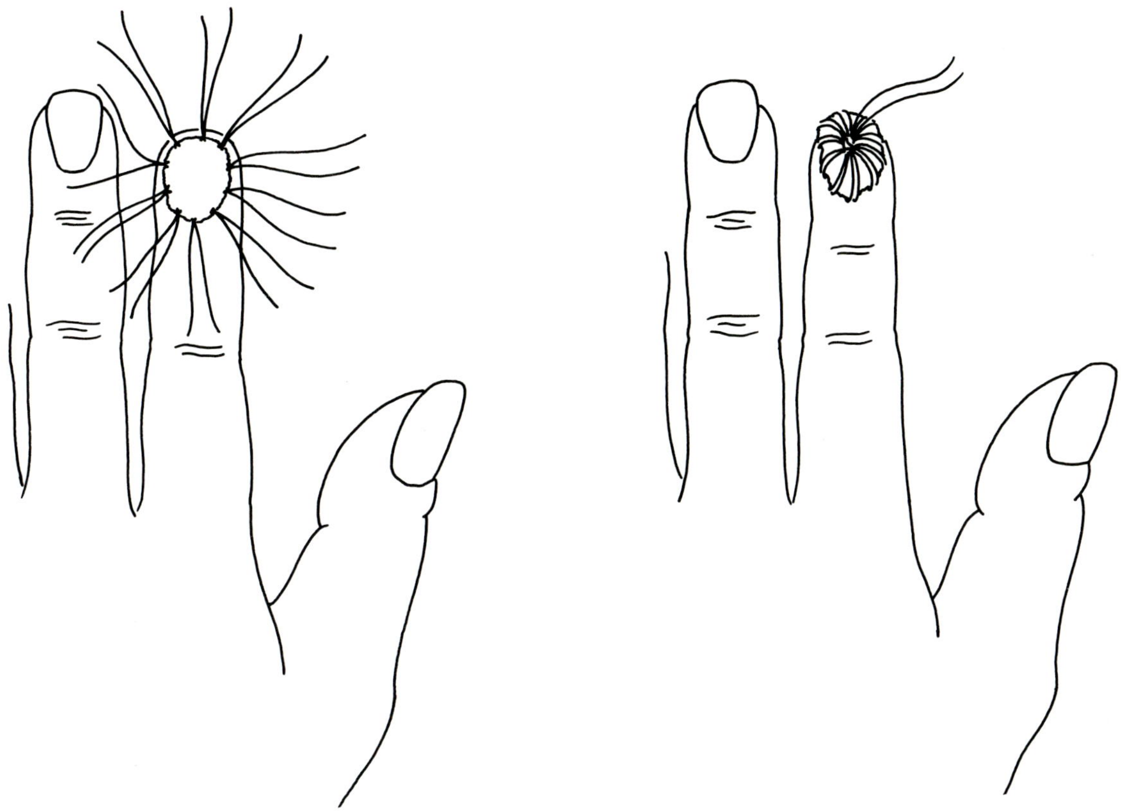

Figure 6-12. *A tied-down dressing (Stent) may be used to immobilize a split- or full-thickness skin graft. Often porous paper strips alone are adequate to secure split-thickness skin grafts.*

A wide variety of donor sites are available for the removal of split-thickness skin grafts. The hypothenar eminences and the soles of the feet provide excellent color matches for palmar skin replacement in people with dark pigmentation. The most useful area for large grafts is generally the buttocks; this suffers the least conspicuous donor site defect and provides good skin coverage. The thighs and abdominal wall may also be used but, primarily because of cosmetic objections, are less preferable. Actually it is usually easier to remove skin from the anterior thighs than from either the buttocks or abdomen.

After the recipient bed has been adequately prepared with proper hemostasis and reasonable vascularity is assured, the graft is applied directly to the bed and held in place with a continuous suture of non-absorbent material around the edges. The graft is covered with non-adherent gauze such as Adaptic or Xeroform and silk tie-over sutures which have been placed at the edge of the wound are used to secure a moistened fluffed gauze.

The donor wound is dressed with a non-adherent gauze such as Adaptic or Xeroform and a bulky absorbent dressing including moistened gauze and abdominal pads with an outer wrapping of adherent stretch gauze. All of the dressing is removed down to the layer of non-adherent gauze on the first postoperative day and the wound is left exposed to the air for drying. The gauze will become detached as epithelialization occurs underneath it (about 10 to 14 days for medium-thickness split grafts).

Postoperatively, immobilization and elevation are the keys to successful split-thickness graft as with full-thickness skin graft. Casts and splints as well as bulky dressings should be used until maximum adherence is assured. Elevation is achieved by two pillows at the patient's side while in bed, and by having him hold the hand in the elevated position while ambulating. Slings are avoided. Inspection and management of the grafted wound postoperatively are as with full-thickness grafts.

COMPOSITE GRAFTS

The most common composite graft used in the hand is the replacement of amputated soft tissue from fingertips. The replacement of such tissue is not universally successful and should not be attempted unless the injury has been a clean, incisive one.

Composite grafts of portions of earlobes have been used to pad fingertips but tend to remain soft and flabby.[12]

Flaps

Flaps are used in most cases when a recipient bed is unsuitable for the take of the skin graft. They are also used in certain instances where more padding is desired, or with island pedicle flaps where additional sensibility is needed.

LOCAL FLAPS

Local flaps are used where possible, utilizing the simplest flaps possible, the donor area being covered with a split-thickness skin graft. Simple rotation or advancement flaps (subcutaneous pedicles), including Kutler flaps[11] or volar triangular flaps[2] from an adjacent uninjured area of the hand, retain the sensibility of the parts and provide the surest cover when available (Fig. 6-13). Composite local or distant flaps are used to cover areas where there is considerable loss of tissue and to replace sites of marked scar formation. They may also be used to furnish a fatty areolar bed to aid in the gliding of tendons and to protect nerves.

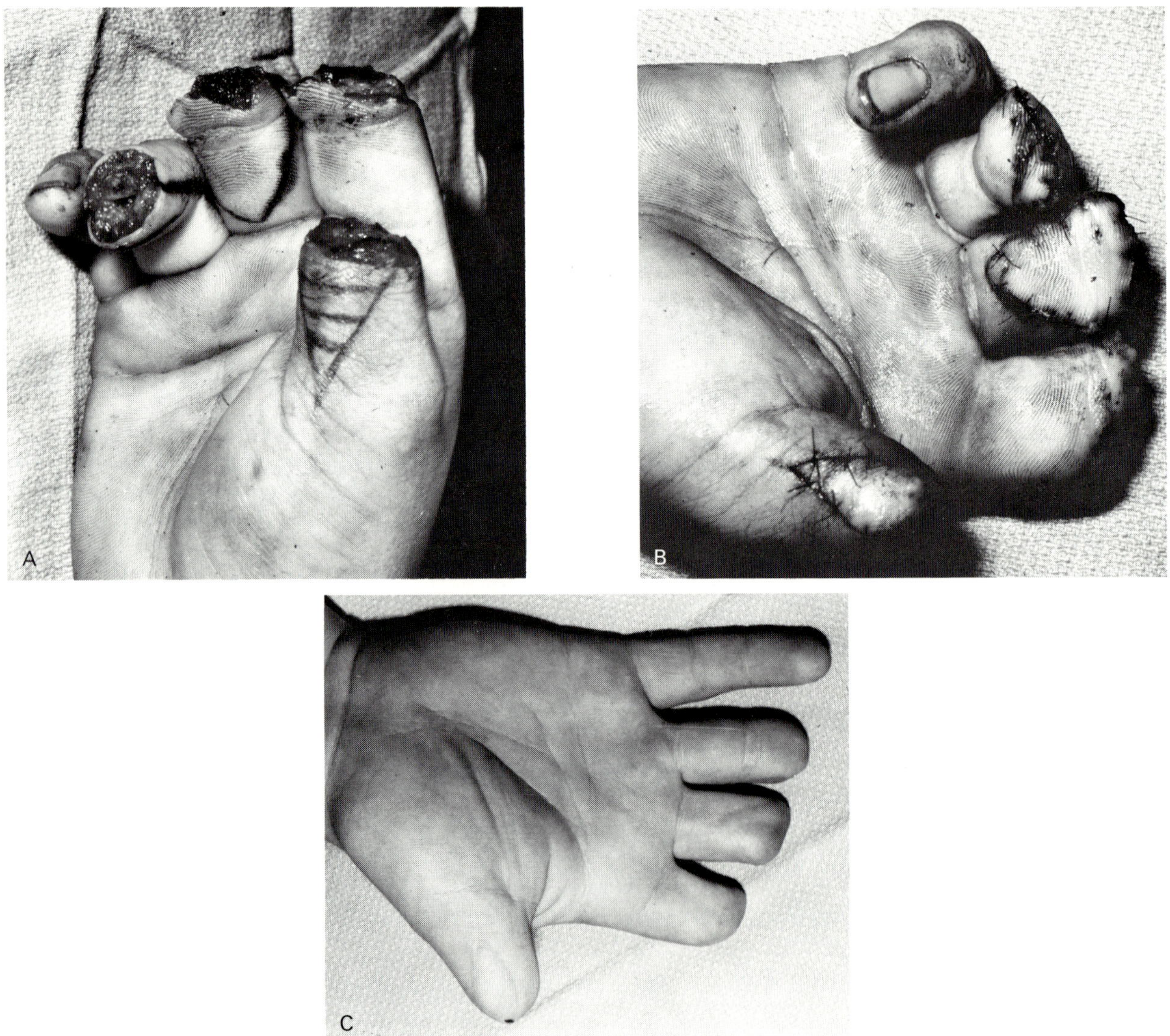

Figure 6-13. *A variety of wound closures were used for these injured fingers: the classical Kutler flaps (lateral advancement) on the thumb and the volar triangular advancement flap for the long finger.*

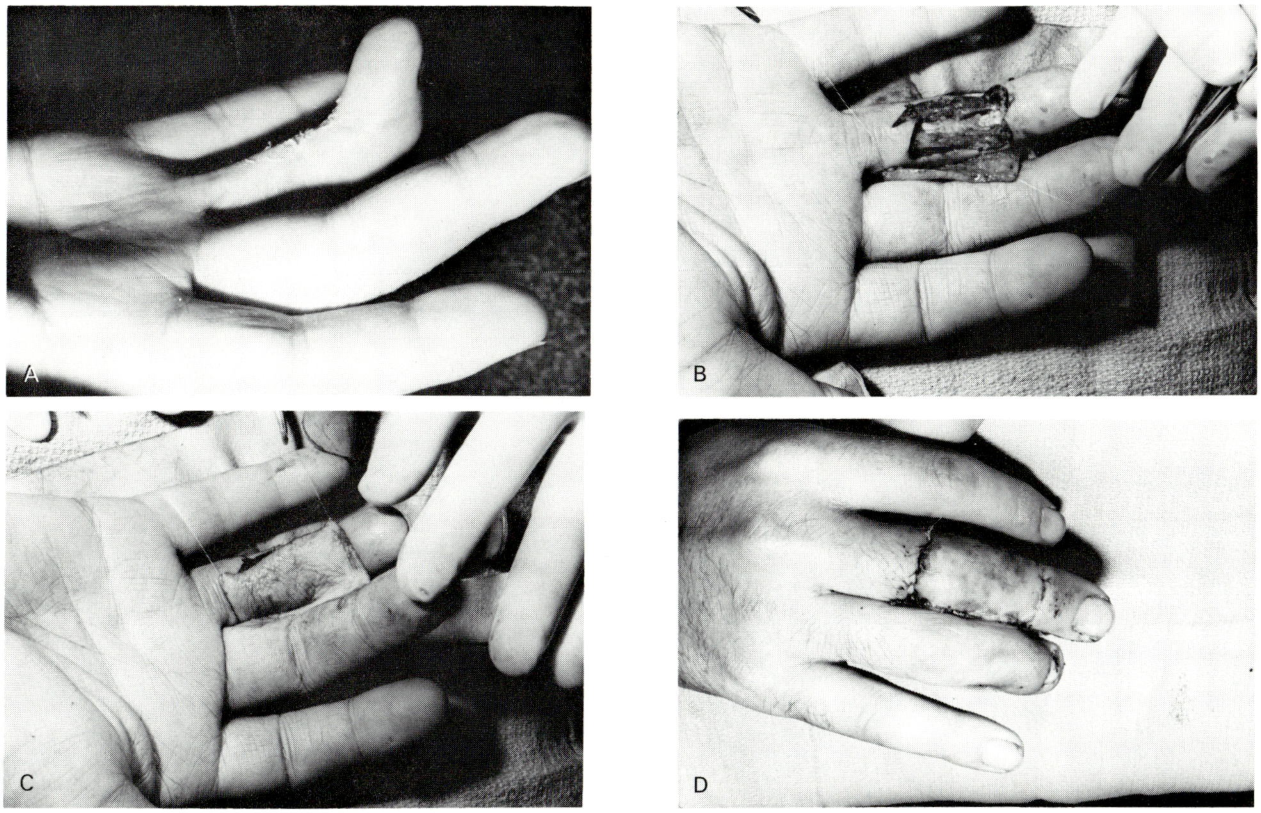

Figure 6-14. *A dorsal cross-finger flap was used to correct this volar skin deficiency of the ring finger.*

Cross-finger flaps provide a good method of coverage on the fingers. These are taken from the dorsum of an adjacent finger with the pedicle based on the midlateral line. These flaps may be used for fingertip amputations and volar surface defects of the fingers (Figs. 6-14, 6-15).

Palmar or thenar flaps with the pedicle based proximally or distally provide excellent coverage in fingertip injuries, but have limited usefulness because of the hazard of residual joint stiffness, especially at the proximal interphalangeal joint. The donor defect is closed primarily and the flap severed at 10 to 12 days. Palmar flaps (Fig. 6-16) are designed so that they are based with the flexed fingertip pointing toward the scaphoid. The incisions for elevating these flaps are never carried distal to the distal palmar crease. Thenar flaps are designed so that the flap is taken from the area immediately proximal to the metacarpophalangeal joint of the thumb.[4]

DISTANT FLAPS

Distant flaps are available as cross-arm flaps or trunk flaps. With all flaps consideration must be given to the disfigurement and disability of the donor site, including such potential problems as shoulder stiffness.

Thin pliable skin is most desirable for replacing integument lost from the hand. This tissue is best obtained from the hand itself, with the arm and chest the areas of second choice. Abdominal flaps tend to be bulky, and to have continuing fatty deposition.

Flap Design. After the recipient site has been defined the design of the flap is accomplished with a pattern either actually drawn out or in mind. Ratios of greater than $1\frac{1}{2}$ to 1 length to width should rarely be exceeded if the flap is expected to survive. The flap is cut with very little fat left on the undersurface, but with care used to preserve the subdermal plexus of circulation. If there is any question about viability, it is wise to return the flap to its original bed as a delay procedure and execute the transfer at 12 to 18 days following. If there is no question about viability, the flap may be transferred to the recipient area and sutured into place. The area from which the flap came is then closed with a split-thickness skin graft. If the donor area is sufficiently small it may be closed by direct

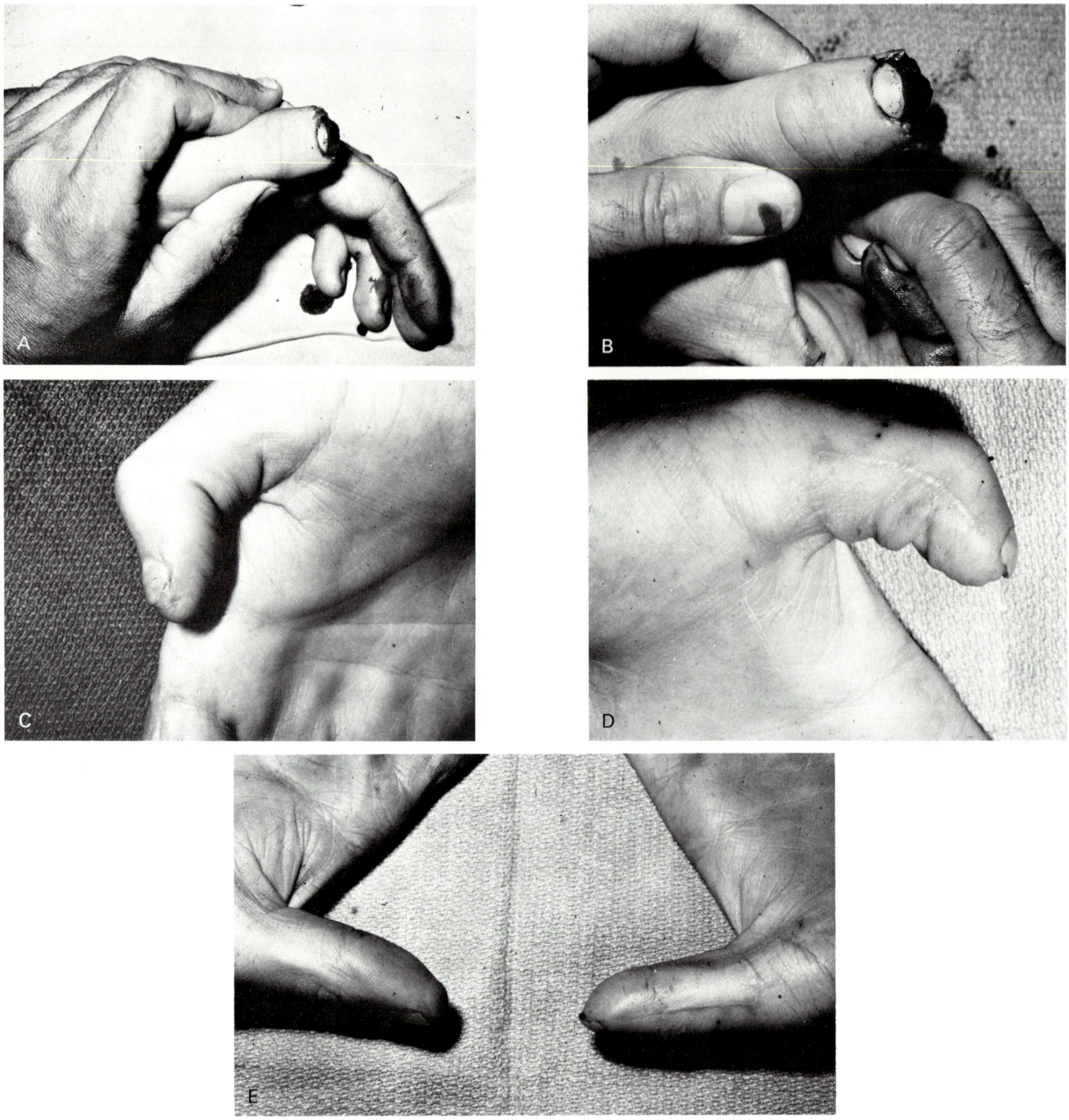

Figure 6-15. *This patient suffered similar injuries simultaneously to both thumbs* **(A, B).** *The right thumb was resurfaced by a cross-finger flap from the side of the index finger* **(C).** *The left thumb was reconstructed with a volar advancement flap* **(D).** *The result proved better with the cross-finger flap* **(E).**

approximation of the edges. The flap itself may be closed by tubing the pedicle or by turning back a hinge of tissue from the edge of the recipient wound. This provides lining for the flap and gives a closed wound. Rigid immobilization, usually with plaster, is necessary while the flap is attached to both the donor and recipient areas.[9]

The pedicle is divided and the flap set in usually at 21 days after transfer. This period may be reduced if the recipient bed is a particularly vascular one. Twelve to 14 days may be long enough. The flap may be tested by a variety of methods, clinical judgment remaining the best. The flap can be divided in stages, with about one-third of the base of the flap divided at daily intervals until it is severed, as long as there is no evidence of stasis or restriction of blood supply. Alternatively, a tourniquet may be placed around the base of the flap to note

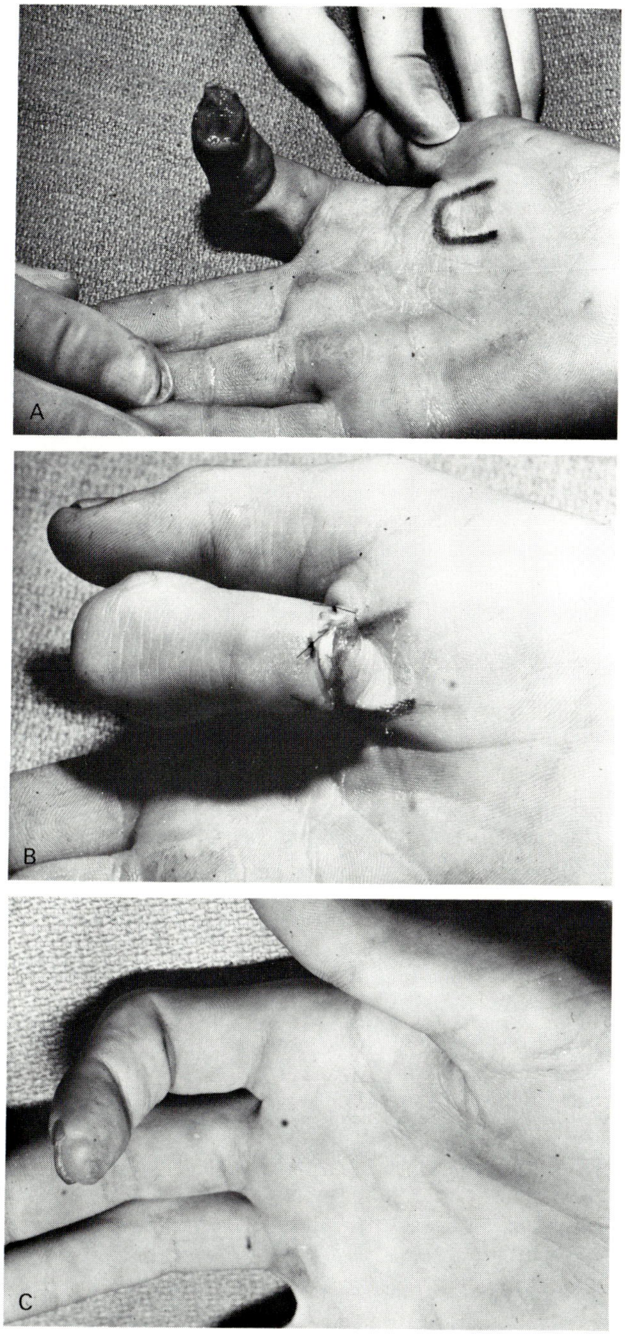

Figure 6-16. *The palmar flap can usually be divided at 10 to 12 days. The donor site on the palm is not grafted* **(C).**

the effect on the distal circulation. After insetting the flap, tailoring is often necessary for appropriate cosmetic effect and sometimes for functional effect as well. This can be done in one or two stages several months following insetting of the flap.

When deciding upon the donor area for distant flaps, age, similarity of the skin to that of the recipient site, and hair-bearing characteristics are important considerations. Other than tissue from the hand itself, the thorax, opposite arm and groin provide the most acceptable tissue, while the abdomen or thoracicoabdominal area is useful because of its availability and comfort as a donor site (Fig. 6-17).

Flaps may be tubed where possible, to decrease the open wound surface. If tubing is impossible, the raw surface of the flap may be covered with a split-thickness skin graft or simply dressed with gauze.

Crane flaps[14] are occasionally useful in hand reconstruction; fatty tissue bed is transferred to the hand without its overlying skin. Most often a deltopectoral or tubed abdominal flap is used to transfer subcutaneous tissue. At 14 to 21 days the flap is transferred back to its original donor site, leaving its subcutaneous tissue on the extremity to be grafted with a free split-thickness skin graft. This permits the surgeon to tailor the subcutaneous fat to the desired thickness and to cover the wound with thinner skin than that from the abdomen.

ISLAND PEDICLE FLAPS

Island flaps are used most often to provide sensibility to an area where there is total loss, but occasionally for a combination of sensibility and improved vascularity. These isolated segments of skin, subcutaneous tissue, and a neurovascular pedicle are usually obtained from a donor site where sensibility and vascularity are least important, as for example the ulnar side of the ring finger.

The recipient defect is prepared and the donor-skin fat pedicle outlined with methylene blue. Dissection then proceeds from proximal to distal (Fig. 15-10) to assure that the vascular pedicle is of adequate size and length. The fatty areolar tissue around the neurovascular bundle must be carefully preserved and all minute vascular branches ligated with very fine nylon (6-0). Zigzag incisions are used in opening the donor and recipient digits in the palm in order to avoid contracture. The donor wound is closed by direct approximation of those edges where there is simple dissection of the neurovascular pedicle, and by a split-thickness graft for the distal skin-subcutaneous defect. The island pedicle of skin and subcutaneous tissue should be slightly larger than the defect at the recipient site. Dissection of the neurovascular ped-

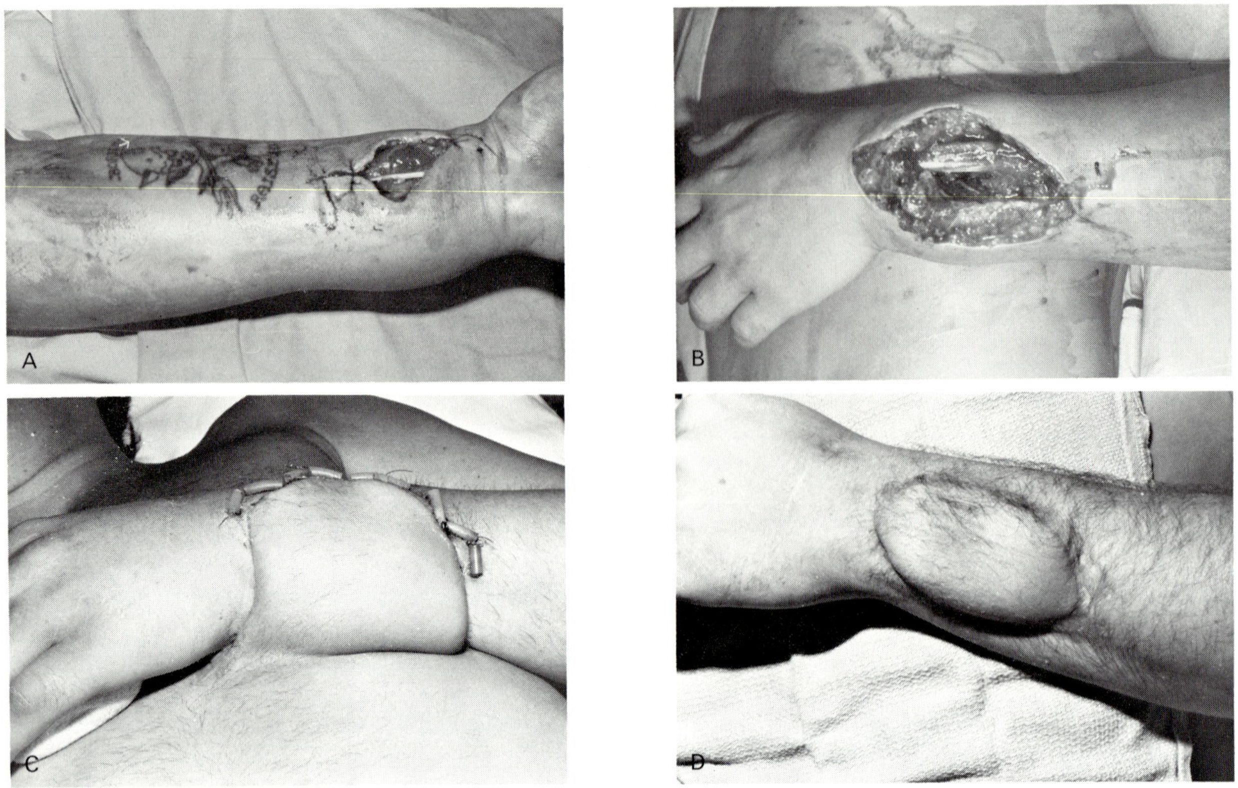

Figure 6-17. *This through-and-through gunshot wound was initially debrided and then closed 48 hours after injury. A split-thickness skin graft was used on the volar aspect* **(A)** *and an inframammary flap for the dorsal wound* **(B).** *The flap* **(C)** *was divided at 3 weeks and several revisions have been done subsequently* **(D).**

icle is done with magnification and under pneumatic tourniquet control of bleeding. The digit artery to the adjacent digit must be ligated with the epineurium of the common digital nerve split proximally, freeing the pedicle for transfer. A subcutaneous tunnel sufficiently large to allow passage of the island flap is created to the recipient site, and the flap is transferred through the tunnel after ascertaining that there are no constricting bands or areas of acute angulation. To facilitate the passage of the pedicle through the subcutaneous tunnel, a moistened Penrose drain is used as an envelope into which the pedicle is threaded and the drain with the pedicle inside is withdrawn into the recipient area. The island flap is sutured into the recipient site with 5-0 nylon and the skin grafting of the donor site is handled as previously described. At times it may be easier to avoid the use of a subcutaneous tunnel and to interconnect the donor and recipient wounds. This avoids any risk of twisting the pedicle and minimizes the chances for congestion of the flap. Immobilization and elevation are critical in the postoperative period. Very occasionally the island pedicle can be retrieved from an otherwise irreversibly damaged digit and transferred acutely to a neighboring injured finger.

Protective sensibility can be expected to be transferred immediately but with perception of the stimulus as arising from the original donor site. The brain usually achieves reorientation with correct cortical representation of the new location of the island pedicle. Normal two-point discrimination is probably rarely achieved but protective sensibility is adequate almost immediately and improves with time. A few patients will never recognize stimuli as coming from the new locus.

References

1. Ashbell, S.T.: The scalloped dorsal metacarpophalangeal skin incision. J. Bone Joint Surg., 51A; 787, 1969.
2. Atasoy, E., Ioakimidis, E., Kasdan, M.D., Kutz, J. and Kleinert, T.H.: Reconstruction of amputated finger-tip with triangular volar flap: New surgical procedure. J. Bone Joint Surg., 52A:921, 1970.
3. Beasley, R.W.: Principles and techniques of resurfacing operations for hand surgery. Am. J. Surg., 92:88, 1957.

4. Beasley, R.W.: Local flaps for surgery of the hand. Orthop. Clin. North Am., 1:219, 1970.
5. Bruner, J.M.: The zig-zag volar-digital incision for flexor tendon surgery. Plast. Reconstr. Surg., 40:571, 1967.
6. Byrne, J.J.: *The Hand, its Anatomy and Diseases.* Charles C Thomas, Springfield, 1959.
7. Carter, S.T., Berman, S.O. and Mersheimer, W.L.: Treatment of digital tenosynovitis by irrigation with peroxide and oxytetracycline. Ann. Surg., 163:645, 1966.
8. Graham, W.P.: Incisions, amputations, and skin grafting in the hand. Orthop. Clin. North Am., 1:213, 1970.
9. Kelleher, J.C., Sullivan, J.G., Baibak, G.J. and Kean, R.K.: The distant pedicle flap in surgery of the hand. Orthop. Clin. North Am., 1:227, 1970.
10. Kilgore, E.S., Jr., Adams, D.R. and Newmeyer, W.L., III: A preferred incision for dorsal finger exposure. Plast. Reconstr. Surg., 47:194, 1971.
11. Kutler, W.: A new method for finger-tip amputation. J.A.M.A., 133:29, 1947.
12. Lewin, M.D.: Digital flaps in reconstructive and traumatic surgery. Clin. Orthop., 15:74, 1959.
13. Littler, J.W.: Principles of reconstructive surgery of the hand. Am. J. Surg., 92:88, 1957.
14. Millard, D.R.: The Crane principle for the transport of subcutaneous tissue. Plast. Reconstr. Surg., 43:451, 1960.
15. Poten, B.: Grafted skin: Observation on innervation and other quality. Acta Chir. Scand., Suppl. 257, 1960.
16. Tanzer, R.C.: Compression neuropathies. In: *Hand Surgery* (Flynn, J.E., Ed.). Williams and Wilkins, Baltimore, 1966.

7 Dermatology

The hands are the most likely of all human functional anatomical units to contact injurious physical, chemical or infectious agents. In addition to the direct effects of these agents, physical trauma or inflammation, the isomorphic or Koebner response in the skin can unmask or elicit certain inherent diseases, e.g. psoriasis.

Palmar and dorsal skin are dissimilar in their capacities to react. Palmar skin is about 4 mm thick and dorsal skin 1 to 2 mm. Sweating by the eccrine glands of palmar skin is controlled by both temperature and emotional mechanisms. Both skin thickness and dermatoglyphics functionally enhance friction for grasp and protection from injury. By virtue of its corrugations, the palmar skin has a greater surface area for absorption than the dorsal skin. The thin dorsal skin with many hair follicles has the reactive potential of thin skin of the trunk, neck and elsewhere on the extremities, but with an even increased susceptibility because of its greater exposure to the environment. The nails are specialized epidermal appendages that protect the fingertips and provide a mechanism for picking up and scratching.

The skin reacts in a few distinct ways to physical injury, infection, antigens, metabolic derangement and neoplasia. Thus, several different etiological agents may cause disease states which appear identical.

Common useful topical theraputic agents (lotions, creams and ointments) are listed in Tables 7-2, 7-3, and 7-4.

The Red Scaly Hand: Eczema and Other Scaling Dermatoses (Table 7-1)

Perhaps the most common reaction pattern of the skin of the hand is redness, roughness and scaling associated with symptoms of itching, burning or simply dryness.

The differential diagnosis rests on the topographical distribution of the lesions. The palmar surface alone, the dorsal surface alone or both are involved.

PRIMARY IRRITANT ECZEMATOUS CONTACT DERMATITIS (PICD) (FIG. 7-1)

This common condition ranges in severity from the mildest of "dry" hands to severe chemical burns. Of all the common scaling dermatoses, irritant contact dermatitis is most likely to involve both palmar and dorsal surfaces. These eruptions are caused by direct irritation of epidermis and dermis by small molecules which gain entry through the usually protective stratum corneum.

Penetration may be simply the result of the solubility or concentration of the molecule in question, or of some alteration of the epidermal stratum corneum by hydration (maceration), drying (from previous exposure to fat solvents), friction or antecedent dermatosis. Ordinary causes of

Table 7-1. *The Red Scaly Dermatoses of the Hands*

	HISTORY	PHYSICAL FINDINGS (HANDS)	DISTRIBUTION	TREATMENT	PROGNOSIS
Irritant dermatitis	Recent onset, work-related	Red scaly palms	Hands and arms	Avoid irritants, lubrication	Good
Allergic dermatitis	Sudden onset	Red, scaly or vesicular (dorsum of hands)	Localized to areas of contact	Topical and systemic steroids	Good if allergen identified and avoided
Atopic dermatitis	Recurrent dermatitis, hay fever, asthma	Red scaly hands	Flexures of extremities, hands, face	Avoid irritants and soap; steroids	Expect recurrences
"Ids"	Fungal infection or stasis ulcer elsewhere	Vesicles of hands (palms)	Palmar	Treat precipitating disease; steroids	Good
Dyshidrosis	Itching and blisters in hot weather or from stress	Excoriated papules and blisters	Hands and feet (interdigital areas common)	Steroids	Expect recurrences
Nummular eczema	40-60 year old Caucasian male	Coin-shaped red oozing lesions	Trunk, legs and dorsum of hands	Steroids (tetracycline often helpful)	Expect recurrences
Psoriasis	Frequently a family history	Sharply marginated red plaques with scale	Scalp, elbows, knees, lumbosacral areas, nails	Topical steroids	Expect recurrences

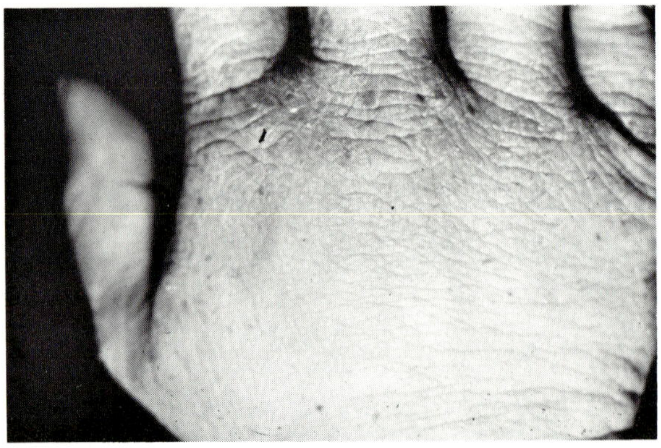

Figure 7-1. *Primary irritant eczematous contact dermatitis (PICD).*

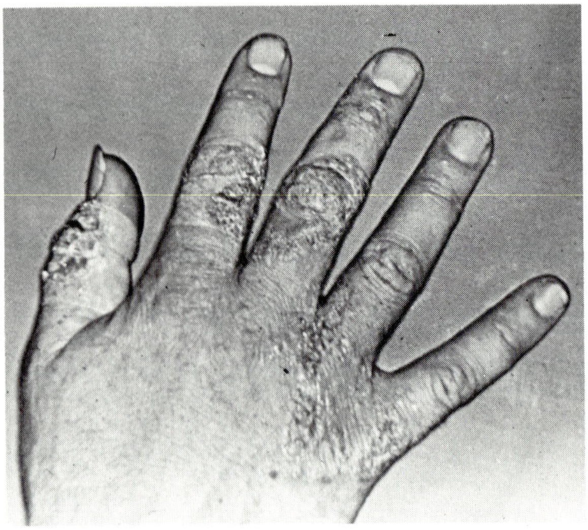

Figure 7-2. *Allergic eczematous contact dermatitis (AECD).*

irritant contact dermatitis are soaps, detergents, frequent hand washing, industrial solvents, chemical reagents and over-the-counter skin medications.

In all skin eruptions of the hands, it is crucial to stop exposure to all irritants. This alone is often curative in primary irritant contact dermatitis. The patient should clean his hands without soap and water, simply by using a bland, non-scented hand lotion. Topical corticoids in ointment or cream bases may be intensively used for several days, but the hallmark of therapy is avoidance of all irritants.

ALLERGIC ECZEMATOUS CONTACT DERMATITIS (AECD) (FIG. 7-2)

True allergic contact dermatitis of the skin of the hands is relatively uncommon and often shows a different pattern from primary irritant contact dermatitis. The palmar surface is much less likely to be involved than the dorsal surface, and the eruption is much more likely to be acute, e.g. vesicular or wet. When the condition is chronic, a more nondescript red scaly dermatitis may occur and may spread onto the palms. This allergic dermatitis is likely to be specifically localized to an area of topical contact with the involved antigen, e.g. to the proximal phalanx of the ring finger in a patient allergic to the metal of a ring. Note, however, that localization here can be PICD caused by trapping of a detergent or chemical under a ring.

Poison ivy or oak dermatitis, a classic example of AECD, often shows linear streaks and patches. Neomycin-containing antibiotic ointments may cause AECD around a cut, or AECD may be superimposed on a preexisting dermatitis. Phenothiazine and sulfonylurea-induced AECD have occurred on the hands of nurses handling these drugs.

Many different patterns of localization of AECD may occur, and only clinical suspicion and a good history will lead to the culprit allergen. Standard contact patch tests to suspected allergens may then identify the offending agent. Once this is determined, the patient can be educated to avoid the allergen in all its environmental guises. At the beginning, the process may be treated with topical and systemic steroids.

The red scaly hand is also seen as a result of *phototoxic* and *photoallergic* dermatoses (Fig. 7-3).

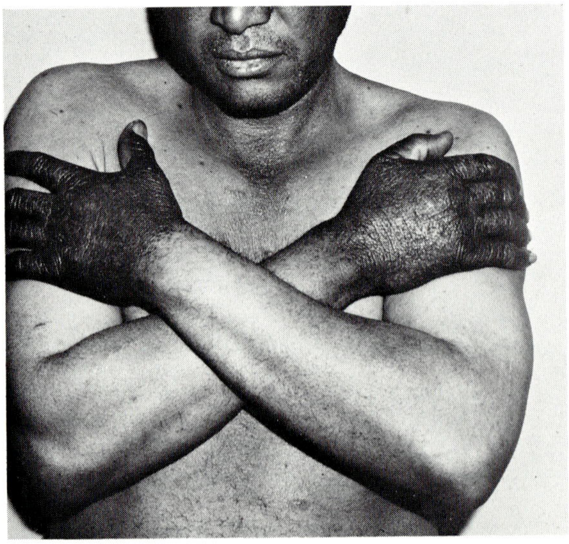

Figure 7-3. *Phototoxic dermatitis.*

These eruptions are limited to the skin commonly exposed to light, namely, the hands, face and neck. They may result either from topical contact to such agents as soap and cosmetic additives or from internally administered drugs such as phenothiazines, diuretics, sulfonamides and antibiotics. The palms are rarely affected. The diagnosis rests on the pattern of redness and scaling limited to areas of skin exposed to light, including the dorsum of the hands.

ATOPIC ECZEMA

This manifestation of the red scaly hand clinically resembles PICD or AECD, but the history often includes childhood eczema of the body flexures, allergic rhinitis or asthma and a family history of one or more of these three conditions. Atopic hand eczema, which may have been dormant since childhood, will commonly surface in women who begin keeping house or caring for a newborn infant. Irritants undoubtedly play an important role, but the pattern is usually patchy and not as widespread as in PICD. The distribution is in the flexural surfaces of the extremities and may become generalized. Treatment consists of the avoidance of irritants, allergens and emotional exhaustion. Steroids may be helpful. Recurrences are common.

"ID" REACTIONS

The greater the appreciation of the prevalence of PICD and AECD, the less commonly is an "id" reaction postulated as the cause of eczema. Nevertheless, every practicing dermatologist sees id reactions with sufficient frequency to make this a constant consideration in the differential diagnosis of hand eczema. The most clear-cut examples of id reactions are those accompanying marked tinea pedis, stasis dermatitis and ulcers of the lower extremities. The reaction of the hands (Fig. 7-4) consists of a pebbly, vesicular eruption which progresses to a chronic eczematous red scaly hand. Thus, in all cases of hand eczema, the legs and feet must also be examined and any precipitating skin disorder there must be treated. Steroids may be of value in treating the eruption on the hands.

DYSHIDROSIS (POMPHOLYX)

Dyshidrosis clinically resembles an id reaction in that it begins as a pebbly vesicular eruption along the lateral borders of the fingers (Fig. 7-5) and the palms and may occur on the feet as well. As a nosologic entity it is now in limbo, as the vesicles have been shown not to be associated with the eccrine sweat pore as was previously believed. Thus, dyshidrosis must presently be considered a diagnosis of exclusion, the cause of which is uncertain. It is treated with steroids.

NUMMULAR ECZEMA (FIG. 7-6)

As the name suggests,* this condition consists of eczematous (red and vesicular or red and scaly) patches which are coin shaped. These may occur on areas of the body other than the hands. Nummular eczema tends to be extremely pruritic and persistent. In some cases there is a strong atopic background, while in others it may precede typical psoriasis by a number of years. It is treated with steroids, and in many instances antibiotics (e.g. tetracycline) have been helpful.

* *Nummus* (Latin)-coin

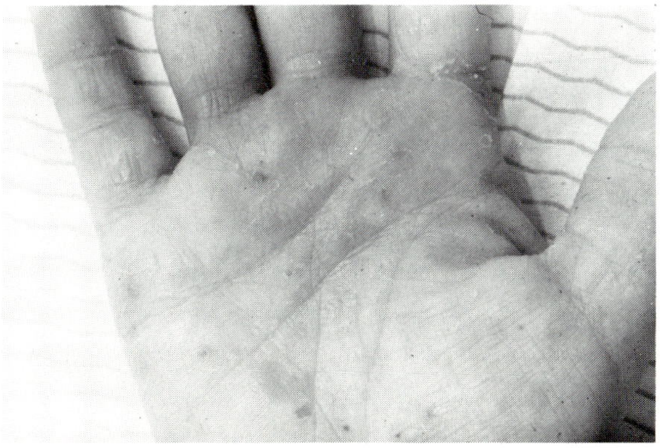

Figure 7-4. *Id reaction.*

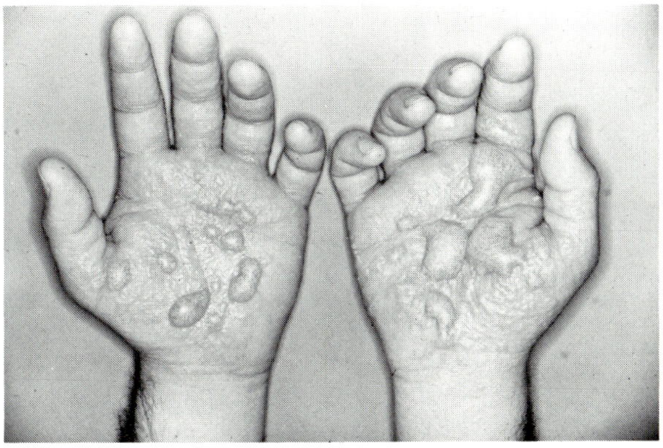

Figure 7-5. *Dyshidrosis.*

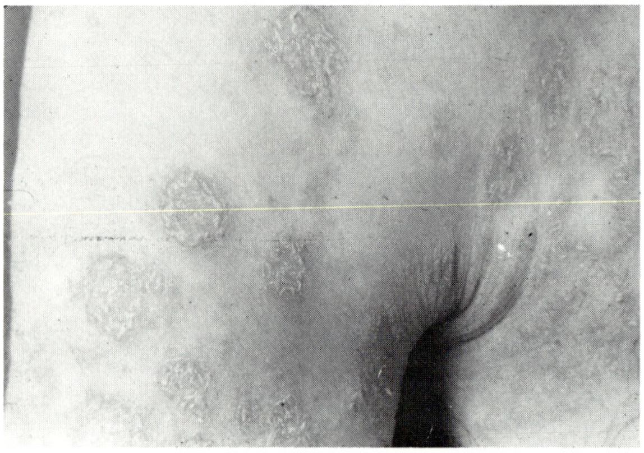

Figure 7-6. *Nummular eczema.*

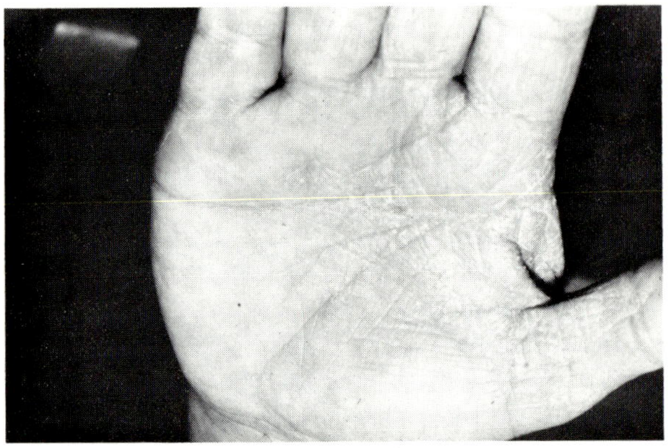

Figure 7-8. *Scaling palms involved with psoriasis.*

PSORIASIS

Psoriasis is a chronic, recurrent inherited skin eruption with a predilection for the hands and nails. It varies in extent and severity from instances of only one transient red scaly patch to those in which the whole skin surface is involved for many years, leading to thermodynamic and protein-losing problems of great magnitude (psoriatic exfoliative erythroderma) (Fig. 7-7).

The history and examination of the patient with red scaly hands must include a search for the presence or absence of scaling lesions of the scalp, elbows and knees, and careful examination for pitting or onycholysis of the nails. Such nail changes are the hallmark of psoriasis. Typical psoriasis on the trunk manifests as red patches with accumulated scale. The patches have distinct borders, and when a scale is picked off there is pinpoint bleeding (Auspitz's sign). On the dorsum of the hand, patches or plaques of this type are found. On the palms, the involvement is ordinarily more diffuse and resembles PICD and AECD (Fig. 7-8).

A variant of hand psoriasis is chronic pustular psoriasis. In this form, which may be located exclusively on the palms, rather firm pustules associated with marked peeling, which may involve all the fingertips and spread proximally, may be seen. Although frequently existing by itself, in more severe form pustular and peeling psoriasis of the fingers and palms may be associated with psoriatic arthritis of the hands. Such arthritis is usually more severe in the distal interphalangeal joints (Fig. 7-9). Psoriatic arthritis is differentiated from rheumatoid arthritis by radiological characteristics and by serological tests showing a negative rheumatoid factor or a non-IGM-containing rheumatoid factor. When the skin and joint changes of psoriasis coexist with urethritis and conjunctivitis, Reiter's syndrome must be considered.

The presence of nail changes in a patient with otherwise non-specific redness and scaling of the hands will help clinch the diagnosis of psoriasis. The most common change consists of small discrete pits (Fig. 7-10) as though caused by sticking

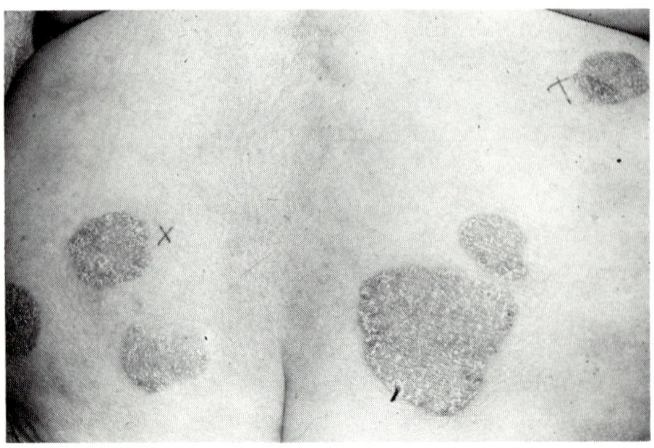

Figure 7-7. *Classic patches of psoriasis.*

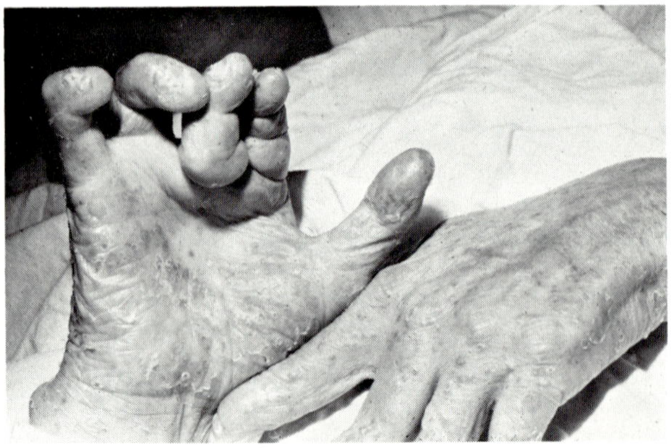

Figure 7-9. *Severe deformities secondary to psoriatic arthritis.*

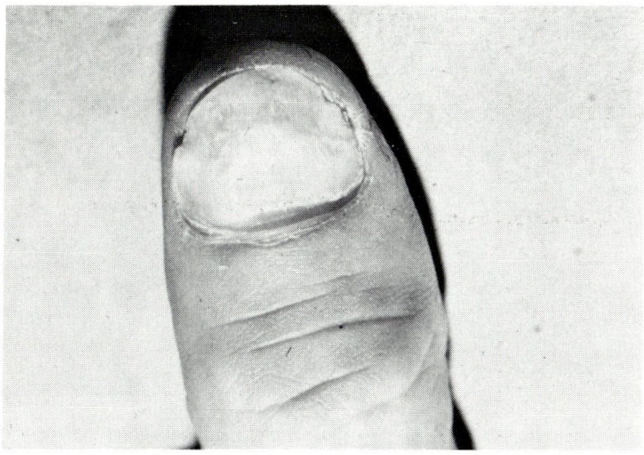

Figure 7-10. *Typical involvement of the fingernails by psoriasis.*

with a pin. Similar pits may occur in other skin diseases such as lichen planus and alopecia areata, but these diseases are not usually considerations in the differential diagnosis of hand disorders. Other nail changes in psoriasis are discolored areas resembling oil spots on paper and heaping up of keratinous debris beneath the tip of the nail so that the nail is lifted from the nail bed. Not all of these nail changes occur in every patient.

Therapy of psoriasis is best handled by a dermatologist, especially if the hand involvement is only part of a widespread or severe eruption. If limited to the hands, and if other conditions have been excluded, therapy may be initiated along the lines suggested under the eczemas. Coal tar derivatives have a time-honored and valuable role in psoriasis therapy. Pustular variants may respond to broad-spectrum antibiotics (although pustules are usually sterile) or to ultraviolet or "soft x-ray" therapy.

The Erythemas

This group includes diverse hand and generalized conditions in which the clinical picture is that of redness and edema without scaling (except perhaps in the healing phase). Most of these conditions are allergic.

SUNBURN (CHAP. 19)

The prevention of sunburn is provided by protective cover and sun-blocking agents. One of the best tincture sunscreens is 5 per cent para-aminobenzoic acid in 50 per cent ethanol. A good soothing cream in the event of sunburn erythema is rose-water ointment (cold cream) (Table 7-3).

URTICARIA

Urticaria (hives, wheals, nettles) is a typical example of a reaction in which erythema may or may not be present. It is a manifestation of the end-result of the release of histamine and other mediators from dermal mast cells and can result from many causes. Although some cases of urticaria are familial and chronic, most are in one way or another associated with an allergic cause. Common among these are reactions to medications, foods, infections or immunological diseases. Acute giant urticaria generally responds to subcutaneous injection of epinephrine, 1 : 1,000. Chronic urticaria may often be controlled with antihistamines. Repeated attacks of acute urticaria or the persistence of urticaria over many weeks warrant investigation to determine specific etiology.

ERYTHEMA MULTIFORME (FIG. 7-11)

Erythema multiforme is another erythema reaction pattern which has a predilection for the hands. Although there are many known precipitating events, including herpes simplex infection, vaccination, mumps, histoplasmosis, typhoid, syphilis, collagen vascular disease and drug eruptions, many erythema multiforme reactions are of unknown cause. A typical sequence is the development of herpes simplex lesions on the lip simultaneously with, or followed by, the lesions of erythema multiforme. These lesions consist initially of papules which spread out to form bull's-eye or target forms with red edges and purplish centers. The palms and dorsum of the hands, wrists, forearms and feet are the usual sites in the milder cases. No specific therapy is required in most instances, as the lesions fade within two weeks. A possible cause should be sought, however, because in the case of

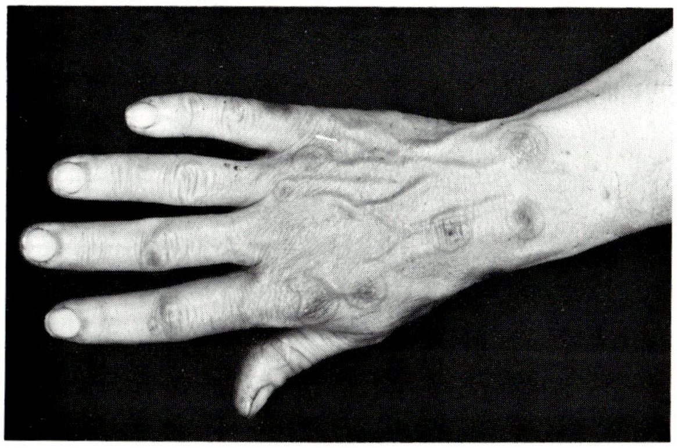

Figure 7-11. *Erythema multiforme.*

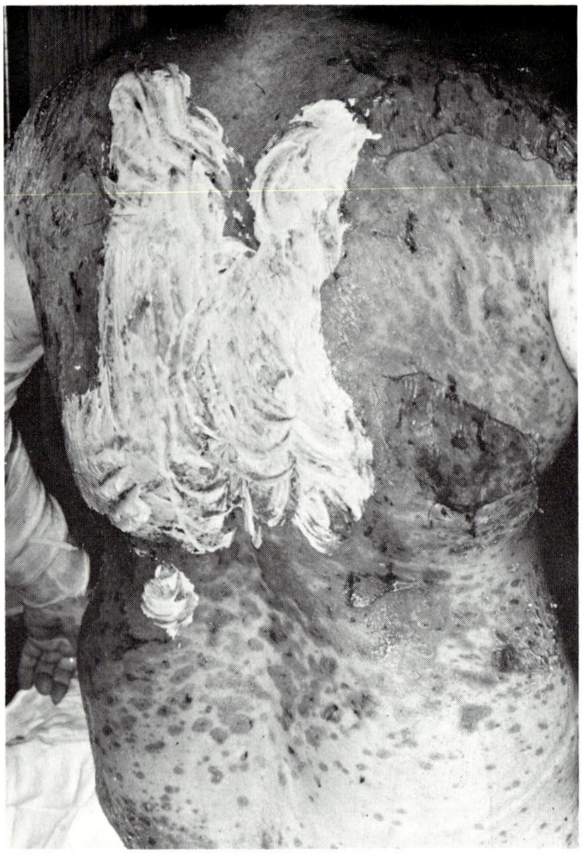

Figure 7-12. *Stevens-Johnson syndrome. This severe reaction to penicillin occurred in a middle-aged male. Silver sulfadiazine was used as a topical antibacterial agent.*

drug reactions the eruption can proceed to a bullous form or to the sometimes fatal Stevens-Johnson syndrome in which mucous membranes are involved (Fig. 7-12).

DRUG ERUPTIONS (FIG. 7-13)

Drug eruptions can mimic nearly any skin disorder. The most typical eruption is that of a symmetrical erythematous rash consisting of macules (flat) and papules (raised) which may look very much like measles. Unlike measles, drug eruptions tend to itch. Such a rash appearing in any patient taking drugs should always suggest the possibility of drug eruption. The penicillins, sulfonamides, diuretics, oral antidiabetic agents and barbiturates are the most common offenders, but nearly any drug can be and has been responsible for a drug eruption. Since drug eruptions can proceed to several types of serious secondary reactions if the offending agent is continued, it is wise to discon-

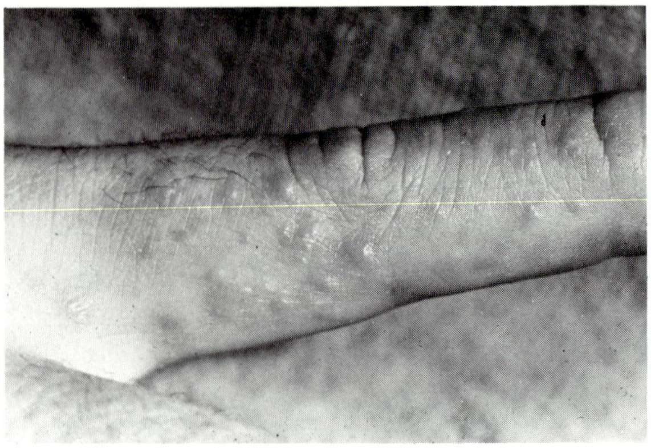

Figure 7-13. *Drug eruption.*

tinue all but the most essential medications at the first thought of drug eruption as a diagnostic possibility.

Fungal Infections of the Skin

Many of the entities described hereunder occur exclusively on the hands or have such a distinctive morphological appearance when they *are* present on the hands that they warrant separate discussion.

DERMATOPHYTOSIS—TINEA OF THE HANDS AND NAILS (FIG. 7-14)

Tinea or dermatophytosis of the hands is more common than generally appreciated. There are three major forms of which the classical ringworm,

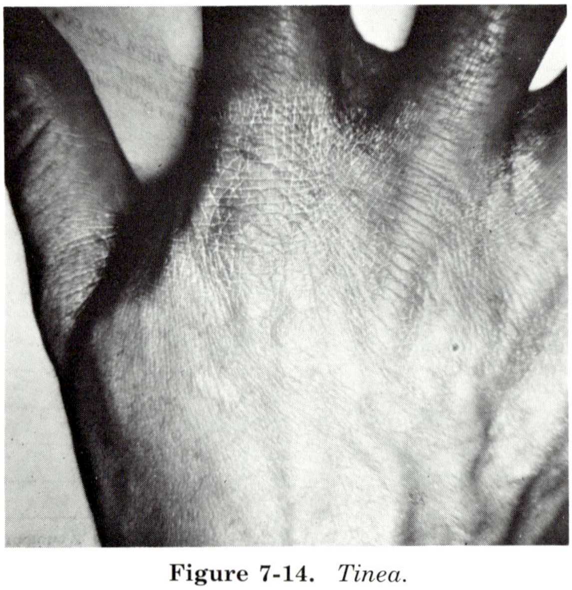

Figure 7-14. *Tinea.*

seen most often in children and acquired most often from pets, is the easiest to diagnose and treat. These lesions are round with a raised, red, irritated border. There may be a tendency to clearing in the center of lesions larger than 1 cm in diameter. This form occurs mainly on the dorsum of the hand. The simplest way to make the diagnosis is to scrape some scale from the active border with a surgical blade, put it on a slide with a drop of 20 per cent potassium hydroxide, apply a coverslip, and examine microscopically. The potassium hydroxide dissolves the cell walls and the fungal hyphae stand out as translucent slender threads.

The classical ringworm of children does not respond well to topical medications and generally requires a short course (1 to 2 weeks) of oral griseofulvin in a dose dependent on age and body weight.

Chronic, erythematous scaling tinea of the palms (Fig. 7-15) (often just one palm) may be associated with a similar infection of the feet. This combination occurs so often in clinical practice that it is referred to as the "two-foot, one-hand syndrome."

A final type of tinea of the hands is the chronic, recalcitrant eczematous tinea of the dorsum of the hands. As with other types, the diagnosis should always be confirmed by microscopic examination of scrapings. In the chronic forms, scale should be cultured on Sabouraud's agar at room temperature. By confirming the diagnosis in chronic forms, the physician may be sure he is not committing his patient to a long and costly course of griseofulvin unnecessarily. Chronic forms of tinea often require one to several months of griseofulvin therapy. Mild desquamating agents such as 3 per cent salicylic acid ointment or sulfur and salicylic acid soap often speed resolution. There is little evidence that topical fungicides are useful. Relapses are common, and some patients require intermittent griseofulvin therapy for years.

Onychomycosis or tinea of the nails usually results by contiguous spread of fungal infection from adjacent skin. One or all of the fingernails may be involved. They may simply discolor (yellow or ivory) or become thickened and fragile. Whereas in psoriasis the involvement is generally symmetrical in each hand, in onychomycosis the nails are involved in a random manner.

Since nails are slow growing (3 months for fingernails and 6 months for thumbnails, on the average) therapy will need to be carried out for many months. Before a patient is committed to such a long course, the diagnosis should be confirmed by direct microscopy and culture. Although frequent trimming and use of topical fungicides are recommended, only griseofulvin (0.5 to 1.0 gm/day) is curative. Surgical removal of nails is worthwhile in resistant cases and has augmented the resolution by griseofulvin in some other cases with marked nail deformity.

CANDIDIASIS (MONILASIS) (FIG. 7-16)

Candidiasis thrives in the body folds—axillae, groins, vulvae, intergluteal cleft, submammary area and interdigital webs. Those whose work requires frequent or prolonged immersion of the hands in water—domestics, bartenders, nurses, doctors, housewives—are common victims. Diagnosis is largely based on clinical appearance: red, raw interdigital webs with distinct, often pustular borders and occasional satellite erythematous papules or pustules. A smear of the epithelial border stained with any available laboratory stain will reveal the thick, short pseudohyphae. Since Can-

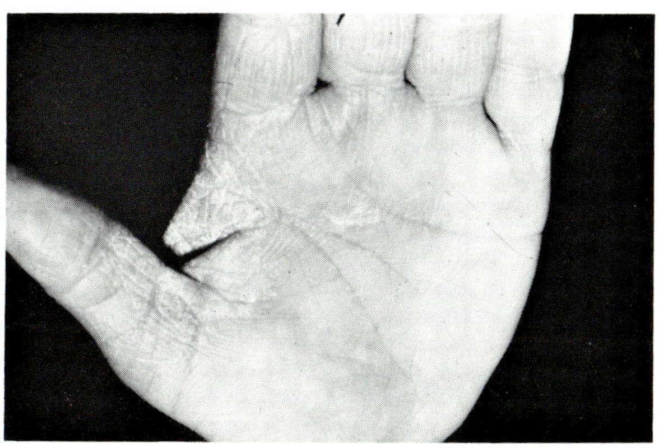

Figure 7-15. *Scaling tinea of the palms.*

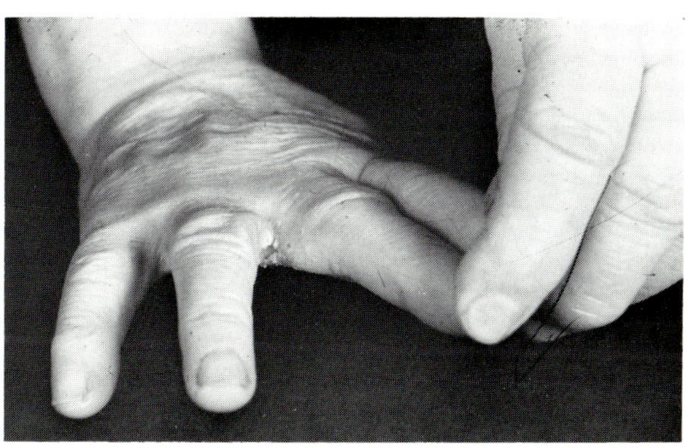

Figure 7-16. *Monilia intertrigo.*

dida albicans is a common minor contaminant of skin, culture is not as helpful as the microscopic examination of a smear. The organism is found only in the epithelium, not the pus.

Treatment should include scrupulous avoidance of water and irritants, drying of the areas involved and application of simple antiseptic agents such as aqueous gentian violet or Vioform lotion. For some cases, nystatin powder or amphotericin-B lotion may be required.

CHRONIC PARONYCHIA (FIG. 7-17)

Chronic paronychia usually occurs because of repeated minor trauma to the cuticle and periungual tissues. It is often the result of frequent wetting and drying of hands, nail-biting or improper manicure. It may be a manifestation of covert emotional stress. There is general agreement that chronic paronychia is more common in diabetics and in those with "cold hands."

Chronic paronychia may begin as a candidal infection in which case pseudohyphae and spores are often found in scrapings from the nail fold. As the condition progresses, inflammation of the nail fold tissue sets the stage for secondary infection with staphylococci, streptococci, Pseudomonas, etc. Although antimicrobial therapy is indicated and often combined with removal of the nail, the hallmark of successful treatment is keeping the hands dry. Those who cannot or will not keep their hands out of water may be doomed to years of chronic paronychia with intermittent acute episodes.

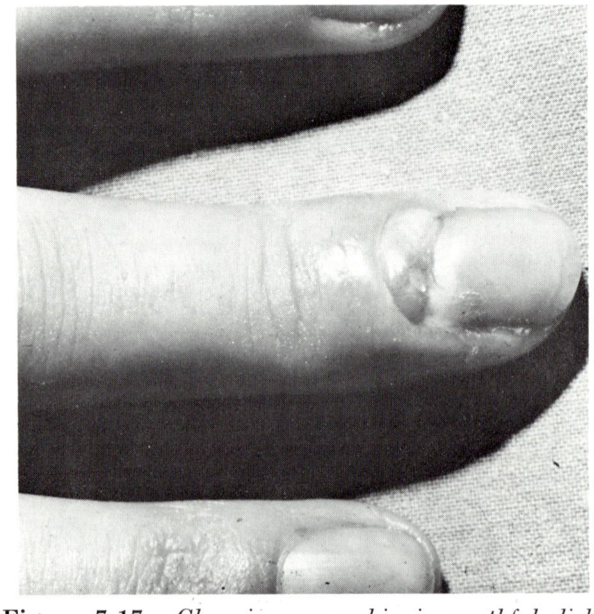

Figure 7-17. *Chronic paronychia in youthful dishwasher.*

There is sometimes a place for systemic therapy in chronic paronychia when smears of pus mainly reveal cocci. Topical applications should be frequent. Early and vigorous treatment with creams combining antibiotics and antimonilial agents are often curative. Treatment must be continued beyond the point of resolution of inflammation and until the cuticle is entirely healed. The patient must be educated to prevent both self-induced and work-induced trauma to the cuticle.

Acute paronychia is a bacterial infection of the periungual tissues of the proximal nail fold (Chap. 20).

SPOROTRICHOSIS (FIG. 20-13A,B)

Sporotrichosis is a fungal disease often caused by inoculation of the causative organism, Sporotrichum schenckii, by the prick of a rose thorn, contamination of a cut by sphagnum moss or other wood products. It is seen, therefore, most often in gardeners, florists, and those in the lumber and construction trades.

Clinically, a chain of several firm, round, crusted or ulcerated lesions may be seen, often along a lymphatic channel and causing epitrochlear or axillary adenopathy. The first lesion is often on the hand or wrist. The organism is rarely demonstrated in scrapings or even tissue sections. Culture on Sabouraud's agar is necessary to confirm the diagnosis. Sporotrichosis rarely responds to griseofulvin but it is sensitive to potassium iodide, which remains the systemic treatment of choice. Fifteen to 30 drops of saturated potassium iodide in a glass of milk or juice is taken three times daily until the lesions have been cleared for 4 to 6 weeks.

Bacterial Infections of the Skin

The bacterial infections described below (and in Chap. 20) are not exclusively limited to the hands, but are frequently found there.

IMPETIGO

Impetigo is a superficial contagious infection of the skin with streptococci, staphylococci or both, which generally manifests itself as multiple distinct oozing and crusting areas. The palms are uncommonly involved. In widespread infections there may be regional adenopathy and fever, although this is not the rule. Since the crusts are infectious, they should be removed when treatment is begun. Topical application of appropriate antibiotic creams is rapidly effective. For widespread infections, systemic antibiotics are indicated. Inasmuch as acute glomerulonephritis has been reported following epidemics of impetigo associated with certain nephritogenic strains of streptococci, cases occurring in epidemics should be empirically treated with systemic antibiotics until the strain responsible is identified as non-nephritogenic. Unfortunately, such systemic antibiotics are no guarantee against renal damage.

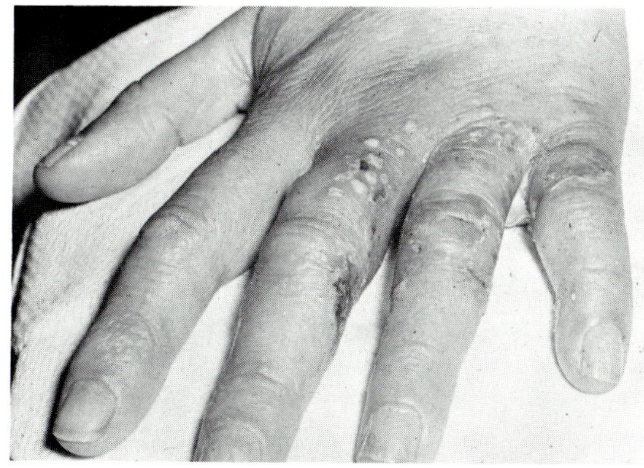

Figure 7-18. *Infected eczematoid.*

INFECTED ECZEMATOID DERMATITIS (FIG. 7-18)

Infected eczematoid dermatitis is a catchall term for several clinical situations which include a secondarily infected eczema and a bacterially caused dermatitis. In both situations there is a more diffuse and less superficial appearance of the involved area than is seen in impetigo. Because of this and because of the disability it can cause in the hand, systemic antibiotics are required. Staphylococci are almost always responsible and are usually sensitive to tetracycline or erythromycin in non-hospital-acquired cases. Topical treatment should consist of simple compresses or soaks in the initial phase, followed by mild anti-inflammatory and anti-infective creams.

BACTERIAL ULCERS

Bacterial ulcers, while relatively rare, can and do occur in the hands. Both primary syphilis (indurated, non-tender), and chancroid (soft, painful) ulcers may be seen. Clinical suspicion will aid the diagnosis. Darkfield examination of tissue fluid squeezed from a true chancre can be performed in any dermatological or public health facility and serological follow-up is indicated. If chancroid is suspected, a cotton-tipped applicator should be rolled across the ulcer and then across a glass slide, which is then dried and stained. The causative Ducrey's bacillus appears in parallel rows of gram-negative rods in such preparations. Diphtheritic ulcers are occasionally reported as occurring on the hands and, with the gradual waning of group immunity and the recent steady increase of diphtheria of all types in the southern part of America, they may be expected more often. In the skin, diphtheria begins as a small pustule which forms an eschar, or an overhanging ulcer with a membranous base. While systemic symptoms are less common in cutaneous than in mucous membrane diphtheria, early diagnosis may help prevent involvement of other tissues and organs.

Ulcers of the hands caused by M. tuberculosis are extremely rare, being limited almost exlusively to morticians, pathologists, and medical students. Another form of skin tuberculosis, Mycobacterium balnei, is being recognized increasingly, and causes indolent, progressive granulomatous lesions of the fingers and hands (Fig. 7-19). This infection is sometimes called "swimming-pool granuloma," since it frequently dates from an injury incurred in a pool and the organism has been cultured from pools. It is also seen in those hobbyists who keep aquariums. When suspected, the diagnosis is dependent on positive culture which usually requires a biopsy. The organism is sometimes seen by

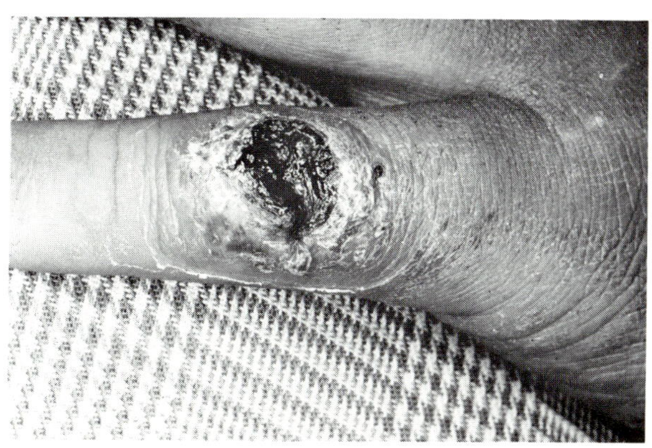

Figure 7-19. *Infection of a finger by M. balnei (swimming-pool granuloma).*

Ziehl-Neelsen stain. Cultures are best submitted to public health or university bacteriology laboratories and may require weeks or months to become positive. The response to the usual antimycobacterial drugs such as streptomycin and isoniazid is erratic, but the response to heat therapy is often dramatic.

Streptococcal ulcers occur in two forms. The acute, progressive gangrenous ulcer (streptococcal gangrene) is associated with marked systemic symptoms and constitutes a surgical emergency. There is, however, a chronic, indolent streptococcal ulcer often seen in warmer climates, especially following insect bites in children. This chronic type usually responds rapidly to topical and systemic antibiotics (e.g. penicillin).

ERYSIPELAS

Erysipelas and streptococcal cellulitis require immediate treatment with penicillin or erythromycin to prevent the compromise of lymphatic drainage which often predisposes to recurrent episodes as well as the immediate complications of abscess formation and septicemia. The hand is red, hot, extremely painful and swollen. Fever and prostration are common.

ERYSIPELOID

Erysipeloid is an uncommon but characteristic infection of the hand seen most often in butchers, fish handlers, fishermen, and farmers. The bacterium is Erysipelothrix rhusiopathiae, the gram-positive organism which also causes hog erysipelas. It gives rise to an acute inflammatory induration of the hand. It differs from erysipelas by the relative mildness of accompanying constitutional symptoms, and by the fact that there is nearly always a visible portal of entry, e.g. a puncture wound or superficial laceration. Vesicles or small blisters may be present at the periphery of the erythema and induration.

An occupational history is crucial in making the diagnosis of erysipeloid. Treatment consists of penicillin or tetracycline for a week to 10 days in addition to any necessary debridement and compress (e.g. with zinc oxide ointment) of an abscess at the portal of entry. Part of the inflammatory process may be a local allergic response to animal, poultry and fish protein introduced at the site of a puncture or cut.

Infestations

Scabies is a cutaneous infestation with Sarcoptes scabiei, a whitish hemispherical mite with four pairs of legs. After years of relative rarity, scabies is assuming nearly epidemic proportions in some areas. The mite is acquired through close contact (not necessarily sexual) with infected persons. The fertilized female burrows into the superficial layers of the epidermis where she lays her eggs. It may take a month before a person develops a large enough population of the mites (and the hypersensitivity to its products) to become symptomatic.

The rash consists of burrow tracks, vesicles, papules and excoriations. Favored areas are the interdigital webs of the fingers, palms, wrists, buttocks and genitalia. Pruritus may be severe, particularly at night.

Diagnosis is difficult unless there is a reasonable index of suspicion. The diagnosis may be confirmed by scraping a layer of skin above a burrow and examining it microscopically. The mite, the eggs or excreta, all of which are characteristic, may be seen. Therapy consists of 1 or 2 neck-to-toe applications of gamma benzene hexachloride or benzyl benzoate lotions.

Viral Infections of the Hand

HERPES SIMPLEX (FIG. 7-20)

Herpes simplex may occur on the hand as it may anywhere on the body. The typical manifestations are those of pain and grouped blisters on an erythematous base, with or without regional lymphadenopathy. The existence of recurrent episodes should alert the physician to the possibility of this diagnosis.

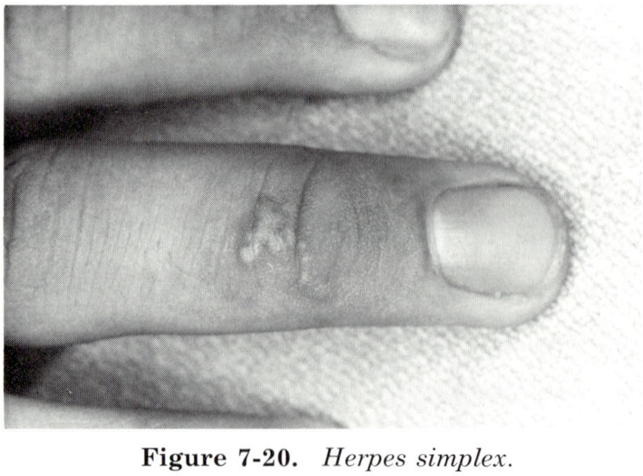

Figure 7-20. *Herpes simplex.*

When it occurs about the nail fold or distal fat pad of the digit, as it may in nurses and dentists who may acquire it from the saliva of herpes-secreting patients, it may be confused with acute or chronic paronychia or a felon. Pain is often severe and out of proportion to the extent of redness or induration. Incision for drainage should be avoided if the tissues are not under tension or there is no obvious abscess.

A Giemsa stain of scrapings from the base of a vesicle may reveal giant multinuclear cells typical of viral infection. Treatment is largely symptomatic as there is no consistently effective antiviral agent. A recent treatment of some promise combines the application of photoactive dyes (neutral red, proflavine) with exposure to incandescent light for 15 minutes daily. Activation of the dye by light is virucidal.

The vesicles may be unroofed, the bases cleansed, and epinephrine, 1 : 1,000 on a cotton ball, applied. Antibiotic powders are prescribed to keep the area dry and to prevent secondary bacterial infection. Recurrences of herpes are triggered in some individuals by stress, heat, fever, sunlight, trauma or the hormonal changes of the menstrual cycle.

HAND-FOOT-AND-MOUTH DISEASE

This syndrome is unrelated to the bovine disease of similar name. Isolated tender vesicles are found on the hands, the oral mucosa and feet. The disease is caused by several Coxsackie type A viruses and may occur in epidemic form.

WARTS (VERRUCA VULGARIS) (FIGS. 7-21, 7-22)

Over 50 per cent of all warts occur on the hands. Warts of the hands are extremely common in children, but they are found in persons of all ages. There are three types of warts of the hands: the common raised wart, the flat wart and the uncommon palmar wart or myrmecium. Since warts are infectious, the more warts a patient has, the more he is likely to get. This would seem to argue for aggressive therapy; however, one-half of all warts will go away in a year if no treatment at all is given. For a disease with a 50 per cent spontaneous cure rate (without scarring), aggression is ill-advised. However, many patients (or their parents) do want their warts treated. The cardinal rule should be: Do no harm!

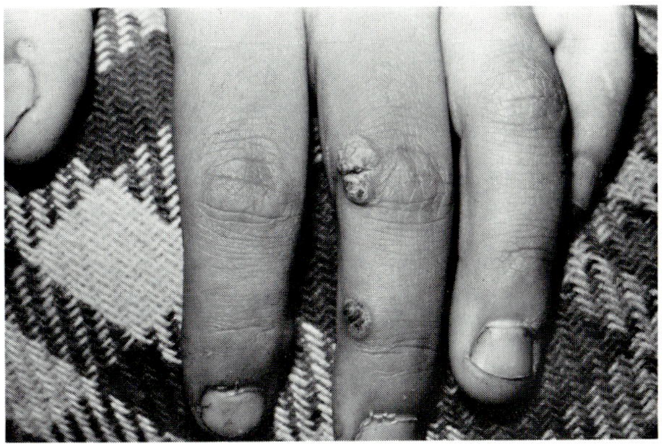

Figure 7-21. *Verruca vulgaris.*

Among the simplest therapies is the use of formalin. Formalin, aqueous (10 per cent) or in petrolatum (20 per cent), may be applied twice daily for several weeks. The drying effect alone (or combined with regular paring) may cause involution. This is also true of 40 per cent salicylic acid plasters which are cut to the shape of the wart and applied. Plasters may be replaced and the warts pared daily, or occlusion may continue for a week before paring.

Cryotherapy with liquid nitrogen (−190° C) is preferred by many dermatologists. The nitrogen is easily obtained in insulated, pressurized tanks and a single day's supply may be kept in a vented thermos in a refrigerator. A cotton-tipped applicator is dipped into the nitrogen and pressed firmly against the wart for 15 to 20 seconds. The wart will turn white as it freezes, will thaw in 30 seconds,

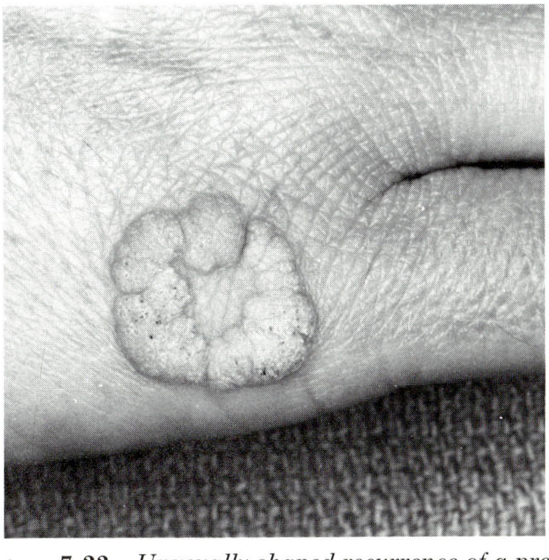

Figure 7-22. *Unusually shaped recurrence of a previously fulgerated verruca vulgaris.*

and may blister in 24 hours. If successful, the wart peels off at 2 to 3 weeks. Repeated treatments are possible. Deep or prolonged cryotherapy may damage digital nerves or permanently injure the nail matrix, resulting in permanent nail dystrophy.

Another effective non-surgical approach is the use of cantharidin, a blistering agent, in collodion. This is particularly useful in fearful children. The cantharidin-collodion mixture is applied carefully to the wart, allowed to dry, and covered by impermeable tape for 24 hours or until a blister results. The wart will exfoliate with the blister in 7 to 10 days. This therapy is particularly effective for extensive periungual warts.

The preferred and most definitive therapy is curettage immediately after electrodesiccation under local anesthesia without epinephrine. Neither the electrodesiccation nor the curettage should be excessive. It should cease when the curettage is flush with the skin. The spark of the current should be very small. It is better to desiccate in stages at weekly intervals than too deeply at once, with damage to nerves or nail beds. Careful and staged desiccations result in negligible scarring.

Multiple flat warts (verruca plana) occur on the dorsum of the hands and may spread to the face. They may be treated with liquid nitrogen, but only very lightly for 5 to 10 seconds. Frequently, simple drying and peeling agents are effective. Salicylic acid, 2 per cent in bay rum or isopropanol applied twice daily, is a useful solution. In recalcitrant cases, careful, limited surface electrodesiccation may be required.

Palmar warts are much less common than plantar warts, but may be equally painful when pressure is applied to them. They should be treated carefully to avoid a painful scar. Here again, the application of a 40 per cent salicylic acid pad for a week, the application of liquid nitrogen used lightly on repeated visits, or repeated minimal electrodesiccation are effective methods of treatment. Simple repeated paring of the "white" (not "pink") tissue to the point of enucleation of the hard core should follow in 1 or 2 weeks. Occasionally the lesion should be excised.

MOLLUSCUM CONTAGIOSUM

These viral papules or warty lesions are commonly found on the hands, although they may occur anywhere on the skin. They may be numerous but respond much more completely to simple therapy than do common warts. Characteristically, molluscum papules have a central dell within which is the virus-rich core. Spraying with ethyl chloride provides temporary mild anesthesia and also accentuates the dell so that the core can be quickly excised with a small curette. With the core gone, the lesion rapidly involutes. Superficial electrocauterization of the delled center is also effective. In the case of infants and frightened young children, painting the lesions with cantharidin in collodion without occlusion is a painless alternative.

Nail Changes

PITTING

A pitting of the fingernails represents the most common asymptomatic nail abnormality. When more than one nail is involved and there are multiple pits, the diagnosis of psoriasis must be considered. The pits often precede cutaneous manifestations of the disease by years. Alopecia areata and lichen planus may also be accompanied by nail pits.

ONYCHOLYSIS (FIG. 7-23)

Onycholysis (lifting of the nail from the nail bed) is manifested by a whitish translucence often starting at the distal portion of the nail (hyponychium). It most commonly results from psoriasis. If caused by fungal infection, diagnosis is readily proven by microscopic examination of the subungual debris in a drop of 20 per cent potassium hydroxide. The nail plate is only secondarily involved; therefore, it is important to establish an

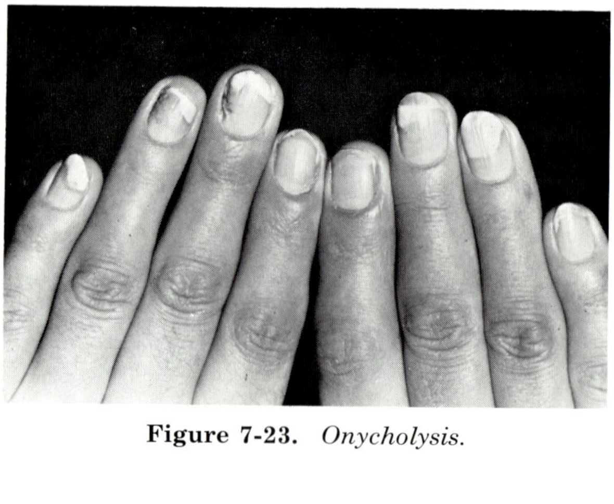

Figure 7-23. *Onycholysis.*

early diagnosis of fungal etiology. Systemic griseofulvin in early cases of fungus involvement is usually curative. Psoriasis, on the other hand, is often intractable.

The lysis may involve much of the nail, but is often only at the sides. The primary lesion is a brownish macule seen through the nail plate; this is not often noted as the macule is quickly replaced by lysis. Other less frequent causes of onycholysis include nail polish and nail hardener irritancy and allergy, systemic drug phototoxicity (such as Declomycin) and self-manipulation by the patient.

BEAU'S LINES (TRANSVERSE GROOVES) (FIG. 7-24)

One or more transverse grooves are called Beau's lines. These occur after a systemic insult (such as high fever, coronary infarction, severe injury, etc.). They may occur in one extremity or one digit after local injury or surgery. Beau's lines are caused by a partial arrest in keratinization by the cells which produce the nail. With knowledge of normal nail growth (0.1 mm/week), the onset of the insult causing Beau's lines can be dated.

PIGMENTED NAILS

A pigmented lesion under a nail raises the question of a malignant melanoma. However, 99.9 per cent of brown or black spots of the nail bed are due to melanin from benign cellular nevi (moles). Although pigmented racial groups such as Negroes have a significant incidence of such benign nevi, no racial group is completely free of them.

Suspicion of a malignant melanoma should be raised only when spread, tumefaction, pain, bleeding or pigment change develops. Whenever there is any question, enough nail should be removed to allow a biopsy. No diagnosis of melanoma should be accepted without an adequate biopsy.

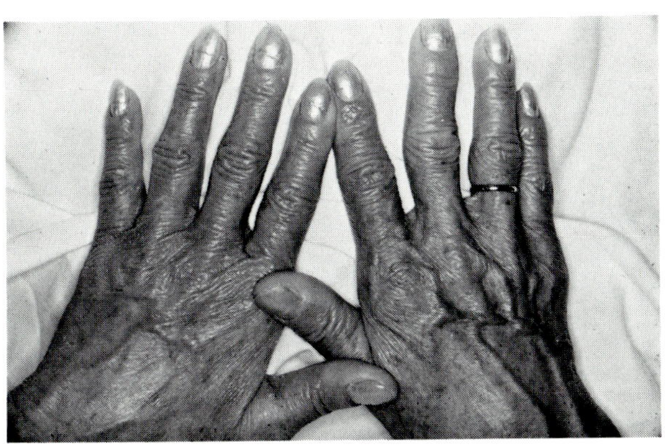

Figure 7-24. *Beau's lines.*

Pigmentations and Cutaneous Tumors

Ephelides or freckles are found primarily on the sun-exposed dorsum of the hand in blondes and redheads. They darken with exposure to the sun, and they tend to decrease with age. Senile lentigo is a sun-induced mottled brown macule which is most often found on the cheeks and the backs of the hands of those over the age of 40. Approximately 90 per cent of persons aged 60 or over have one or more. They rarely transform into a melanoma (Hutchinson's melanotic freckle); however, any rapid change in size or shape or elevation above the surface of the skin warrants an incisional biopsy. The melanoma arising in a Hutchinson's freckle is not as virulent as nodular melanoma and only rarely metastasizes.

Pigmented nevi or moles of the flat or junctional type are present in 2 to 5 per cent of newborns, 40 per cent of 20-year-olds, 10 per cent of 40-year-olds, and 5 per cent of 80-year-olds. Most nevi begin as brown or black flat spots (junction nevus) and gradually become raised (compound or intradermal nevus). They may involute by fibrosing, by accumulating lipid or by forming a white halo around themselves and resorbing. Nevi with junctional activity, that is, the perfectly flat or slightly raised or halo nevi, have a malignant potential of one in a million. There is no evidence that nevi on the palms or nail beds have a greater malignant potential than those at any other site.

Simple nevi are removed only for cosmetic reasons. A history of change in size or shape of a lesion, or the finding of spontaneous disruption of the surface, may constitute justification for simple excision and microscopic examination. When the diagnosis of melanoma is considered, the biopsy specimen should, if possible, be examined by more than one pathologist or dermatopathologist before definitive surgery is undertaken.

Several common clinical entities appear as flat pigmented spots on the hands. Cafe-au-lait spots are best known for their association with neurofibromatosis. In 75 per cent of cases of neurofibromatosis there are six or more cafe-au-lait spots. Larger spots with irregular borders are seen in

Albright's syndrome, which includes precocious puberty in females and polyostotic fibrous dysplasia. Despite their association with these conditions, 10 per cent of the entire normal population has one or more cafe-au-lait spots. Thus, a diagnosis of one of these serious diseases is not warranted on the basis of one pigmented macule.

Melanoma (Chap. 15) (Fig. 7-25) is certainly the most malignant of skin tumors and one of the most feared of all tumors. As already stated, nevi on the palms and nail beds have no greater malignant potential than those anywhere else; however, more than the expected number of melanomas occur on the hands and subungual areas. This is probably because sun exposure increases the incidence of melanoma. Among light-skinned populations in sunny climes, e.g. Texas and Australia, there is a higher incidence of melanoma in the hands and nail beds. Some melanomas arise from skin that was previously normal in appearance, others appear in birthmarks (large, pigmented disfiguring moles), and some arise from a Hutchinson's freckle.

Clinically, melanoma may resemble nearly all of the pigmented lesions we have described plus many non-pigmented ones, since not all melanomas are pigmented. The differential diagnosis includes pigmented nevi, traumatized warts, traumatized papillomas, seborrheic keratoses, subungual hematoma, pigmented basal cell epitheliomas, traumatic tattoos, etc. The physician should be alerted by: (1) a reliable history of *change* of size, shape, elevation or color of any lesion; (2) the rapid de novo appearance of a pigmented lesion; (3) irregularity of pigmentation; (4) irregularity of surface contour; (5) peripheral spread of pigment from a raised lesion; (6) satellite papules or color spots; and (7) ulceration of pigmented lesions.

Granuloma annulare (Fig. 7-26*A*,*B*) is a palisading granuloma (necrobiosis) of the skin which is most often seen on the dorsum of fingers, hands and forearms and predominantly affects children and young adults. The incidence in females is twice that in males. The etiology is unknown and it is often self-limited, although a lesion may take months to recede and is subject to recurrence.

The condition typically manifests itself as single or multiple slowly developing symptomless rings, 1 to 5 cm in size, of closely set firm papules. These are colorless or faintly erythematous. Occasionally, there are associated deeper plaques and, rarely, ulceration. The major histological change occurs in the dermal collagen, which shows areas of necrosis and homogenization. No form of treatment is significantly predictable. Remission may seem to follow the trauma of biopsy or the local injection of steroid or procaine, or even saline.

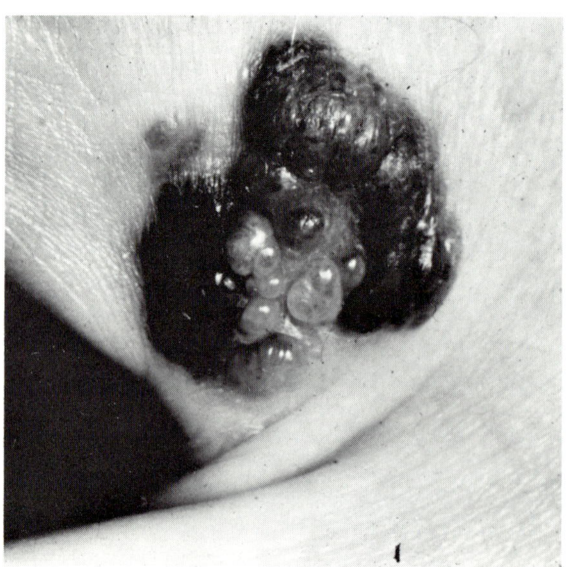

Figure 7-25. *Nodular melanoma.*

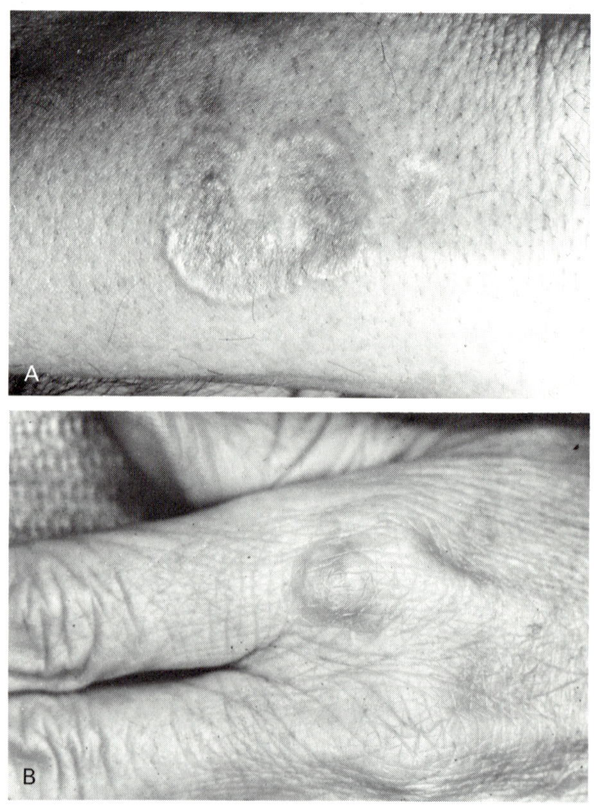

Figure 7-26. *Different manifestations of granuloma annulare.*

Epithelial Precancers, Pseudocancers, and True Cancers of the Hands (Chap. 22)

ACTINIC (SOLAR, SENILE) KERATOSES (FIG. 7-27)

Actinic keratoses are caused by excessive sun exposure of the dorsum of the hand and forearm over many years. The lighter the skin, the more likely it is that actinic keratosis will develop. Keratoses begin as simple persistent hyperkeratotic spots. They proceed to warty growths and, in a small percentage of cases, to frank squamous cell carcinoma. Actinic keratoses are not to be confused with seborrheic keratoses (basal cell papillomas) which often have a pitted surface and are not premalignant.

Early actinic keratoses will respond to topical corticosteroids. Cryotherapy with liquid nitrogen is also effective. Widespread superficial actinic keratosis will clear after the daily use of 5-fluorouracil topically for several weeks. A brisk inflammatory reaction will precede the involution. Actinic keratoses with a firm or tender base should be biopsied for histopathological examination, for without this they are frequently impossible to distinguish from early or invasive squamous cell carcinomas.

If the histopathologist feels there is an actinic keratosis or an early in situ carcinoma, this excisional biopsy is adequate. It is seldom that squamous cell carcinomas of the hands arising from actinically damaged skin are aggressively infiltrating or metastasizing. Thus, radical surgery is not indicated in simple squamous cell carcinoma of actinically damaged hands. There are, however, situations in which squamous cell carcinoma of the back of the hands may have a metastatic potential (Chap. 22, Tumors)—those arising in scars, burns, chronic ulcers, lupus erythematosus (Fig. 7-28*A*,*B*) and poikiloderma. But even here, it must be established that the histopathology is truly squamous cell carcinoma and not pseudocarcinomatous hyperplasia, as may be seen in chronic ulcers (Chap. 15).

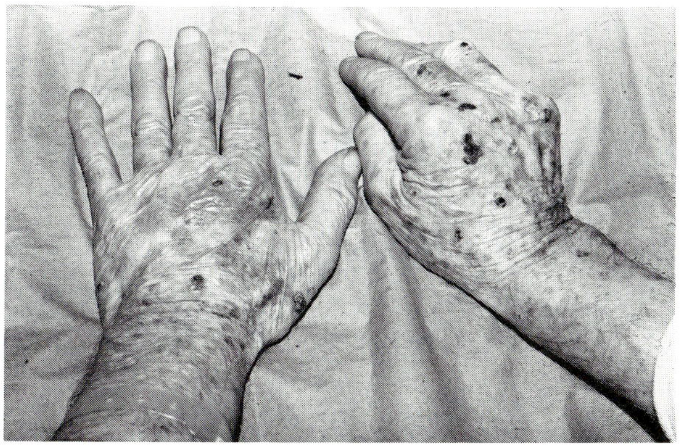

Figure 7-27. *Actinic keratoses.*

BOWEN'S DISEASE (FIG. 7-29A–C)

Bowen's disease, or carcinoma in situ of the skin, may appear as a verrucous plaque of the hands or fingers. Many cases arise spontaneously, but there is a much higher percentage in patients in whom there is a history of arsenical ingestion, either from therapeutic agents such as Fowler's solution or from arsenic-contaminated well water. Many proceed to frank squamous cell carcinoma if not treated. Patients with Bowen's disease have a distinct predilection to skin malignancies, and 25 per cent are said to develop or have internal malignancies. The extent of cutaneous involvement of Bowen's disease can be easily determined by paint-

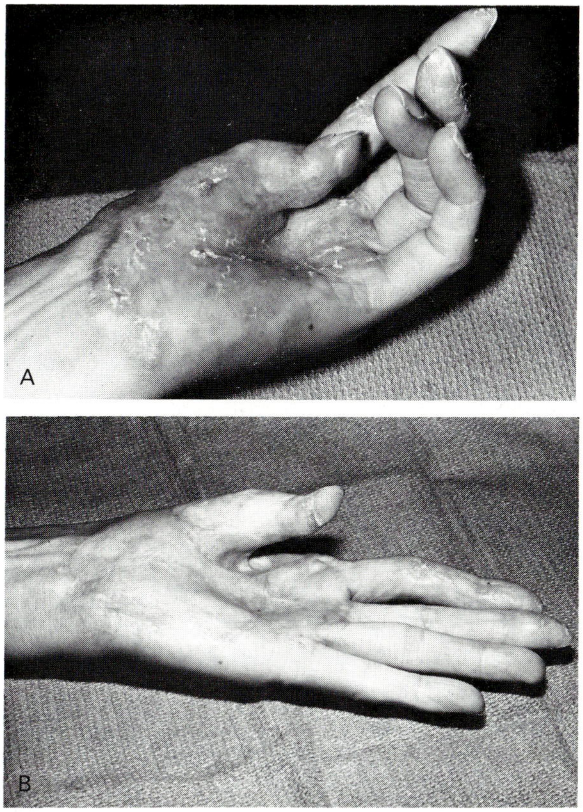

Figure 7-28. *Severe involvement of palmar skin by discoid lupus erythematosus* **(A),** *treated by excision and grafting with split-thickness skin* **(B).**

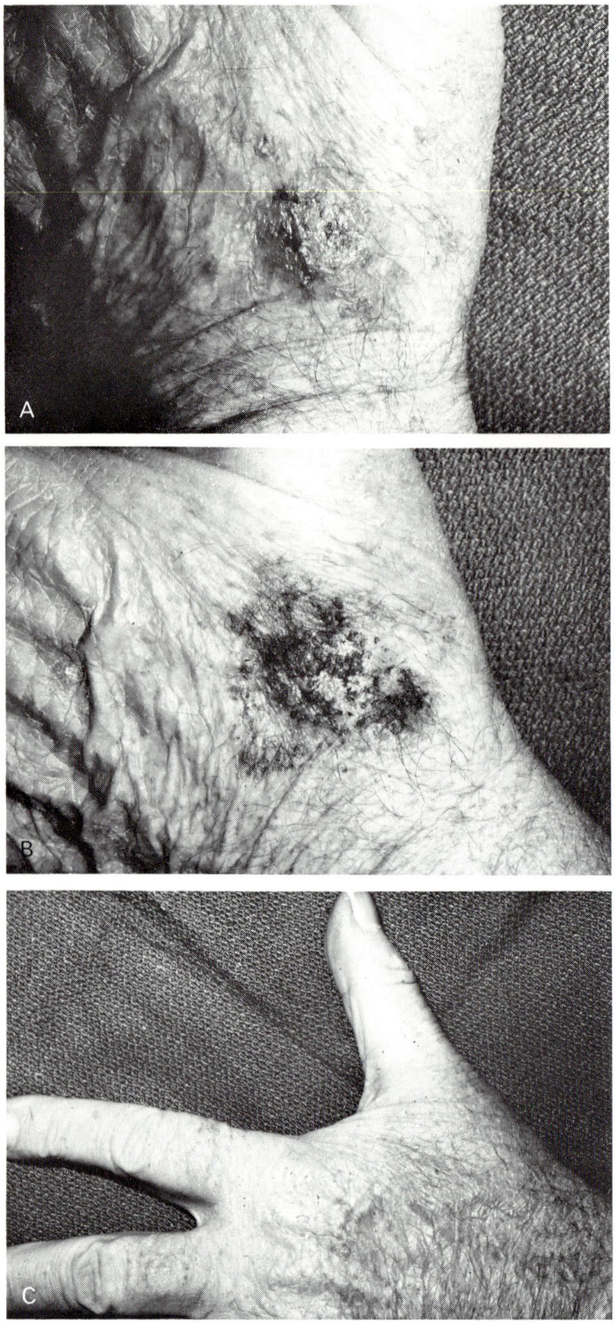

Figure 7-29. **A:** *Bowen's disease.* **B:** *Application of toluidine blue staining.* **C:** *Six months after treatment with topical 5-fluorouracil.*

ing the area with 1 per cent toluidine blue and rinsing it with 1 per cent acetic acid. The blue color remains in the areas of Bowen's disease. Small plaques are easily curetted and desiccated or excised. Larger plaques may require excision and grafting. An alternative therapy is topical 5-fluorouracil or high doses of a superficial x-ray (grenz ray). Patients with Bowen's disease should have regular follow-up checks of the treated site as well as of their entire skin for other lesions, and regular complete physical examinations to detect early internal malignancies.

KERATOACANTHOMA (FIG. 7-30)

Keratoacanthoma is a pseudocancer which both clinically and histologically may resemble squamous cell carcinoma. It occurs most frequently on the dorsum of the hand. Typically, the keratoacanthoma resembles a volcano with a keratin plug in its crater. It arises and grows rapidly to maximum size in about six weeks, remains for about six weeks, and often involutes in another six weeks. The rapid growth, however, nearly always leads to its removal before natural involution.

BASAL CELL CARCINOMA (EPITHELIOMA—BCE)

Basal cell carcinoma is not nearly so common on the hands as on other sun-exposed areas of the head and neck. The reasons for this discrepancy are not clear, inasmuch as basal cell epitheliomas are as definitely related to sun exposure and skin color as are actinic keratoses. The most common clinical appearance of a basal cell epithelioma occurring on the hand is the classical rodent ulcer—a raised ulcer which is partially undermined. Nonulcerated basal cell epitheliomas are typically

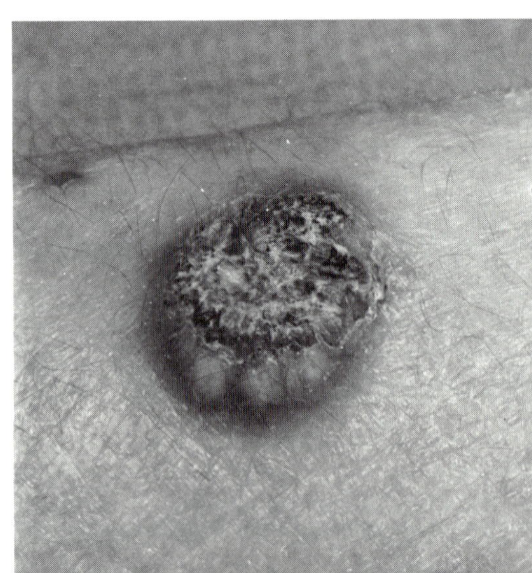

Figure 7-30. *Keratoacanthoma.*

gray-pink with slightly raised borders and small telangiectatic vessels. If there is good reason clinically to suspect a basal cell epithelioma, an excisional biopsy and histopathological evaluation should be done. Basal cell carcinomas, while they are locally invasive, metastasize with extreme rarity. Very large or infiltrating basal cell carcinomas may require excision and grafting of the wound with split-thickness skin.

Table 7-2. *Lotions (may be mixed with ointment bases for prolonged action)*

CALAMINE LOTION (soothing and drying)

Prepared calamine	8
Zinc oxide	8
Glycerin	2
Magma of bentonite	25
Lime water, gs ad	100

Add 1% phenol for antipruritic effect

Uses: Apply t.i.d. or q.i.d. for acute dermatitis
Avoid excessive drying by prolonged use

STARCH LOTION (antipruritic, soothing and drying)

Cornstarch	24
Zinc oxide	24
Glycerin	12
Lime water, gs ad	120

Uses: Apply b.i.d. for acute dermatitis

COAL TAR LOTION (soothing, drying and keratoplastic)

Solution of coal tar	12
Zinc oxide	24
Starch	24
Glycerin	36
Water gs ad	120

Uses: Apply h.s. but not over hairy or infected area
Use for subacute dermatitis

Table 7-3. *Ointments and Creams*

ROSEWATER OINTMENT (cooling and soothing) (cold cream)

Spermaceti	12.5
White wax	12.0
Expressed almond oil	56.0
Sodium borate	0.5
Rose water	5.0
Distilled water	14.0
Rose oil	0.02

ALUMINUM ACETATE OINTMENT (soothing and helpful for receding inflammatory ("1-2-3") process)

Aluminum acetate solution	10.0
Lanolin	20.0
Zinc oxide paste	30.0

STEROID OINTMENT OR CREAM (to be applied as thin film b.i.d. and may be combined with coal tar or antibiotics)

Hydrocortisone	(0.25, 1.5, 1 and 2.5 per cent)

STEROID OINTMENT OR CREAM (for localized eczema or psoriasis and applied h.s. and covered with thin plastic such as Saran Wrap)

Triamcinolone	(0.025 or 0.1 per cent)
Fluocinolone	(0.01 or 0.25 per cent)
Betamethasone valerate	(0.1 per cent)
Fluocinonide	(0.05 per cent)
Desonide	(0.05 per cent)

HALOPROGIN CREAM (1 per cent Halotex)* (for athletes' foot apply b.i.d.)

*Halotex: Westwood Pharmaceuticals, Buffalo, New York

Table 7-4. *Ointment Bases*

ACTIONS: Keep skin moist by trapping moisture
Draw fluid and moisture out of lesions when ointment is hydrophilic
Hold medicinal additives against the skin

CONTRAINDICATIONS:

Acute, oozing inflamed lesions
Hairy skin (except hydrophilic ointment)

White petrolatum	—Inert and retards penetration of contained medication
Hydrophilic petrolatum (3 per cent cholesterol in petrolatum white wax and stearyl alcohol)	—Hydrophilic and favors penetration of contained medication
Hydrous lanolin	—Favors penetration and adheres well to skin. Occasional sensitization
Anhydrous lanolin	—Hydrophilic and favors penetration Occasional sensitization
Zinc oxide (20 per cent ZnO_2 in liquid petrolatum, white petrolatum, lanolin, wax)	—Hydrophilic, adheres well to skin and gives body to ointment

8 Non-specific Inflammatory and Constrictive Conditions

A variety of non-specific inflammatory and constrictive conditions affect the *musculotendinous* and ligamentous tissues of the upper extremity (Table 8-1). Sometimes vague symptoms and an insidious onset make the diagnosis difficult. As a rule, however, the history alone yields the obvious diagnosis. In the differential diagnosis specific etiological factors must always be considered, particularly gout. Rheumatoid disease must also be ruled out, as occasionally must the other collagen disorders (Chap. 24). In the case of tenosynovitis, tuberculosis must be considered.

Table 8-1. *Non-specific Inflammatory States*

DESMITIS
TENDONITIS
Tendonitis without synovitis
Tendonitis with simple uncomplicated synovitis
Tendonitis with villonodular tenosynovitis
MYOSITIS
Myositis crepitans
EPICONDYLITIS
Medial
Lateral (tennis elbow)
BURSITIS
Calcific
Non-calcific

Acute and excessively repetitious strain may give rise to these disorders, but frequently they develop spontaneously. The usual treatment consists of rest and the local injection of triamcinolone. Rest consists of abstinence from stressful activity or if necessary the use of a splint or circumferential cast. However, splinting should never exceed 3 to 4 weeks without reevaluating the patient's tolerance to effort.

The triamcinolone is injected slowly into the painful area with a small needle with the patient recumbent. The injection should never be under pressure or into nerves or vessels. Intraneural injection can be avoided by repeated questioning about distal radiation of pain or paresthesias as the needle is advanced. Intravascular injection is avoided by repeated aspiration. The volume of the injection must be entirely adapted to the amount the tissues will accommodate without distension. Five to 10 mg of triamcinolone per cc of saline is injected weekly for 1 to 4 weeks.

In lieu of local triamcinolone, systemic anti-inflammatory agents may be used until relief is obtained or for 2 to 6 weeks (Table 8-2). Failing a satisfactory response to these conservative measures, a surgical solution to the problem may be considered.

Inflammatory States

Desmitis

This precise but seldom used term is specific for inflammation of a ligament. Usually the ligaments of the wrist and digital joints are involved, most

Table 8-2. *Anti-inflammatory Medications for Non-specific Disorders*

DRUG	DOSE	DURATION
Aspirin	600 mg every 4 hours	3 to 6 weeks
Buffered phenyl-butazone	200 mg t.i.d. with meals for 6 doses, then 100 mg t.i.d. with meals and/or antacids	1 to 2 weeks
Indomethacin	25 to 50 mg b.i.d. or t.i.d.	3 to 6 weeks
Prednisone	2.5 to 5.0 mg t.i.d.	2 to 4 weeks

commonly on the radial and ulnar sides. Desmitis frequently occurs spontaneously but is also seen following trauma or repetitive stress. Underlying hypertrophic osteoarthritis is a common factor in the differential diagnosis of this disorder in the older individual.

Swelling and redness are infrequent. Pain and tenderness may be minimal to severe and are usually well localized. They are elicited by pinpoint direct pressure and by tensing the affected ligament. Roentgenograms are generally not helpful as calcification is rarely seen.

Local steroid injections generally bring prompt relief, but recrudesences are not uncommon. Nocturnal splinting and avoiding of the precipitating stress are obvious adjuncts.

Tendonitis

Isolated tendonitis most commonly involves one of the wrist flexors or extensors; the active process may blend with desmitis in the juxtaposed ligament. Active and passive tension of the tendon accentuates the pain, which is usually pinpoint in its localization. Some redness and swelling, though infrequent, are more likely to be present than with desmitis alone. Tenderness is a common finding, whereas calcific deposits on roentgenography are rare. The process often arises de novo but is seen following stress of an isolated or repetitive nature. The response to local injections of triamcinolone is usually immediate and lasting.

A form of tendonitis is seen along isolated flexor tendons within the digital flexor sheath without concomitant evidence of synovitis. The findings are pain and tenderness of minimal to slight degree with localization in most instances through the region of the metacarpophalangeal joint. This is the same area of involvement as that of the usual "trigger finger" but there is no associated jog in the rhythm as the tendon glides. The treatment with locally injected triamcinolone is the same as that for trigger finger.

TENDONITIS WITH SYNOVITIS

Tendonitis with uncomplicated synovitis is free of gross synovial thickening (the matted synovium seen in villonodular tenosynovitis). Frequently no precipitating factors can be recognized. At other times a history of excessive repetitive stress is correlated with onset. Usually this stress is a high-frequency amplitude of tendon gliding; at other times it is a repetitive percussive activity. The primary mechanism is one of friction between the tendon and its sheath, leading to an effusion. If the stress is not contained, the effusion may become hemorrhagic. Eventual villonodular thickening of the synovium and ischemic rupture of tendons may result, as may acute carpal tunnel syndrome when the flexor sheaths are involved at the wrist level.

The most commonly recognized form of uncomplicated tenosynovitis involves the extensor tendon sheaths. A soft, non-tender diffuse subcutaneous swelling is seen over the base of the hand which is confined to the limits of the synovium not contained under the extensor retinaculum. Occasionally a dumbbell deformity is seen, reflecting the proximal and distal limits of the extensor synovium on either side of the extensor retinaculum. This is differentiated from a ganglion of joint origin by the fact that its contour shifts and margins pucker with active extension. The same form of synovitis undoubtedly occurs along the flexor synovial sheaths but is not recognized because of the tethered skin and generous fatty padding of the palm.

Uncomplicated synovitis responds well to rest, injections of triamcinolone and a change of occupation or of technique in performing an assigned task.

TENDONITIS WITH VILLONODULAR SYNOVITIS

The villonodular synovium becomes so thickened that it is tumorous and palpable. Its bulk may obstruct the excursion of joints. The fingers are fattened by the exuberant hypertrophy of the flexor synovial sheaths. The dorsal and volar aspects of the base of the hand and distal forearm are characteristically bulbous (Fig. 8-1). As a rule tenderness is negligible or absent.

When rapid in onset, this process is a consequence of uncurtailed repetitive stress and is usually highly vascular and hemorrhagic. When insidious in onset, the synovium has less vascularity and is not hemorrhagic. Unlike the uncomplicated synovitis which can be decompressed with aspiration, there is little free synovial fluid and aspiration is usually negative. Rice bodies (hyalinized fibrin) may occur (Fig. 8-2).

Local triamcinolone is ineffective. These patients require synovectomy, which is performed with the same technique as that described for rheumatoid synovectomy (Chap. 24). The condition and its etiology are not related to rheumatoid synovitis. All instances of the insidious form should be cultured for the different forms of mycobacteria.

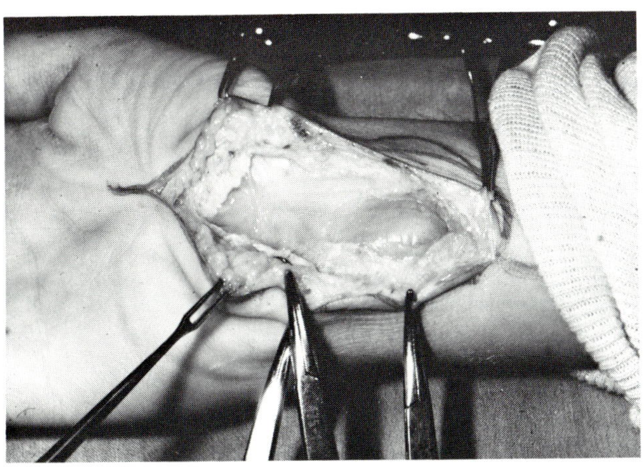

Figure 8-1. *This elderly woman had a carpal tunnel syndrome with both flexor and extensor synovitis. Biopsy at the time of synovectomy confirmed the diagnosis of villonodular tenosynovitis.*

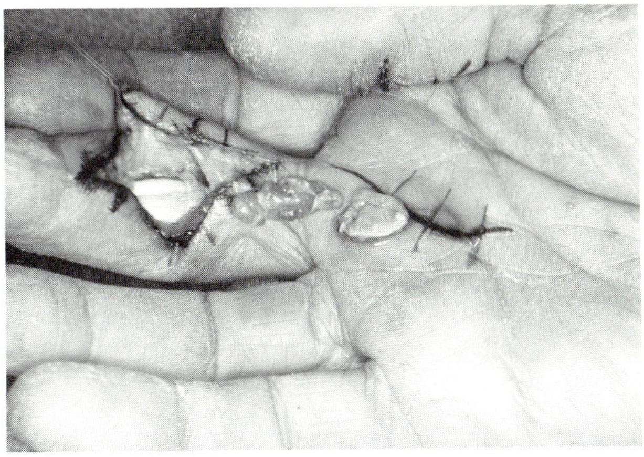

Figure 8-2. *Typical rice bodies are formed from fibrin deposits in synovial spaces affected with chronic inflammatory changes.*

Myositis

Everybody has experienced at one time or another muscle soreness following effort to which he is not conditioned. However, medical aid is sought infrequently unless the problem is overwhelming, as occurs in myositis crepitans.

Myositis crepitans results from stressful repetitive muscle contraction by an unconditioned muscle. The most common muscles involved are the abductor pollicis longus and extensor pollicis brevis. The second most commonly involved muscle groups are the wrist and digital extensors. The typical example of this is the experience of the suburban springtime gardner who develops swelling, local hyperthermia, tenderness, pain and crepitation of the involved musculature on motion after a solid Sunday's hedge clipping. The crepitation, which is palpable, is even more dramatic when heard with a stethoscope. The edematous muscle fractures the interstitial fibrin during contraction, causing the crepitation.

If the acute case responds to a single early injection of triamcinolone, splinting may not be needed. Patients who have been untreated or are chronically symptomatic for several days usually require 1 to 2 weeks of forearm splinting or casting. In either instance the etiological activity must be temporarily curtailed. Intractability is rare.

Lateral Epicondylitis (Tennis Elbow)

This is a non-specific inflammatory condition producing pain in the region of the lateral humeral epicondyle. The locus of maximum tenderness on or near the epicondyle may vary from examination to examination. The affliction may be sufficiently disabling to require the patient to give up certain activities that aggravate it, e.g. tennis. The pain may radiate down the dorsum of the forearm into the hand. Usually it can be reproduced by tensing the extensor musculature against resistance.

No single etiology has been offered to explain this problem. Occasionally it follows a direct blow to the area. At other times there is a history of strain of the extensor musculature. It may also appear spontaneously. Upon operation, there are no objective findings save occasional hypertrophy of the synovium between the radial head and the capitulum.

The suggested causes of this problem are small tears of the extensor muscle origin, pain arising from the annular ligament from degenerative changes and pinching of the hypertrophied synovium in the radiohumeral joint.[1]

The process usually responds promptly to injection of triamcinolone. It may subside spontaneously or become indolent. No form of treatment is totally predictable. Occasionally the condition is impossible to cure and the patient must learn to tolerate it.

In the acute phase the elbow, forearm and wrist should be kept at rest in a sling or splint while analgesics and anti-inflammatory agents are administered. When the disabling symptoms continue in spite of the foregoing treatment, radiation may be given. This is administered as superficial therapy (low voltage, 125 kvp) delivering 100 rads twice a week for a total of 600 rads through a small 8- to 10-cm field. The patient should be advised of the risks of radiation for benign conditions and only in unique situations should such therapy be recommended.

Failing any response to the above treatments, the only alternative is surgical. This should be done only upon the patient's demand with his willingness to accept the risk that results are uncertain and with his knowledge of the potential for aggravating his symptoms.

The usual operation consists of detachment of the extensor muscle origin from the lateral epicondyle and the partial resection of the annular ligament. Hypertrophic synovium if present is also resected. This is done under general anesthesia with an upper-arm tourniquet through a longitudinal incision over the lateral epicondyle. The radiohumeral joint is defined by pronation and supination of the forearm. Bosworth[1] recommends that the anterolateral portion of the orbicular or annular ligament be resected, freeing the attachment of the radial collateral ligament to it (Fig. 8-3). The aponeurotic origin of the extensor muscles is not resutured. Postoperatively the extremity is placed in a well-padded long arm cast with the elbow flexed at 90° and the forearm in neutral. Motion is started in 2 to 3 weeks. According to Tupper,[5] about 80 per cent of patients with this problem will respond to conservative non-operative treatment, whereas only half of patients who eventually have surgical treatment experience relief.

Medial epicondylitis is no different from its counterpart on the lateral aspect of the elbow. Fortunately it is less common and less recalcitrant to non-operative treatment. In addition to direct

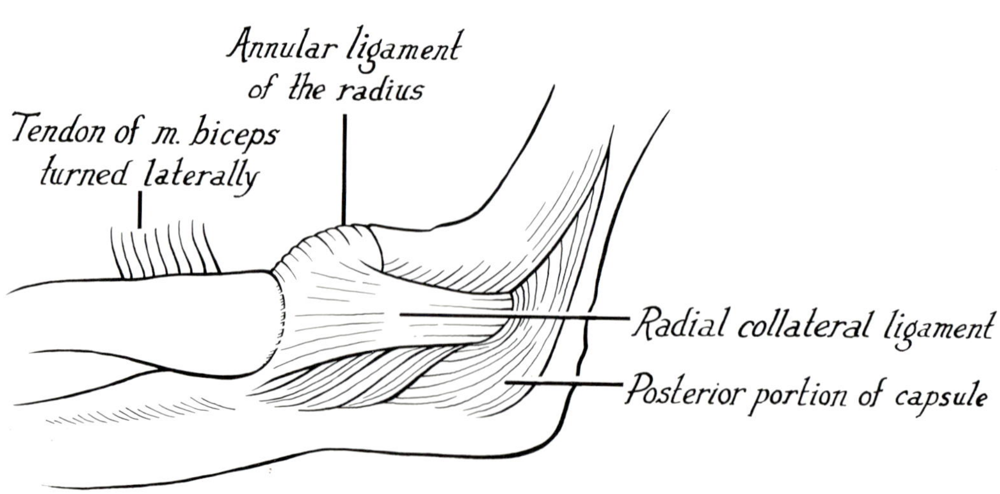

Figure 8-3. *Lateral aspect of the elbow illustrates the orbicular (annular) ligament. The attachment of the collateral ligament to the orbicular ligament may need to be resected.*

tenderness, pain can be elicited by forceful pronation of the thumb. Rest and the local instillation of triamcinolone usually suffice as treatment.

Bursitis

Minor trauma to muscles, tendons or joint capsules can result in calcium deposits which are evident on roentgenograms. At times no etiology for either calcific or non-specific bursitis can be found. Many patients manifest pericapsular calcifications without any related symptomatology, especially when the supraspinatus tendon at the shoulder is involved. In contrast, such deposits within the hand may be acutely uncomfortable. Certain of the collagen disorders (scleroderma) seem to have a propensity for the deposition of calcium within the hands and elsewhere in the subcutaneous tissues.

Basically the treatment is one of surgical excision of the offending calcium deposit when it is present in the hand and is producing symptoms.[3] The non-specific bursitis from stress (more often desmitis) may respond to rest, local heat, local steroids and/or systemic anti-inflammatory agents.

Constrictive States

The constrictive states exist as a consequence of the disproportion in the size of the canal and the volume of nerves or tendons that occupy the canal (Table 8-3). The pressure upon nerves causes paresis and paralysis. Tendons are trapped and their glide impaired. Severe physical constriction alters tendons and nerves which are narrowed at the point of constriction and bulbous proximal or distal thereto.

The etiologies for this are developmental, post-traumatic edema and cicatrix, degenerative thickening, use hypertrophy and rheumatoid synovitis. In all instances, the fluid content of the fibrous ring and the tendons and nerves within it plays a major role. Accordingly, mechanical and medical measures to control waterlogging are effective in many patients.

Table 8-3. *Constrictive States*

STENOSING TENOSYNOVITIS
Trigger finger
De Quervain's
Extensor pollicis longus
NEURAL ENTRAPMENT
Median nerve
Carpal tunnel
Pronator tunnel
Superficialis muscle (anterior interosseous nerve)
Ulnar nerve
Olecranon groove
Flexor carpi ulnaris (cubital tunnel)
Ulnar tunnel at wrist (Guyon's canal)
Dorsal interosseous nerve
Arcade of Frohse (supinator)

Stenosing Tenosynovitis

This state can be invoked upon any tendon passing through any pulley system. Most commonly it involves the flexor tendons at the level of the pulley over the metacarpophalangeal joint, the abductor longus and extensor brevis over the radial styloid and the extensor pollicis longus at Lister's tubercle. The problem is mechanical and parallels that of pulling a knotted thread through the eye of a needle.

Developmentally the pulley appears too snug for the tendon. This is most frequently seen as a locked thumb in the newborn and often mistaken for a defect in extension or joint function. The excessive size of the sesamoid bones contained in the sides of the pulley undoubtedly plays a part in this instance.

The post-traumatic condition is a function of edema and possibly cicatrix of the pulley or localized swelling and cicatrix (e.g. callus formation) within the tendon itself, which can result from blunt or open trauma. It can also result from highly repetitive motions.

Most of these problems are seen in women after middle life, occurring spontaneously with the onset of stiffness in other joints of the body. The symptoms are most common upon first arising and after excessively vigorous resistive effort. These periods correspond to moments of maximal tissue edema. The condition may be bilateral but shows no predilection for the dominant hand. Clinically, however, the pulleys appear thicker and tougher than they do at a younger age. Both tendons and their pulleys hypertrophy in response to strain, leading to an inevitable encroachment of the two. This obstruction may become symptomatic. In the case of the rheumatoid disease there may be specific involvement of either or both the pulley or the tendon with a rheumatoid nodule within its substance. An inescapable trigger phenomenon follows.

The average adult trigger finger is manifested as a painful blocking of flexion and extension of the involved digit. The patient withholds movement because of the fear of pain and usually believes the snapping to be intrinsic to the joint. At times he complains exclusively about the proximal interphalangeal joint, which is the site of referred pain from the proximal flexor pulley (Fig. 8-4). This may occur in those few cases in which triggering is not demonstrable by any maneuver. Hence, this entity must be suspected in all cases of proximal interphalangeal joint pain, particularly when clinical examination of the joint fails to demonstrate an intrinsic source for the pain. The examination should then focus on the proximal flexor pulley, which is usually discretely tender.

In most instances active closing of the fist reproduces the locking. At times the only way to reproduce the trigger in the finger is to have the maximum superficialis muscle contraction precede the profundus muscle contraction (Fig. 8-5). This advances the bulge in the superficialis tendon so that it will be impinged upon by the bulge in the profundus within the proximal pulley, causing locking on attempted extension.

When the swelling of the tendon precludes any passage beneath the pulley, the position of the swelling in relation to the pulley governs the attitude of the digit. If it lies proximal to the pulley, the digit will be flexed and cannot be extended. If the swelling is distal to the pulley, the digit can be passively but not actively flexed.

De Quervain's stenosing tenosynovitis involves the abductor pollicis longus and extensor pollicis brevis in the first dorsal wrist compartment. It is infrequently associated with a trigger phenomenon. The patient's complaint is of pain over the radial aspect of the wrist with radiation proximally and distally. There is localized tenderness over the radial styloid where the pulley may appear and feel thickened. The pathognomonic tests produce pain by tensing the involved tendons actively (by thumb abduction-extension) or passively (by clutching the thumb in the palm and deviating the wrist ulnarward—Finkelstein's test) (Fig. 8-6).

Stenosing tenosynovitis of the extensor pollicis longus at Lister's tubercle is an infrequent problem. The jog in excursion of the tendon may be referred along the thumb so that it is mistaken for a joint abnormality. Tenderness is localized to Lister's tubercle where rupture may occur more

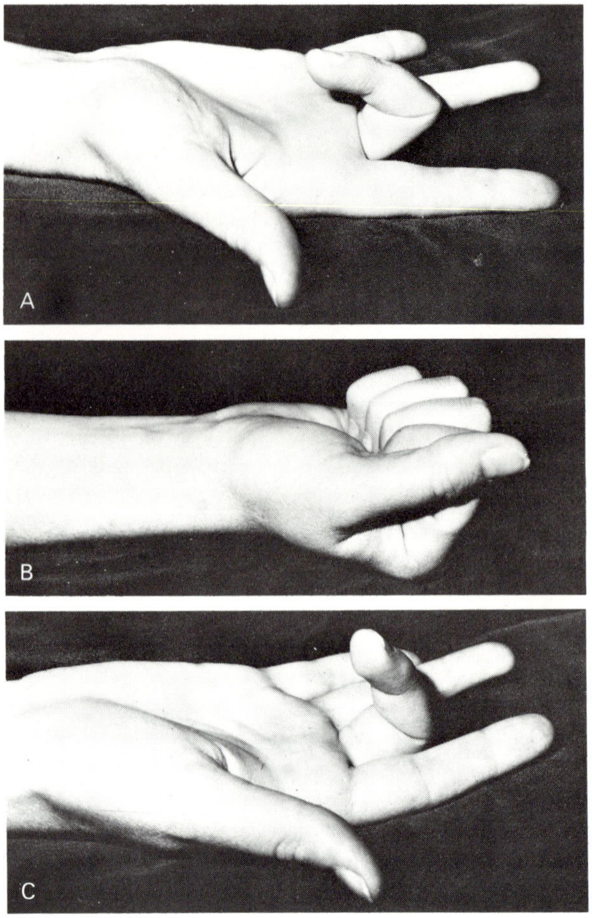

Figure 8-5A: *In demonstrating triggering, it is sometimes necessary to flex the superficialis tendon first.* **B:** *The profundus tendons are then completely flexed.* **C:** *An attempt at extension following the above produces triggering or locking in flexion.*

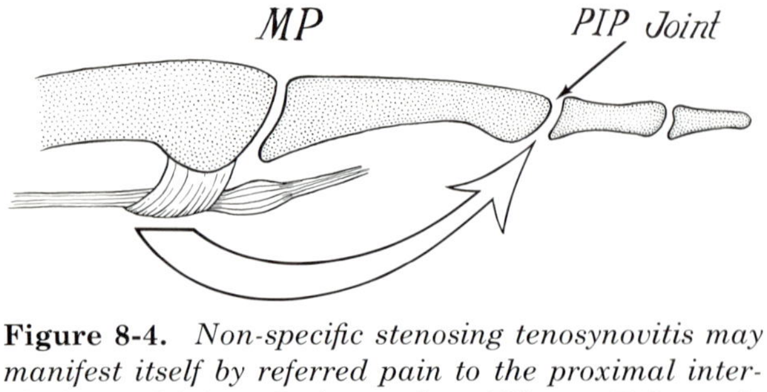

Figure 8-4. *Non-specific stenosing tenosynovitis may manifest itself by referred pain to the proximal interphalangeal joint. (Redrawn from Kilgore, E.S. et al.: The painful hand. In:* Symposium on the Hand *(Cramer, L. and Chase, R. Eds.). C.V. Mosby, St. Louis, 1971.)*

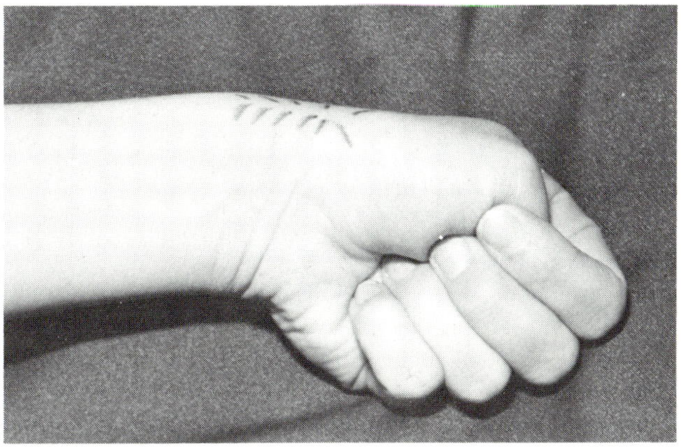

Figure 8-6. *Finkelstein's test produces exquisite pain over the abductor pollicis longus tendon in its dorsal compartment as the wrist is deviated ulnarward while the thumb is clasped.*

readily than in the other stenotic states described above, hence the need for early surgery.

The decision to treat these problems by injection rather than by surgery rests on the degree of locking and the tendon involved. All acute cases of trigger finger and De Quervain's tenosynovitis and all chronic mild cases where symptoms and signs are slight should be treated with local triamcinolone. Up to four injections (5 to 10 mg each) should be given at weekly intervals, and if no lasting relief is obtained surgery is undertaken.

The injections must spare the digital nerves in the palm and the branches of the radial nerve at the wrist. The patient should be supine and the injection given with a 26- or 28-gauge needle. It is important to enter the skin and flexor sheath in the midline of the latter to avoid the nerves. As long as the tip of the needle lies within the pulley or tendon, it is impossible to inject. Therefore advancing or withdrawing the needle with simultaneous pressure on the syringe plunger will produce a sudden soft impulse along the distal extension of the injected sheath. This impulse can be detected by the soft touch of the examiner's other fingers on the more distal portion of the sheath. There may be almost complete relief of the patient's pain even though the trigger phenomenon is still present. The patient should be warned of the probable ensuing anesthesia, which may last 1 to 2 hours. He should also be warned of a potential "flare" of pain which sometimes occurs when the lidocaine wears off. This may require analgesics for relief. Fortunately such a flare usually has a favorable prognosis in terms of the subsequent resolution of the patient's misery.

OPERATIVE TREATMENT

Trigger Finger. With few exceptions this is done as an outpatient operative procedure, but only with ideal surgical facilities. It is done with magnification (2-power loupe) under local anesthesia so that the cooperation of the patient can be enlisted to test the adequacy of the release. Tourniquet ischemia is indispensable to avoid the complications of iatrogenic neuromas and tendon injuries. The preferred incision for a single finger is longitudinally in the fat pad of the distal palm in the midline of the involved metacarpal. This does not cross flexion creases. If two adjacent fingers are involved, a transverse incision parallel to the distal palmar crease is preferred. The approach to the thumb is through an incision paralleling the proximal flexion crease; this is necessary to avoid a hypertrophic scar in the thenar area. In this location the surgeon must be extremely careful to avoid cutting the digital nerves which lie close to the skin near the midline.

The fat and neurovascular structures are retracted with lid or small right-angle retractors. A small nick is made transversely or longitudinally at the proximal lip of the pulley. The pulley is then elevated with a fine hook. Fine blunt-nosed scissors are used to cut the pulley longitudinally without traumatizing the tendon. The adequacy of the tenovaginotomy is tested by passing a probe into the residual sheath proximally and distally and by having the patient actively flex and extend while palpating for a remnant of the trigger phenomenon. The surgeon should be guided by his discretion regarding the need for biopsy of the pulley and sheath.

An alternative method is to lengthen rather than completely divide the pulley. This is done by notching the pulley on opposite sides so that the depth of each notch exceeds half the width of the pulley. Thereby no pulley fiber is left uninterrupted. The pulley is then stretched by the insertion of a mosquito hemostat and its opening expanded to allow free passage of the tendons. This technique is akin to that used to lengthen shortened musculotendinous units by staggered tenotomies.

A padded dressing is applied for 3 to 7 days. The fingers are free for motion at all times. The minimal duration of disability for normal use of the hand is 10 to 14 days.

De Quervain's Tenosynovitis. The greatest hazard of surgery in this area is an iatrogenic neuroma of the sensory branch of the radial nerve, which in an individual with a low pain threshold can be crippling (Fig. 8-7). Therefore the most meticulous attention must be directed at guarding the branches of this nerve during dissection and retraction. The incision may be longitudinal, transverse or oblique. The transverse incision favors a hairline scar while the longitudinal favors the protection of the nerve, but tends to become hypertrophic.

As with the trigger finger, tourniquet ischemia is an indispensable aid to the procedure, which may be done under local anesthesia. The nerve is avoided during dissection by elevating the skin edges with fine hooks and separating the subcutaneous tissues along the axis of the nerve with careful spreading down to the tendon sheath. The soft tissues are then gently retracted (Fig. 8-8). The rest of the procedure follows the technique used for trigger finger. The surgeon may find multiple tendons (e.g. 4 to 6) within the sheath. These are not anomalous. One of them is the extensor pollicis brevis, which may lie in a separate canal and must also be freed. The others belong to the abductor pollicis longus. If the operation is done under local anesthesia, its adequacy can be tested in the fashion described for trigger finger.

In the event of demonstrable tendon luxation after this release, the pulley may be primarily or secondarily reconstructed using a distally based tendon flap from the adjacent extensor carpi radialis longus.

A padded forearm cast is used for immobilization for 7 to 10 days postoperatively. The fingers are left free for motion from the beginning. The minimal recovery time for normal use of the hand is 2 to 3 weeks.

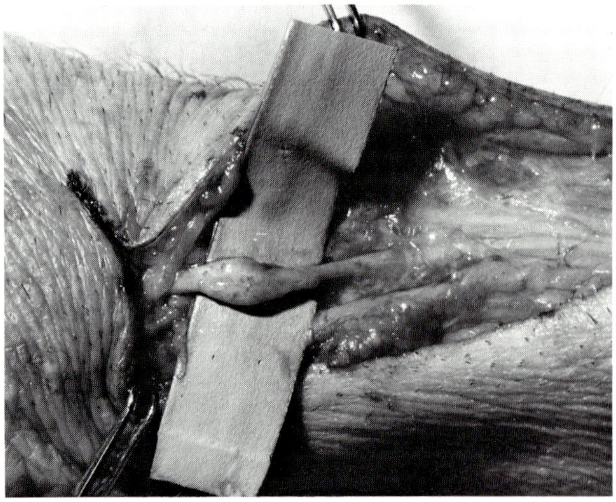

Figure 8-7. *Painful neuroma of the radial nerve developed after release of a De Quervain's tenosynovitis.*

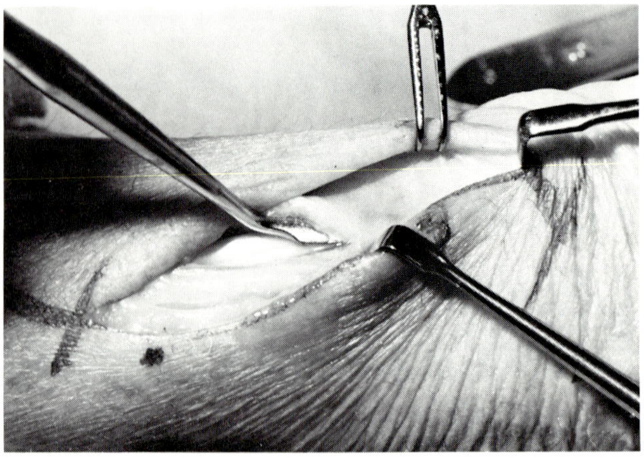

Figure 8-8. *The elevator lies beneath the thickened pulley, protecting the underlying tendons as the tunnel is released. Extreme care must be taken during this procedure to avoid injury to the dorsal sensory branches of the radial nerve.*

Extensor Pollicis Longus Tenosynovitis. The incision preferred is a longitudinal or serpentine incision over the dorsum of the wrist near the midline. This is extended to the extensor retinaculum by the technique described for De Quervain's tenosynovitis. The sheath of the tendon is opened by an incision along its ulnar limit and the extensor pollicis longus is allowed to luxate. The tendon canal can then be obliterated using a flap of the extensor retinaculum. The wrist is splinted for 8 to 10 days with the thumb free for motion.

Neural Entrapment

All of the sites of nerve entrapment, their causes, treatment and prognoses are discussed in Chapter 15.

Secretan's Disease[2,4]

Secretan termed the very firm dorsal induration which seemed to follow minor trauma to the hand as "hard edema." Characteristically the patient gives a history of a relatively minor contusing injury to the dorsum of the hand. Ecchymosis may or may not have occurred, but over the ensuing week or two a gradual increase in the amount and firmness of the dorsal subcutaneous swelling occurs. The patient enters a protracted course of dorsal swelling, limitation of flexion and vague aching discomfort in the hand. Usually little local warmth or erythema occurs. Many patients experience secondary gain from this disability and, regardless of the mode of non-operative treatment (analgesics, physiotherapy, anti-inflammatory drugs), the induration usually resolves over 4 to 8 months.

Exploration of the induration usually reveals a dense peritendinous fibrosis with no evidence of infection. Often when drainage of a suspected abscess or surgical exploration is carried out healing may be protracted (Fig. 8-9).

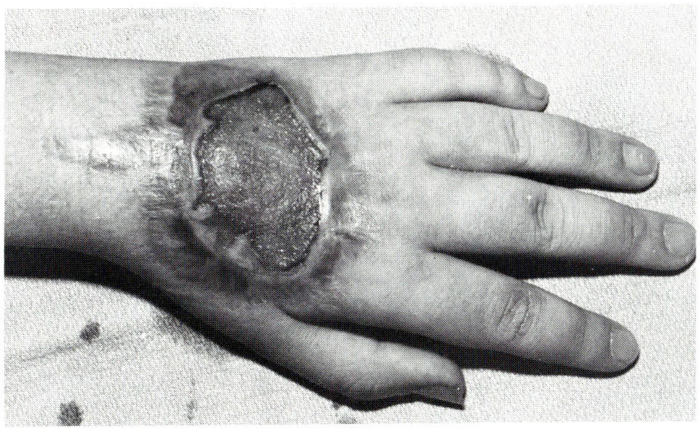

Figure 8-9. *This 22-year-old right-handed girl had had four previous procedures for Secretan's disease, including skin grafting. She was suspected of inducing repeated injury to the dorsum of her left hand for secondary gain.*

References

1. Bosworth, D.M.: The role of the articular ligament in tennis elbow. J. Bone Joint Surg., 37A:527, 1955.
2. Boyes, J.H.: *Bunnell's Surgery of the Hand,* 4th ed. J.B. Lippincott, Philadelphia, 1964.
3. Phalen, G.S.: Calcification adjacent to the pisiform bone. J. Bone Joint Surg., 34A:579, 1952.
4. Secretan, H.: Hard edema and traumatic hyperplasia of the dorsum of the metacarpus. Rev. Med. Suisse Romande, 21:409, 1901.
5. Tupper, J.W.: Experiences with epicondylitis. In: *Symposium on the Hand* (Cramer, L.M. and Chase, R.A., Eds.). C.V. Mosby, St. Louis, 1971.

9 Wounds, Foreign Bodies and Iatrogenic Injuries

Wounds

Rank and Wakefield[1] have standardized the categorization of hand wounds by dividing them into tidy and untidy injuries. Although the so-called golden period has been extended by virtue of today's more acute appreciation and management of the hand wound, it is the wound itself rather than the surgeon's skill that dictates the course of therapy. However, a tidy wound may be converted by inappropriate initial treatment into an untidy one, and under proper circumstances an untidy wound can be made tidy.

Basically a tidy wound has minimal contamination and the injured tissues are not contused or mangled. An untidy wound may result from the nature and degree of contamination or from considerable local tissue injury with the potential for ischemia.

A tidy wound which is carefully cleansed and irrigated with a physiological salt solution need not be closed immediately. If necessary the closure may be delayed 24 to 48 hours provided the patient receives systemic antibiotics and the wound is protected and the extremity splinted.

On the other hand, the untidy wound must be debrided and cleansed as soon as possible, since the nature of this wound makes its susceptibility to infection high. Undue delay risks the establishment of an infection which may extend beyond the originally injured area to affect the whole hand. Delayed closure may be indicated in treatment of an untidy wound.

The general principles of wound management include:

1. Assessment and evaluation
   - An accurate history
2. Cleansing
   - The wound with physiological saline solutions and the surrounding skin with an antibacterial (povidone-iodine)
3. Debridement*
   - Removal of foreign and potentially non-viable material
4. Planning the closure
   - Delay
   - Primary suture
   - Grafting—free graft or pedicle
5. Anticipating rehabilitation

INCISED WOUND

The clean knife or glass cut usually needs little trimming and toilet. However, certain circumstances such as the risk of contamination by virulent organisms (streptococci, Erysipelothrix rhusiopathiae, etc.) may warrant wound cleansing and delayed closure. This type of contamination occurs most frequently in the meat and fish-handling industries. Depending upon the circumstances the deeper structures may not be repaired but treated secondarily (Fig. 9-1).

AVULSED WOUNDS

Wounds in which tissue is torn away may suffer a sufficient loss of substance that grafting is needed for closure. The amount of contamination and the

*Originally from the French root meaning to unbridle, hence decompress or release; it now commonly refers to wound toilet.

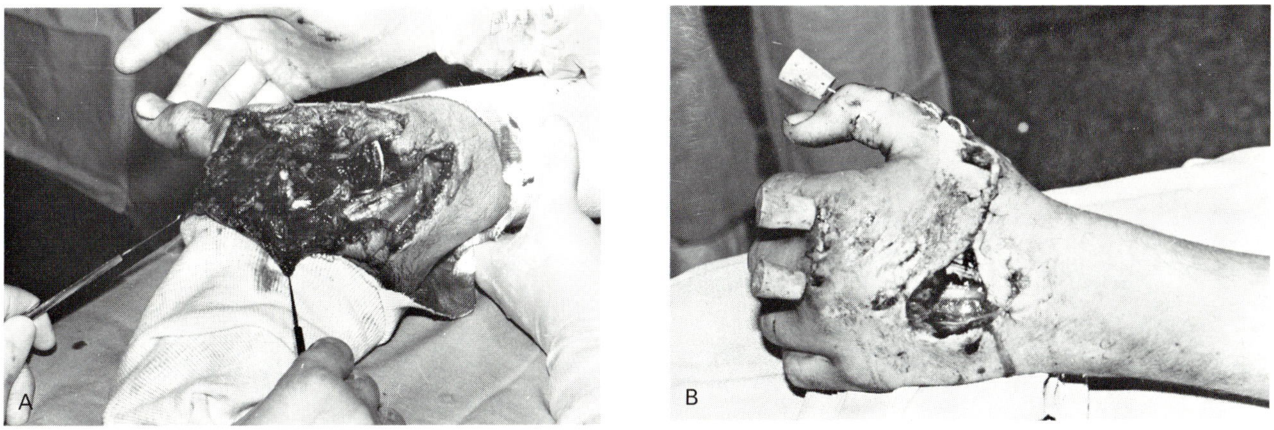

Figure 9-1. *A 17-year-old boy sustained an avulsion injury and multiple metacarpal fractures in a motorboating accident. Split-thickness skin grafts were applied to the open wounds 48 hours after initial treatment.*

underlying injuries dictate whether or not the closure will be primary or secondary.

Small avulsions of skin and subcutaneous tissue are treated by free grafting with split-thickness skin grafts. Larger areas may also be grafted, but may require the transfer of pedicle tissue if joints, tendons or nerves are uncovered. The decision to use a pedicle, either local or distant, should be based upon essential need rather than technical feasibility. A free graft can often be replaced or revised by the use of a pedicle flap whereas revision and replacement of an unsatisfactory pedicle flap might prove more difficult (Figs. 9-2, 9-3).

BLAST WOUNDS

When the hand has been forcefully penetrated by a foreign object, the extent of the injuries is difficult to assess. Early closure of such wounds may seal in necrotic bone, muscle and foreign matter. The initial debridement must be adequate, but precise. Nerves bridging gaps may be only contused (neurapraxia) rather than internally disrupted (axonotmesis) and thus capable of recovery. Their wanton resection would only diminish the function of the mangled hand further. A second look at 36 to 72 hours after injury can be taken and, after final debriding, wound closure concluded.

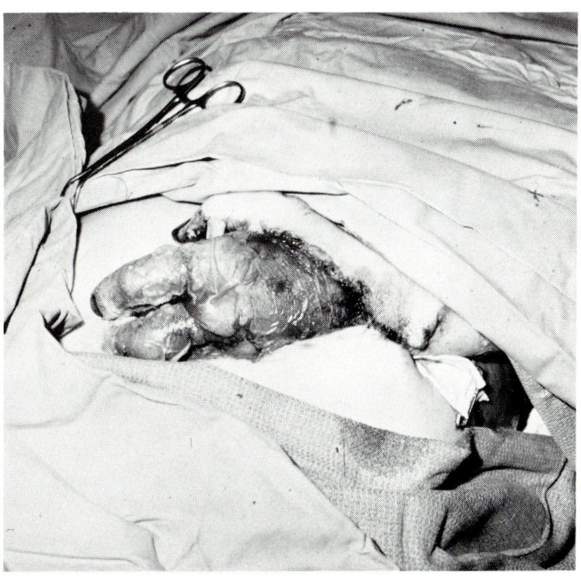

Figure 9-2. *This 35-year-old lithograph pressman had a severe crushing injury to his minor hand. An immediate abdominal pedicle flap was placed. Further necrosis of the injured tissues resulted in the need for digital amputation and revision of the initial treatment plan.*

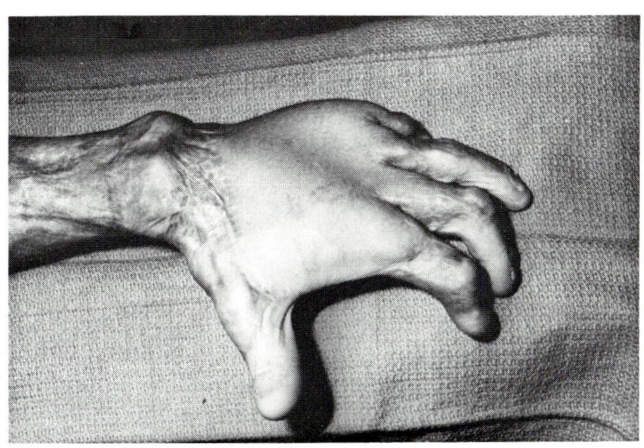

Figure 9-3. *The initial unstable grafts on the dorsum of this boy's hand were replaced by an abdominal pedicle flap for better padding and eventual reconstruction of his extensor tendons some months after his burn injury.*

INJECTION INJURIES

The inoculation of the hand by a highly irritating chemical substance of varying temperature under pressure can occur in many industries. Neglect leads to disaster, with extensive loss of tissue and infection.

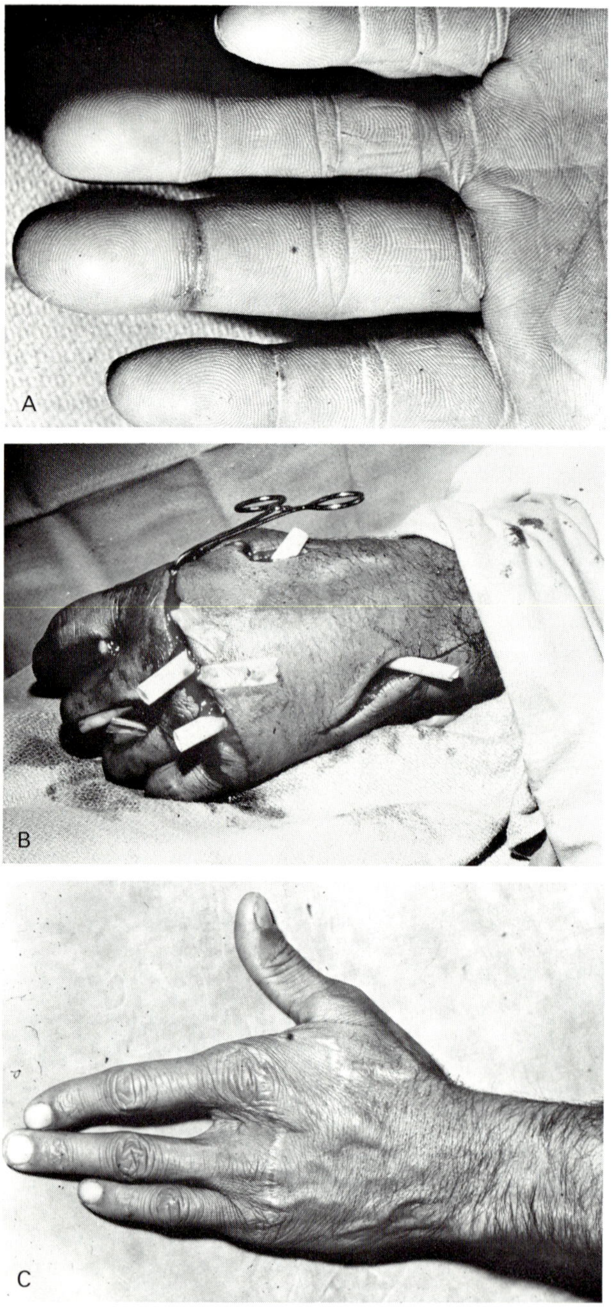

Figure 9-4. *This man experienced an injection of paint thinner at the distal interphalangeal joint of the long finger* **(A).** *Extensive decompression and drainage were performed* **(B).** *Early amputation of the irreversibly ischemic long finger was necessary* **(C).**

The digits, hand and forearm must be opened extensively without delay (Chap. 16). Potentially the most severe of the untidy injuries, these accidents to the hand often result in amputation and frequently in permanent stiffness with dysesthesias and paresthesias (Fig. 9-4).

Certain drugs if accidentally given intra-arterially or others that escape extravascularly will produce severe loss of tissue. All potentially toxic medications designed for intravenous use should be given through an established intravenous infusion rather than with a needle and syringe.

CRUSHING INJURIES

Always the twin specters of congestion and ischemia lurk in the crushed extremity. The surface wound may be deceptively misguiding with respect to the potential severity of the underlying injury. Adequate venous and arterial circulation must be maintained in crushing injuries. Usually wound closure is delayed or modified to accommodate the circulatory needs of the extremity (Fig. 9-5).

Foreign Bodies

The most common foreign bodies entering the hand are usually slivers of glass, metal or wood. Many of these are inert and may not produce any reaction or symptoms. At times their location,

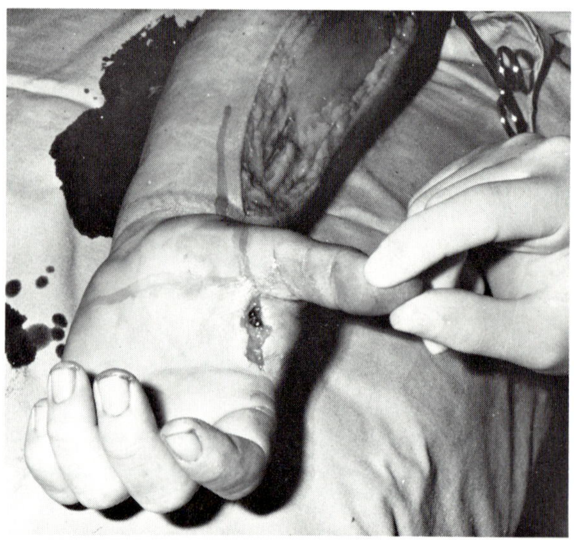

Figure 9-5. *An extensive fasciotomy was needed to decompress this man's forearm following a severe crushing injury.*

rather than their composition, leads to the patient's awareness of their existence.

Roentgenographic examination may be helpful in locating those foreign bodies that are radiopaque, but not always useful in finding the others.

GLASS

Glass foreign bodies may be radiopaque or radiolucent, depending upon the presence of lead in them. If they are tiny they do not require removal. The larger ones tend to migrate and become symptomatic as a fibrous reaction envelops them.

Most glass fragments enter the hand during a fall upon the outstretched palm. There may be no injury except for the cutaneous laceration. Often there is considerable local hemorrhage, a factor which obscures the foreign body and makes identification of important structures difficult. Many surgeons like to splint the injured hand and wait several days before exploring it for glass or other relatively inert materials. Obviously an expanding hematoma necessitates immediate surgery. Likewise a large glass fragment among tendons and nerves or within muscle should be removed before any motion is allowed.

At times the smaller fragments will become encapsulated and gradually delivered to the surface (Fig. 9-6). When this occurs it is much easier to remove the fragment and its capsule than it would have been to find it at the time the initial injury occurred. Patience can be rewarded.

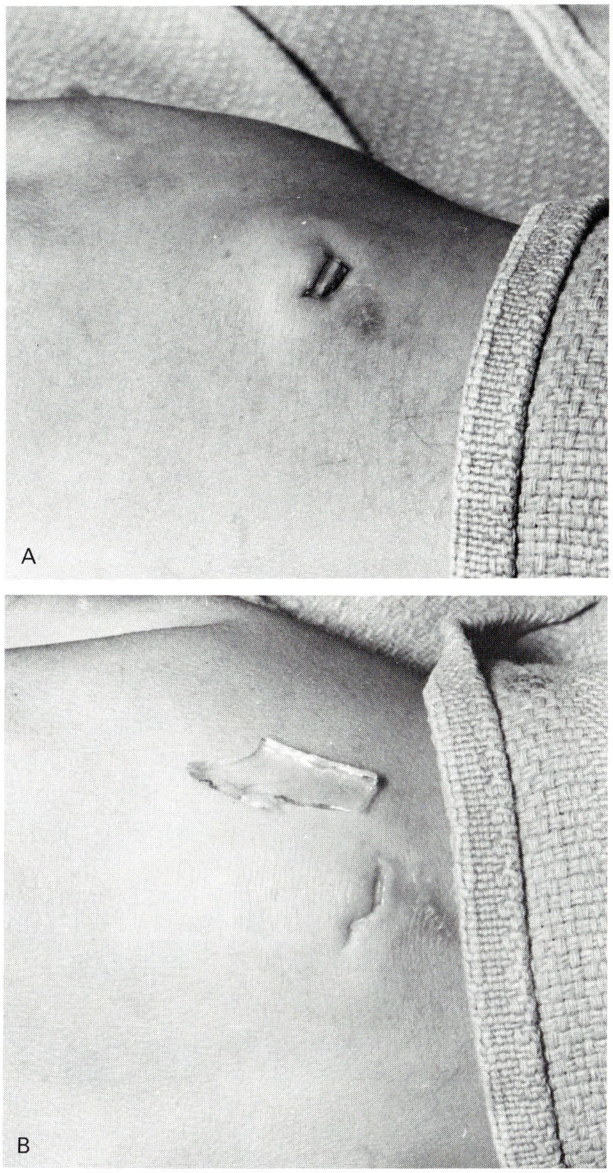

Figure 9-6. *Six months previously this adolescent girl had injured her hand in a fall through a glass door. The laceration of the dorsum of the hand had been sutured primarily without inspection in her physician's office. Months later this glass sliver spontaneously extruded.*

METALLIC FOREIGN BODIES

Aside from the shrapnel effect of blast injuries most metallic foreign bodies that become embedded within the hand are slivers of metal and may remain totally inert and asymptomatic (Fig. 9-7). It is especially important to realize that many metallic foreign bodies may remain within the hand without any cause for alarm.

Asymptomatic metallic foreign bodies require no action by the surgeon. Those which do cause discomfort should be allowed to develop a surrounding capsule which in a bloodless field can be readily identified and removed.

WOODEN FOREIGN BODIES

The carpenter and the weekend repair man are most prone to acquire wooden splinters within the hand. Probably more than any other worker, the carpenter not only has foreign bodies driven into his hand but also acquires inclusion cysts from the deeper implantation of dermal and epidermal elements.

Most wooden foreign bodies are radiolucent and therefore are difficult to localize by roentgenography. Fortunately most are inert, except for those that are stained with toxic dyes (aniline), saturated with creosote or have a high concentration of nat-

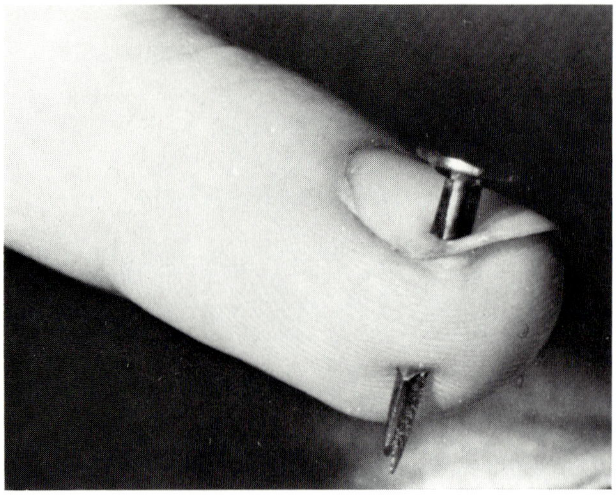

Figure 9-7. *This young woman inadvertently drove an upholstery tack through the tip of her index finger. This type of injury often leads to the development of an inclusion cyst and at times infection with oral bacteria, as when the upholsterer holds tacks in his mouth prior to use.*

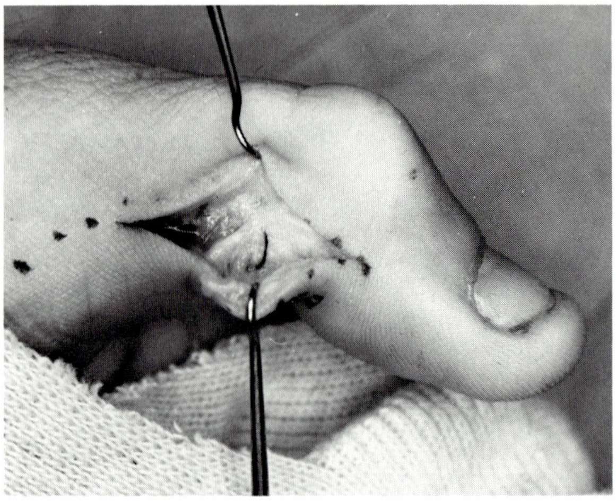

Figure 9-8. *Nylon ligature neatly surrounds neurovascular bundle. This was placed blindly by the patient's physician in an attempt to control hemorrhage from a small laceration. Dysesthesias and parathesias were relieved by its removal.*

Table 9-1. *Iatrogenic Injuries of the Hand*

COMMISSION:

Too-tight constricting dressings or casts
Intra-arterial injection of vasospastic substances
Extravascular injection of tissue with toxic substances
Suture of palmaris longus to median nerve
"Intricate" surgery without tourniquet ischemia
Blind suture ligation of ulnar artery and ulnar nerve in a bloody field
Improperly designed incisions
Improper drainage of infected spaces
Indwelling arterial lines
Anatomical fracture reduction at the expense of other tissues
Preservation of non-viable tissues
Inappropriate use of complicated flaps for wound coverage
Surgery beyond the skill and training of the physician
Poorly chosen free graft sites
Thoracic outlet surgery for carpal tunnel syndrome and vice versa
Immobilization in a compromising attitude
Probing exploration in the emergency room
Irrigation of wounds with tissue toxic antiseptics

OMISSION:

Failure to operate in a bloodless field (tourniquet ischemia)
Failure to drain purulent collections early
Failure adequately or properly to decompress impending Volkmann's contracture
Failure to recognize human bite injuries
Failure to recognize ligamentous tears (gamekeeper's thumb)
Lack of appreciation of unstable fractures or dislocations
"Skillful neglect" of fingertip injuries
Inadequate, late or inappropriate cutaneous decompression of burn eschars
Improper, inadequate, or insufficient immobilization
Failure to relieve congestion

ural oils and resins (redwood). Tremendous inflammatory responses follow the implantation of such materials. The resulting chemical cellulitis, if not relieved by removal of the foreign body and thorough drainage of the wound, may lead to incapacitating fibrosis and induration. Most carpenters who work with these woods are cognizant of their toxic properties and may be better informed than their physicians concerning the potential problems associated with them.

Iatrogenic Injuries

Physician-induced injuries of the hand result from sins of commission and omission. The lists of each are long and discouraging, often a result of honest ignorance of the intricacies of surgery of the hand (Table 9-1). Virtually all of these problems are discussed in ensuing chapters, but their significance is so great that it is appropriate to list them here to ensure their recognition. Perhaps the greatest errors committed by physicians are operating without the use of a proximal tourniquet and failing to prevent or relieve congestion (Fig. 9-8).

References

1. Rank, B.K., Wakefield, A.R. and Hueston, J.R.: *Surgery of Repair as Applied to Hand Injuries*. 3rd ed. Williams and Wilkins, Baltimore, 1968.

10 Vascular Injuries and Disorders

The radial and ulnar arteries supply the hand through the deep and superficial palmar arches, to which the contributions of the ulnar artery are usually the more substantial. The normal communications between the two arches may be absent.[16] Although major terminal arterial anastomoses are not present in the digits, fortunately sufficient transverse communications are present so that the interruption of one digital artery usually does not jeopardize the circulation except possibly in the thumb.

Profound alterations in the vascular status of the hand occur in response to changes in posture, temperature and physical activity, and in metabolic, psychological and chemical influences. Greater vasodilatation of the digital arteries occurs after general warming of the body than after local application of heat. The blood flow is capable of increasing 100 times above the resting state.[14]

Important factors influencing the vascularity of the hand include such generalized problems as diabetes, allergies, syphilis, rheumatic heart disease, arteriosclerosis, hypertension, arthritis and neuritis. Congenital abnormalities may be present. There may be a history of exposure to tobacco, alcohol, ergot, lead, arsenicals or other toxic substances. An occupational history of continued exposure to cold, dampness or repeated trauma may be important. Those factors which produce the patient's symptoms may give clues to the etiology of his complaints.

The time of onset and the nature of any pain present are important aids in diagnosing vascular problems. The presence of skin or muscle wasting suggests a chronic process. Alterations in sensibility can occur with acute vascular accidents, develop insidiously with metabolic disturbances or reflect long-standing ischemia. Cardiac irregularities and angina or previous myocardial infarctions can lead to embolization from mural thrombi in the heart.

The patient with a long-standing vascular disorder of the upper extremity should be examined in a warm quiet room (72° F). The patient is disrobed sufficiently to permit complete examination of all four extremities as well as the heart and chest. Inspection is an essential first step: observing the hand at rest, its color and position, the condition of the skin, nails, and hair. Is there any evidence of previous trauma and has muscle atrophy occurred?

The patient should move the extremity through all possible range of motion which should be compared with the normal side. Changes in color of the skin and nails produced by elevation should be noted. A sensory assessment and palpation of all the pulses should be done. Temperature gradations can be measured with a thermistor or estimated by comparison with the other hand. The presence of sweating is important and may require a magnifying loupe to detect.

Special Tests for Vascular Disorders

ALLEN'S TEST[3]

Intermittent occlusion of the radial and ulnar arteries permits assessment of their individual contributions to the hand. After both arteries have been palpated at the wrist they are occluded by direct pressure. The patient pumps his hand to exsanguinate it. One artery is released and the distribution of its reactive hyperemia and the time of its appearance in the palm and fingertips are observed. The process is repeated with release of the opposite artery. This test indicates the relative contribution of each artery to the hand and the adequacy of communications between the two arches. A comparable assessment can be made of each digital artery.[4]

ADSON'S TEST[1]

The radial pulse can be obliterated through compression of the subclavian artery by the scalenus anticus muscle against a cervical rib or a high-riding first rib. Adson's maneuver involves palpation of the radial artery at the wrist with arm extended, the head turned to the affected side and the neck extended. A positive test produces obliteration of the radial pulse. Diminution or even obliteration of the radial pulse by this maneuver does occur in normal individuals. If aneurysmal poststenotic dilatation of the subclavial artery has occurred, a bruit may be present in the supraclavicular area.

ANGIOGRAPHY[14,20]

Complete examination of the circulation of the extremity is impossible without angiography, but it is not necessary in all instances. The brachial or axillary artery may be injected with 10 to 15 cc of an iodinated contrast material after placement of a Cournand needle or 18-gauge short-beveled needle. Catherization from the groin or opposite arm may be preferable in studying the entire extremity. Magnification studies can be helpful in discovering disturbances in the fine circulation of the digits. Films taken 5 seconds after the injection will show the venous phase of the circulation when the circulation is normal.

CERVICAL SYMPATHETIC BLOCK (CHAP. 26)

If excessive sympathetic nervous tone is contributing to vascular changes in the hand, a sympathetic block may help to determine the eventual value of sympathectomy. A Horner's syndrome should be produced if the block is satisfactorily complete. A definite rise in skin temperature should result, with good filling of the superficial veins.

INTRA-ARTERIAL RESERPINE

Vasospastic states may be diagnosed and relieved temporarily by the intra-arterial injection of reserpine. One milligram is injected intra-arterially via a small (25-gauge) needle and the distal extremity is observed for improvement in color and skin temperature. The effects of a single injection may last several hours and result in a diminution of painful symptoms for a considerable period.

Other tests which may have special value for specific problems include: oscillometry (Collen's oscillometer), plethysmography,[14] reflex vasodilatation, circulation time and capillary microscopy.

Causes of Arterial Vascular Problems

The major causes of arterial vascular problems are listed below and discussed further in this section.

- Traumatic causes
  - Division
  - Thrombosis
  - Aneurysm
  - Arteriovenous fistulae
  - Intra-arterial injection
- Congenital arteriovenous fistulae
- Arterial occlusive disease
  - Embolus
  - Arteriosclerosis
  - Thromboangitiis obliterans
- Vasospastic states
- Volkmann's contracture

Trauma

Either blunt or penetrating trauma may produce direct vascular injury or cause reflex vasospasm. Repeated trauma may sufficiently sensitize an area so that a Raynaud's phenomenon may be produced. Intimal or intramural vascular damage can lead to thrombosis.[27]

VASCULAR REPAIR[9,12,21,22,47,49]

Arterial division requires precedence in repair when the distal circulation is dangerously diminished (Fig. 10-1). The damaged portion of the vessel should be removed and either a simple arteriorrhaphy should be done or a segment of vein or

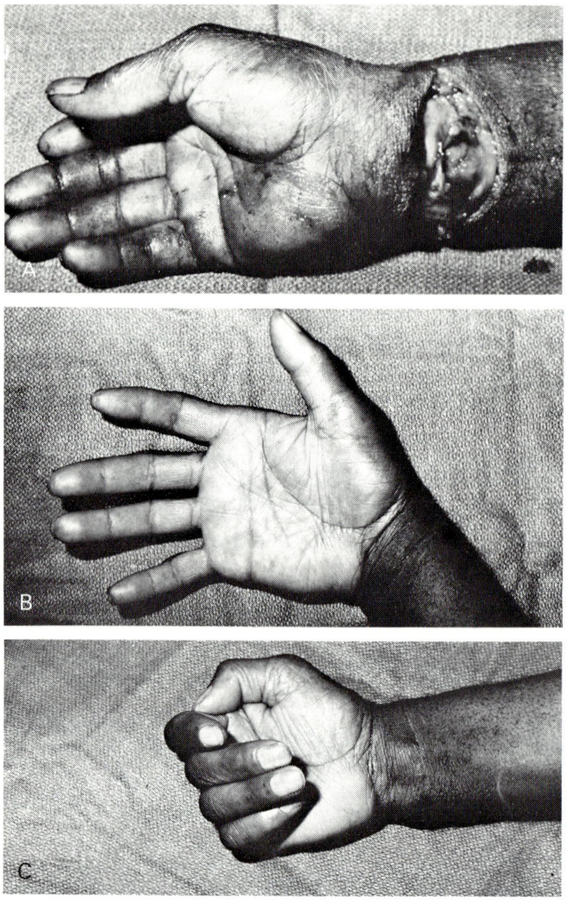

Figure 10-1. *This 63-year-old male divided both the ulnar and radial arteries as well as ten flexor tendons and the median and ulnar nerves. Primary arteriorrhaphies and repair of six tendons were done. Active extension and flexion are demonstrated six months after his injury.*

artery should be interposed as a graft. Meticulous attention must be given to the technique (Fig. 10-2). Prerequisites of vascular repair are as follows:

- Adequate anesthesia
- Good light
- Magnification (2–4 X loupe may be sufficient). For digital vessels the operating microscope may be needed
- Capable assistance
- Restoration of blood volume, absence of shock and other major life-endangering conditions
- Proper instruments

Underlying fractures should first be stabilized and vessels should be carefully identified by gentle irrigation with isotonic electrolyte solutions.[22] Minimal handling of the vessels is important to avoid intimal injuries. A small band of adventia (1 to 2 mm) should be removed about the site of the arteriorrhaphy. If both the radial and ulnar arteries have been divided and the circulation to the hand still appears adequate, the ulnar artery at least should be reanastomosed.

Most traumatic circulatory problems in the hand are a result of diminished venous drainage rather than of arterial supply. Repair of the dorsal veins should be planned if they have been extensively divided.

Reexploration is necessary if thrombosis of the repair occurs. Low-molecular-weight dextran, sympathetic blocks and anticoagulation help to reduce microthrombi occurring from sludging. Aspirin, 600 mg q 4 hours, can reduce platelet adhesiveness. These adjuncts are no substitutes for careful technique—only properly done arteriorrhaphy and venorrhaphy will remain patent providing congestion can be minimized.

Bridging arterial gaps with vein grafts is often necessary. A colored (blue, green or yellow) background of moistened rubber sheeting from a child's balloon aids in the repair. Incisions to decompress the digits or the hand should be made in anticipation of future swelling.

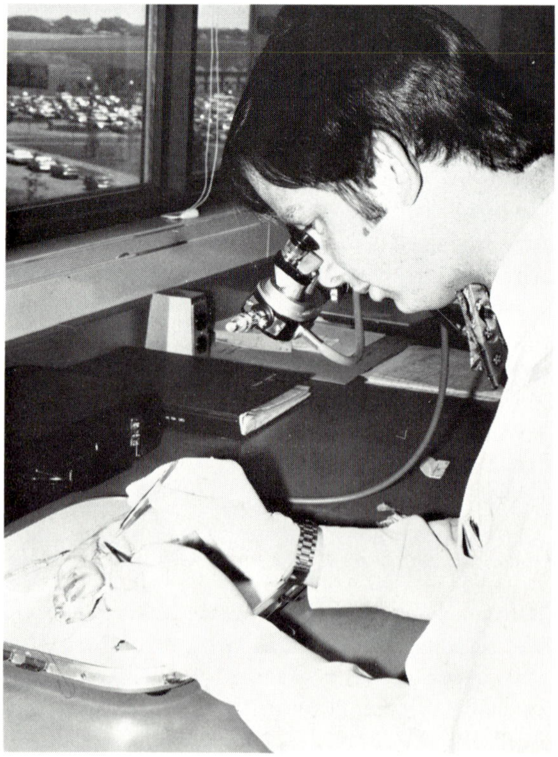

Figure 10-2. *Practice of microsurgical techniques by the novice surgeon can be provided in the laboratory initially on pig's feet and later on rats or rabbits.*

In general arteries and veins can be repaired to the middle phalangeal level, although those beyond the superficial arch require extremely precise microsurgical techniques, as outlined:

- Proximal control of bleeding to clear the field
- Removal of all debris, clots, and devitalized tissue
- Stabilization of associated fractures
- Identification of the divided dorsal veins and injured arteries
- Heparinization of the patient and instillation by gentle irrigation of dilute heparin into the vessels
- Removal of clots proximally and distally by a small Fogarty catheter if feasible
- Repair of the dorsal veins (1 or 2) and the arteries using 8-0 to 10-0 non-absorbable synthetic suture
- Placement of initial vascular sutures about $\frac{1}{3}$ of the circumference apart to avoid accidently suturing the repair closed. Interrupted sutures are generally used

The smaller vessels are the more difficult to keep open. The venous anastamosis is of great importance, for many excellent arterial reconstructions fail because of inadequate venous return. Furthermore, venous compression can result from edema, necessitating cutaneous relaxing incisions to restore or maintain venous return. Principles of treatment following microvascular repair may be listed as follows:

- Elevation of the injured hand on 1 or 2 pillows above the level of the heart
- Immobilization in the position of function
- Continuation of heparinization (2 weeks)
- Administration of systemic antibiotics
- Careful observation for Volkmann's ischemia
- Consideration of sympathetic block
- Cooling of the extremity by iced bags applied around the cast (72 hours)
- Administration of low-molecular-weight dextran
- Administration of aspirin, 600 mg p.o. q 6 hr
- Administration of Persantine 25 mg q 6 hr (dipyridamole)

FREE ARTERIAL FLAPS

The description of the unique arteriovenous circulation of the groin noted by McGregor and Jackson[24] has provided the reconstructive surgeon with an additional tool, the direct transfer of free composite tissue. Occasionally, injuries to the hand or upper extremity will lend themselves to such reconstructive efforts either for coverage or the creation of a new thumb.[19]

The vascular pedicle of the "groin flap" is the superficial circumflex iliac artery and vein. Since the artery often divides at the medial border of the sartorius muscle into a deep and superficial branch, dissection of the composite flap must be beneath the fascia of that muscle to ensure adequate circulation. In most instances the superficial circumflex iliac vein forms a common trunk with the superficial epigastric vein before entering the saphenous bulb. The authors have not had occasion to utilize this flap in the upper extremity, but have used it successfully about the foot (Fig. 10-3).

The base of the flap should lie over the femoral artery. The central axis of the flap lies on a line drawn from 2.5 cm below the inguinal ligament on the femoral artery laterally to the anterior iliac spine. The flap is outlined to correspond to the size of the recipient defect (or slightly larger). Dissection is done from lateral to medial and deep to the fascia, and the venous confluence of the superficial circumflex iliac vein and the superficial epigastric vein is identified. The recipient bed is then prepared and the recipient vessels are readied. The flap is freed and the microvascular anastomosis carried out as outlined above, after the flap is secured at its margins. Generally 10-0 suture is used, approximating the vessels by triangulation. If end-to-side anastomosis is done, the recipient vessel is slit and an oval excised from each side with the curved microscissors. During the repair the vessel ends should be repeatedly flushed with heparinized Ringer's lactate solution (100 U/cc) to avoid drying of the vessels. Twisting or rotation of the vessels will impair subsequent flow.

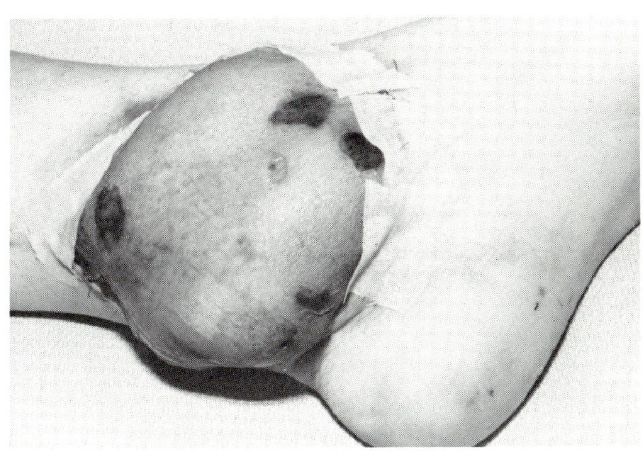

Figure 10-3. *This free vascular flap based upon the superficial circumflex iliac vessels was anastomosed to the posterior tibial vessels at the ankle. A prolonged ischemia time ($2\frac{1}{2}$ hours) contributed to considerable skin necrosis.*

The flap margins must not be sutured too snugly or congestion may result. The ischemia time of the flap should not exceed 90 minutes. Usually the donor area can be approximated primarily, although if it is greater than 12 cm in width a skin graft will usually be required.

ARTERIOVENOUS FISTULAE

Although congenital arteriovenous fistulae do occur in the hand, the majority seen are the result of trauma. The possibility should be suspected when a penetrating wound has occurred near a major neurovascular bundle.[5,15]

The congenital variety may persist into adulthood, with pain and ulceration. Usually these arise from cavernous hemangiomas and are extremely difficult to remove totally. Angiography can delineate multiple communications and is usually most helpful with the recurrent variety or with those in which previous radiation therapy has been given. Careful resection of all of the abnormal vasculature may be impossible with extensively infiltrating hemangiomas. If a single digit is involved, amputation may be the preferred solution. Disturbances in growth are not unusual and gigantism can occur.

A history of injury is invariably obtainable with post-traumatic arteriovenous fistulae. There may be pain and local warmth at the site of the fistula. If the vessels are sufficiently large, a bruit can be heard or felt. Occlusion of the proximal arterial flow eliminates the bruit. Varices may develop distal to the point of communication.

The treatment is simple division of the communication and restoration of arterial continuity. The veins can be ligated if necessary.

ANEURYSMS[29]

Most aneurysms of the upper extremity follow vascular trauma. They may be either true aneurysms with an intact vascular wall or false aneurysms ("pulsating hematoma"). Compression of the subclavian artery at the thoracic outlet can lead to a distal aneurysmal dilatation. The turbulence of blood swirling through this area produces mural thrombi which eventually may embolize distally with disastrous consequences. If a distal subclavian arterial aneurysm has been demonstrated, the preferred surgical approach is resection of the medial clavicle and release of the scalenus anticus muscle. End-to-end repair of the artery without an interposed graft is usually possible after resection of the aneurysm. Abduction of the arm is prevented for three weeks after surgery. The removal of the clavicle generally poses no disability.

The ulnar artery may develop post-traumatic aneurysms at the distal border of the transverse carpal ligament (Fig. 10-4). These are painless, pulsatile slowly enlarging masses located just at the junction between the hypothenar and thenar musculature, and are treated by excision. Angiography is usually not needed in the evaluation of simple traumatic aneurysms. An Allen's test is performed preoperatively to assess the radial arterial communications with the distal ulnar artery. When the aneurysm has been dissected out and small vascular clips have been placed proximally and distally, the tourniquet is deflated to assess the adequacy of remaining circulation. Arterial repair

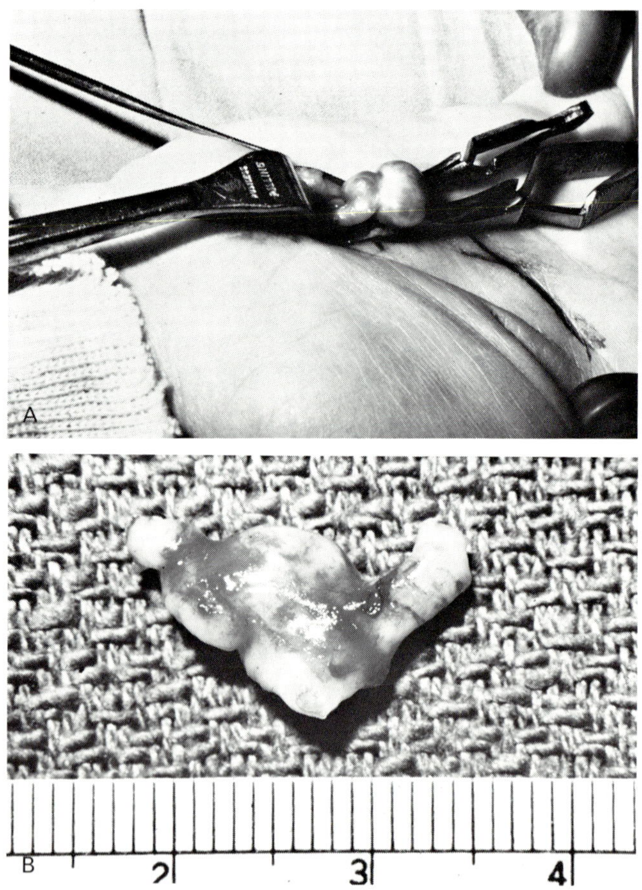

Figure 10-4. *This lady had a window fall on her outstretched hand, which contused the proximal palm. Several months later a pulsatile mass appeared, which proved to be an aneurysm of the ulnar artery. A resection of the aneurysm and arteriorrhaphy were done.*

after removal of the ulnar artery aneurysm is not imperative, but is advisable. Often a short vein graft is needed to bridge the defect.

Occasionally an aneurysm of the superficial radial artery may occur after a blow over the thenar eminence. In this area the radial artery lies unprotected between the abductor pollicis brevis and the opponens pollicis muscles. A third point of true aneurysm formation is within the deep palmar arch. Arteriosclerotic aneurysms do occur in the hand, but are quite rare.

THROMBOSIS DUE TO INTRA-ARTERIAL INJECTIONS

The inadvertent instillation into an artery of a substance which is chemically irritating will produce vasospasm. This spasm can be sufficiently severe or the effect on the intima so extensive that thrombosis follows. The accidental intra-arterial injection of such drugs as hydroxyzine hydrochloride has resulted in substantial loss of tissue. Drug addicts have lost whole hands as the result of the intra-arterial administration of a contaminated or noxious substance (Fig. 10-5).

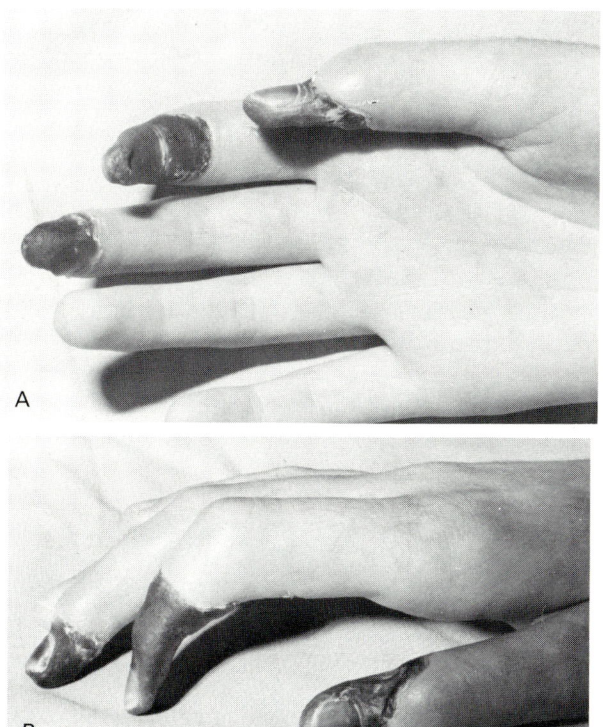

Figure 10-5. *A 20-year-old girl inadvertently injected her radial artery with pentobarbitol. Despite treatment with anticoagulants, intra-arterial reserpine and sympathetic nerve blocks, considerable digital loss occurred.*

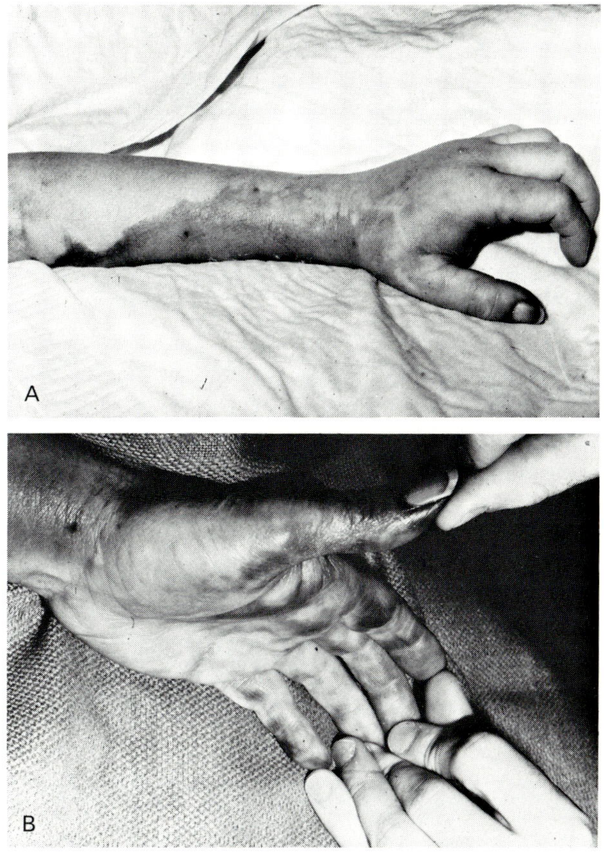

Figure 10-6A. *A young woman suffered loss of her thumb and a portion of her index finger as well as considerable radial forearm skin after cardiac surgery in which catheterization of the radial artery was done.* **B.** *This man eventually had a midforearm amputation following radial artery thrombosis secondary to radial artery catheterization.*

If the material injected produces a chemical vasculitis, often little can be done to improve the condition of the extremity. If there is delay in the treatment and the tissues have begun to demarcate, the management of the problem becomes that of salvaging the extremity and providing wound closure. Often a neuritis accompanies the vasculitis, and this chemical neuritis plus the ischemic neuritis secondary to the vascular injury may produce a state of causalgia. The combination of neuritis and vasculitis leads to stiffness and diminished function, seriously limiting the hand.

The current use of indwelling arterial catheters for monitoring patients after major surgical procedures results occasionally in ischemic injury of the hand[6,18] (Fig. 10-6). If hypotension is prolonged or hypertonic solutions are administered by the arterial line, thrombosis may occur. Substantial losses of tissue may result. Occasionally multiple peripheral emboli may complicate this problem. Conservatism in the use of arterial cannulation and limitation of the duration of use to the acute postoperative period can minimize this risk.

The treatment of acute accidental intra-arterial injection is outlined as follows:

- Administration of intra-arterial lidocaine and tolazoline HCl (Priscoline)
- Systemic anticoagulation and low-molecular-weight dextran
- Sympathetic block
- Arteriography
- Vascular exploration and thrombectomy if demonstrable by angiography
- Decompression of hand and digits
- Elevation and cooling of the extremity

Arterial Occlusive Disease

EMBOLISM

Acute occlusion of the arterial circulation of the upper extremity usually is the result of an embolus from a central source. Cardiac disease, old myocardial infarcts, atrial fibrillation and subacute bacterial endocarditis may be the etiological factors. If the embolus has lodged beyond the bifurcation of the brachial artery, it may be possible to extract the clot through the antecubital space with a Fogarty catheter. Flushing the distal artery with dilute heparin and lidocaine (0.5 per cent) for the prevention of vasospasm may be beneficial. Caution must be observed if sufficient time has passed to permit ischemic necrosis of the flexor muscle mass to begin—the first stage toward the development of a crippling Volkmann's contracture if it is neglected. Fasciotomy may be required. The absence of sensation in the distribution of the median nerve or the appearance of throbbing pain suggests this as a possible complication.

ATHEROSCLEROSIS

Chronic thrombotic occlusion is the result of long-standing atherosclerosis.[13] Often sufficient collateral circulation has developed over the years to reduce the specific symptoms of main arterial occlusion. The hand and arm may manifest fatigue or claudication with extensive use.[17] This problem requires the same systemic therapy and attention to maintaining the circulation as does peripheral vascular insufficiency of the lower extremities.

THROMBOANGIITIS OBLITERANS (BUERGER'S DISEASE)

It is likely that this specialized form of occlusive arterial disease is really a variation of the more common atherosclerosis. Although the special type of phlebitis described by Buerger does exist, it is uncertain as to whether or not a specific arterial lesion accompanies it.[14]

Raynaud's Phenomenon and Vasospastic Disorders

Vasomotor instability in Raynaud's phenomenon is manifested by acute changes in the skin, varying from cyanosis to deep blue-red, and by hyperemia with a burning sensation. Many causes can produce this phenomenon: exposure to cold, vascular disorders with a neurogenic component and emotional reactions[2,7] (Fig. 10-7). The early vasomotor effects of this disability may progress to changes within the arteries, digital ulceration and gangrene (Fig. 10-8). The possibility of underlying collagen disorders such as lupus, scleroderma or rheumatoid arthritis must be investigated in the evaluation of the patient with Raynaud's phenomenon (Fig. 10-9).

The prognosis is quite good, and protection of the hands and feet in warm dress is the only precaution. For severely symptomatic individuals, oral Priscoline may be beneficial. Reserpine can also help by its ganglionic blockade and the production of a chemical sympathectomy.[8]

For the patient with Raynaud's phenomenon

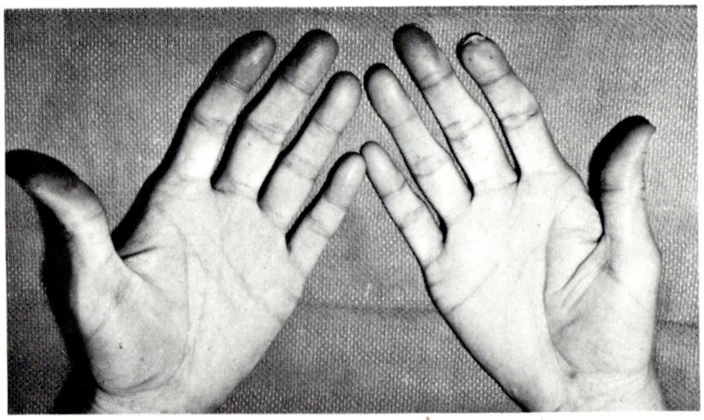

Figure 10-7. *Severe Raynaud's phenomenon.*

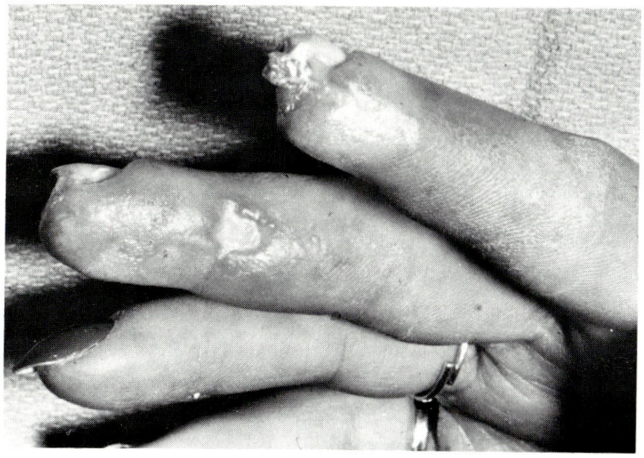

Figure 10-8. *A young woman with scleroderma developed progressive gangrene after her family physician attempted to drain a non-existent felon of her index finger.*

and progressively increasing symptoms, a sympathectomy may be justified. Alcohol, reserpine, methyldopa and steroids may benefit some patients. If gangrene occurs, conservative management with systemic antibiotics to reduce the risk of infection is important.

Volkmann's Contracture

Prevention or early recognition is essential in the treatment of Volkmann's contracture. Once the muscle necrosis has occurred, treatment has started too late. The presence of peripheral pulses can be deceptive.[14,23] The key in anticipating this problem is the appearance of *pain.* Accompanying the pain will be digital swelling and paraesthesias. If these are not relieved by removing the dressing or cast, the fascial compartments should be opened surgically and the lacertus fibrosis and two heads of the pronator teres divided to free the median nerve. The wound should be left open, and may be closed secondarily or skin grafted as seems appropriate (Fig. 10-10).

If relief is not provided, three elements will emerge in the established Volkmann's contracture. The forearm is pronated and the digits and wrist are flexed. Intrinsic muscle paralysis without con-

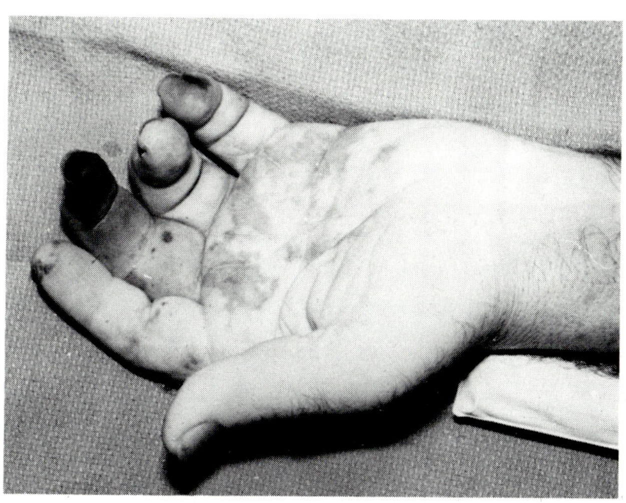

Figure 10-9. *Severe vasculitis progressing to gangrene associated with rheumatoid arthritis. (See also Figure* **24-2A–E.**)

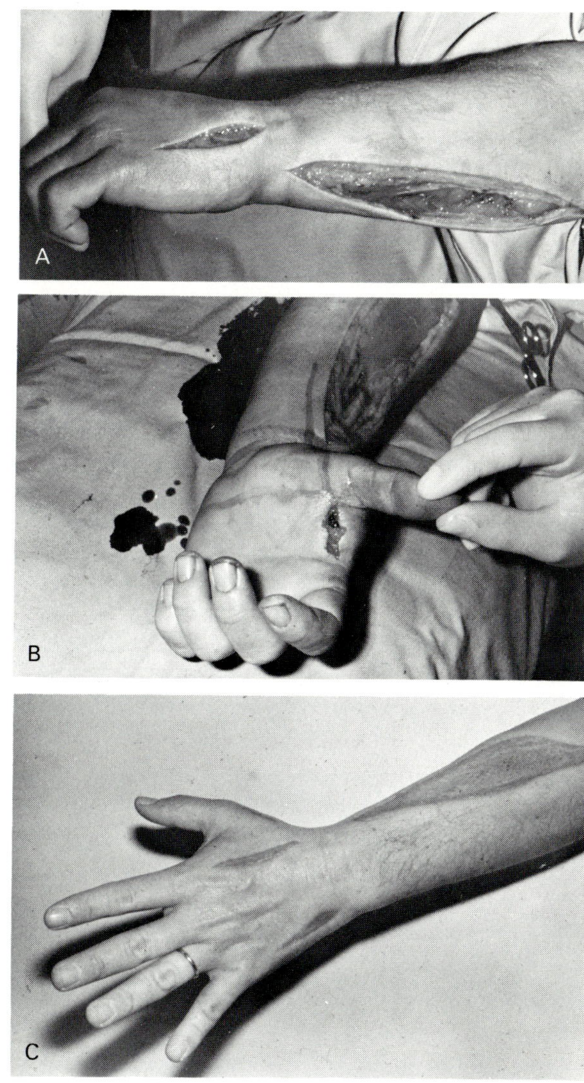

Figure 10-10. *Crush injury of the hand and forearm which was immediately decompressed and subsequently grafted 48 hours later with a mesh skin graft. (From Graham, Miller, et al.: Trauma: Treating wringer injuries. Pa. Med., 78:67, 1975. Used by permission of the publisher.)*

tracture occurs and a diminution of median and usually ulnar sensibility is found. The crucial factor is that of lack of sensibility. Attention must be directed at freeing the nerves before they are irreversibly damaged within the constricting fibrotic compartment. The incision to decompress the flexor muscle compartment extends from the medial aspect of the elbow to the musculotendinous junction of the forearm. The brachial artery is examined and the median nerve completely freed. The ulnar nerve should be examined at the same time.

A non-adhering single layer of gauze (Xeroform, Furacin, or Adaptic) or an allograft is placed directly on the skin defect. A fluffy gauze dressing is applied next and a splint incorporated in the dressing to extend the wrist and abduct and extend the thumb. The fingers are allowed to flex into a comfortable position. If a supracondylar fracture is present, a Kirschner wire is inserted through the olecranon and overhead traction exerted on the arm, with the hand and forearm supported at a right angle. After the fracture has become somewhat stable ($2\frac{1}{2}$ to 3 weeks), the traction can be discontinued and reduction maintained with a long-arm cast positioning the wrist in extension and the forearm midway between supination and pronation. Revision of the final forearm wound can be performed electively well after full recovery if an unsatisfactory scar has resulted.

Seddon[26] has advised freeing the median nerve, excising the flexor muscular infarct and splinting the hand in a functional position in treating the established contracture. Once sensation has begun to return, muscle transfers can be done. Some return of nerve function can be expected even after a year. To restore digital flexion, the extensor carpi radialis longus is transferred around the radial border of the forearm into the four profundus tendons. Increasing tension is provided by an oblique insertion of this tendon so that the flexor tone is increased across the palm from the index to the little finger.

Should the muscles of opposition not recover, then the abductor digiti minimi is transferred across the palm into the insertion of the tendon of the abductor pollicis brevis. The usual extrinsic muscles utilized for restoration of opposition are not available after a Volkmann's contracture.

Independent flexion of the thumb can be achieved by use of the extensor indicis proprius and fusion of the interphalangeal joint. The extensor indicis proprius is routed around the radial border and into the carpal tunnel or around the border of the palmaris longus using it to create a pulley.

Following tendon transfers, the wrist and fingers must be splinted for five weeks, with careful passive motion applied to the digits by the physician every other day after two weeks.

Disorders of the Veins and Lymphatics

The venous and lymphatic drainage of the hand is from volar to dorsal. The major vessels are superficial so even a minor constriction due to clothing or a snug dressing can produce distal edema. Persistence of edema produces limitation of motion and facilitates fibrosis; consequently it is imperative that no impediment to proximal venous and lymphatic flow be present. Elevation and active movement are the best safeguards against the formation of edema.

Congenital Problems

Angiomas of both venous and lymphatic vessels (Figs. 10-11 and 22-32) occur in the extremity. Often the areas involved with these vascular anomalies develop marked overgrowths. Since local removal of the vascular abnormality can be difficult, if not impossible, amputation has been suggested if one or two fingers are involved. The tendency for the cavernous hemangiomas to recur may necessitate repeated operations as symptoms develop. Usually pain is not a feature but dull aching and at times cutaneous ulceration with hemorrhage and infection may result. If massive involvement of the extremity is present in a small child, thrombocytopenia can be produced.

The surgical removal of these growths is not easy

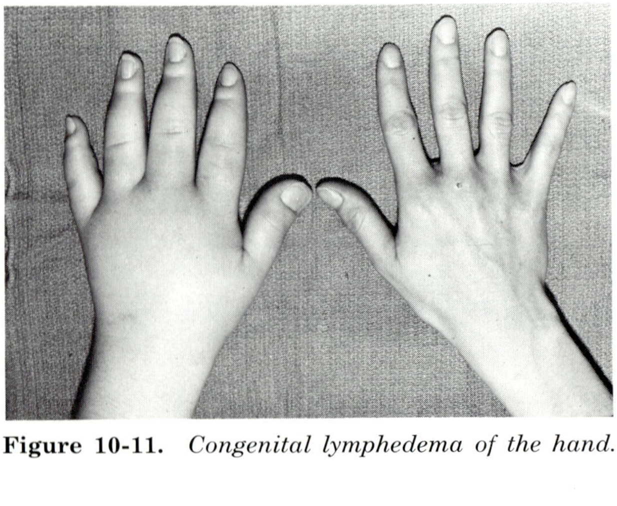

Figure 10-11. *Congenital lymphedema of the hand.*

and the anticipated problems should be explained to the patient or his family (Chap. 22). The injection of sclerosing materials is not useful.

Recurrence is the rule and, with progressively proximal involvement, repeated ulceration, cellulitis and pain, amputation may be the only solution. Elastic compression bandages may be helpful in reducing the bulk of a hemangioma and controlling its growth (Chap. 22).

Trauma

Disruption of proper venous and lymphatic drainage from the distal extremity can occur from a variety of traumatic insults. Often the underlying nerve, muscle or bony injuries are so great that the problems of proper drainage of the extremity are neglected. Circumferential full-thickness or deep partial-thickness burns can occlude the venous return sufficiently to produce distal gangrene and a Volkmann's type of contracture. Division of the eschar produces dramatic resolution of the distal congestion. Similar obstruction can result if circumferential skin grafting is done without interruption of the margins of the graft.

Venous thrombosis may occur after blunt trauma to the extremity. With this type of injury, however, in a short while the vessels either recannulate or collateral channels dilate, and persistent edema is seldom present unless the thrombotic process has been massive. Thrombosed veins may remain as firm movable subcutaneous nodules and even become calcified (Fig. 22-20).

The most common cause of chronic edema of the upper extremity is the effect of the treatment of breast cancer—surgery and/or irradiation. Injury to the axillary vein, postoperative cellulitis, overly tight wound closure and the local effects of irradiation can all be incriminated as contributory to chronic lymphedema. Should the lymphedema develop years after the initial treatment, a recurrence of the breast carcinoma should be suspected. Ulceration and breakdown of the skin of the chronically lymphedematous limb years after the initial treatment lead to the suspicion of the occurrence of a lymphangiosarcoma (Chap. 22).

The initial treatment of potential lymphedema following axillary surgery is preventive. The patient must be educated to move the extremity repeatedly through its entire range of motion. If lymphedema begins despite good active motion of the extremity, a custom-fitted elasticized sleeve and glove can be utilized. Periodic use of pneumatic alternating-pressure sleeves may also be of benefit. Swimming is a superb form of active physiotherapy for this problem.

If the weight of the extremity becomes cumbersome and incapacitating, the development of a dermal skin flap can be considered[31,32] (Fig. 10-12). A section of skin is removed with the dermatome from either the medial or lateral aspect of the arm. The excess fat is removed from beneath this area and the leading margin of the denuded skin is rotated into the underlying deep muscles and sutured there. The other edge of the wound is undermined to resect the excess subcutaneous fat. The skin edge is advanced and sutured to the denuded dermal area. Suction drains are placed beneath the flaps and a bulky compressive dressing is applied. The dressing is changed after 4 or 5 days, at which time the drains are removed. The dressing is continued for a total of two weeks, when a fitted elasticized glove and sleeve are applied. These compressive devices may have to be worn indefinitely.

At times a thoracic pedicle flap can be inserted into the axillary area to facilitate better lymphatic drainage from the extremity. Tubes of omentum have also been tunneled from the abdomen beneath the skin of the chest wall and across the axilla in an effort to enhance lymphatic egress

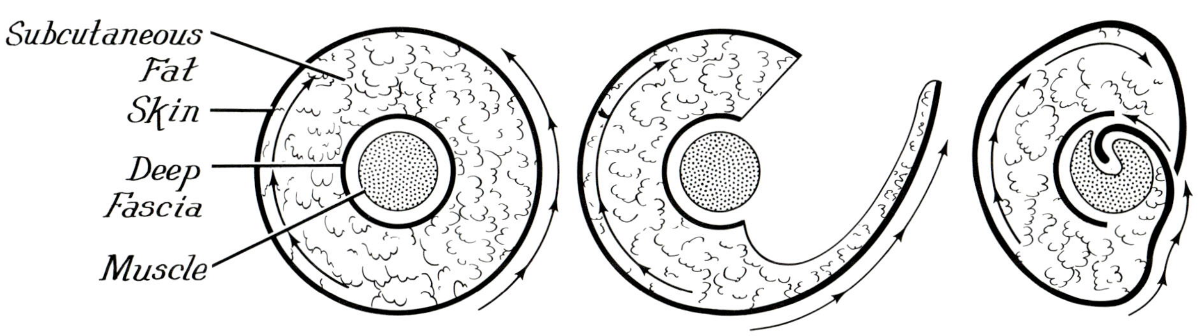

Figure 10-12. *Thompson's technique for utilizing the subcutaneous transposition of superficial lymphatics into the deep compartment of a limb by burying a deepithelized skin flap. (Redrawn from Thompson, N.*[31]*)*

from the arm. None of these procedures is assured of success, and the patient must be made aware of the shortcomings and the risk of failure before any of them is undertaken.

Infections

It is rare for chronic lymphedema to affect the upper extremity following a single episode of infection. A combination of venous and lymphatic obliteration attends the habitual use of adulterated solutions by the drug addict, resulting in "puffiness" particularly of the dorsum of the hand. Neviaser and his associates[25] have shown this brawny edema to be secondary to fibrotic replacement of the subcutaneous tissue. Lymphangiography in these patients shows an absence of normal dermal channels and extravasation of the contrast media within the arm[32] about the areas of repeated injection. Whether the lymphatic drainage will improve following the cessation of drug abuse is not yet known.

Treatment requires a high index of suspicion and management of the addiction. Elevation of the extremity and the use of systemic antibiotics when cellulitis is present will hasten improvement.

References

1. Adson, A.W.: Surgical treatment for symptoms produced by cervical ribs and the scalenus anticus muscle. Surg. Gynecol. Obstet., 85:687, 1947.
2. Allen, E.V., Barker, N.W. and Hines, E.A.: *Peripheral Vascular Diseases.* W.B. Saunders, Philadelphia, 1962.
3. Allen, E.V. and Brown, G.E.: Thromboangiitis obliterans. Ann. Intern. Med., 1:535, 1928.
4. Ashbell, T.S., Kutz, J.E. and Kleinert, H.E.: The digital Allen test. Plast. Reconstr. Surg., 39:311, 1967.
5. Barker, W.J.: *Peripheral Arterial Disease. Major Problems in Clinical Surgery.* W.B. Saunders, Philadelphia, 1966.
6. Bedford, R.F. and Wollman, H.: Complications of percutaneous radial artery cannulation: An objective prospective study in man. Anesthesiology, 38:228, 1973.
7. Blain, A., Coller, F.A. and Carver, G.B.: Raynaud's disease. Surgery, 29:387, 1951.
8. Boyes, J.H.: *Bunnell's Surgery of the Hand.* J.B. Lippincott, Philadelphia, 1964.
9. Buncke, H.J., Corbett, J.R., Smith, J.W. and Tamai, S.: *Techniques of Microsurgery.* Ethicon, Inc., Somerville (New Jersey), 1969.
10. Buncke, H.J. and Schulz, W.P.: Experimental digital amputation and reimplantation. Plast. Reconstr. Surg., 36:62, 1965.
11. Corbett, J.R.: Microvascular surgery. Surg. Clin. North Am., 47:521, 1967.
12. Corbett, J.R.: Microvascular surgery. In: *Plastic Surgery* (Grabb, W.C. and Smith, J.W., Eds.). Little, Brown & Co., Boston, 1968.
13. Darling, R.C.: Peripheral arterial surgery. N. Engl. J. Med., 280:26, 1969.
14. Deterling, R.A.: Vascular disorders of the hand. In: *Hand Surgery* (Flynn, J.E., Ed.). Williams and Wilkins, Baltimore, 1966.
15. Dumanian, A. and Kelikian, H.: Vascular complications of orthopedic surgery. J. Bone Joint Surg., 51A:103, 1969.
16. Edwards, E.A.: Organization of the small arteries of the hand and digits. Am. J. Surg., 99:837, 1960.
17. Garrett, H.E., Morris, G.C., Howell, J.F. and DeBakey, M.E.: Revascularization of the upper extremity with autogenous vein bypass graft. Arch. Surg., 91:751, 1965.
18. Graham, W.P., Blakemore, W.S., Waldhausen, J.A. and Zinsser, H.F.: Tissue necrosis from vascular complications of the upper extremity after arterial catheterization. Rev. Lat. Am. Chir. Plast., 17:37, 1973.
19. Harii, K. and Ohmari, K.: Direct transfer of large free groin skin flaps to the lower extremity using microvascular anastomoses. Chir. Plast., 3:1, 1975.
20. Imparto, A.M.: Management of vascular injuries of the upper extremities. Orthop. Clin. North Am., 1:383, 1970.
21. Jacobson, J.H. and Suarez, E.L.: Microsurgery in anastomosis of small vessels. Surg. Forum, 11:243, 1960.
22. Kleinert, H.E., Kasdan, M.L. and Romero, J.L.: Small blood vessel anastomosis for salvage of severely injured upper extremity. J. Bone Joint Surg., 45A:788, 1963.
23. Littler, J.W.: Principles of reconstructive surgery of the hand. In: *Reconstructive Plastic Surgery* (Converse, J.M., Ed.). W.B. Saunders, Philadelphia, 1964.
24. McGregor, I.A. and Jackson, I.T.: The groin flap. Br. J. Plast. Surg., 25:3, 1972.
25. Neviaser, R.J., Butterfield, W.C. and Wieche, D.R.: The puffy hand of drug addiction. J. Bone Joint Surg., 54A:629, 1972.
26. Seddon, H.: *Surgical Disorders of the Peripheral Nerves.* Williams and Wilkins, Baltimore, 1972.
27. Shires, G.T. and Patman, R.D.: Vascular injuries. In: *Care of the Trauma Patient* (Shires, G.T., Ed.). McGraw-Hill, New York, 1966.
28. Smith, J.W.: Microsurgery: Review of the literature and discussion of microtechniques. Plast. Reconstr. Surg., 37:227, 1966.
29. Smith, J.W.: True aneurysms of traumatic origin in the palm. Am. J. Surg., 104:7, 1962.
30. Smith, J.W. and Jacobson, J.H.: Microsurgical repair of blood vessels and peripheral nerves. In: *Hand Surgery* (Flynn, J.E., Ed.). Williams and Wilkins, Baltimore, 1966.
31. Thompson, N.: The surgical treatment of chronic lymphedema of the extremities. Surg. Clin. North Am., 47:445, 1967.
32. Thompson, N.: Surgical treatment of chronic lymphedema of the lower limb, with preliminary report of new operation. Br. Med. J., 2:1566, 1962.
33. Whitaker, L.A. and Graham, W.P.: Management of hand infections in the narcotic addict. Plast. Reconstr. Surg., 52:384, 1973.

11 Fractures of the Hand

Fractures in the hand are common, but they represent more than "just a broken finger." A metacarpal or phalangeal fracture, indifferently treated, can have a serious impact—rendering the laborer or watchmaker jobless, the housewife unable to care for her family or the athlete permanently sidelined. These fractures are a significant cause of disability and economic loss; the importance of prompt proper therapy can hardly be overstated.

The general principles in the care of hand fractures are those of good treatment of fractures of any bone: gentle examination and reduction, adequate roentgenograms, proper handling of soft tissue coverage, accurate assessment and appropriately timed treatment of associated nerve, tendon and vascular injuries, and immobilization by either external or internal techniques. The indications for, and use of, tetanus toxoid or antitoxin and antibiotics in open fractures in the hand are the same as those in other areas.

Specific considerations in the treatment of hand fractures are critical and demand emphasis. A thorough comprehension of the exquisitely balanced extensor and flexor tendon systems passing across the series of interrelated joints is essential. Local anatomy and biomechanics determine the deformity once the bone has fractured, and must be utilized to obtain and maintain the reduction. These biomechanics will be described for each type of fracture.

Regardless of the site of fracture, the adjacent joints must be given careful observation. To maintain the reduction at the expense of adjacent joint motion and hand function is a Pyrrhic victory indeed. The reduction must be accurate with a minimum of soft tissue trauma. Immobilization of the fractured ray must be in the general attitude of the position of function—wrist extended 20°, metacarpophalangeal joints flexed 45 to 60° (index to little), and interphalangeal joints flexed a few degrees. The thumb should be in the "fist position," with the basal joint in 20° of radial abduction and 30° of palmar abduction. The dressing should be well molded and contoured, and supported by external plaster with gentle anterior-posterior support (Fig. 11-1).

Percutaneous Kirschner wires can often be used to great advantage following closed reduction to eliminate the need for extreme positions of immobilization and to preserve position of otherwise unstable fragments.[4,9,54,56] This is considered an integral part of many closed reductions. Obviously it must be done with the aseptic technique of an open reduction. It is an internal suture, and the reduction and wire must be protected with a plaster cast which holds the hand in a position of function until the fracture unites and the wire is removed.

For a satisfactory functional result following treatment of a fracture, normal tendon excursion over the healed fracture is mandatory. This essential gliding can be compromised by soft tissue edema and fibrosis or by adhesion to the callus. The latter is particularly true in fractures of the proximal phalanx, a bone enveloped on all sides by tendinous structures directly adjacent to the periosteum. Fortunately, during the reduction and

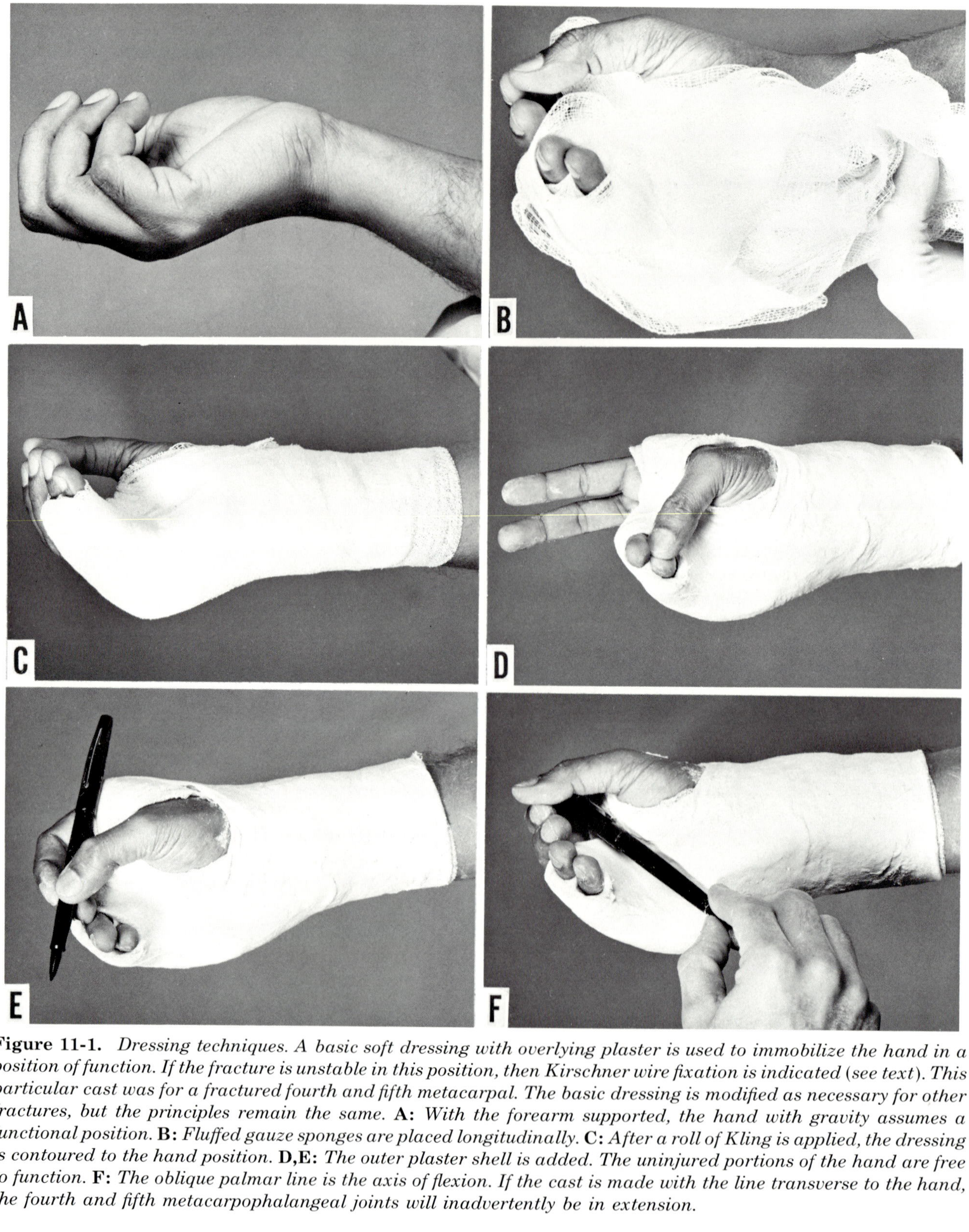

Figure 11-1. *Dressing techniques. A basic soft dressing with overlying plaster is used to immobilize the hand in a position of function. If the fracture is unstable in this position, then Kirschner wire fixation is indicated (see text). This particular cast was for a fractured fourth and fifth metacarpal. The basic dressing is modified as necessary for other fractures, but the principles remain the same.* **A:** *With the forearm supported, the hand with gravity assumes a functional position.* **B:** *Fluffed gauze sponges are placed longitudinally.* **C:** *After a roll of Kling is applied, the dressing is contoured to the hand position.* **D,E:** *The outer plaster shell is added. The uninjured portions of the hand are free to function.* **F:** *The oblique palmar line is the axis of flexion. If the cast is made with the line transverse to the hand, the fourth and fifth metacarpophalangeal joints will inadvertently be in extension.*

immobilization the proximity of these structures to the fracture can be utilized to help control the inherent forces of displacement.

In assessing fractures, roentgenographic technique is important. The usual posteroanterior and oblique views of the hand, a routine in most radiology departments, are inadequate. A true lateral, as well as the posteroanterior, of the fractured digit both before and after reduction is essential to determine the alignment of the fragments. Meaningful lateral views can be obtained with careful positioning of the non-injured fingers. If necessary, laminograms can be obtained in difficult cases, e.g. certain complex fractures of the proximal portion of the proximal phalanx, when overlap of adjacent phalanges obscures detail.

The closed reduction of hand fractures is well suited to block anesthesia—median, ulnar or radial at the wrist, and digital (Fig. 11-2). The infiltration of anesthetic agents into a fracture site is to be condemned. The adjacent delicate soft tissues, with their tendency to become fixed to the fracture, are already edematous and contused by injury. Local injection into the area of injury causes further tissue distension and damage and, by opening a closed fracture, is a potential portal for infection. The occasional septic fracture caused by this technique is an unjustified disaster.

Traction techniques are rarely used. No matter how precisely applied, they are difficult to maintain accurately, especially for uncooperative patients (addicts, alcoholics) or for active students, busy housewives or vigorous children. Countertraction against a splint may be applied through delicate soft tissue, and may cause scarring of adjacent gliding structures. In these difficult cases, a more certain and predictably good functional result is obtained either by gentle closed reduction with percutaneous Kirschner wires as an "internal suture" or by careful gentle open reduction.

Metacarpal Fractures of the Fingers (index, middle, ring, little)

The longitudinal and transverse arches of the hand are essential to normal hand function. They must be restored in the reduction, and maintained during the period of immobilization.

The transverse distal carpal arch, combined with the longitudinal immobile second and third metacarpals, forms the "fixed component" of the hand, a rigid stock from which the rest of the hand is suspended. The metacarpal heads in the distal transverse arch are interconnected by the intermetacarpal ligaments. These might be more accurately termed the intervolar plate ligaments.[14] These ligaments, combined with the hypothenar muscles and the ligaments of the two ulnar carpometacarpal joints, tether the fourth and fifth metacarpals, permitting considerable mobility of the distal transverse arch.

Metacarpal fractures result from axial compression applied to the metacarpal head, from a direct perpendicular force or from torque. The first causes a transverse or short oblique shaft fracture or an impacted fracture through the metacarpal neck ("boxer's fracture"). The second generally produces a transverse simple or comminuted shaft fracture, and the third a spiral fracture.

The longitudinal pull of the flexor tendons and intrinsic muscles may produce telescoping or flexion at the fracture site. The intervolar plate ligament does give some rotational stability to proximal fractures, especially the long and ring metacarpals. If malrotation is present, it must be recognized and corrected (Fig. 11-3). Shortening, when present, is usually not disabling, particularly if it involves the ray of index or little finger.

For reduction and immobilization of metacarpal shaft fractures, the deforming forces are controlled by flexion of the metacarpophalangeal joints,[8,20,54] thus relaxing the extrinsic and intrinsic flexors. Note that this is the position of function for this joint. Once reduced, these fractures are frequently stable in this position and plaster immobilization for 4 to 5 weeks will maintain the reduction (Fig. 11-4).

If the reduction of the diaphyseal fracture is unstable, internal fixation should be used. A percutaneous intramedullary Kirschner wire may be inserted (Fig. 11-5), and the fixation must be protected by plaster mobilization for 4 to 5 weeks. At that time the wire can be removed and gentle, active motion encouraged.

In general, closed treatment of metacarpal shaft fractures is preferred. This will leave the periosteal blood supply relatively undisturbed and minimize scarring and fibrosis of the interosseous muscles and extrinsic tendons. Occasionally, in comminuted fractures, in fractures more than a few days old or in certain oblique fractures with unacceptable shortening or uncontrolled rotation, open reduction and internal fixation with Kirschner wires may be necessary. In such cases, a gently

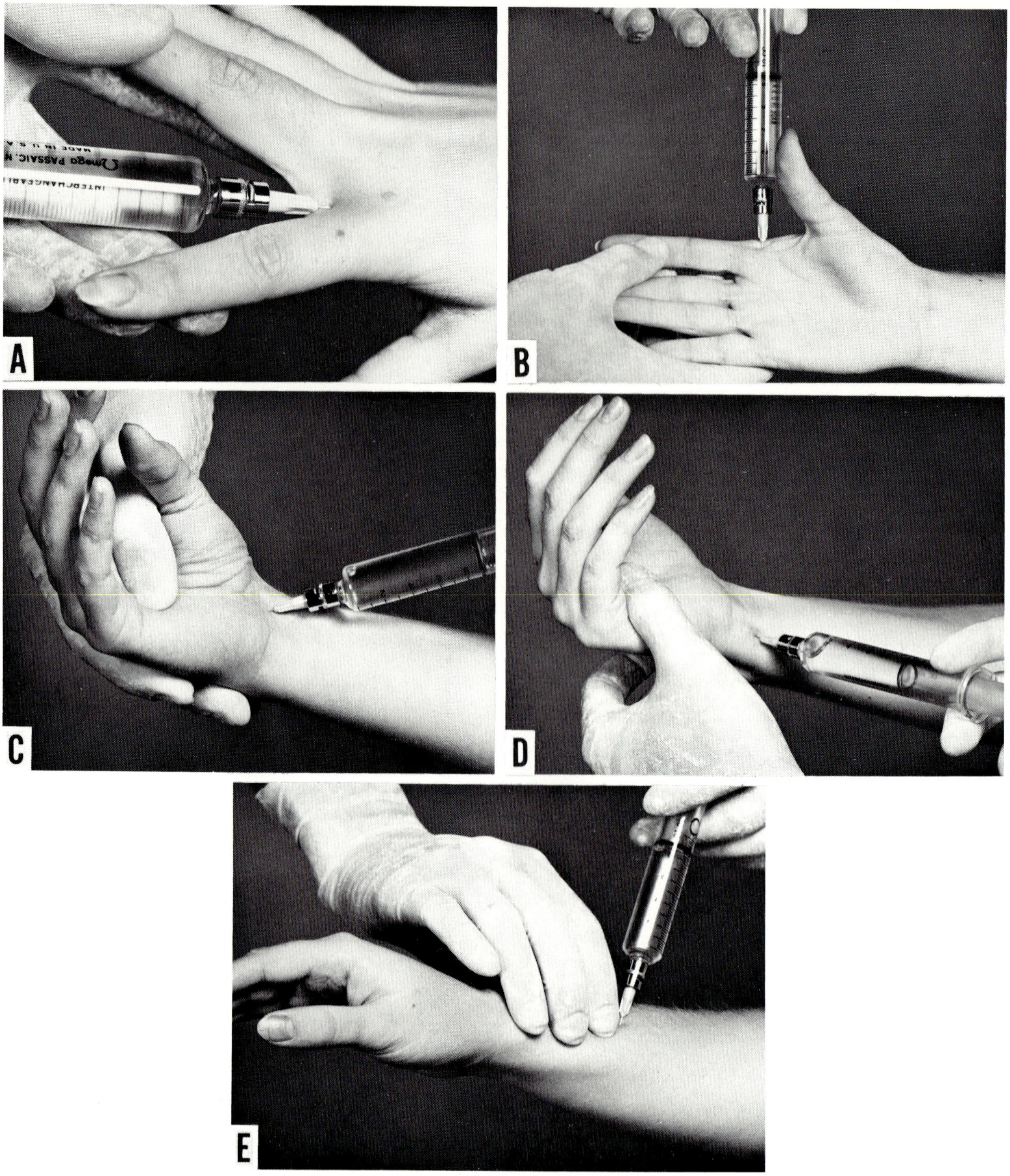

Figure 11-2. *Anesthetic techniques. These techniques are simple and reliable. The block should be performed 15 to 20 minutes before the planned procedure. The authors use 3 to 5 cc of 1 per cent carbocaine without epinephrine, and a 25-gauge needle. No attempt is made to elicit paresthesias.* **A:** *The digital block is best performed introducing the needle just dorsal to the web in the plane of the palm, into the lumbrical canal for 1 to 1.5 cm. This technique is safer and less painful than the traditional "ring block."* **B:** *To block the radial digital nerve to the index finger, the tissues are infiltrated just volar to the metacarpophalangeal joint.* **C:** *The median nerve is blocked at the wrist radial to the palmaris longus. The needle is inserted 1 cm in a dorsal-ulnar-distal direction. Care should be taken not to inject directly into the substance of the nerve.* **D:** *The ulnar nerve is anesthetized 1 cm dorsal and deep to the flexor carpi ulnaris tendon, with the syringe and needle in the plane of the distal radial ulnar joint. Aspiration prior to injection is essential, to be certain the needle is not in the ulnar artery.* **E:** *The main branch of the radial sensory nerve can easily be blocked as it emerges from beneath the brachioradialis, 6 to 8 cm above the radial styloid.*

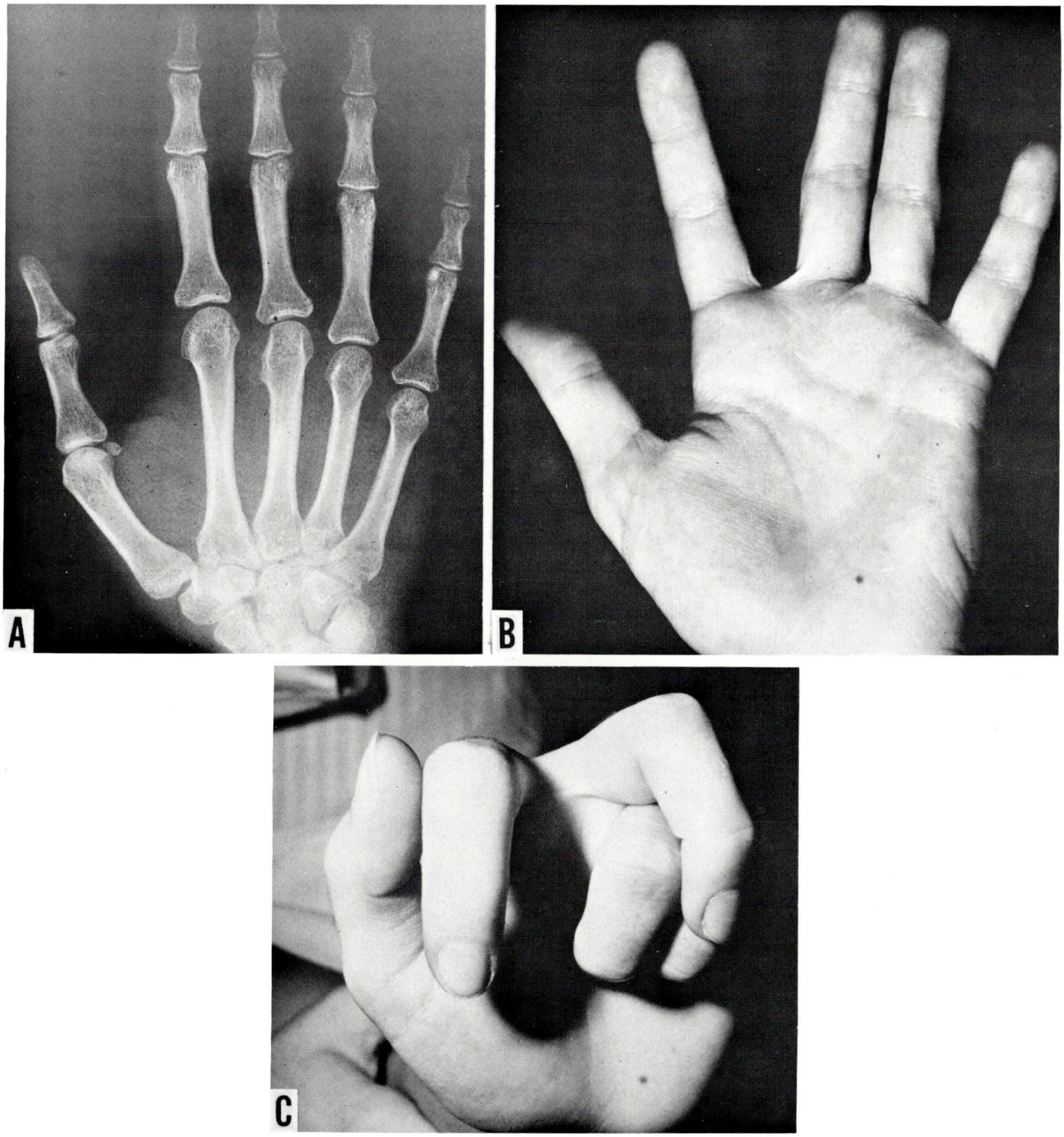

Figure 11-3. *Malunion of the third metacarpal in a 22-year-old female.* **A,B:** *Normal alignment is suggested in extension.* **C:** *The deformity is obvious with flexion.*

curved dorsal longitudinal parametacarpal incision, with lateral subperiosteal exposure, minimizes extensor tendon fixation.

An often unrecognized problem accompanying fractures of the base of the ring and little metacarpals is injury to the motor branch of the ulnar nerve, resulting in intrinsic paralysis of all but the hypothenar musculature. This is most frequently seen as an accompaniment of crushing injuries with the added insults of congestion and ischemia. Many times the nerve injury will not become apparent until the initial edema and induration have subsided and active motion is started.

One type of metacarpal fracture is quite common—the impacted neck fracture or "boxer's fracture." It is often overtreated. Rotational malalignment must be meticulously corrected, yet up to 40° of volar angulation can be accepted, especially

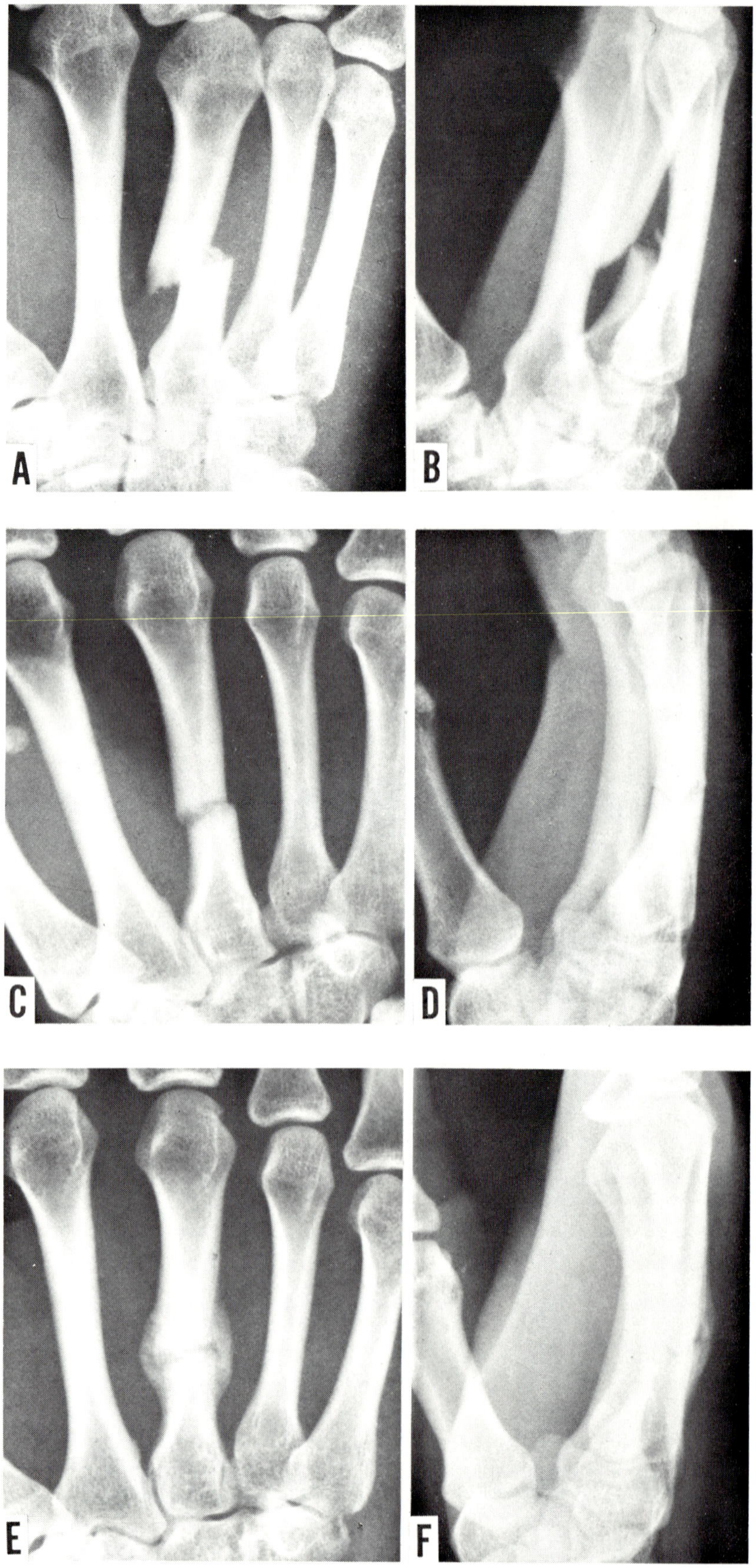

Figure 11-4. *Metacarpal fracture in a 25-year-old female treated with closed reduction.* **A,B:** *Initial x-rays.* **C,D:** *In this case, closed reduction was stable because of the irregularity of the transverse fracture surface, best seen on lateral view.* **E,F:** *Clinical union was present at 6 weeks. As in phalangeal fractures, functional union often precedes loss of "fracture line" on roentgenogram.*

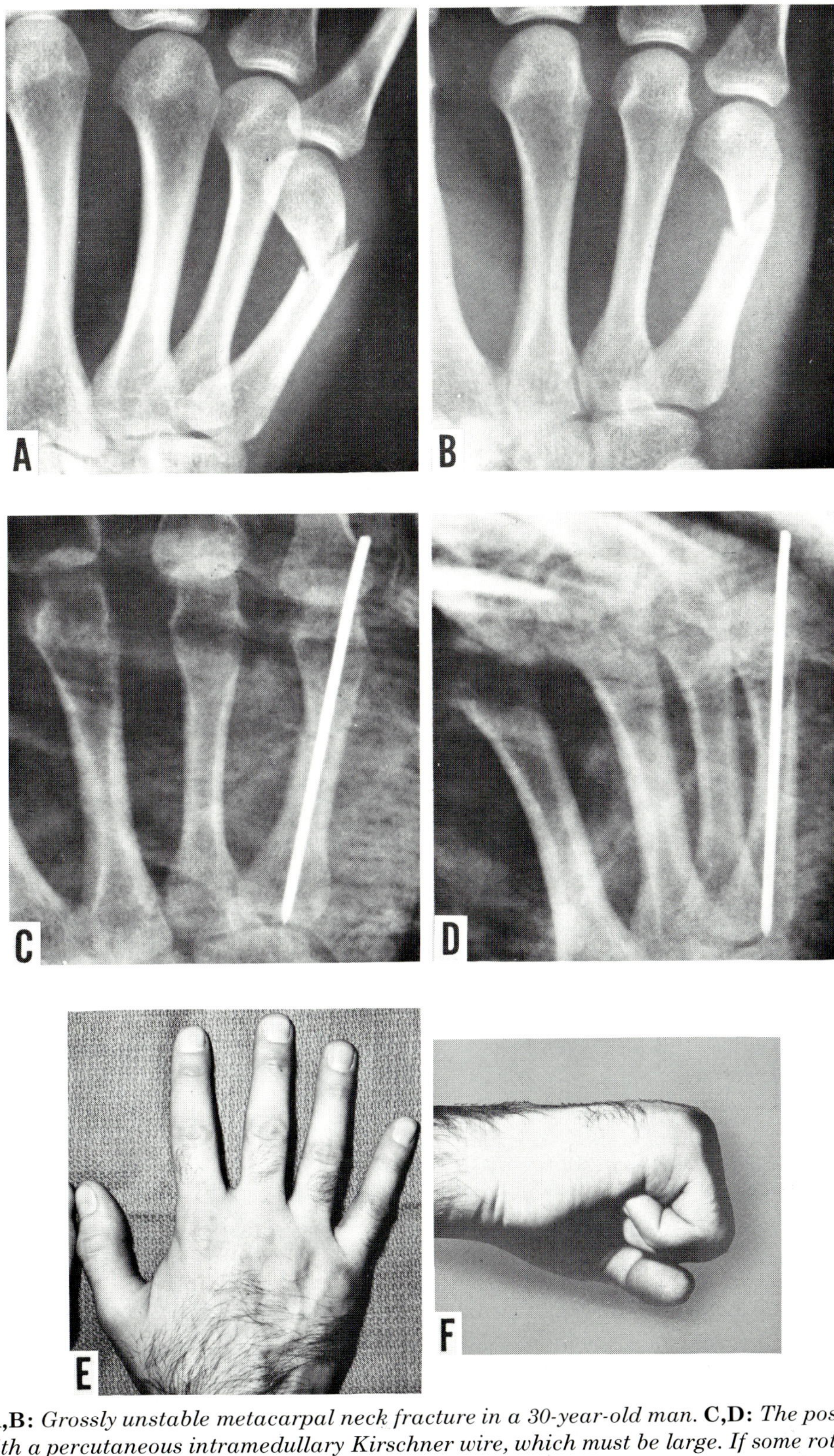

Figure 11-5. **A,B:** *Grossly unstable metacarpal neck fracture in a 30-year-old man.* **C,D:** *The post-reduction x-rays show fixation with a percutaneous intramedullary Kirschner wire, which must be large. If some rotational instability remains, the fixation may be augmented with a smaller oblique percutaneous wire. Note that a plaster dressing is used for external support as well.* **E,F:** *The final range of motion at two months was excellent.*

in the more mobile fourth and fifth metacarpals.[15] It is important to remember that this is an impacted fracture, especially when it is not severely angulated. The less the deformity, the more stable is the fracture. With greater deformity, the reduction is easier but is proportionately less stable. These fractures require four weeks' immobilization in a gauntlet cast with the wrist in 20° extension and the metacarpophalangeal joint in 50 to 60° flexion, leaving the interphalangeal joints free. In order to maintain rotational reduction, it may be necessary to include the adjacent ray in the cast. Only minimal padding is placed between these two digits or the dressing will cause malrotation. If the fracture is unstable, percutaneous Kirschner wires should be used. During immobilization, pressure on the dorsum of the flexed proximal interphalangeal joint to maintain a reduction is contraindicated, for this frequently produces a full-thickness skin slough and varing degrees of boutonniere deformity, as the lateral bands drop volar to the flexion axis of the proximal interphalangeal joint. Such an extreme position has no place in the management of this simple, usually non-disabling fracture. If the fracture is grossly unstable when the hand rests in a position of function, percutaneous Kirschner wires should be used to achieve stability.

The intra-articular metacarpal head fracture can be treated by either open or closed techniques, depending on the details of the particular injury. The congruity of the articular surface with the base of the proximal phalanx must be restored. If closed reduction is attempted, the attachments of the collateral ligaments and volar plate (Chap. 12) can be used to advantage in the manipulation. It should be remembered that a grossly incongruous joint may commit the patient to future arthroplasty or arthrodesis.

There are multiple complications of metacarpal fractures. The metacarpal shaft is embedded within the interosseous muscle and is covered dorsally by the common extensor mechanism. A crush injury to this area sufficient to create fractures may either produce interosseous muscle fibrosis through hemorrhage or ischemia or cause damage directly to the extrinsic extensor mechanism. The extensor mechanism may thus be restrained by either intrinsic muscle tightness or fixation of the extrinsic extensor mechanism to the metacarpal callus. The fractures may thereby cause disastrous loss of flexion at either the metacarpophalangeal or interphalangeal joints. This loss of motion may be further compounded by secondary collateral ligament tightness from malposition. These complications can be minimized by gentle and appropriate reduction, careful application of dressings and casts and adequate elevation during the phase of tissue edema.

Malrotation or dorsal bony prominences can occur if fractures are not well treated. Malrotation may well require osteotomy and bone grafting (Fig. 11-3). The dorsal bony prominence may cause tenting of the extensor mechanism, with binding at the fracture site, and loss of flexion at the metacarpophalangeal joint with alteration of the entire flexion-extension balance in the ray. Moderate prominence of the metacarpal head in the palm does not cause appreciable symptoms, even with power grasp.

Non-union may be the case following fractures associated with sepsis, segmental bone loss, insufficient immobilization of an unstable fracture or inadequate soft tissue coverage. In the latter, resurfacing with an abdominal pedicle may be needed before attempting to restore bony stability. After adequate debridement a gap may exist between the metacarpal head-neck distally and the metaphysis proximally. This may be filled with an iliac bone graft or a bone spacer fashioned from one or more Kirschner wires.

"Bone spacing" is accomplished by proximal and distal transfixion, the interposition of crossed Kirschner wires or a single wire bent to prevent collapse with loss of length. When the soft tissue coverage is adequate and the circulation sufficient, bone grafting can be done. An iliac bone graft is recommended using the technique described by Littler.[26]

Proximal Phalangeal Fractures of the Digits

Fractures of the proximal phalanx are potentially the most disabling in the hand, and, unfortunately, are often tragically underestimated in importance. Unless they are thoughtfully assessed, anatomically reduced and properly immobilized, function of the entire longitudinal unit may be severely compromised.

The proximal phalanx enters into critical proximal and distal articulations. Restricted movement of either is serious; restriction of both is a disaster. Maximum attention must be given to the details of reduction and immobilization.

The phalanx is ensheathed on the dorsal and lateral surfaces by the exquisitely balanced extensor mechanism and on the volar aspect by the flexor tendons. The flexor and extensor tendon systems are immediately adjacent to the periosteum, and thus may readily become adherent to even small amounts of callus from a less-than-perfect reduction. When this occurs, tendon fixation at the fracture site may disrupt the flexor-extensor balance, resulting in a significant loss of joint movement. The post-reduction immobilization must be in the position of function. If this position must be compromised to maintain a reduction, internal stabilization with Kirschner wires is advisable. As discussed below, this may be percutaneous or at open reduction.

Malrotation is a common problem in proximal phalangeal fractures and must be specifically checked. In flexion, the fingertips should cascade in slight overlap, pointing toward the proximal scaphoid.

The mechanism of the midshaft and distal fractures may be a torque resulting in a spiral fracture (Fig. 11-6) or a direct blow causing a transverse fracture. Another common type of fracture is the transverse or short oblique fracture of the base of the proximal phalanx, which develops a characteristic hyperextension deformity (Fig. 11-7).

The deforming forces of the intrinsic and extrinsic systems must be recognized and utilized in controlling these fractures. The proximal fragment is flexed by the intrinsics. The longitudinal pull of the extrinsic flexors and extensors creates a compression force which extends the distal fragment and results in angulation with a volar apex.

If the fracture is oblique or spiral, additional problems may occur. The spike of the proximal fragment may slide under a collateral ligament or into the volar retrocondylar fossa, severely disrupting the proximal interphalangeal motion (Fig. 11-8). Furthermore, the oblique spiral fracture under axial compression will rotate as the spiral fracture surfaces override, resulting in malrotation as well as shortening (Fig. 11-6).

Fractures near the proximal interphalangeal joint are often grossly unstable. The distal fragment frequently cannot be adequately stabilized by a cast. The reduction must be maintained by Kirschner wires (Fig. 11-9).

In hyperextension fractures of the base, the reduction may be relatively simple and often can be maintained by flexion of the distal fragment and metacarpophalangeal joint. However, when obliquity or loss of dorsal cortical fragments compro-

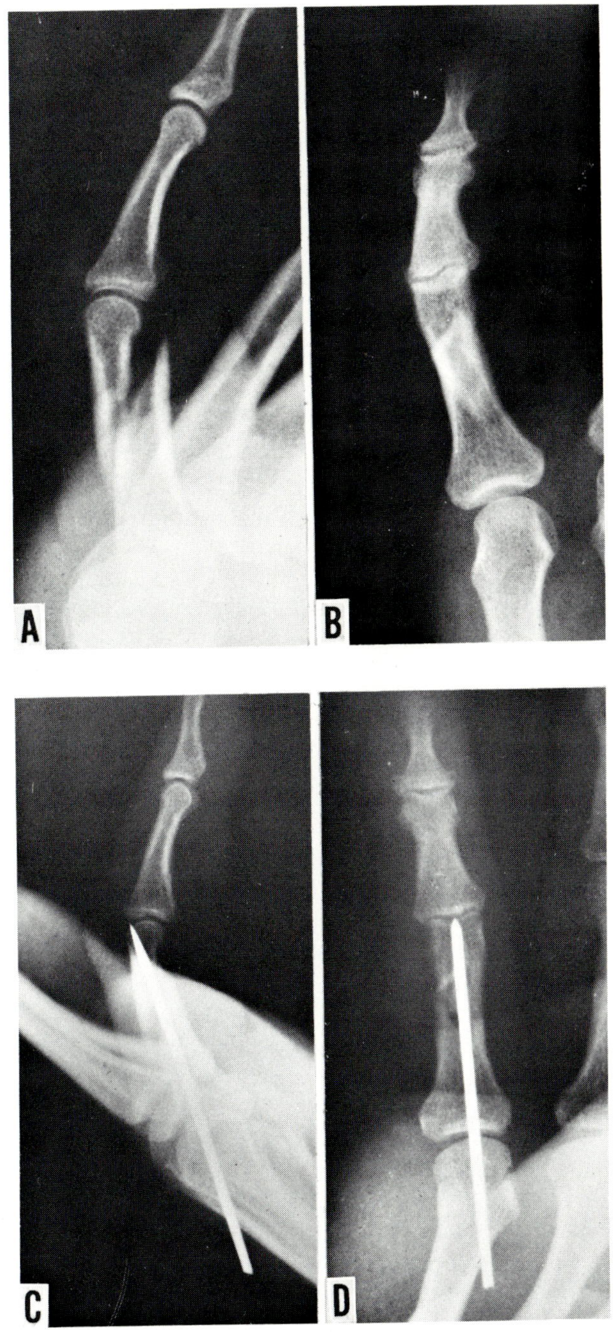

Figure 11-6. A,B: *Grossly unstable spiral fracture of the proximal phalanx treated by closed reduction and percutaneous Kirschner wire fixation.* **C,D:** *Note the reduction with maintenance of length and alignment by the single longitudinal wire, which must be introduced the full length of the phalanx. It is critical that the hand be immobilized in a position of function. Note that less-than-perfect reduction was accepted, as length and alignment were restored and the distal spike of the proximal fragment well removed from the critical retrocondylar area (see text and Fig. 11-8). The excellent result is shown in Figure 11-6***E–I.**

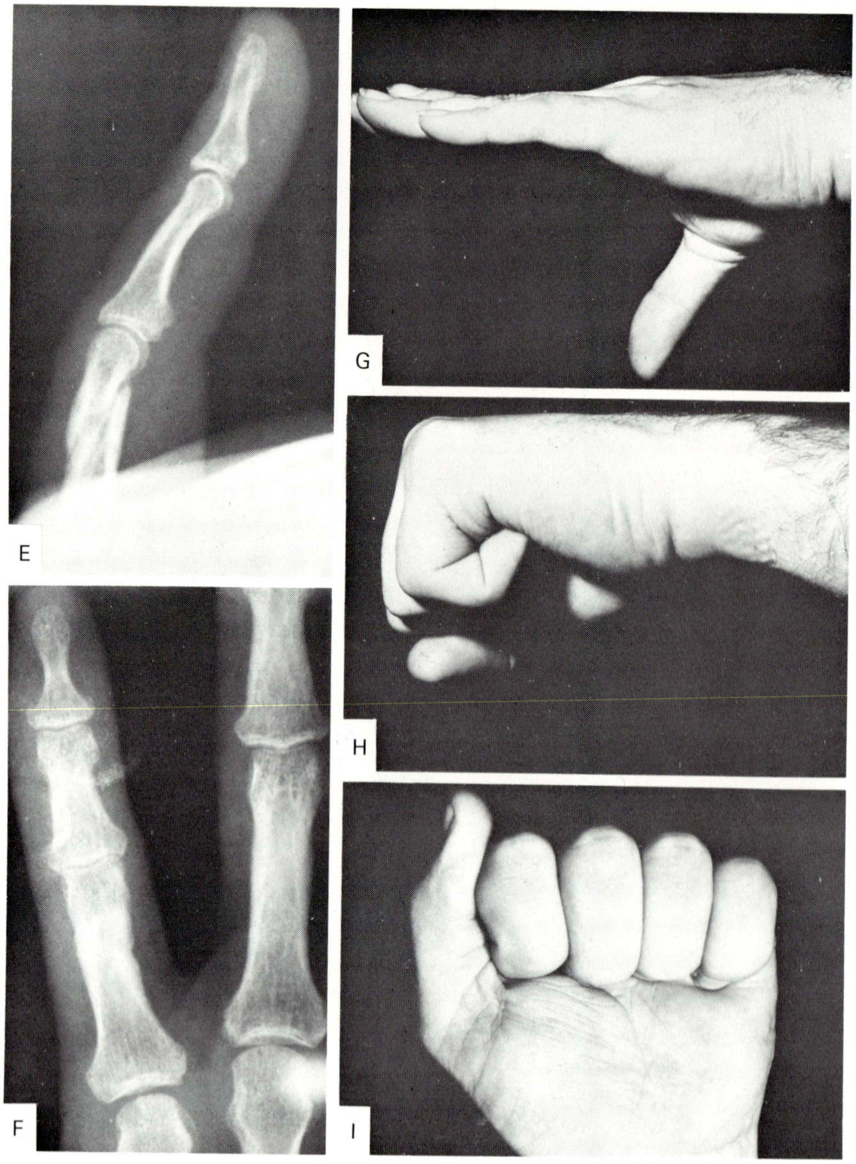

Figure 11-6. E,F: *Bony union occurred without loss of position.* **G,H,I:** *Full range of motion was achieved four months after injury.*

mises stability, percutaneous internal fixation may be necessary (Figs. 11-7, 11-10).

The technique of closed reduction of all these fracture types is similar. First, length is regained by longitudinal traction applied with the metacarpophalangeal joint slightly flexed. With the traction still maintained, the finger is then flexed 90° at the metacarpophalangeal joint to remove the deforming force of the intrinsics. Such flexion also tightens the metacarpophalangeal collateral ligaments, effectively stabilizing the proximal fragment.[33] The finger is also flexed 90° at the proximal interphalangeal joint to relax the extrinsic flexors.[8,20,54] With this maneuver, aided by the circumferential support of the closely enveloping extensor mechanism, reductions may be remarkably anatomical. However, should position be lost with release of proximal interphalangeal flexion and traction, the reduction must be maintained with percutaneous Kirschner wires, placed either longitudinally (Figs. 11-6, 11-7), obliquely (Fig. 11-9) or transversely (Fig. 11-11).

As mentioned, a phalangeal fracture must be reduced accurately. This can often be achieved with the above closed technique. If not, then a careful open reduction should be done.

The surgeon must fully appreciate the delicate anatomy, since a well intended but poorly executed incision may increase the functional loss. As has been detailed in the literature, the intrinsics and the extrinsic extensors are a dual system for the extension of the interphalangeal joints. Simple

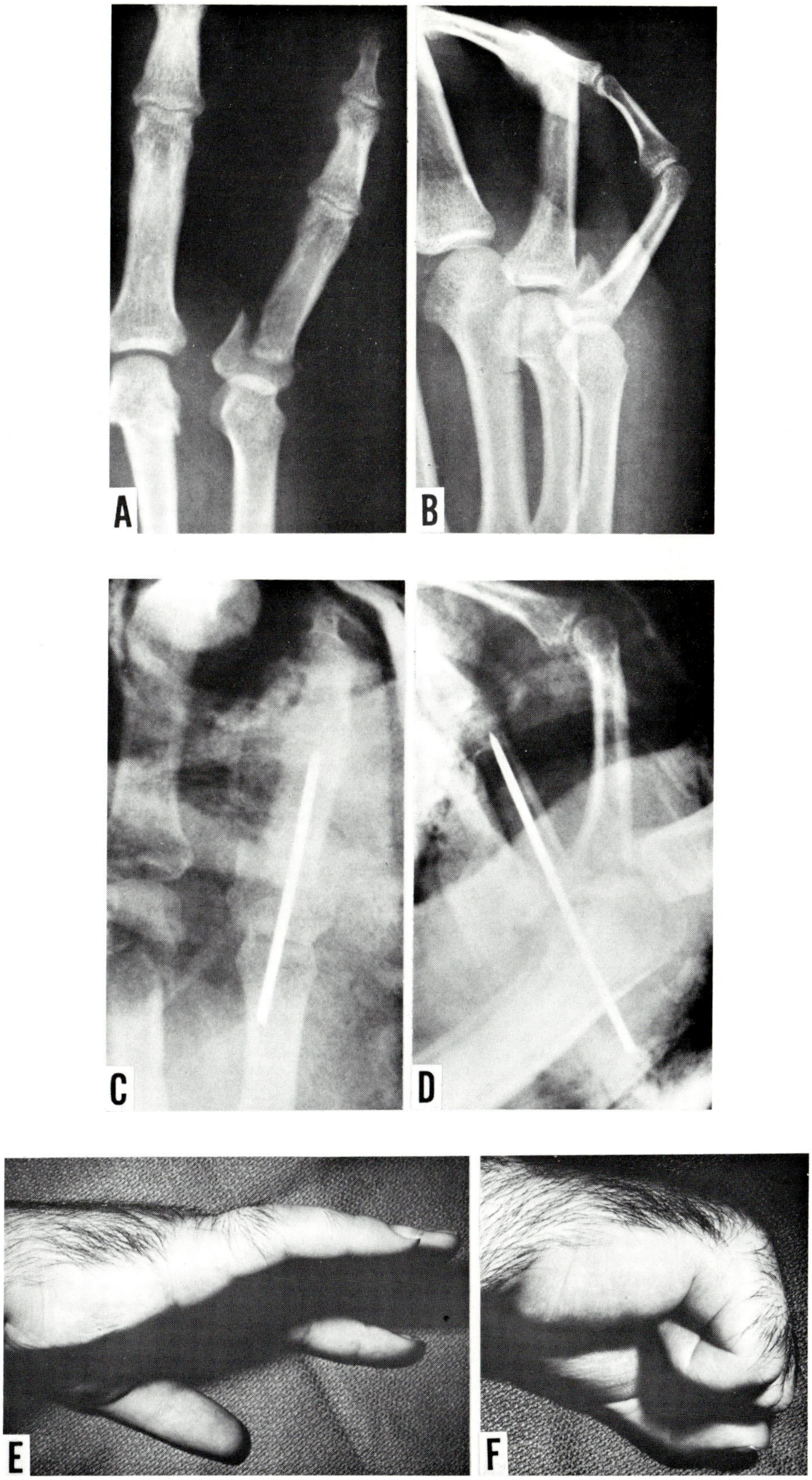

Figure 11-7. A,B: *Fractures of the base of the proximal phalanx are often quite unstable.* **C,D:** *Excellent fixation of the closed reduction may be obtained with a percutaneous Kirschner wire inserted through or next to the metacarpal head and down the full length of the phalanx.* **E,F:** *The pain-free functional range of motion with union is seen two months following injury.*

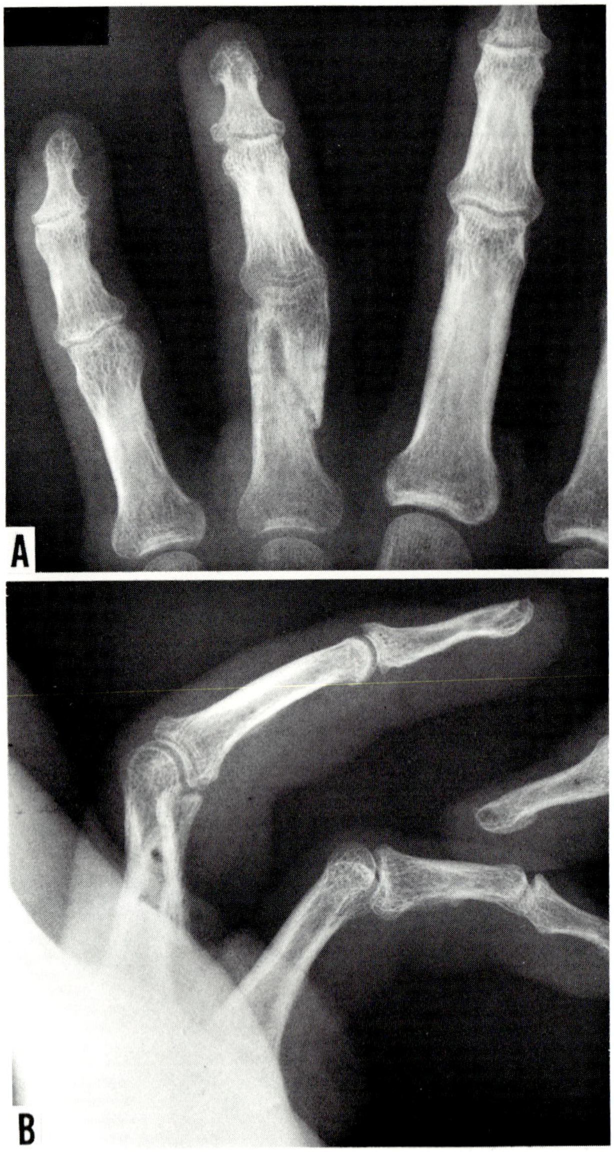

Figure 11-8. *A 30-year-old male with a malunion of proximal phalangeal fracture. The bony block to proximal interphalangeal joint flexion is seen on the lateral roentgenogram. The distal spike of the proximal fragment has healed in the retrocondylar area. The results of joint reconstruction are less satisfactory than those from proper primary care.*

incision through these structures causes additional fixation to the underlying callus and bone, compounding the functional loss from the injury. A portion of either should be excised to achieve optimal exposure, but limits of the tissue removed must be exact. It should be noted that, once exposed, the fracture is often deceptively difficult to reduce anatomically. It is helpful to proceed through the maneuvers normally used for a closed reduction while the fracture fragments are under direct vision. Frequently, with this atraumatic maneuver to relax the deforming structures, an anatomical reduction can be obtained.

The reduced fracture is immobilized in plaster for 3 to 4 weeks, with the adjacent joints maintained in a physiological position. Then the wires are removed and active range of motion exercises are started. It is advisable to tape the injured ray to an adjacent one for protection for an additional 2 to 3 weeks.

Complications of a fracture of this phalanx are numerous. The most frequent, and the most difficult to treat, are those with scarring of the extensor mechanism and proportionate loss of motion. Intrinsic or extrinsic releases can be done, but are inferior substitutes for proper primary care. Adherent flexor tendons will disrupt hand function and may cause secondary changes in adjacent joints. Flexor tendon releases can be done, but results are unpredictable. If the tip of a proximal oblique fracture fragment heals in a position under the collateral ligament or in the retrocondylar fossa of the proximal-interphalangeal joint (Fig. 11-8), restoration of full joint motion is unlikely. Attempts to release collateral ligaments and the volar plate and to remove bony blocks are no substitutes for good primary care. Should the fracture heal with rotational malalignment, correction through a proximal phalangeal or metacarpal osteotomy may be considered. The amount of correction of rotational deformity obtainable by metacarpal osteotomy is limited by the transverse intervolar plate ligament, especially in the long or ring ray.

Non-unions are found in open fractures with infections, and in poor reductions with inadequate immobilization. Treatment is with bone grafting and Kirschner wire fixation. The prognosis for a fully functional finger is poor indeed. It is fortunate that non-unions are rare if the above program is followed.

Fractures of the Middle Phalanx

The middle phalanx, acted upon by a much less complicated flexor-extensor tendon system, poses a less complex anatomical problem than does the proximal phalanx. However, as this phalanx is composed principally of cortical bone, fractures may be more difficult to transfix with Kirschner wires, and may be longer in healing.

The mechanisms and types of fracture are simi-

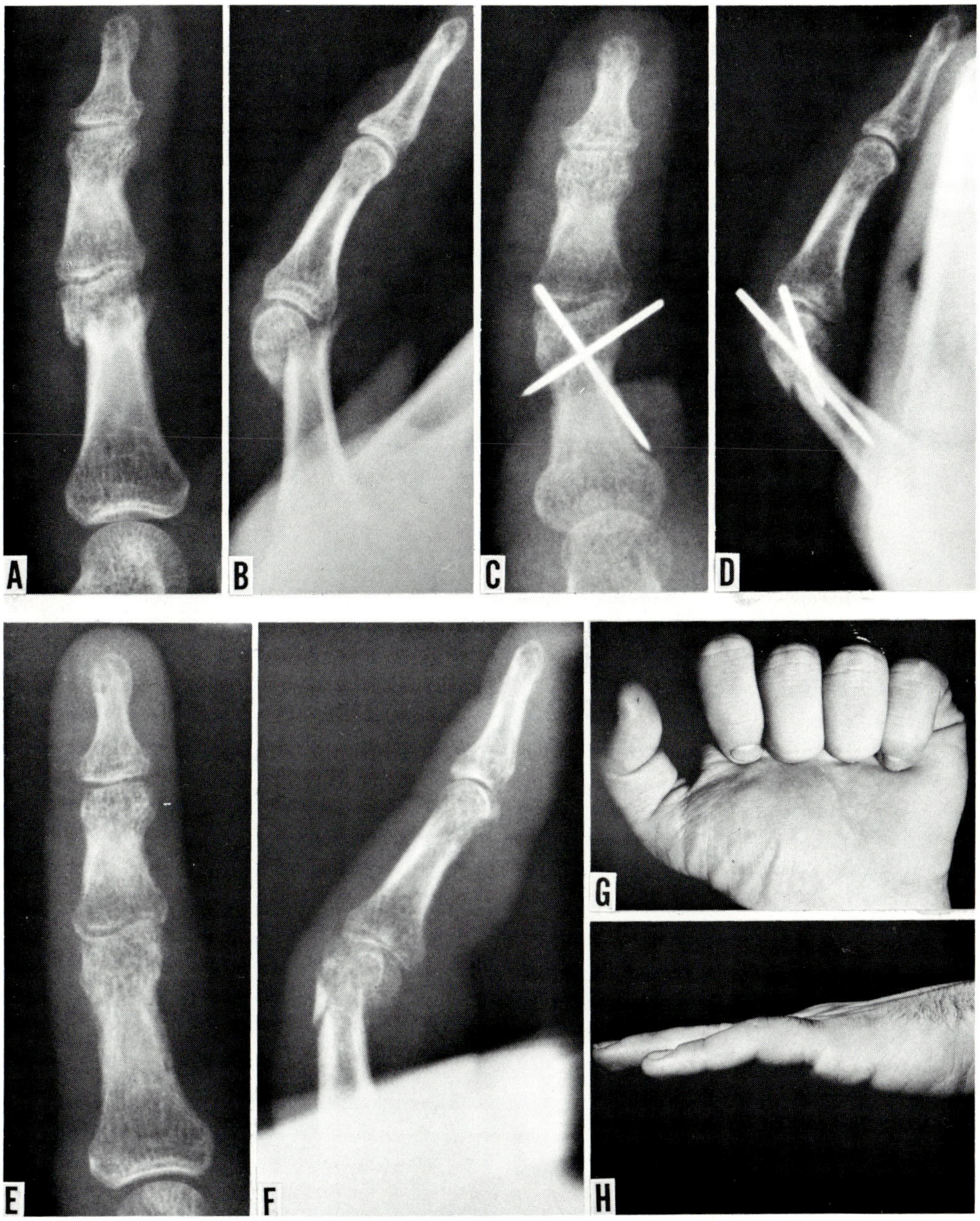

Figure 11-9. *Fracture of the distal portion of the proximal phalanx.* **A,B:** *This grossly unstable fracture in the small finger could not be controlled by external support.* **C,D:** *Closed reduction and percutaneous Kirschner wire fixation were followed by plaster immobilization in a position of function.* **E,F:** *Solid union has occurred by two months.* **G,H:** *Pain-free range of motion was nearly normal at four months after injury.*

lar to those of the proximal phalanx. However, since it is a more distal bone, it is relatively less protected by adjacent rays. The proximal interphalangeal joint absorbs much of the energy delivered to this phalanx, often dislocating and thus sparing the phalanx from fracture. Middle phalangeal fractures are usually in the narrow midshaft portion and may be either transverse or oblique.

The flexor superficialis insertion into the volar base of the middle phalanx exerts a strong flexor force on the proximal fragment, overpowering the extensor force of the central tendon. The extensor mechanism distal to the fracture includes the dorsally converging lateral bands and the oblique retinacular ligaments, passing volar to the axis of rotation at the proximal interphalangeal joint and dorsal to that of the distal interphalangeal joint. These distal structures have no insertion on the

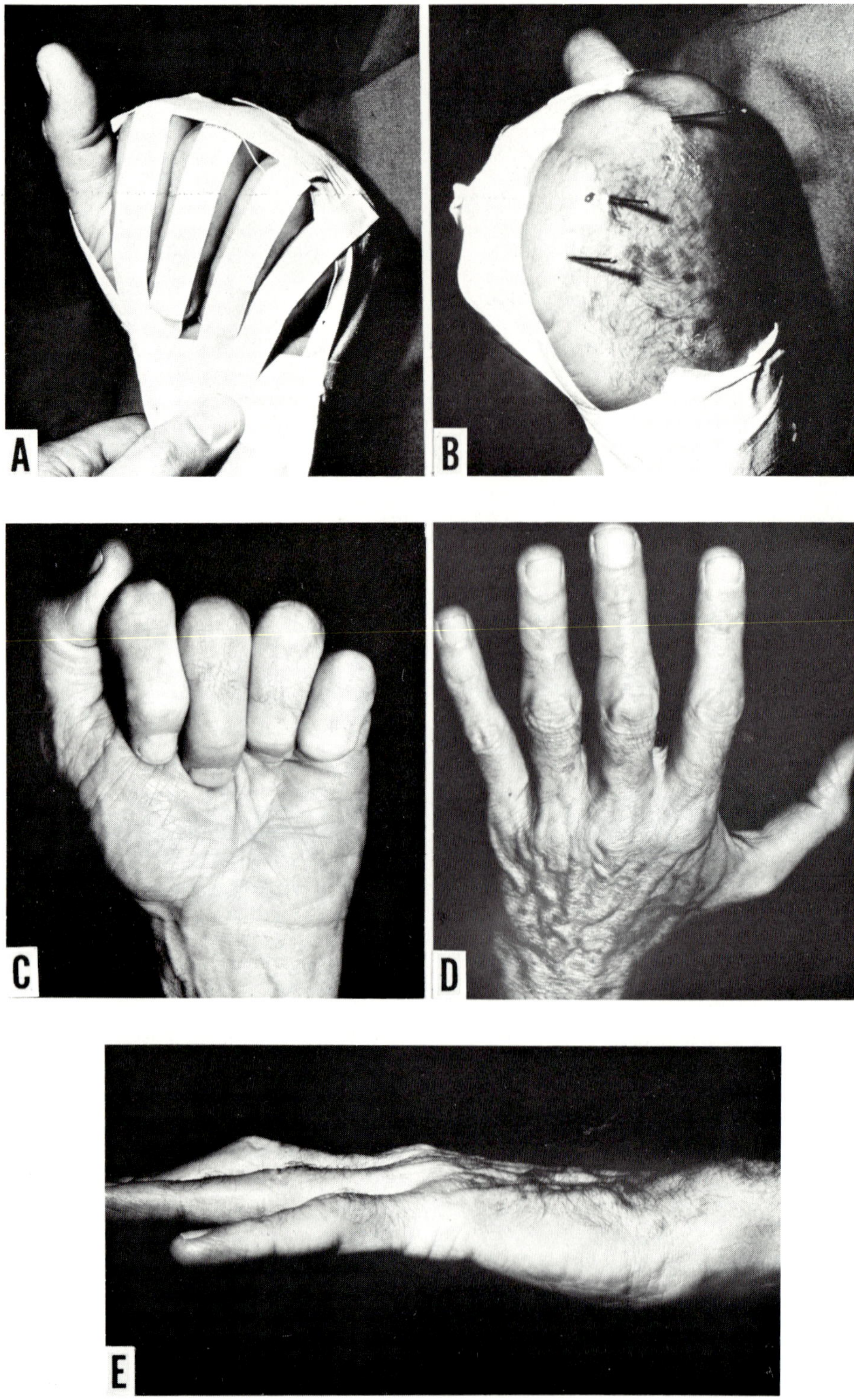

Figure 11-10. *Technique of Kirschner wire fixation. A 55-year-old professional pianist had sustained fractures of the medial three proximal phalanges which were grossly unstable.* **A,B:** *The closed reductions were held temporarily with adhesive tape dressing while roentgenograms were taken to confirm position. Kirschner wires were then introduced, the tape was removed and the hand was immobilized in a position of function.* **C,D,E:** *Normal hand function resulted.*

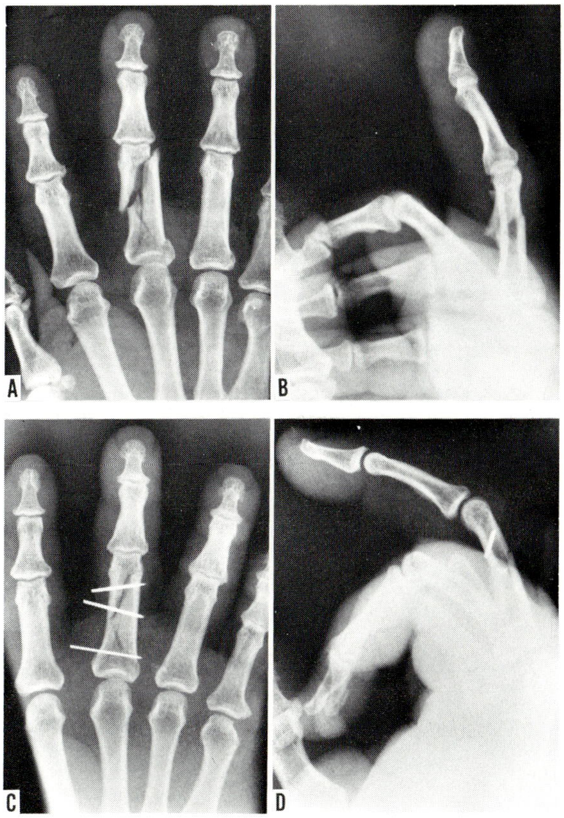

Figure 11-11. A–D. *Comminuted fracture of proximal phalanx. This comminuted unstable fracture required open reduction and Kirschner wire fixation. An excellent functional result was obtained, as accurate bony coaptation will minimize scarring of the extensor mechanism to the underlying callus (see text).*

middle phalanx and exert their force on the distal fragment via the distal interphalangeal joint. The resultant deforming forces produce flexion of the proximal fragment and extension of the distal fragment (Fig. 11–12). Axial compression by the profundus tendon and the extensor tendons may cause overriding or further angulation at the fracture site.

Closed reduction (Fig. 11-12) is almost always possible, providing ample longitudinal traction precedes flexion of the distal fragment to align it with the proximal fragment. Gentleness is important to spare any intact periosteum. These fractures heal slowly and every attempt should be made to maintain as much periosteal continuity as possible so that the healing will not be further delayed. The periosteum may also provide a delicate hinge against which to reduce the fracture as well as protecting the extensor mechanism from callus entrapment. Immobilization is for 4 to 6 weeks, with the interphalangeal joints flexed 15° to 20° and the metacarpophalangeal joints 50°.

If the transverse fracture is unstable, longitudinal or oblique percutaneous Kirschner wires should be inserted. If the unstable fracture is spiral or oblique the major problem may be malrotation, by the same mechanism as in the proximal phalangeal fractures. In such cases, transverse Kirschner wires should be used either percutaneously or at operation, after accurate reduction has been accomplished. Occasionally in comminuted or certain compound fractures, open reduction must be performed.

Fractures of the Distal Phalanx

These fractures are very common. The mechanism is usually a crush or a high-speed shearing force.

The distal anatomy is rather simple. The flexor and extensor tendons insert just distal to the distal interphalangeal joint. Beyond these tendons, the bone is covered by the nail matrix dorsally and the pulp volarly.

Treatment of these injuries, if the fracture is undisplaced, is primarily directed to the adjacent soft tissues. A subungual hematoma may be very painful, and usually should be drained early. Following cleansing of the nail, a red-hot paper clip is touched to the nail, promptly melting a sterile drainage tract to the hematoma.

Note that the phalanx is just beneath the nail matrix. This technique must be aseptic as such drainage creates a compound fracture. The pulp may be taut with edema or hematoma and very painful. The finger should have a gentle supportive dressing with a splint protection for comfort.

Non-union and significant deformities of the distal phalanx may be found with displaced fractures (Fig. 11-13). The most common such complication is interposition of the nail matrix between the fracture fragments. This is often masked by a partially avulsed nail. The interposed matrix flap displaces the distal fragment volarward. The result is an unsightly bulbous fingertip with a chronic granulomatous mass arising through the nail bed from the open fracture site. Osteomyelitis may occur. The problem will persist until the interposed matrix is removed and the fracture fragments are realigned. Reduction usually must be maintained with a longitudinal Kirschner wire.

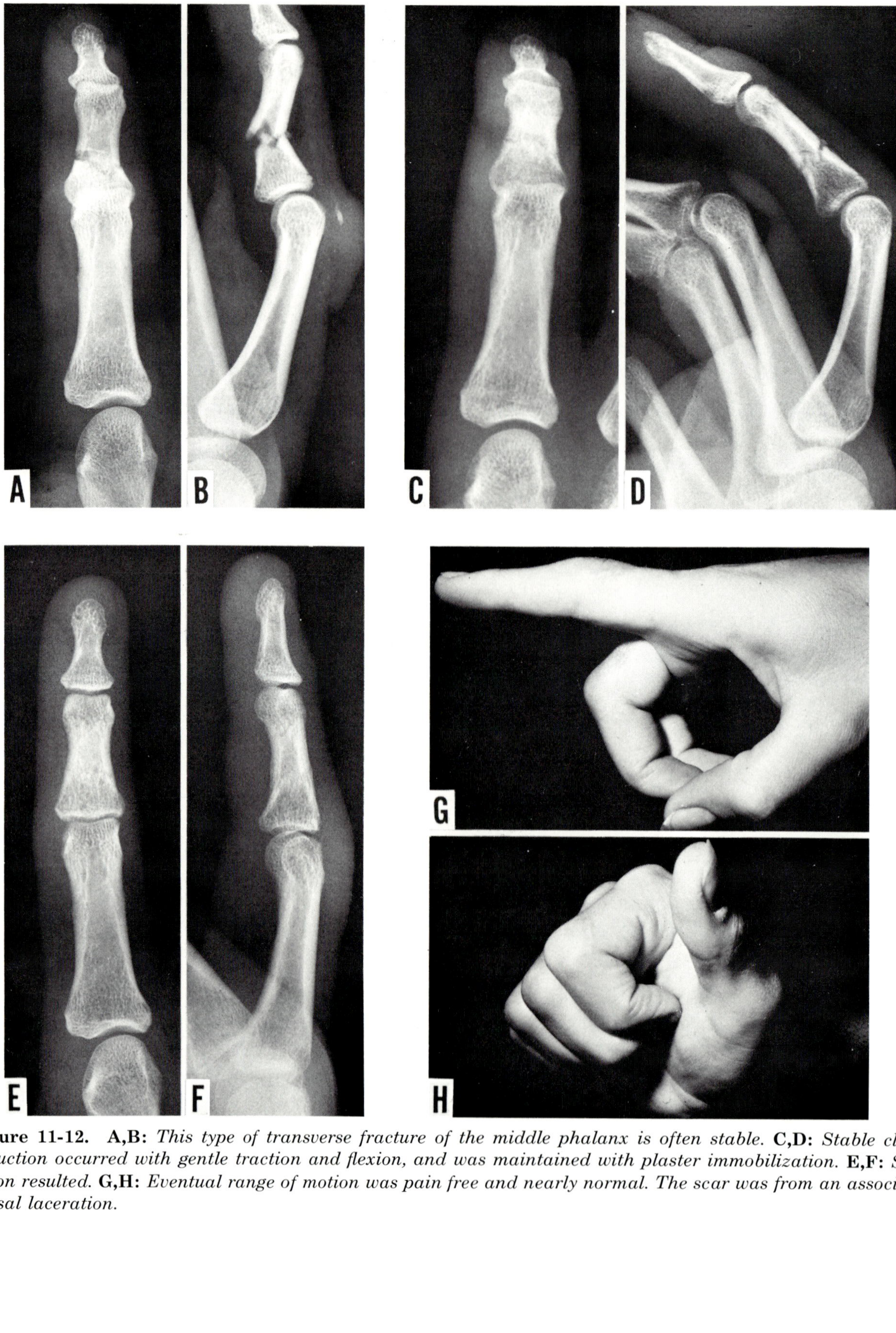

Figure 11-12. **A,B:** *This type of transverse fracture of the middle phalanx is often stable.* **C,D:** *Stable closed reduction occurred with gentle traction and flexion, and was maintained with plaster immobilization.* **E,F:** *Solid union resulted.* **G,H:** *Eventual range of motion was pain free and nearly normal. The scar was from an associated dorsal laceration.*

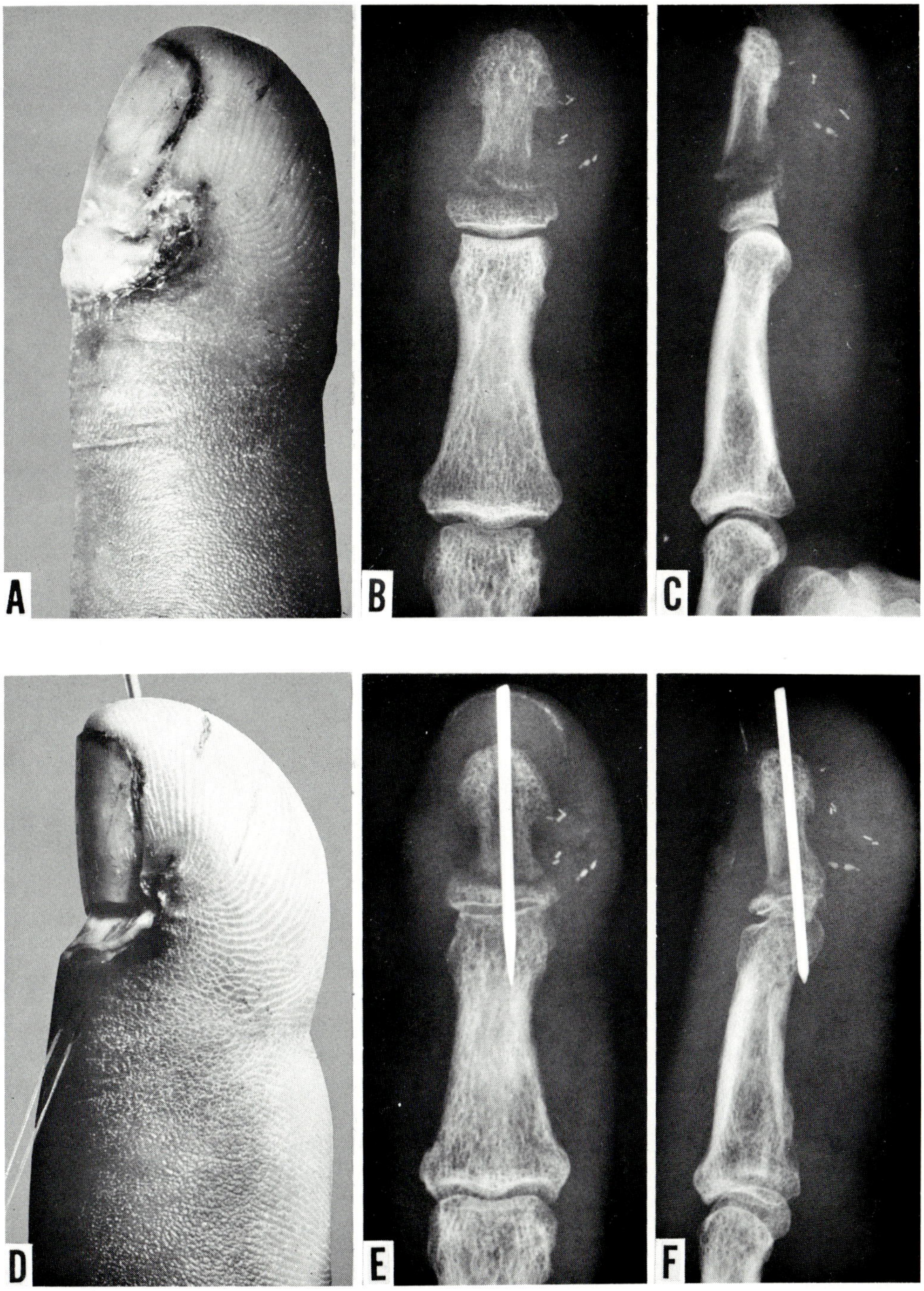

Figure 11-13. *Fracture of distal phalanx with interposed nail matrix. Non-union and chronic infection occur in open fractures of the distal phalanx if nail matrix is allowed to remain interposed.* **A:** *Appearance of such a fingertip is characteristic.* **B,C:** *Roentgenograms demonstrate the changes from interposed matrix, infection and non-union.* **D:** *Note the marked change in contour of fingertip with reduction.* **E,F:** *Reduction should be secured for three weeks with a single Kirschner wire. With adequate debridement, accurate reduction, rigid fixation and appropriate antibiotics, the infection quickly resolves.*

Fractures of the Proximal Phalanx of the Thumb

The treatment of this injury is easier than that for fractures of the proximal phalanx of a finger. The motion of the adjacent joints is not as essential to the function of the ray. The extensor mechanism, although analogous, is not so complex, there being only a single distal joint.

These fractures are usually the result of a direct blow or crush injury. A torque or angulation force will usually be absorbed by the mobility of the thumb or will disrupt the metacarpophalangeal joint, sparing the proximal phalanx. The intrinsic muscles tend to deform the fracture by flexing the proximal fragment. However, this may be minimal since, unlike the fingers, the thumb often has a separate extensor acting on the proximal phalanx. The axial pull of the extrinsic flexor and extensor tendons will telescope, angulate or (if the fracture is oblique-spiral) rotate the fragments.

Closed reduction is usually successful. The thumb is immobilized for four weeks with each joint in a neutral position. If the reduction is unstable, more often the case with oblique or spiral fractures, percutaneous pins or open reduction may be necessary.

Fractures of the Thumb Metacarpal (excluding Bennett's fracture)

The proper projection of the thumb is essential to hand function. Because of the independence and mobility of the thumb with its unique basal joint, more deformity can be accepted in thumb metacarpal fractures than in other metacarpal fractures without compromising hand function.

Fractures of the thumb metacarpal are less common than those of the fingers. Though the thumb is more exposed and therefore receives more trauma, its mobility dissipates much of the force. Fractures of the shaft are usually the result of direct blows or crushing. Distally applied torque or angulation will cause metacarpophalangeal dislocation before metacarpal fracture.

Thumb metacarpal shaft fractures are subject to more complex deforming forces than other metacarpals. Although not all of the intrinsic mechanism spans the fracture, the adductor pollicis, abductor pollicis brevis, and flexor pollicis brevis muscles flex the distal fragment. The long flexors and extensors will cause some telescoping and angulation of the fragments, although this is considerably limited by the bulk of thenar muscles. The abductor pollicis longus may rock the proximal fragment of a shaft fracture into abduction. There are no adjacent metacarpals for internal splints and no intervolar plate ligament to control rotation. However, the bulk of the thenar muscles will usually prevent excess displacement and will also decrease the scarring of tendons to the fracture callus.

The reduction of transverse shaft fractures can usually be performed closed and, with well-applied plaster, may be maintained without percutaneous wires. If the fracture surface forms an oblique spiral, however, shortening may be accompanied by a rotational malalignment. In such cases, percutaneous Kirschner wires may be needed. In the evaluation of the reduction, it is the projection of the thumb that is critical. The arcs of abduction-adduction, flexion-extension and opposition must not be comprised in the final result.

Fractures of the proximal metacarpal (Fig. 11-14) are more difficult to treat. The proximal fragment with its intact articular surface is stabilized by the ligaments of the carpometacarpal joint. The distal fragment will be pulled proximally by all of the extrinsic and intrinsic muscles of the thumb. This distal fragment will also ride laterally and be supinated by the combined pull of the extrinsic extensors.

If seen promptly after injury, reduction is simple with traction, abduction and pronation of the distal fragment. Maintenance of the reduction, however, is not easy and usually requires percutaneous fixation with two oblique Kirschner wires. These are passed proximally ulnarward, and dorsally first through the distal fragment, then through the proximal fragment and into the carpi. If treatment is delayed, however, closed reduction and percutaneous wire fixation are diffcult. The massive swelling which accompanies this fracture may obscure the landmarks and make accurate palpation of the fracture site very difficult.

Bennett's Fracture

Bennett's fracture[1,2,3] distinctly differs from the proximal shaft fractures. It is an intra-articular fracture-dislocation, in effect an avulsion injury with the small medial beak fragment remaining attached to the deep ulnar ligament. Reduction

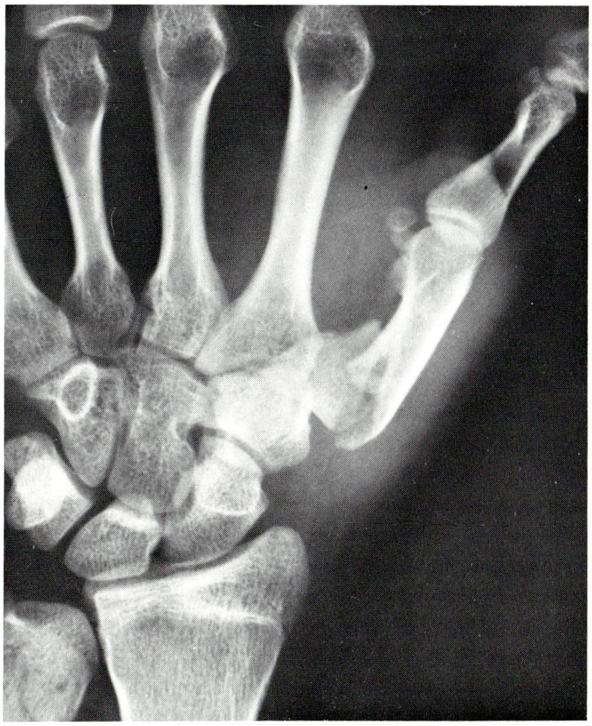

Figure 11-14. *Fracture of proximal thumb metacarpal. This fracture should be compared to the Bennett's fracture seen in Figure 11-15. Note that the articular portion of the thumb metacarpal remains in its normal relationship to the greater multiangular. Closed reduction can be performed in these cases with percutaneous Kirschner wire fixation. Because the articular surface of the basal joint and its ligamentous attachments remain normal, an excellent functional result without resultant osteoarthritis or instability can be anticipated.*

must be perfect, for it is an articular surface which is being reconstituted.

The deforming forces are the extrinsic extensors and the abductor pollicis longus, combining to cause a lateral and proximal subluxation of the major portion of the metacarpal, which will be supinated as well.

Occasionally, an anatomical joint surface can be restored by closed reduction and maintained with percutaneous Kirschner wires passed from the distal fragment into the carpus. An accurate roentgenographic evaluation of this reduction is difficult. Superimposition of the carpal bones and the thumb's projection make the important true posteroanterior and lateral views somewhat elusive.

Open reduction (Fig. 11-15) is indicated where satisfactory restoration of the metacarpal articular surface has not been achieved. With the basal joint exposed, the technique of Gedda and Mobert[18,19] is used. A Kirschner wire passed through the base of the thenar eminence transfixes the small fragment. Then the major distal fragment is reduced and the wire advanced into the large metacarpal fragment.

After reduction, the hand must be immobilized for 4 to 5 weeks. The pins are then removed and gentle active range of motion exercises started. The thumb should be protected between exercise periods for another three weeks.

Carpal Fractures

With severe trauma to the wrist, the most common injuries to the carpus are the lunate and perilunate dislocations and fractures of the scaphoid.[5] A detailed discussion of car-

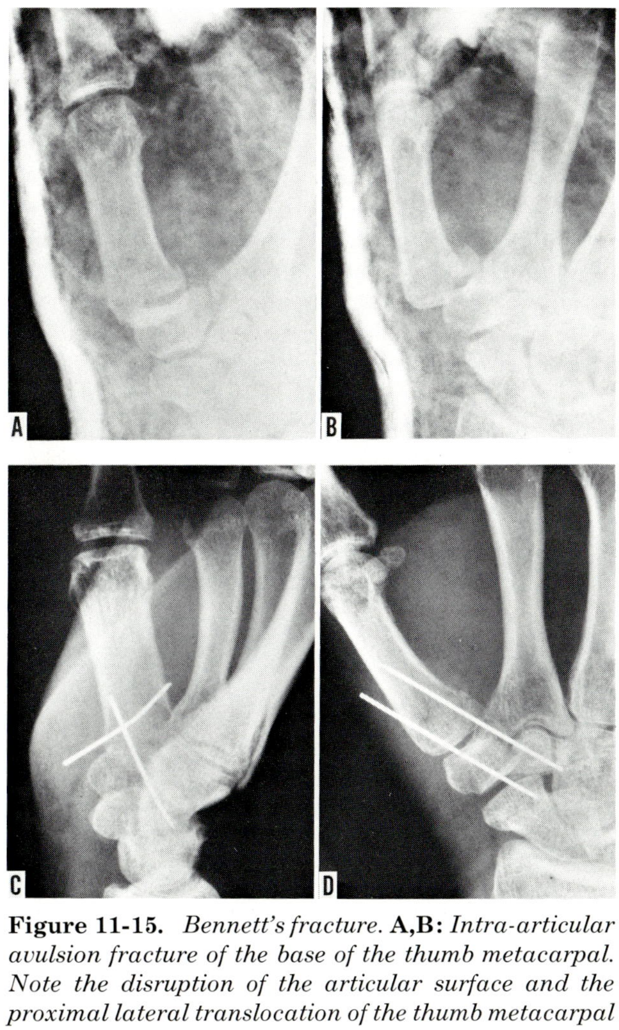

Figure 11-15. *Bennett's fracture.* **A,B:** *Intra-articular avulsion fracture of the base of the thumb metacarpal. Note the disruption of the articular surface and the proximal lateral translocation of the thumb metacarpal shaft.* **C,D:** *Excellent reductions are possible by open reduction. Restoration of the articular surface is essential (see text).*

pal injuries is beyond the scope of this chapter. The writings of Verdan[52,53] and others[5,10,11,16,23,24,34,43,45,47,48,49,51,55] provide an ample review of these complex injuries.

One fracture, the scaphoid, occurs with such frequency that its management should be emphasized. The scaphoid has a notorious reputation for delayed union and non-union, probably caused more by delayed or inadequate treatment than by the fracture itself. Postmortem studies have demonstrated the role of pronation and extension in the mechanism of the fracture and the necessity to control pronation and supination in order to immobilize the fracture.[52,53] Failure to do this will permit excessive motion and jeopardize the precarious blood supply to the fracture site and the proximal fragment.

Any patient with a history of trauma to the wrist who on physical examination has tenderness in the anatomical snuffbox on direct pressure, or pain in this area on pronation or supination, must have not only posteroanterior and lateral roentgenograms but also "scaphoid views." The posteroanterior view is best taken with the wrist in some extension and ulnar deviation and with the x-ray tube angled to avoid any superimposition of the radius on the navicular. Oblique views in 25° and 45° of pronation are also helpful. Even if a fracture cannot be seen on roentgenography, the patient with these well-localized specific findings should be immobilized from the interphalangeal joint of the thumb to above the elbow. A roentgenogram should be taken in the cast to check the position of the fragments. If the alignment is not anatomical, the displacement is usually caused by the rotational position of the forearm disrupting the fracture site via the radiocarpal ligaments. Fluoroscopic examination of the displaced fracture in various positions of supination or pronation may be necessary to determine the best position for immobilization.

The cast may be cut low in the antecubital area to allow some elbow flexion-extension, but must be high enough medially and laterally to control forearm rotation. The patient should be treated with 6 to 10 weeks of immobilization, the first four in the cast as described, the remaining weeks with a short-arm cast.[2,3] At the end of this time most of these fractures will be healed.

If no fracture was visible on the initial roentgenogram, the cast should be removed in two weeks and roentgenograms repeated. Bone resorption at the fracture site will then usually permit detection of a minimal fracture. If the roentgenograms remain normal and the local tenderness has subsided, a scaphoid fracture is not present. Should definite pain and tenderness remain, the cast must be reapplied and the roentgenograms and examination repeated in two more weeks.[24] An occasional fracture will not be demonstrated radiographically until four weeks after injury.

With those fractures which have progressed to establish non-union with sclerotic margins and cystic changes, the patient should undergo debridement of the fracture site and bone grafting. The anterior technique of Russe[42] spares the blood supply and has been most effective in our experience.

General anesthesia is necessary because of the need to obtain an iliac bone graft. A 4-cm longitudinal incision is made along the radial border of the flexor carpi radialis tendon, which is then retracted ulnarward. The radial artery must be carefully protected. The scaphoid is exposed after the joint capsule has been incised. Extension of the wrist aids in visualizing the site of the non-union. The sclerotic margins of the fracture are minimally curetted. A trough is made across the two fragments, and the sclerotic bone removed from inside the bone, especially proximally.

A segment of cancellous bone 1.0×2.0 cm is removed from the patient's iliac crest and is cut into many slender struts. These are placed from one fracture fragment into the other around the perimeter. The medullary cavity is tightly packed with small bone chips.

Roentgenograms are taken before packing the scaphoid to determine the size of the defect and afterward to verify the completeness of the graft. The capsule is carefully closed. The tourniquet is usually removed to allow identification of any severed veins and the wound is closed with fine nylon sutures.

The hand and forearm are casted with the thumb completely immobilized and the forearm in neutral. The cast initially extends to above the elbow, but is open anteriorly to allow flexion without rotation. The sutures are removed at two weeks and the long-arm cast continued for two more weeks. At four weeks postoperatively the cast is reduced to a short-arm cast. The total period of immobilization depends upon roentgenographic evidence of healing and ranges from 12 to 14 weeks. The procedure is 85 to 90 per cent successful. Pain is relieved and grip strength is improved; there may, however, be some residual limitation of full wrist motion.

Open Fractures

The treatment of open fractures embraces the same principles in the hand as elsewhere—debridement, irrigation, stabilization, antibiotics, tetanus prophylaxis, and soft tissue coverage. A few specific problems do occur with open fractures of the phalanges and should be briefly discussed.

An open fracture, with damage to the neurovascular bundles and other soft tissue, is in effect an incomplete amputation. The question arises in each case whether to reattach the digit or to do a primary amputation. Firm rules are meaningless. The pertinent factors to be considered are the finger involved, dominant hand and occupation of the patient. The magnitude of associated systemic injuries may preclude staged reconstruction of a single digit. Associated injuries to the hand may require that the subtotally amputated digit be filleted for resurfacing of more essential areas. In considering staged reconstruction of a salvaged digit, the surgeon must remember that the restricted motion in otherwise normal adjacent digits during repeated periods of immobilization may seriously diminish eventual function of the hand.

The level of the compound fracture is critical, particularly for the index finger. In this ray, if the fracture is proximal to the midshaft of the middle phalanx, an attempt should be made to salvage the distal segment, since a short index finger is more of a functional liability than an asset. An index finger amputated proximal to the middle phalanx has little use in pinch. The patient very swiftly learns to bypass the index, developing an extended, out-of-the-way attitude in the short index finger. In due time this digit loses range of motion. If this occurs, a ray resection through the metacarpal base may become the ultimate treatment.

Hand Fractures in Children

In children, the same general principles exist as have been outlined above for adults.

In addition, there is the problem of epiphyseal injury. Fractures and dislocations occur through the epiphyseal plate and the implications for altered growth are the same here as elsewhere.[44] Remodeling of fractures will occur and some angulation can be accepted, but only at that portion of the bone near the growth plate. No rotational correction will occur with growth, however, and displacement in this plane must never be accepted.

Usually it is possible to achieve excellent closed reductions in children. Their tough periosteal support not only aids the reduction but assists in the immobilization. Once reduced, the fracture is often so stable within its periosteal sleeve that there is no need for Kirschner wires. Open reduction in a child is seldom necessary.

References

1. Bennett, E.H.: Fractures of the metacarpal bones. Dublin J. Med. Sci., 73:72, 1882.
2. Bennett, E.H.: On fractures of the metacarpal bone of the thumb. Br. Med. J., 2:12, 1886.
3. Bennett, E.H.: Fracture of the metacarpal bone of the thumb. Trans. Acad. Med. Ireland, 15:309, 1897.
4. Berkman, E.F. and Niles, G.J.: Internal fixation of metacarpal fractures exclusive of the thumb. J. Bone Joint Surg., 25:816, 1943.
5. Borgeskov, S., Christiansen, B., Kjaer, A. and Balsley, I.: Fractures of the carpal bones. Acta Orthop. Scand., 37:276, 1966.
6. Boyes, J.H.: *Bunnell's Surgery of the Hand,* 5th ed. J.B. Lippincott, Philadelphia, 1970.
7. Bradford, C.H. and Dolphin, J.A.: Fractures of the hand and wrist. In: *Hand Surgery* (Flynn, J.E., Ed.). Williams and Wilkins, Baltimore, 1966.
8. Burnham, P.J.: Physiological treatment for fractures of the metacarpals and phalanges. J.A.M.A., 196:663, 1959.
9. Butt, W.D.: Rigid wire fixation of fractures of the hand. Henry Ford Hosp. Med. Bull., 4:134, 1956.
10. Campbell, R.D., Thompson, T. C., Lance, E.M. and Adler, J.B.: Indications for open reduction of lunate and perilunate dislocations of the carpal bones. J. Bone Joint Surg., 47A:915, 1965.
11. Campbell, R.D., Lance, E.M. and Yeoh, C.B.: Lunate and perilunar dislocations. J. Bone Joint Surg., 46B:55, 1964.
12. Charnley, J.: *The Closed Treatment of Common Fractures,* 3rd ed. E. & S. Livingston, Edinburg and London, 1963.
13. Coonrad, R.W. and Pohlman, M.H.: Impacted fractures of the proximal phalanx. J. Bone Joint Surg., 51A:1291, 1969.
14. Eaton, R.G.: *Joint Injuries in the Hand.* Charles C Thomas, Springfield, 1971.
15. Eichenholtz, S.N. and Rizzo, P.C., III: Fracture of the neck of the fifth metacarpal bone—is overtreatment justified? J.A.M.A., 178:425, 1961.
16. Fisk, G.R.: Carpal instability and the fractured scaphoid. Ann. R. Coll. Surg. Engl., 46:63, 1970.
17. Flatt, A.E.: *The Care of Minor Hand Injuries,* 2nd ed. C.V. Mosby, St. Louis, 1963.
18. Gedda, K.O.: Studies on Bennett's fracture. Acta Chir. Scand., Suppl. 193, 1954.
19. Gedda, K.O. and Moberg, E.: Open reduction and osteosynthesis of the so-called Bennett's fracture in the carpometacarpal joint of the thumb. Acta Orthop. Scand., 22:249, 1953.
20. Jahss, S.A.: Fractures of the metacarpal. A new method of reduction and immobilization. J. Bone Joint Surg., 20:178, 1938.
21. James, J.I.P.: Common simple errors in management of hand injuries. Proc. R. Soc. Med., 63:69, 1970.
22. James, J.I.P. and Wright, T.A.: Fractures of metacarpals

and proximal and middle phalanges of the fingers. J. Bone Joint Surg., 48B:181, 1966.
23. Jorgensen, E.C.: Proximal row carpectomy. J. Bone Joint Surg., 51A:1104, 1969.
24. Hill, N.A.: Fractures and dislocations of the carpus. Orthop. Clin. North Am., 1:275, 1970.
25. Kilbourne, B.C.: Management of complicated hand fractures. Surg. Clin. North Am., 48:201, 1968.
26. Littler, J.W.: Metacarpal reconstruction. J. Bone Joint Surg., 29:1, 1947.
27. Littler, J.W.: Architectural principles of reconstructive surgery of the hand. Surg. Clin. North Am., 31:463, 1951.
28. Littler, J.W.: The hand and wrist. In: *A Textbook of Orthopedics.* (Beckett-Howorth, M., Ed.). W.B. Saunders, Philadelphia, 1952.
29. Littler, J.W.: The physiology and dynamic function of the hand. Surg. Clin. North Am., 40:259, 1960.
30. Littler, J.W.: Principles of reconstructive surgery of the hand. In: *Reconstructive Plastic Surgery* (Converse, J.M., Ed.). W.B. Saunders, Philadelphia, 1964.
31. Littler, J.W.: The hand. In: *The Craft of Surgery* (Cooper, P., Ed.). Little, Brown and Co., Boston, 1964.
32. Littler, J.W.: The finger extensor mechanism. Surg. Clin. North Am., 47:415, 1967.
33. Mansoor, I.A.: Fractures of the proximal phalanx of fingers. J. Bone Joint Surg., 51A:196, 1969.
34. Mazet, R., Jr. and Hohl, M.: Fracture of the carpal navicular. J. Bone Joint Surg., 45A:82, 1963.
35. Milford, L.W.: The hand. In: *Campbell's Operative Orthopedics,* 4th ed. (Greenshaw, A.H., Ed.). C.V. Mosby, St. Louis, 1963.
36. Moberg, E.: Fractures and ligamentous injuries of the thumb and fingers. Surg. Clin. North Am., 40:297, 1960.
37. Moberg, E.: *Emergency Situation of the Hand.* E & S Livingston, London, 1967.
38. O'Donoghue, D.H.: *Injuries of the Hand. Treatment of Injuries to Athletes.* W.B. Saunders, Philadelphia, 1962.
39. Pollen, A.G.: The conservative treatment of Bennett's fracture, subluxation of the thumb metacarpal. J. Bone Joint Surg., 50B:91, 1968.
40. Riordan, D.C.: Hand fractures. Indust. Med. Surg., 37:103, 1968.
41. Robbins, R.H.C.: *Injuries and Infections of the Hand.* Williams and Wilkins, Baltimore, 1961.
42. Russe, O.: Fractures of the carpal navicular. J. Bone Joint Surg., 42A:759, 1960.
43. Russell, T.B.: Intercarpal dislocations and fracture dislocations: A review of fifty nine cases. J. Bone Joint Surg., 31B:524, 1949.
44. Salter, R.B. and Harris, W.R.: Injuries involving the epiphyseal plate. J. Bone Joint Surg., 45A:586, 1963.
45. Speed, K.: Fractures of the carpus. J. Bone Joint Surg., 17:965, 1935.
46. Stark, H.H.: Troublesome fractures and dislocations of the hand. Instructional Course Lectures. Am. Acad. Orthop. Surg., 19:130, 1970.
47. Stewart, M.J.: Fractures of the carpal navicular. A report of 436 cases. J. Bone Joint Surg., 36A:998, 1954.
48. Stein, F. and Siegel, M.W.: Naviculocapitate fracture syndrome. J. Bone Joint Surg., 51A:391, 1969.
49. Swanson, A.B.: Fractures involving the digits of the hand. Orthop. Clin. North Am., 1:261, 1970.
50. Taleisnik, J. and Kelly, P.J.: The extra-osseous and intraosseous blood supply of the scaphoid bone. J. Bone Joint Surg., 48A:1125, 1966.
51. Thompson, T.C., Campbell, R.D. and Arnold, W.D.: Primary and secondary dislocation of the scaphoid bone. J. Bone Joint Surg., 46B:73, 1964.
52. Verdan, C.: Fractures of the scaphoid. Surg. Clin. North Am., 40:461, 1960.
53. Verdan, C. and Narakas, A.: Fractures and pseudarthrosis of the scaphoid. Surg. Clin. North Am., 48:1083, 1968.
54. Von Saal, H.H.: Intramedullary fixation in fractures of the hand and fingers. J. Bone Joint Surg., 35A:5, 1953.
55. Wagner, C.J.: Fracture—dislocations of the wrist. Clin. Orthop., 15:181, 1959.
56. Wright, T.A.: Early mobilization in fractures of metacarpals and phalanges. Can. J. Surg., 11:491, 1968.

12 Ligamentous and Joint Injuries of the Hand

Ligamentous injuries are some of the most common forms of trauma the hand receives. Many serious joint injuries are underdiagnosed and undertreated because they are usually closed and seldom exhibit roentgenological evidence of disruption. The number of stiff, painful chronically swollen joints a physician sees among friends and acquaintances as well as patients should remind him of the magnitude and frequency of such injuries.

Natural healing of joint support structures is unpredictable and frequently imperfect. It is most important, therefore, that they receive optimal treatment at the time of injury. *Ligamentous injury must be ruled out in all joints having a history of significant trauma.* When there has been known displacement or deformity, an accurate assessment of the extent of disruption and the joint's remaining functional stability must be made.

Clinical findings accompanying a ligamentous injury or dislocation include pain, hemarthrosis or tenderness localized to one or both sides of the joint. Deformity and malalignment are not common, since the patient usually applies traction to the angulated finger, quickly reducing it during the brief initial period of hypoesthesia. Once reduced, the extent of ligamentous disruption is difficult to determine, yet the extent of disruption is particularly significant as it relates to the stability of the joint. Most finger dislocations are sufficiently stable after reduction that redisplacement will not occur. However, each joint must be appropriately immobilized to assure optimum ligamentous healing. Stable or non-displacing ligamentous disruptions, being of lesser magnitude, obviously require less immobilization. Excessive immobilization tends to produce stiffness, whereas inadequate immobilization with premature motion produces excessive ligamentous "callus" with subsequent fibrosis and limitation of motion.

Examination of the Injured Joint

The essential feature in the examination of an injured joint is the stability of that joint to (1) lateral stress and (2) active motion. Stability associated with pain on lateral stress suggests a partial tear or sprain, whereas angulation or redisplacement with stress is evidence of extensive ligamentous disruption. Functional stability is evaluated by the active motion test. This test, one of the most useful in evaluating a joint injury, requires that the joint be put through a complete range of motion, i.e. full extension to full flexion. Should pain prevent a *complete* range of motion, the presence of a significant disruption must be ruled out. In this case, a wrist or digital anesthetic block should be administered and the anesthetized digit put through a full range of active motion. This technique provides anesthesia without inducing paralysis. Should doubt exist regarding lateral stability, the stress test should also be done under digital anesthesia (Fig. 12-1). This may bring out instability not detected in the unanesthetized finger.

Roentgenograms in the posteroanterior and true lateral projection should be done on all patients having a history of significant joint trauma. Awareness of an avulsion fracture or old joint injuries is

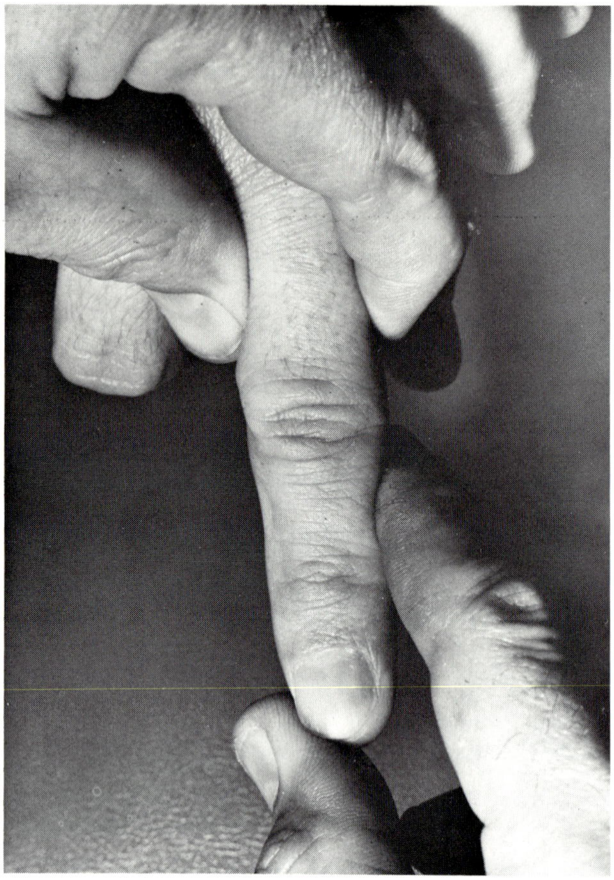

Figure 12-1. *The integrity of each collateral-accessory ligament system may be tested by applying lateral stress to the fully extended joint. Normal interphalangeal joints should permit no more than 5° angulation. The injured joint must be compared to the normal contralateral joint. When doubt exists, the test should be done under digital anesthetic block.* (*From Eaton, R.G.*[3])

useful in determining the duration of immobilization and prognosis and in making the most accurate diagnosis possible. Stress roentgenograms rarely provide information additional to that obtained by clinical test under block. The presence of definite joint instability when compared to the uninjured contralateral joint indicates a significant ligamentous disruption. Specific treatment of these will be discussed in subsequent sections. The diagnosis of an incomplete ligamentous tear or sprain can be made only after thoughtfully eliminating a major ligamentous disruption. An accurate anatomical diagnosis is essential in establishing the proper treatment, particularly in the few specific ligamentous tears which require immediate surgical repair.

Sprains

An incomplete ligamentous tear or sprain implies the injured joint has retained sufficient capsular support to prevent displacement under appropriate stress. Such stability may be present though the disruption involves as much as 99 per cent of the involved ligamentous system. Since the per cent of intact fibers is impossible to estimate, all stable or non-displacing joint injuries must be treated as though a major portion of the ligaments were torn. Fortunately with an incomplete tear there will be almost anatomical realignment of the ligament, the torn structures lying as well apposed naturally as they could be approximated surgically.

An acutely injured ligament requires rest in order to assure optimum healing. For incomplete tears, this is best accomplished by complete immobilization for a minimum of 10 to 14 days. Joints with demonstrable instability to stress must be immobilized 21 days, as will be discussed later. Interphalangeal joints are best splinted in 30 to 35° flexion. Finger metacarpophalangeal joints are splinted in 45 to 50° flexion and the thumb metacarpophalangeal joint in 30°. The necessary immobilization can be achieved by a lightly padded plaster cast or aluminum splint.

Following adequate immobilization, active motion is encouraged. Marked capsular thickening at the completion of appropriate immobilization suggests that the initial damage has been underestimated and additional protection may be needed. Satisfactory "mobile splinting" can be achieved by taping the injured finger to an adjacent one for 5 to 7 days. The possibility of redisplacement is remote. *The major sequelae of disrupted joint structures are not instability and redisplacement, but protracted stiffness, limited motion and pain.*

Digital Interphalangeal Joints

The proximal and distal interphalangeal joints are ginglymus or hinged joints, moving primarily in the sagittal plane around the concentric arc of the proximal condyle (Fig. 12-2). Because of their broad bicondylar diameter, they have remarkable stability in all positions to lateral or angular stress.

Capsular support for these joints consists of tough collateral-accessory ligaments laterally and a fibrous plate volarly. Dorsal support is minimum, made up mostly of the thin semielastic extensor mechanism as it blends with the delicate dorsal

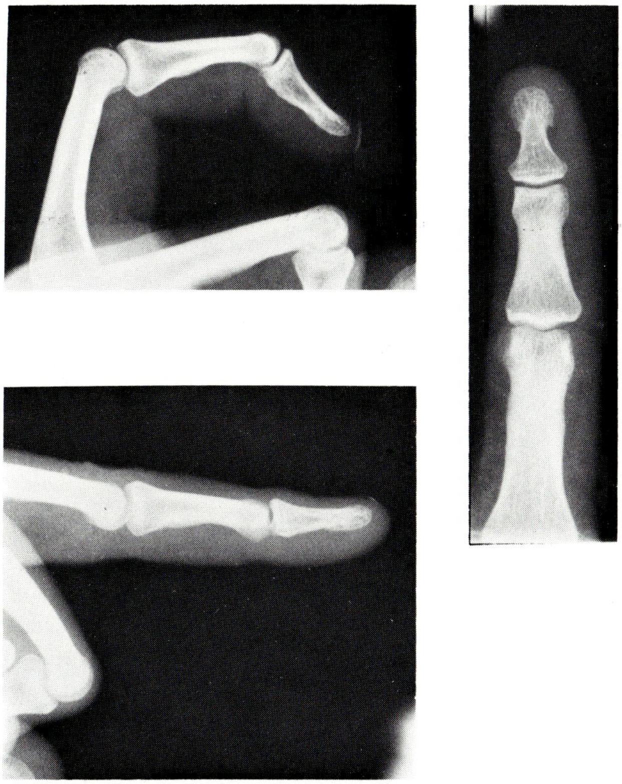

Figure 12-2. *Roentgenogram of the interphalangeal joints. In the lateral views (left) are seen the extremes of motion around the concentric arc of the condyles. In maximum flexion, the base of the middle phalanx seats firmly into the retrocondylar recess, a position of maximum stability. Obliteration of this recess by scar, bone spur or adherence of the volar plate will produce a major restriction in motion. In the posteroanterior view (right), the tongue-and-groove articular contours which contribute stability against rotatory and shearing stress can be observed. (From Eaton, R.G.*[3]*)*

capsule. The collateral-accessory ligaments are thick rectangular straps which arise from a concentric depression on the lateral aspect of the condyle and pass distally and volarly to insert into (1) the opposing volar lateral articular margin and (2) the volar plate (Fig. 12-3). *This three-dimensional junction involving the articular margins, volar plate and collateral ligaments is the key to interphalangeal strength and stability. As long as this junction remains intact significant displacement is impossible.*

Fanning volarward from the condylar origin of the collateral ligaments to insert along the proximal margin of the volar plate is the triangular-shaped accessory ligament. It is continuous with the collateral ligament, completing the lateral wall of the interphalangeal joint capsule. The accessory ligament represents the tapering proximal portion of the collateral ligament which must be membranous in order to fold upon itself in the position of maximal flexion.

With the paired collateral ligaments serving as walls, the volar plate forms the floor of the joint. The volar plate is a square cartilaginous plaque which bridges the volar aspect of the joint. It is 2 to 3 mm thick at its distal insertion and tapers proximally into a thin elastic sheet. Though this proximal margin is membranous in the midline, it is thickened laterally to form a pair of check ligaments[5,6,7] which are firmly anchored to the volar periosteum of the distal proximal phalanx. These ligaments prevent hyperextension, yet are sufficiently flexible that they can fold upon themselves in the position of maximum flexion (Fig. 12-2). The volar plate, therefore, forms a semirigid floor into which the lateral capsule is anchored, thus forming a mobile box around the interphalangeal joint (Fig. 12-4). This open box moves as a unit with the distal portion of the joint as it glides around the condyle, maintaining stability in all positions of flexion and extension.

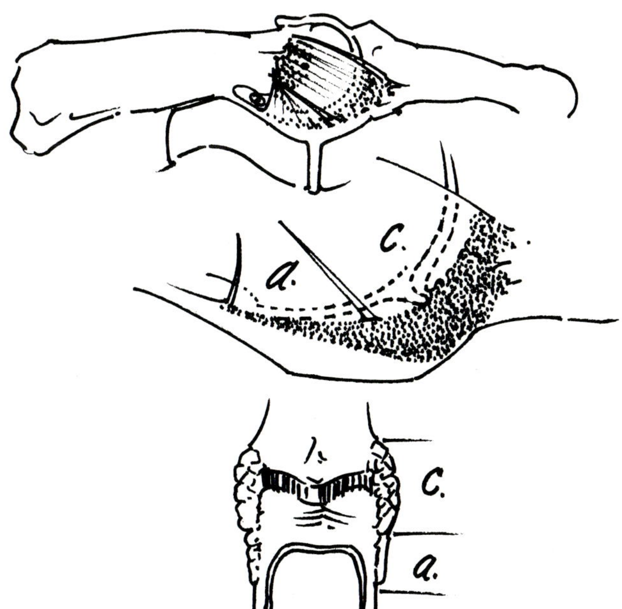

Figure 12-3. *Ligament support for the proximal interphalangeal joint. The quadrangular collateral ligament (c), by inserting on the volar plate and opposite joint margin, overlaps and reinforces the volar plate insertion. The accessory ligament (a) represents a thinning of the proximal portion of the collateral ligament. (From Eaton, R.G.*[3]*)*

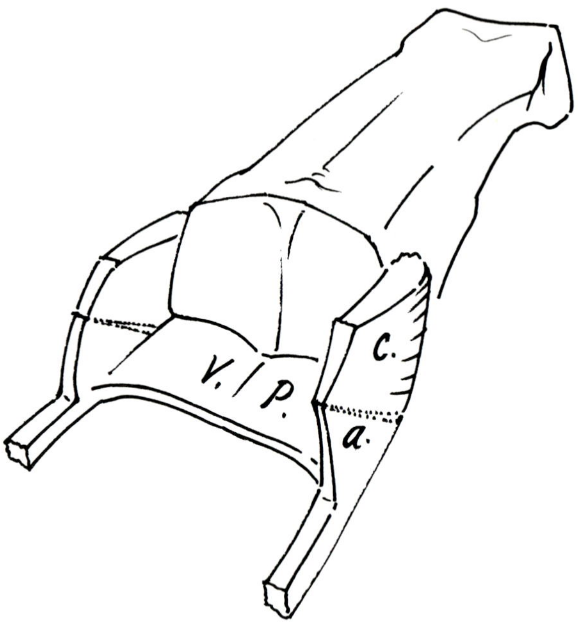

Figure 12-4. *Schematic drawing of the ligament seat or box configuration which supports the interphalangeal joints. The thickest portion of the collateral ligament overlaps and reinforces the insertion of the volar plate into the base of the middle phalanx. The two ligaments firmly inserted around the vertical base of the middle phalanx create a support system of great strength. Displacement of the middle phalanx cannot occur unless two of these insertions are disrupted. The proximal convergence of the volar plate and accessory ligament to form the check ligament can be seen.* (*From Eaton, R.G.*[3])

Mechanism of Interphalangeal Joint Injuries

Interphalangeal joint injuries range in severity from the "stoved finger" to the irreducible dislocation. However, once the joint has been reduced, it may be difficult to distinguish an extensively disrupted capsule from a simple sprain. For purposes of treatment, however, anatomical disruption is significant only as related to loss of joint stability. Initial treatment, duration of immobilization and prognosis are directly related to the post-reduction stability of the injured joint.

Joint stability may be accurately ascertained by the test of active motion and lateral stressing, as previously described. The examination is most valid under digital anesthesia. If reduction is maintained through a full range of active motion, it must be assumed that adequate ligamentous and tendinous support remain; hence 10 to 14 days of immobilization are sufficient. Should redisplacement occur, usually in the last 15° of extension, a major disruption must be assumed; therefore the joint requires immobilization in 30 to 35° flexion for a full three weeks. Roentgenograms before and after reduction are essential, particularly when a question of stability exists. Follow-up roentgenograms are also needed in treating the unstable joint, to be certain that redisplacement does not occur during the early period of immobilization. The most unstable dislocations are those which have a small avulsion fracture of the volar plate insertion. In fact, certain of these may not reduce at all.

Distal Joint

At the distal interphalangeal joint, dorsal or lateral displacement may occur. Because of extensive skin fixation about this joint, dislocations are frequently associated with open wounds, the skin rupturing rather than sliding or stretching during the extreme joint distortion.

Closed reduction is usually simple and is almost always stable despite complete rupture of the volar plate and collateral ligament.* Splinting in slight flexion for three weeks allows healing with minimum permanent restriction in motion.

Proximal Joint

Proximal interphalangeal joint stability is directly related to the three-plane junction of the volar plate with the base of the middle phalanx and collateral-accessory ligamentous system. This complex resembles an armchair, the seat being the volar plate, the back the base of the middle phalanx, and the arms the collateral-accessory ligamentous system (Fig. 12-4). This open-box configuration creates a three-dimensional hinge system of remarkable strength. *For significant joint displacement* to occur, there must be disruption of at least two sides of this box. For example, an isolated radial collateral-accessory ligamentous tear will not permit the joint to angulate ulnarward because of the intact volar plate insertion. However, if both the radial collateral-accessory ligament and the volar plate are disrupted, angulation will occur

*Volar plate tears occur at the proximal margins of the distal interphalangeal and metacarpophalangeal joint levels. Only at the proximal interphalangeal joint does the plate tear away from its distal attachment.

as this joint pivots laterally on the remaining intact collateral-accessory ligament system. Two types of ligament injury may occur: (1) dorsal or sagittal and (2) lateral or jack-knife dislocation.

DORSAL DISLOCATION

In dorsal dislocation of the proximal interphalangeal joint, the major disruption is usually through the distal insertion of the volar plate accompanied by a split extending longitudinally into the collateral ligament (Fig. 12-5). Unrestrained by the volar plate, the middle phalanx may slip into extreme hyperextension or undergo complete dorsal displacement, coming to rest atop the condyles like a bayonet (Fig. 12-6). Occasionally, the compression force will be sufficient to shear a triangu-

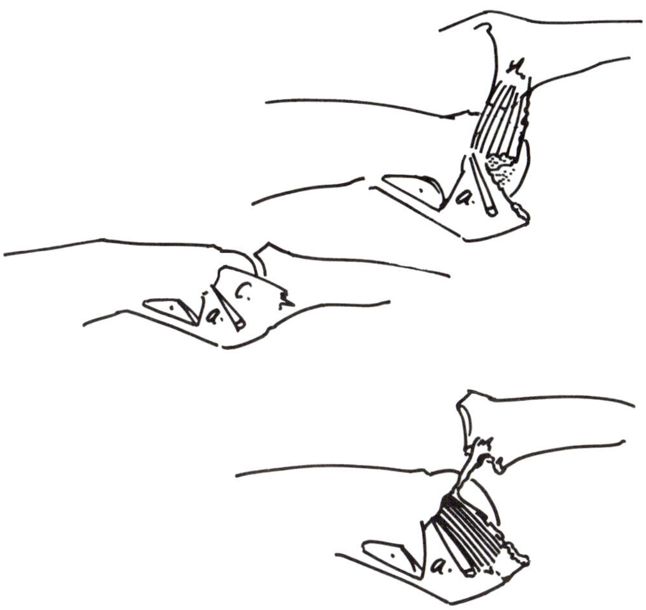

Figure 12-5. *Schema of proximal interphalangeal joint dislocation.* **Left:** *The division of the lateral capsule into collateral (c) and accessory (a) ligaments is hypothetical; no actual separation exists. The tough check ligaments are firmly anchored to the distal portion of the proximal phalanx, bridging the retrocondylar space through which pass the nutrient vessels to the flexor tendons and joint synovium.* **Top:** *Stable dorsal dislocation. The volar plate insertion has been ruptured yet the collateral-accessory ligament attachment to the volar plate retains the normal condyle-volar plate relationship. Closed reduction will reapproximate all structures so that capsular restitution will be satisfactory.* **Bottom:** *Unstable dorsal dislocation. The middle phalanx has dislocated dorsally, leaving a large volar fragment still attached to the volar plate and the major portion of the collateral ligaments. Should a few fibers of the ligament remain attached to the phalanx to facilitate complete reduction, structural restitution may be satisfactory; however, if these ligamentous fibers have been completely torn or are subsequently ruptured, a satisfactory reduction is unlikely.* (*From Eaton, R.G.*[3])

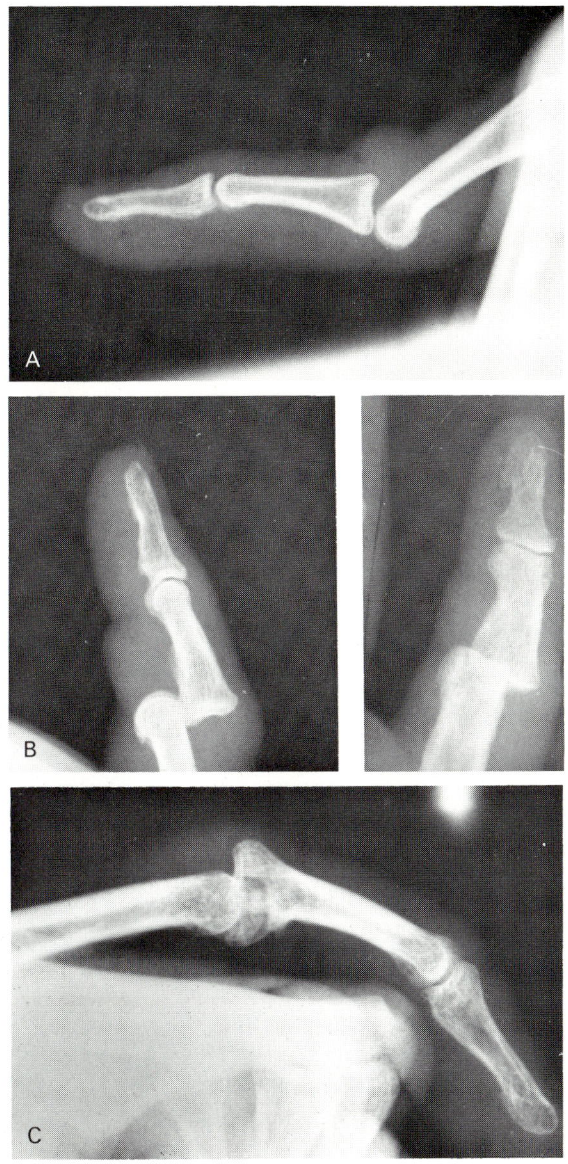

Figure 12-6. *Roentgenograms of proximal interphalangeal dorsal dislocations.* **A:** *Subluxation or severe hyperextension injury. The volar plate insertion has been ruptured, but sufficient collateral ligament remains intact to prevent complete displacement.* **B:** *Complete dorsal dislocation. The volar plate has ruptured and there has been a major split in the collateral ligament.* **C:** *Avulsion fracture of the volar plate and collateral ligament insertions. The larger the fragment, the less ligament remains attached to the middle phalanx.* (*From Eaton, R.G.*[3])

lar fragment of bone from the base of the middle phalanx. Such a fragment may contain the entire collateral ligament insertion as well as that of the volar plate, leaving the middle phalanx almost totally devoid of ligamentous support.

Occasionally the volar plate will rupture proximally, apparently stripping one or both check ligaments. Such a tear is not apparent until later, when a proximal spur may be seen on roentgenogram and a mild boutonniere deformity may be present clinically.[10] Proper immobilization initially may prevent this rare complication. Boutonniere deformity, symmetrical or asymmetrical, may follow any major proximal interphalangeal joint displacement. The degree of deformity is related to the extent of rupture and the position of proximal interphalangeal joint immobilization.[8]

Reduction of dorsal dislocations is simple and is usually quite stable providing some portion of the collateral ligament system remains intact (Fig. 12-5). An accurate reduction depends upon the integrity of the remaining lateral capsule to pivot and guide the middle phalanx back into a congruous relationship with the condyles, much as a medieval knight would swing closed the visor of his helmet. If the collateral ligament insertions are torn or remain on the fragment with the volar plate, the middle phalanx will have no hinge on which to pivot and the reduction may not be congruous or stable (Fig. 12-7).

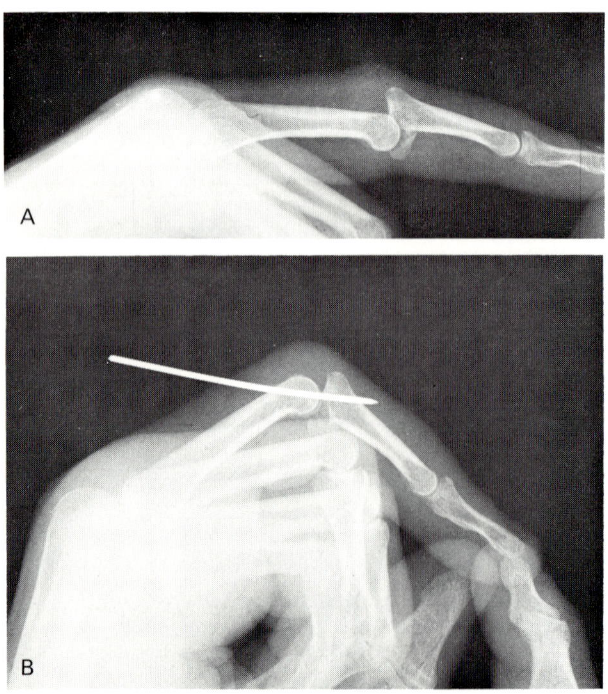

Figure 12-7. *Roentgenograms of an unstable dislocation.* **A:** *This volar plate fragment represents approximately 40 per cent of the articular surface and probably all of the collateral ligament insertion on the middle phalanx.* **B:** *Closed reduction was unsuccessful without the guidance of the collateral ligaments.* (*From Eaton, R.G.*[3])

The larger the volar fragment, the less likely a stable reduction can be achieved, since a greater portion of the collateral ligament will have been disrupted. When 50 per cent of the articular surface has been avulsed, a satisfactory reduction is usually impossible and open reduction will be necessary.

LATERAL DISLOCATION

Lateral displacement occurs when torsion, angular or shearing stress ruptures one collateral ligament and the major portion of the volar plate insertion. With two sides of the ligamentous box disrupted, dislocation will occur, the middle phalanx pivoting laterally on the remaining collateral-accessory ligamentous system. The displaced joint will usually reduce spontaneously, or, if not, the patient may quickly reduce it with longitudinal traction. When a lateral dislocation is suspected, in addition to the test of active motion each collateral ligament must be carefully stressed with the joint in full extension and preferably under digital block. The degree of angulation elicited is a reliable index of the extent of ligamentous disruption. The length of immobilization and the prognosis are directly related to the degree of disruption. If the joint is stable to lateral stress, splinting in 30° flexion for two weeks is sufficient. Joints which are unstable to lateral stress, but are stable to active motion, require a full three weeks of complete immobilization. Open reduction of lateral dislocations is necessary only when reduction cannot be accomplished or the joint redisplaces with active flexion and extension.

Open Reduction

Joints which redisplace with active motion or lose reduction while adequately immobilized require open reduction and ligamentous repair. Most frequently unstable are dorsal dislocations in which a large fragment of bone has been avulsed from the base of the middle phalanx. In these, reduction is rarely satisfactory or redisplacement is almost immediate, making repair mandatory. Restoring a smooth articular surface to the middle phalanx requires accurate replacement of the fragment of bone and is often difficult. Fixation of the fragment with a fine Kirschner wire is standard practice and may be satisfactory providing *anatomical* replacement can be achieved. Not infrequently, however, reduction is imperfect or the fragment is split by the fixation wire, further compromising the articular surface and joint reduction.

A simple effective reconstruction of such unstable dislocations can be achieved by debridement of the fragments of bone and advancement of the volar plate into the defect remaining in the articular surface.[4] The volar aspect of the joint is exposed and the flexor sheath overlying the proximal interphalangeal joint is excised. The volar plate is visualized by retracting the flexor tendons. Extension of the joint will readily expose the disruption at the base of the middle phalanx. The bony fragment, often comminuted, is excised and a lateral margin pull-out wire is inserted in the volar plate (Fig. 12-8). The plate is inserted into the defect by drawing the sutures through drill holes which

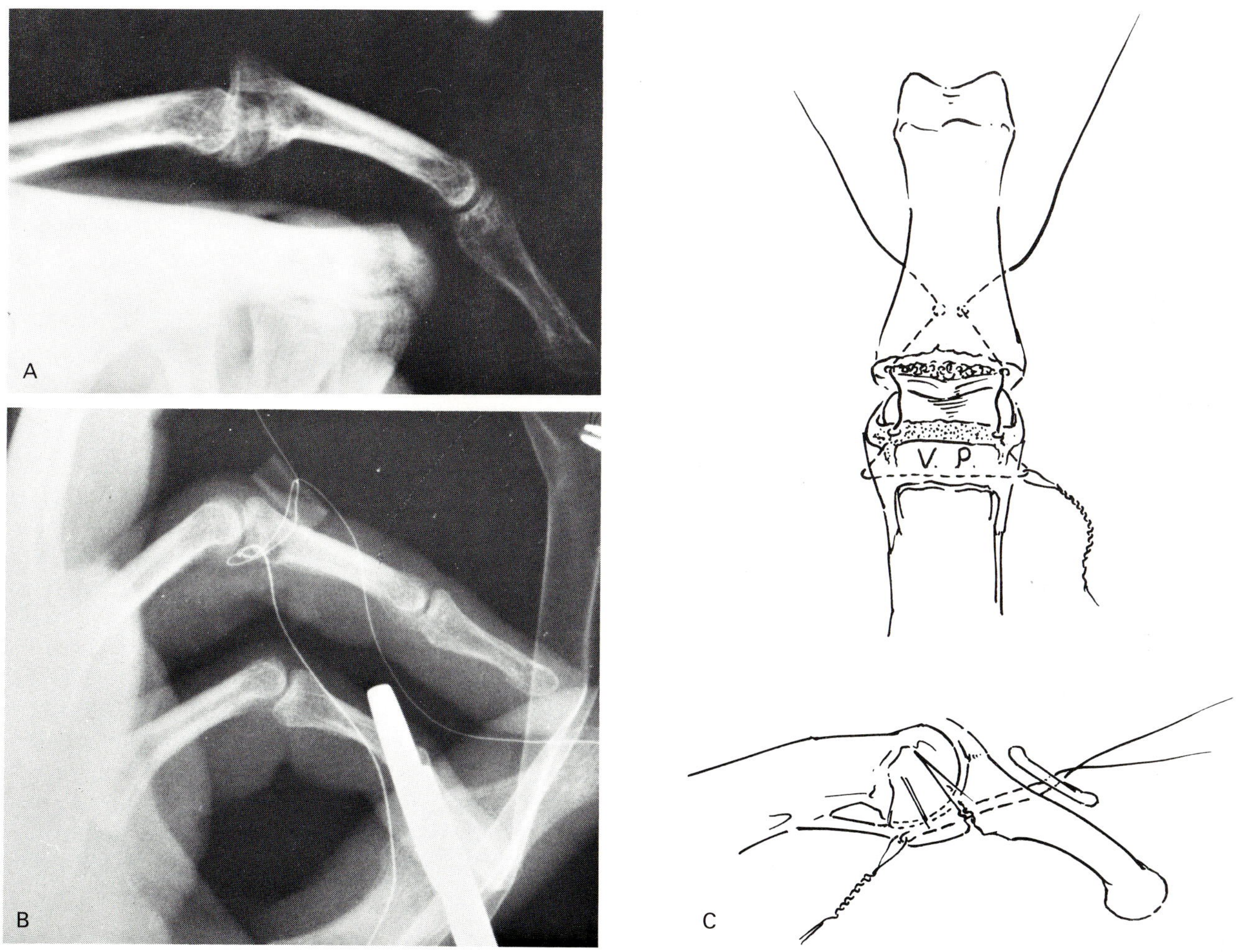

Figure 12-8. *Schema of reconstruction of unstable proximal interphalangeal joint fracture-dislocation by volar plate advancement.* **A:** *The fragments of bone are excised and the volar plate is advanced to resurface the defect in the articular surface. For maximum stability, the pull-out wire suture must maintain the full width of the volar plate. After emerging from the distal corners of the plate, the wires are passed through lateral drill holes in the articular defect to be secured over a button in the dorsal midline of the middle phalanx. Traction on the suture simultaneously reduces the dislocation and draws the volar plate into the articular defect, thereby resurfacing the base of the middle phalanx. With release of its remaining collateral-accessory ligament attachments, the volar plate can be advanced to replace as much as 50 per cent of the articular surface.* **B:** *Roentgenogram of an unstable fracture-dislocation. The base of the middle phalanx is comminuted. A satisfactory reduction could not be achieved.* **C:** *Excision of the fragments and advancement of the volar plate into the resulting defect. The dislocation is reduced simultaneous with resurfacing of the damaged articular surface.* (*From Eaton, R.G.*[3])

emerge on the dorsum of the middle phalanx. Traction on these wires advances the volar plate into the defect while simultaneously reducing the middle phalanx. It is not necessary to flex the middle phalanx more than 35° to achieve this advancement.

Congruous reduction is confirmed by lateral roentgenogram. Through volar plate advancement, *a smooth middle phalangeal articular surface can be restored* and a stable reduction assured (Fig. 12-8). The joint is securely immobilized in 35° flexion for three weeks, at which time the pull-out wire is removed and active flexion is begun. Extension is not permitted until four weeks after repair. Occasionally dynamic extension splints are needed if full extension is not achieved by eight weeks.

Lateral dislocations rarely require open reduction, since they are stable to active motion which is in the sagittal plane, i.e. perpendicular to the instability. The flexor sheath and remaining collateral ligament prevents the volar plate from retracting proximally. With joint realignment, the plate lies in an essentially normal relationship with its middle phalangeal insertion. Satisfactory healing is the rule, though return to a full range of motion may be slow. The stability of the joint comes from restoration of one volar plate-collateral ligament junction. The torn ligament heals to itself once reduced and does not require specific surgical care.

The Finger Metacarpophalangeal Joints

There are major structural differences between the finger metacarpophalangeal and interphalangeal joints. Classified as condyloid joints, the metacarpophalangeal joints have, in addition to a full range of flexion and extension, as much as 30° lateral movement (in extension). Stability despite such movement is possible because (1) *the eccentric nature of the metacarpal condyles* creates a cam effect which produces tightening of the collateral ligaments in passing from extension to flexion, and (2) *the triangular cross section of the metacarpal head* permits relaxation of the collateral ligaments as they cross the more narrow dorsal aspect of the condyles in extension.

The collateral ligaments also differ anatomically from the interphalangeal ligaments. Their triangular shape is well suited to the two-way stretch over the condyles during flexion. These ligaments insert into the base of the proximal phalanx and volar plate and are continuous with the membranous accessory ligament proximally. The volar plate has several differences from the interphalangeal plate. Since there is no flexor sheath proximal to the metacarpal neck, there are no check ligaments for the metacarpophalangeal plate. Lacking these restraints, the metacarpophalangeal joint is capable of varying degrees of hyperextension, the most extreme being the hyperextension seen in a clawhand deformity. These weak proximal attachments permit the volar plate to remain attached to the dorsally displaced proximal phalanx, consequently blocking reduction.*

Another unique feature of the metacarpophalangeal plate is the strong intervolar plate ligament (intermetacarpal ligament) which links all finger metacarpophalangeal joints. This strong ligament is continuous with the lateral margins of the volar plate and is reinforced by the vertical insertion of the collateral-accessory ligaments. These three-dimensional interconnections add considerable stability to the mobile metacarpophalangeal joints.

Treatment of Metacarpophalangeal Dislocations

Dorsal dislocation of the metacarpophalangeal joint has been accurately termed the complex irreducible dislocation. Compared to interphalangeal joints, this particular dislocation is relatively uncommon, presumably because of the intervolar plate ligament and intrinsic muscle support as well as the protected position of these joints within the palmar webspace. Clinically, the involved finger appears shortened and usually lies ulnar deviated in extension. The index finger is most commonly involved. The metacarpal head is prominent in the palm (Fig. 12-9). Roentgenograms show dorsal displacement of the proximal phalanx and widening of the joint space.

Closed reduction fails for two reasons: (1) The metacarpal head is actually buttonholed between the flexor tendons and lumbrical muscle which lies scissorlike around the metacarpal neck. Attempts to extend or flex the proximal phalanx serve only to tighten this "finger-trap" arrangement. (2) The thick volar plate, still attached to the dorsally

*In dislocations at the proximal interphalangeal level, the check ligaments contribute to restraining the volar plate; hence, the rupture predominantly occurs at the distal insertion.

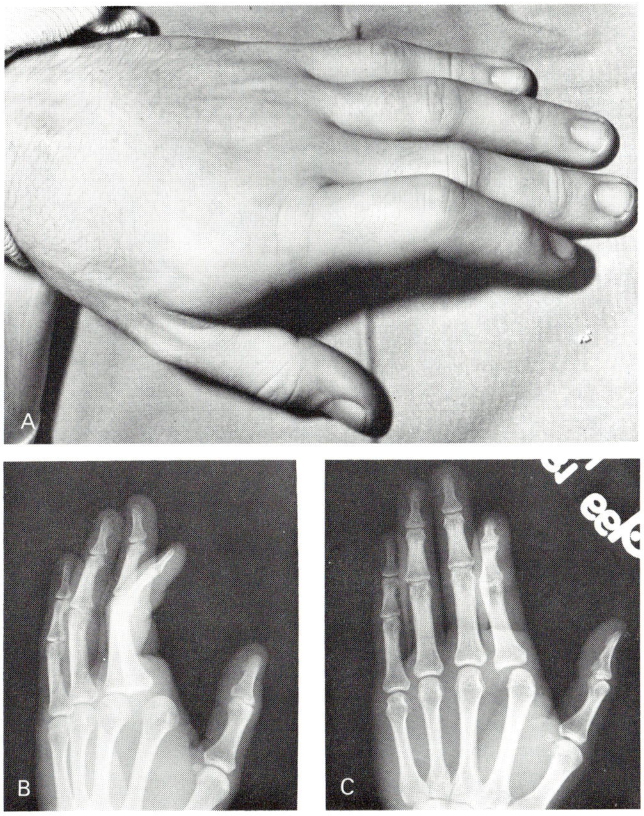

Figure 12-9. *The irreducible dislocation of the metacarpophalangeal joint.* **A:** *Shortening, slight extension and ulnar deviation are the hallmarks of this injury. The volarly displaced metacarpal head is readily palpable in the palm.* **B:** *Roentgenograms reveal a widened joint space where the volar plate, still attached to the proximal phalanx, has become wedged over the dorsum of the metacarpal head.* **C:** *The posteroanterior roentgenogram shows ulnar deviation of the proximal phalanx, suggesting at least a partial tear of the radial collateral ligament.* (*From Eaton, R.G.*[3])

displaced proximal phalanx, becomes interposed between the joint surfaces, blocking attempts to flex. The cam effect of the metacarpal head, augmented by the thickness of the interposed plate,* and sphincterlike encirclement of the metacarpal neck combine to prevent reduction.

Open reduction can be readily accomplished through a volar approach, carefully avoiding the superficially displaced radial nerve.† The flexor tendon sheath, drawn dorsally with the displaced volar plate, is incised longitudinally for 1 to 2 cm. This release permits bowstringing of the taut flexor tendons, thus relaxing the circumferential entrapment. The plate spontaneously slips out of the joint, making possible an atraumatic reduction. Immobilization is in 35° flexion and slight radial deviation for three weeks.

A clear distinction must be made between complete dorsal dislocations and subluxation. In a dislocation, which is *irreducible,* the dorsally displaced phalanx lies like a bayonet, slightly overlapping and parallel to the metacarpal, with little or no contact between the opposing articular surfaces. In the subluxation, which is *reducible,* the proximal phalanx is locked in 60 to 90° hyperextension yet the articular surfaces are at least in partial contact. This distinction is critical because the subluxed joint may be converted into an irreducible dislocation through attempts at reduction which involve a hyperextension maneuver.[9] Extension of the proximal phalanx will draw the incompletely displaced volar plate dorsal to the metacarpal head while forcing the metacarpal head volarly. The presence of shortening, parallel alignment of the proximal phalanx with the metacarpal and a roentgenogram showing a widened joint space are sufficient evidence to conclude that dislocation has already occurred and open reduction is required. Subluxation is easily reduced by simple flexion with traction.

Injuries of Metacarpophalangeal Collateral Ligament and Volar Plate

Most common and creating far more disability are metacarpophalangeal hyperextension injuries. Transient hyperextension may tear several proximal volar plate attachments and, with extreme stress, even the vertical septae and pretendinous portions of the palmar fascia. Individual collateral ligaments may be spared through the transverse linkage of the intervolar plate. Massive ecchymosis and swelling ensue. Roentgenograms are usually negative. Treatment consists of gently compressive dressings with light plaster reinforcement to maintain the metacarpophalangeal joints in 35 to 45° flexion, extending from the proximal interphalangeal joints to midforearm. Immobilization should be for 2 to 3 weeks depending on the degree of swelling. Pain and induration may persist for months, in proportion to the degree of initial soft tissue disruption.

Isolated collateral ligament tears do occur. Precise diagnosis can be made by flexing the metacarpophalangeal joint, thereby placing the ligaments under stretch. Ulnar or radial stress in such

*The presence of a large sesamoid may further thicken the plate and impair even open reduction.

†Alternative technique, page 16.

flexion will usually cause pain localized to the site of injury. Optimal healing follows splinting the joint in slight flexion or taping it to the finger adjacent to the site of injury.

The Thumb

The thumb has three completely different types of joints, each remarkably well suited to the position it occupies in this important cantilever system. Its strength is directly dependent upon the stability of each of these joints for the efficient transmission of power to the terminal phalanx. Because of its exposed position, the thumb is vulnerable to many stresses; hence, injuries to its joints are not uncommon.

Interphalangeal Joint

The interphalangeal joint of the thumb is basically identical to the distal interphalangeal joint of the fingers. The most frequent injuries are dorsal dislocations. Lateral dislocations are less common, apparently because of the stability produced by the proportionately wider transverse diameter of the proximal phalangeal condyles. Dorsal dislocations are frequently associated with open injuries.

Reduction of a dorsal dislocation is usually simple, particularly with a median nerve wrist block. The reduction is quite stable. As with the fingers, the volar plate remains attached to the distal phalanx and may come to lie over the proximal phalangeal condyle. This is well demonstrated in roentgenograms of patients who have a sesamoid bone in the displaced volar plate (Fig. 12-10). For optimal results, the joint should be immobilized in slight flexion for three weeks.

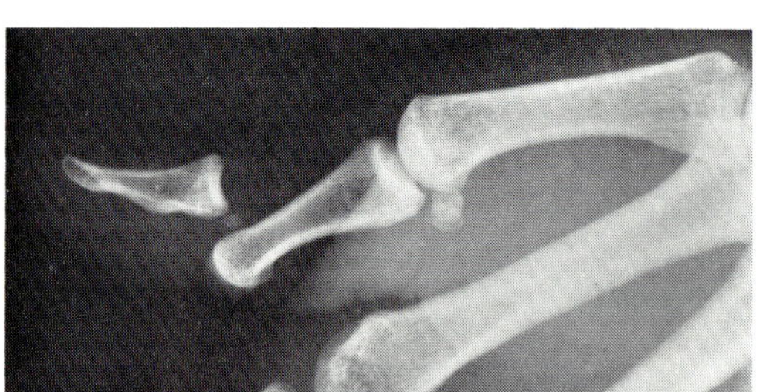

Figure 12-10. *The small sesamoid lying within the substance of the volar plate demonstrates that in dorsal dislocations the volar plate remains attached to the distal phalanx.* (*From Eaton, R.G.*[3])

Metacarpophalangeal Joint

The metacarpophalangeal joint of the thumb has structural features of both an interphalangeal and a metacarpal joint. Because of its condylar form, slight lateral mobility is present in extension. Its motion in flexion and extension, however, is highly variable, ranging from 5 to 100°, with a mean range of 75°. The collateral ligaments are thick and quadrangular, inserting into the proximal phalanx and volar plate. The accessory ligaments insert into the lateral margins of the volar plate and are in continuity with two sesamoid bones. These sesamoids lie within the substance of the volar plate, articulating with the metacarpal condyle. They serve as insertions for the flexor pollicis brevis (radial sesamoid) and oblique head of the adductor pollicis (ulnar sesamoid). This muscular proximal attachment of the volar plate provides strength with some degree of elasticity, in distinction to the fixed check ligaments which restrain the volar plate of the proximal interphalangeal joints. The thumb metacarpophalangeal joint, therefore, has a more mobile ligamentous boxlike support which permits a moderate degree of lateral movement, particularly when in flexion. Further unique dynamic support for the thumb metacarpophalangeal joint is provided by the cone of thenar intrinsic muscles. The dual support of the collateral ligament-volar plate "box" configuration, reinforced by these intrinsic muscles, imparts remarkable stability to this vulnerable and exposed joint.

Thumb metacarpophalangeal joint dislocations are six times more frequent than those of the digital metacarpophalangeal joints.[9] There are two basic types of displacement; dorsal and lateral. Each occurs with approximately equal frequency.[2]

DORSAL DISPLACEMENT

Dorsal dislocations occur when extreme hyperextension or shearing forces cause disruption of the volar supporting structures. Ligamentous disruption is proportional to the extent of joint distortion. Displacement may vary from transient hyperextension to complete displacement of the proximal phalanx which comes to rest in a bayonet position over the metacarpal head.* For such displacement, there must be a complete tear of the

*Actually it is the metacarpal head which is displaced, perforating, volar and proximal to the volar plate, lying between the heads of the adductor and flexor pollicis brevis muscles.

volar plate and part of each collateral ligament system. The disruption is almost always through the membranous proximal volar plate, proximal to the sesamoids. This can be confirmed in a roentgenogram which will show the sesamoids lying 1 to 2 mm proximal to the base of the proximal phalanx (Fig. 12-11).

Despite complete dorsal displacement, closed reduction is almost always successful. This dislocation differs from the irreducible finger metacarpophalangeal dislocation in that no lumbrical is present to complete the "finger-trap" encirclement of the metacarpal neck. Reduction is simplified by initially flexing the metacarpal into the palm, thereby relaxing the thenar muscles. Traction with flexion completes the reduction. Occasionally, the impacted volar plate must be maneuvered out of the joint utilizing the flexor pollicis longus tendon. This tendon lies in the pulley formed in part by the volar plate. (This same pulley is the culprit in the trigger thumb.) By extending the distal phalanx, the flexor tendon is tightened, bowstringing the pulley (and plate) volarly, permitting an easy reduction. Moderate lateral instability may be present after reduction, but unless 40° or more is present simple splinting will be adequate treatment. The joint should be immobilized in flexion for three weeks.

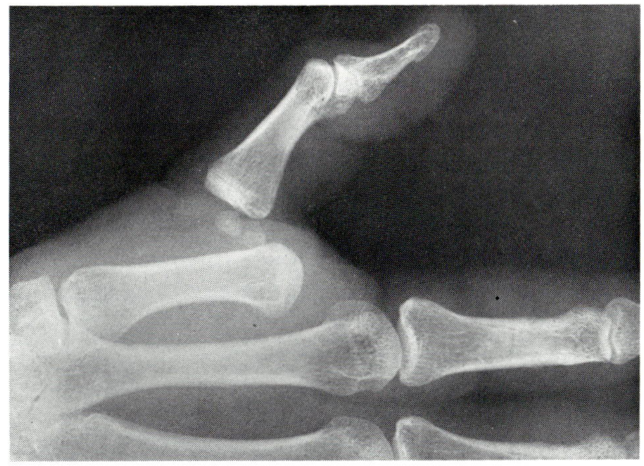

Figure 12-11. *Dorsal dislocation of the proximal phalanx. The sesamoids mark the location of the volar plate. Their proximity to the phalanx suggests the plate has ruptured proximally. The intrinsic muscles, inserting into the sesamoids, have stretched to allow such displacement.* (*From Eaton, R.G.*[3])

LATERAL DISPLACEMENT

Lateral dislocations with their unilateral collateral ligament-volar plate disruptions present a special diagnostic challenge. Following displacement, other than local pain and swelling there is scant physical evidence to indicate the extent of ligamentous disruption, particularly since the joint is usually stable through a full range of active flexion and extension. In suspected thumb injuries, sagittal stability is not the sole criterion, for equally critical is the joint's stability to ulnar and radial stress. Diagnosis of a ligamentous tear is made by the stress test in extension which, unless obvious hypermobility is present, is most valid under regional anesthesia.

Ulnar Ligament

Ulnar collateral ligamentous tears occur ten times more frequently than radial tears.[11] Ulnar ligamentous laxity is particularly disabling since it produces significant weakness in the thumb's ability to resist flexion-adduction stress, as in strong pinch. Partial tears of the ulnar ligament will not permit significant laxity and angulation. However, when lateral stress applied to the joint in full extension elicits more than 40° in angulation, a major disruption has occurred.[3,4] Complete unilateral ligamentous rupture must be present before significant displacement can occur.

Ulnar collateral ligamentous tears present special diagnostic problems. Complete tears may not heal because of interposition of the adductor aponeurosis across the site of ligamentous disruption. This unique interposition occurs as the aponeurosis, attached to the extensor pollicis longus, is drawn distally as the proximal phalanx undergoes angulation. The aponeurosis sweeps across the point of the distal rupture of the ligament. In realignment, the proximal edge of the ligament may slide *beneath* the proximal end of the collateral ligament, displacing it dorsally and preventing realignment or contact with its distal counterpart (Fig. 12-12). The resulting defect in the ulnar capsule heals with scar which provides less rigid support than the tough natural ligament. Stener found such ligamentous displacement in 25 of 39 (64 per cent) patients operated upon for suspected ulnar collateral ligamentous tears.[12]

Because of the frequency of this interposition, all injured metacarpophalangeal joints which exhibit 40° of ulnar ligamentous instability should be explored, since only one out of three could be expected to heal satisfactorily by immobilization alone. When instability of less than 40° is present,

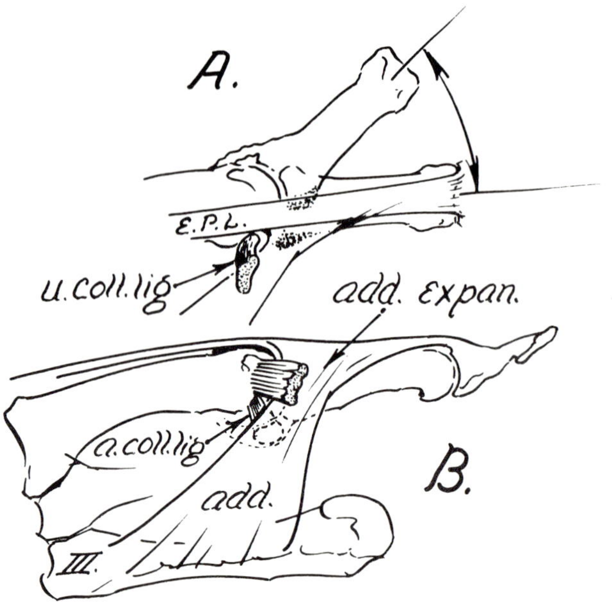

Figure 12-12. *The mechanism of displacement of the ulnar collateral ligament.* **A:** *Forceful abduction tears the ulnar collateral ligament distally and draws the adductor aponeurosis tightly across the site of rupture. With realignment, the ligament is swept proximally by the edge of the extensor mechanism.* **B:** *The torn end of the ligament is prevented from healing in its normal position by interposition of the aponeurosis.*

the ligament will heal satisfactorily with three weeks' immobilization. Ruptures of the radial ligament even when 40° angulation can be demonstrated usually heal adequately with three weeks' immobilization, since there is no such interposition on the radial aspect. (Occasionally slight volar subluxation will accompany radial ligament tears. This suggests a rotatory displacement, for which the ligament should be repaired.)

Repair of a complete ulnar collateral ligamentous tear is through a curved ulnar-dorsal incision. The proximal edge of the adductor aponeurosis is identified and, adjacent to it, the ulnar collateral ligament. When displaced, the ligament is seen reflected dorsally and proximally. It is shortened, thickened and frayed. When explored later than ten days, the ligament may be so shortened and edematous that it cannot be approximated to its distal attachment. In order to achieve optimal exposure, the adductor aponeurosis is divided longitudinally from the extensor tendon, allowing it to be reflected ulnarward. Reattachment of the ligament is most effectively achieved by pull-out wire technique, placing a drill hole at the site of detachment. When ruptured at a point away from the insertion, a simple end-to-end suture is all that is required. The adductor aponeurosis is reattached to the extensor tendon with several fine sutures and the thumb immobilized for three weeks in a slightly overcorrected position. Complete ulnar ligamentous tears initially unrecognized heal imperfectly, leaving considerable lateral instability. When thumb instability and weakness are sufficiently disabling, reconstruction of this ulnar collateral ligament can be done by using a free tendon graft.[4,13]

References

1. Alldred, A.J.: A locked index finger. J. Bone Joint Surg., 36B:102, 1954.
2. Coonrad, R.W. and Goldner, L.: Soft tissue injury of the thumb metacarpophalangeal joint. J. Bone Joint Surg., 50A:439, 1968.
3. Eaton, R.G.: *Joint Injuries in the Hand.* Charles C Thomas, Springfield, 1971.
4. Eaton, R.G. and Littler, J.W.: Dislocations and ligamentous injuries of the hand. Sound-slide presentation, American Academy Orthopedic Surgeons, New York City, January 1969.
5. Gad, P.: The anatomy of the volar part of the capsules of the finger joints. J. Bone Joint Surg., 49B:363, 1967.
6. Kuczuynski, K.: The proximal interphalangeal joint. J. Bone Joint Surg., 50B:656, 1968.
7. Littler, J.W.: Mobilization of the stiffened proximal interphalangeal joint. J. Bone Joint Surg., 46A:917, 1964.
8. Littler, J.W. and Eaton, R.G.: Redistribution of forces in the correction of the boutonniere deformity. J. Bone Joint Surg., 49A:1267, 1967.
9. MacLaughlin, H.L.: Complex 'locked' dislocations of the metacarpophalangeal joints. J. Trauma, 5:683, 1965.
10. McCue, F.C., Honner, R., Johnson, M.C., Jr., and Gieck, J.H.: Athletic injuries of the proximal interphalangeal joint requiring surgical treatment. J. Bone Joint Surg., 52A:937, 1970.
11. Moberg, E. and Stener, B.: Injuries to the ligaments of the thumb and fingers. Diagnosis, treatment, and prognosis. Acta Chir. Scand., 106:166, 1953.
12. Stener, B.: Displacement of the ruptured ulnar collateral ligament of the metacarpophalangeal joint of the thumb. J. Bone Joint Surg., 44B:869, 1962.
13. Strandell, G.: Total rupture of the ulnar collateral ligament of the metacarpophalangeal joint of the thumb. Results of surgery in 35 cases. Acta Chir. Scand., 118:72, 1959.

13 Small Joint Arthrodesis in the Hand

Arthrodesis of one or several carefully selected small joints in the hand, precisely done for specific indications, is a reliable procedure with predictable results that often will be of significant benefit in improving function and decreasing pain.

However, the reliability of arthrodesis does not mean that it should be undertaken lightly. The indications are specific, and the technique must be precise. An ill-advised arthrodesis on an inappropriate joint or in a non-functional position may severely jeopardize hand function, e.g. the thumb basal joint fused in adduction or the proximal interphalangeal joint fused at 0°. Furthermore, the operative technique must be impeccable, for a significant incidence of non-union has been reported.[1,9,15]

Indications

There are several indications for arthrodesis in the arthritic hand, commonly including pain, instability and/or deformity.[8] Frequently, arthrodeses are advised for treating the ravages of idiopathic osteoarthritis at the level of the distal interphalangeal joints or in the basal joint of the thumb, particularly in middle-aged women.[7]

A second group of patients with pain, instability and/or deformity who may benefit from small joint arthrodesis are those with rheumatoid arthritis. The joints most commonly fused are those in the thumb, the distal interphalangeal finger joints and the proximal interphalangeal joints of the index and long fingers (Chap. 24).

In certain situations, small joint arthrodesis is indicated when secondary degenerative changes have followed trauma.

Joints destroyed by infection may also require arthrodesis. In certain situations in the subacute stage of joint infection, arthrodesis will assist in the eradication of the infection and provide a pain-free, stable digit; this is particularly true for a drug addict with septic arthritis at the proximal interphalangeal joint.[14]

Lastly, and perhaps the most complex situation to evaluate preoperatively, is the use of small joint arthrodesis to simplify the digital system in conjunction with tendon transfers.[11,12] For example, in certain types of median and ulnar palsies of the hand, the functional benefit from an opponens tendon transfer will be significantly increased by fusion of either the interphalangeal joint or the metacarpophalangeal joint, depending upon the specific situation.[12]

Contraindications

Generally the advantages of arthrodesis must be weighed against the advantages of implant arthroplasty. When skin cover, musculotendinous function and motivation of the patient are good, arthroplasty is generally considered. An unsuccessful arthroplasty can be converted to a successful arthrodesis, but the reverse is much harder to achieve.

There are specific contraindications to small joint fusion.[4,19,20,21] The most important is severe involvement of an adjacent joint which cannot be treated with implant arthroplasty. In the *thumb,* it is inadvisable to fuse the arthritic metacarpophalangeal joint if that same thumb has a severely involved carpometacarpal joint for which fusion is anticipated.[4] Conversely, it is inadvisable to fuse the carpometacarpal joint of the thumb of a patient with arthritic deformities or stiffness at the metacarpophalangeal joint.[4,21] Arthrodesis of either of these two joints will accelerate the degenerative changes in the other. In this clinical situation, it is best to fuse the metacarpophalangeal joint at the same time that an arthroplasty is performed on the basal joint. The carpometacarpal joint of the thumb should not be fused if the other joints of the trapezium are also significantly involved in the arthritic process.[21]

The metacarpophalangeal joint and the proximal interphalangeal joint in the same digit should not both be fused. In selected cases one joint might be fused and an implant arthroplasty might be performed on the other.[21] In the rheumatoid, it is usually the proximal joint which receives the implant and the distal joint the arthrodesis.

Position of Arthrodesis

The position selected for small joint fusion is critical to hand function. The index finger is involved primarily in pinch, whereas the fingers on the ulnar side of the hand are involved in grasp. Therefore, the radial fingers function in a straighter position than do the ulnar digits.

For the distal interphalangeal joint, an arthrodesed position between 10 and 25° is recommended. The index finger is usually fused nearly straight, whereas the distal joint of the little finger is fused at approximately 25°.

Similarly, at the proximal interphalangeal joint, the index and long fingers are fused at 25 to 30° and the ring and little fingers at 35 to 45°. Note that extension of the distal interphalangeal joint depends upon the position of the proximal interphalangeal. As the proximal interphalangeal joint flexes it becomes increasingly difficult to extend the distal interphalangeal joint.[13] Very forceful, active distal interphalangeal motion will not remain after proximal joint arthrodesis.[13] Therefore, proximal interphalangeal arthrodesis is not to be undertaken lightly, and the position must be accurate since it will affect both interphalangeal joints.

Should it be necessary to fuse a finger metacarpophalangeal joint, the index finger is best fused at 25°, with gradually increasing flexion passing to the ulnar side of the hand, fusing the fifth metacarpophalangeal joint at 45°. The metacarpophalangeal joints of adjacent fingers should not be fused.

The thumb interphalangeal joint is best fused at 10° flexion and 10° pronation. The metacarpophalangeal joint of the thumb is best fused at 10 to 15° flexion, neutral abduction, and approximately 10 to 15° pronation.

The carpometacarpal thumb joint should be fused in the "fist position" (Fig. 13-7).

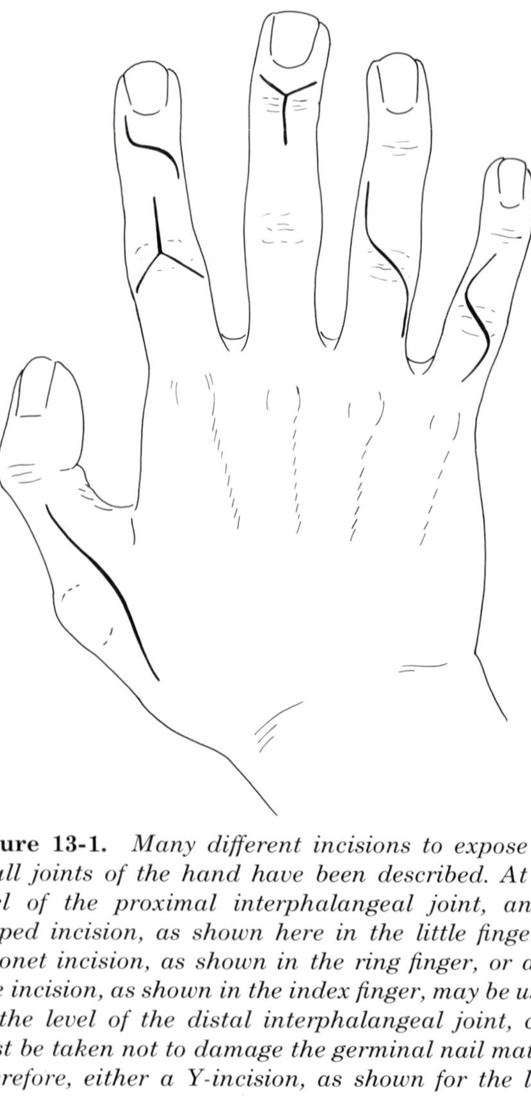

Figure 13-1. *Many different incisions to expose the small joints of the hand have been described. At the level of the proximal interphalangeal joint, an S-shaped incision, as shown here in the little finger, a bayonet incision, as shown in the ring finger, or a Y-type incision, as shown in the index finger, may be used. At the level of the distal interphalangeal joint, care must be taken not to damage the germinal nail matrix. Therefore, either a Y-incision, as shown for the long finger, or a gently curved incision, as shown in the index, is preferred. In the burned hand a transverse incision may be all that is needed.*

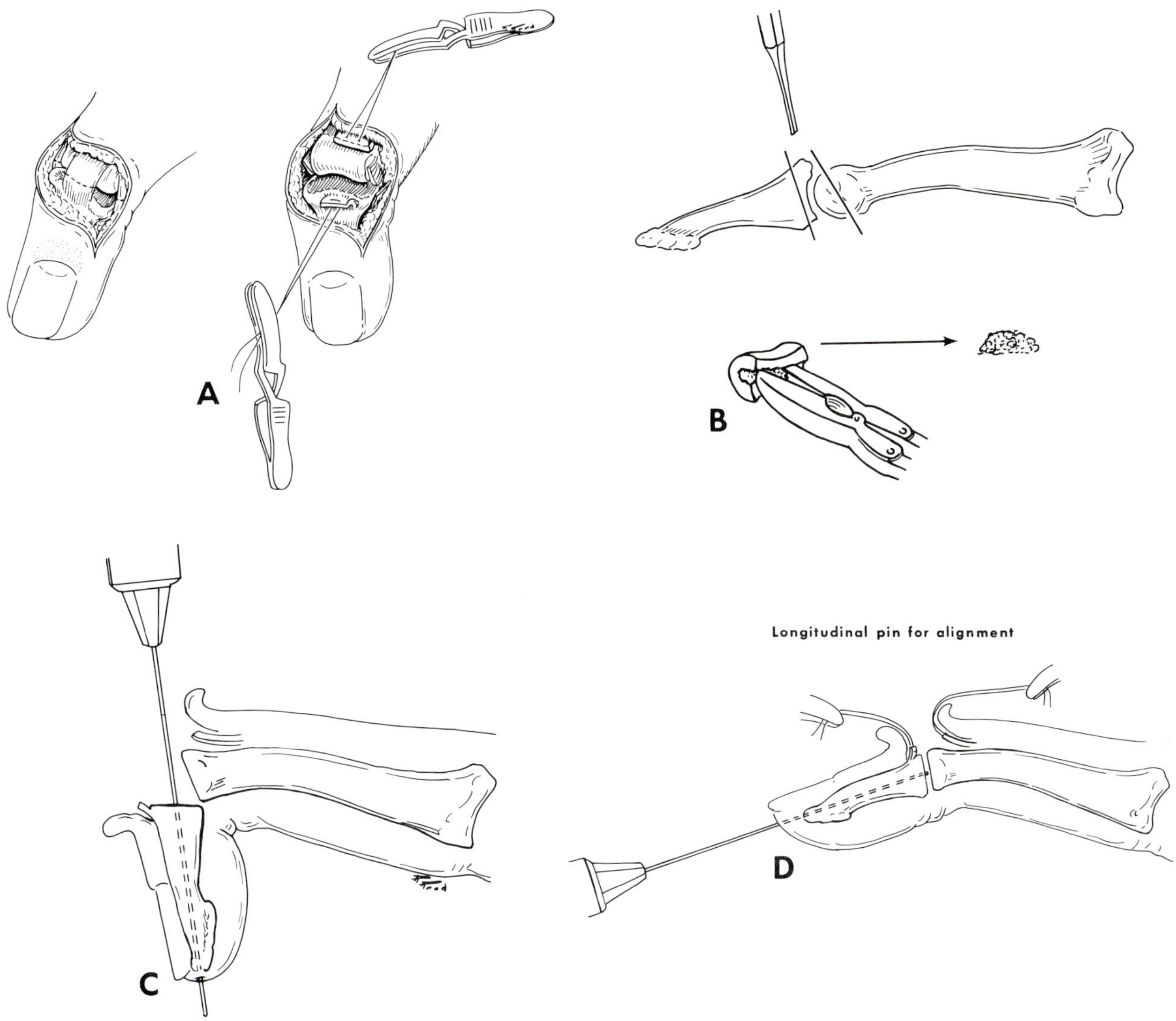

Figure 13-2. **A:** *Once the dorsal aspect is exposed, the extensor tendon is visualized. This may be transected. The collateral ligaments are released from their proximal attachments, and the joint is exposed by flexion.* **B:** *Bone is removed from the head of the middle phalanx at an angle, so that when the arthrodesis site is coapted it will be in the desired amount of flexion (see text). As shown in the insert, a surprising amount of medullary bone chips can be removed from the condylar portion, utilizing a small rongeur. The subchondral bone is removed from the base of the distal phalanx in a plane perpendicular to its shaft. Often a large osteophyte is present dorsally. The removal of this may include the extensor tendon insertion.* **C:** *A longitudinal Kirschner wire is then driven down the shaft of the distal phalanx.* **D:** *The arthrodesis site is then reduced, and the wire is driven proximally into the middle phalanx. The .045 double-ended Kirschner wires are very useful for this.*

Technique of Arthrodesis

The technique of small joint arthrodesis must be precise. Failure to be precise will result in a significant incidence of pseudarthrosis. Many techniques have been described.[2,3,5-7,9,10,15-19] The techniques preferred by the author are summarized in the legends of Figures 13-1 through 13-7. The following generalities bear emphasis and are pertinent to each of the joints.

First, the technique must be gentle, with great care being taken to protect and not damage the adjacent flexor and extensor systems.

Second, an exact fit of the coapted arthrodesis is mandatory. If the fit of the two surfaces is not perfect, then small medullary bone chips should be added.

Third, the Kirschner wires are used to provide accurate longitudinal alignment and to maintain coaptation and control rotation. They are not a

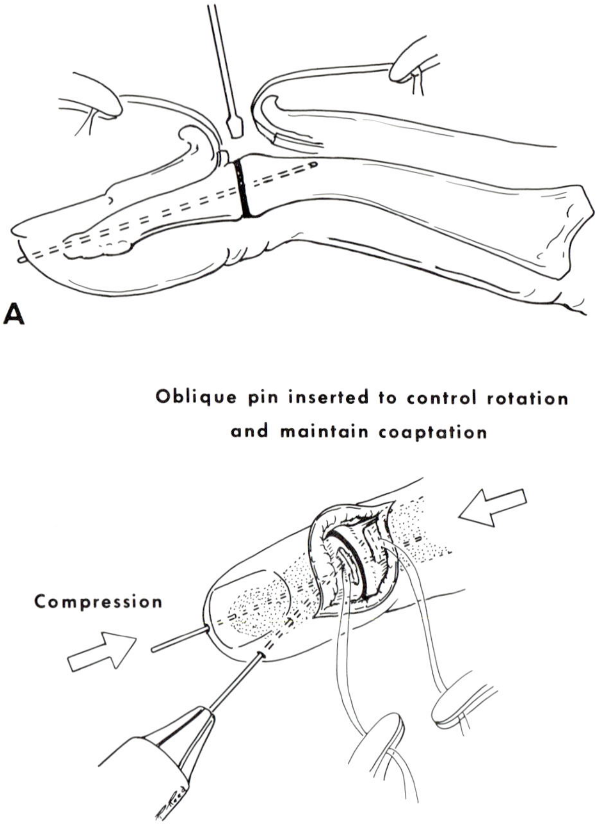

Figure 13-3. A: *The bony apposition must be perfect. If any slight irregularities exist, the medullary bony chips from the condylar specimen are impacted into the arthrodesis site.* **B:** *The arthrodesis site is then coapted under pressure, and an oblique Kirschner wire is introduced to control rotation and maintain coaptation.*

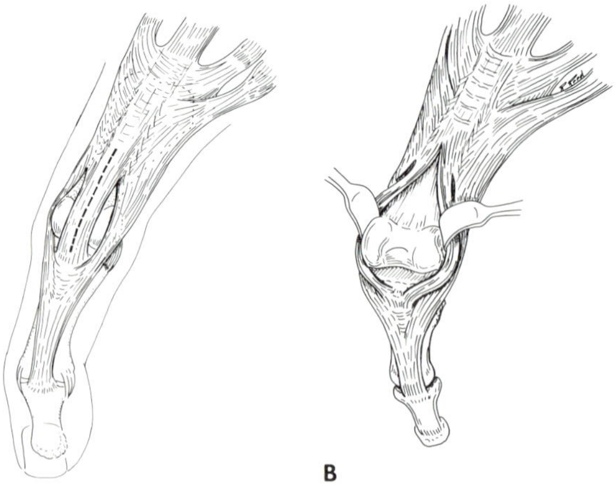

Figure 13-4. A: *The extensor mechanism is split longitudinally.* **B:** *The joint is exposed by flexion and retraction of the extensor mechanism. Collateral ligaments are released from their proximal attachments.*

substitute for external immobilization but are merely used as an adjunct to the external support.

Fourth, following finger surgery, the operated portion of the hand and wrist is immobilized for approximately three weeks in a supportive soft dressing with an overlying plaster shell in a position of function. At that time, the oblique pins are removed and the longitudinal pins are left in position. The patient uses a finger dressing with a splint during the subsequent time. The single longitudinal pin and the splint are maintained until fusion is demonstrated roentgenographically, usually at 7 to 10 weeks.

For either the metacarpophalangeal joint or the carpometacarpal joint of the thumb, immobilization of the thumb and wrist in plaster is continued until arthrodesis is demonstrated roentgenographically. This usually takes 6 to 8 weeks for the metacarpophalangeal joints and 9 to 10 weeks for the basal joint.

Fifth, if the patient is a rheumatoid in whom finger interphalangeal joint fusion has been done in conjunction with arthroplasty of the metacarpophalangeal joint, at approximately one week postoperatively the external plaster may be removed and the exercise program started for the metacarpophalangeal arthroplasty. The interphalangeal joint arthrodesis is protected both by the internal fixation with Kirschner wires and by accurate and carefully applied finger splints.

If a rheumatoid thumb has a simultaneous arthrodesis of the metacarpophalangeal joint and arthroplasty of the basal joint, six weeks of external immobilization is required to protect the capsular repair of the arthroplasty. Exercise of the basal joint is then started and the Kirschner wires at the metacarpophalangeal joint are left in place for two more weeks or until the fusion is healed.

The techniques preferred by the author for arthrodesis of the distal interphalangeal joint, proximal interphalangeal joint, metacarpophalangeal joint, and the interphalangeal joint and the metacarpophalangeal joint of the thumb are all quite similar (Figs. 13-1 through 13-6).

To fuse the carpometacarpal joint of the thumb, the technique of Eaton and Littler is recommended[7] (Fig. 13-7). Using a dorsal longitudinal incision, care is taken not to damage the sensory branches of the radial nerve. The joint is exposed by reflecting the margin of the abductor pollicis longus insertion. Bone is removed from the base of the thumb metacarpal in a plane perpendicular to its long axis. The thumb is then placed in a fist position and a cut is made through the trapezium

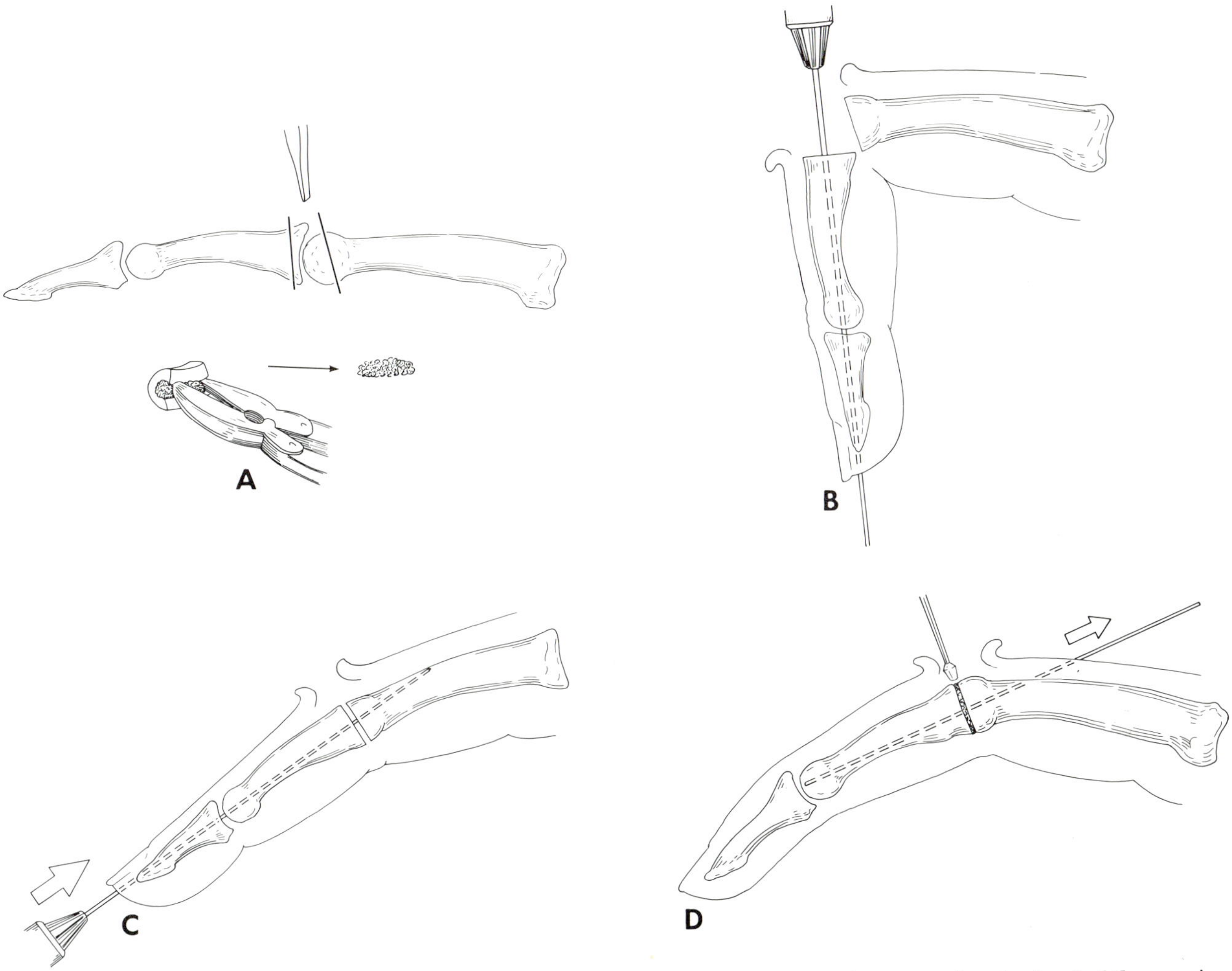

Figure 13-5. **A:** *In a fashion similar to that of the distal joint (Fig. 13-2), bone is removed at the level of the proximal interphalangeal joint (see text regarding position).* **B:** *The distal two phalanges are then flexed, and the pin is driven down the shaft of the two phalanges. The pin is then withdrawn so that the proximal end is flush with the base of the middle phalanx.* **C:** *The arthrodesis site is reduced, and the pin is driven proximally into the proximal phalanx.* **D:** *The pin is withdrawn so that the distal end lies just within the substance of the head of the middle phalanx. Again, as for the distal interphalangeal joint, bony apposition must be perfect. If it is not perfect, medullary bone chips from the condylar specimen are impacted, as for the distal interphalangeal joint in Figure 13-3.*

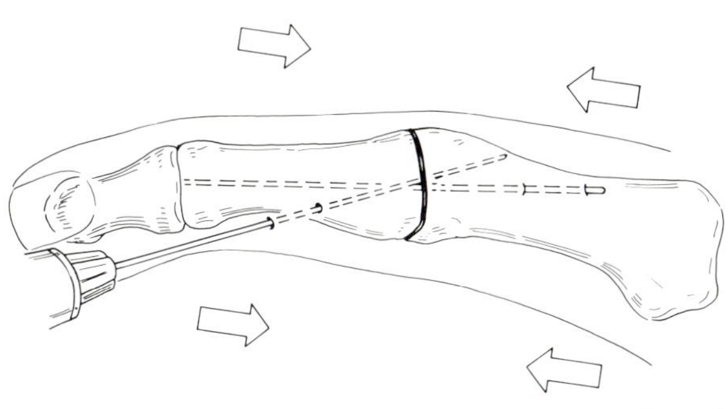

Figure 13-6. *The arthrodesis site is coapted under pressure, and an oblique Kirschner wire is introduced to maintain coaptation and control rotation.*

in a plane parallel to that of the base of the thumb metacarpal. Care must be taken to remove the bony projection from the ulnar margin of the trapezium toward the index metacarpal. This is important, for it allows a more accurate apposition of the arthrodesis site and, more importantly, it increases the motion at the other trapezial joints to allow for better mobility at the basal joint area of the thumb. With the bony surfaces coapted under pressure and the thumb in a fist position, crossed Kirschner wires are then introduced across the arthrodesis site to maintain coaptation. A third Kirschner wire is introduced from the thumb

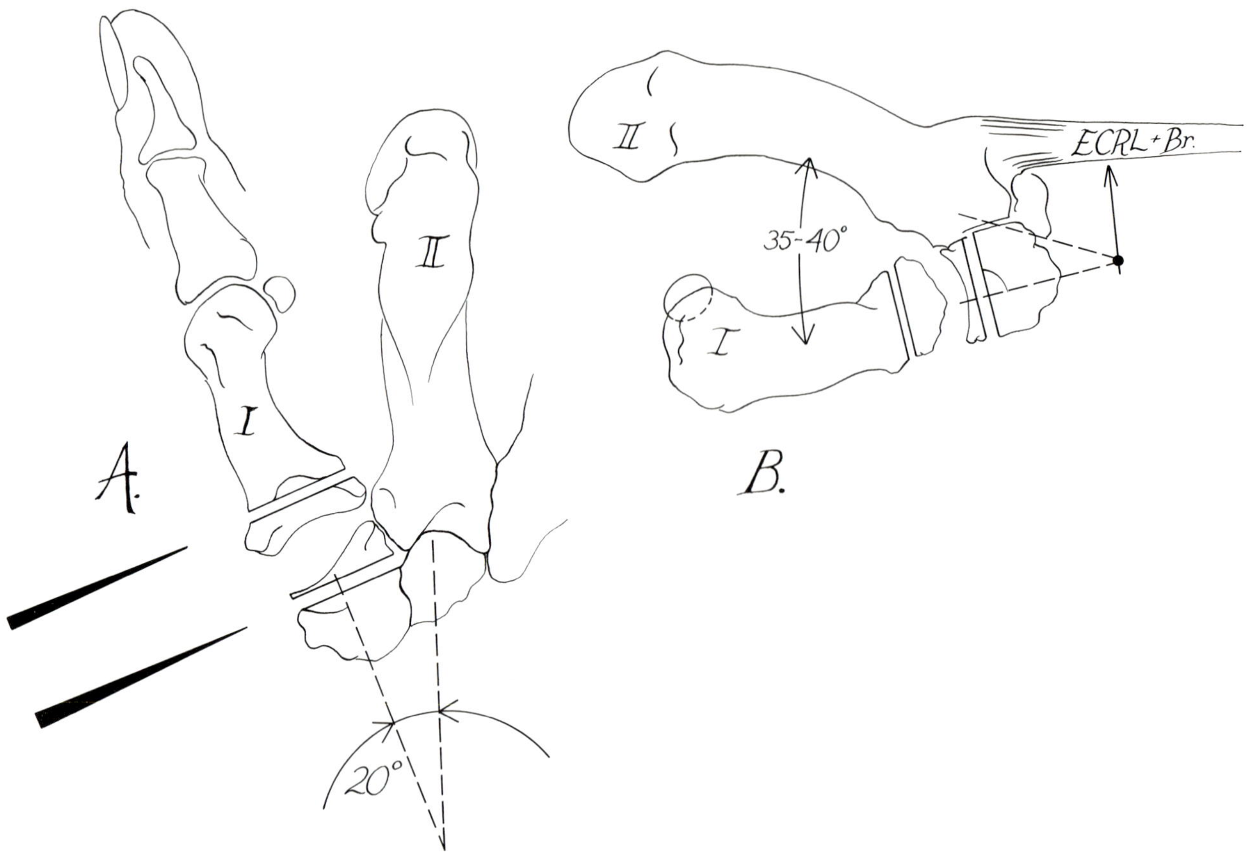

Figure 13-7. *Arthrodesis of the carpometacarpal joint of the thumb. Position is critical and has been described as the "fist position" or projection of the thumb metacarpal when the fingers and thumb are clenched in a fist. The bone is first removed from the metacarpal in a plane perpendicular to its long axis and then from the trapezium with a parallel cut. Fixation is obtained with Kirschner wires (see text). (Redrawn from Eaton, R.G. and Littler, J.W.*[7])

metacarpal into the index metacarpal. When fusion is demonstrated roentgenographically, these pins are removed and a gentle exercise program is begun. For the arthritic with arthrodesis in the proper position, good pain-free thumb function, including opposition, is obtained.

In summary, arthrodesis of selected small joints in the hand is often indicated in the arthritic or palsied hand for relief of pain, to gain stability, to reduce deformity or to simplify the disrupted linkage of a multiarticulated system. The results are predictable and gratifying if the procedure is carefully done for the proper indication.

References

1. Anderson, G.R.: Arthrodesis of the distal interphalangeal joints. (Abstract.) J. Bone Joint Surg., 52B:800, 1970.
2. Brittain, H.A.: *Architectural Principles in Arthrodesis,* 2nd ed. Williams and Wilkins, Baltimore, 1952.
3. Bunnell, S.: *Surgery of the Hand.* J.B. Lippincott, Philadelphia, 1948.
4. Burton, R.I.: Basal joint arthrodesis of the thumb. Orthop. Clin. North Am., 2:331, 1973.
5. Campbell, D.: Experiences of a hand surgery service. Br. J. Plast. Surg., 9:23, 1956.
6. Carroll, R.E. and Hill, N.A.: Small joint arthrodesis in hand reconstruction. J. Bone Joint Surg., 51A:1219, 1969.
7. Eaton, R.G. and Littler, J.W.: A study of the basal joint of the thumb. J. Bone Joint Surg., 51A:661, 1969.
8. Flatt, A.E.: *The Care of the Rheumatoid Hand,* 2nd ed. C.V. Mosby, St. Louis, 1968.
9. Granowitz, S. and Vainio, K.: Proximal interphalangeal joint arthrodesis in rheumatoid arthritis. Acta Orthop. Scand., 37:301, 1966.
10. Leach, R.E. and Bolton, P.E.: Arthritis of the carpometacarpal joint of the thumb. J. Bone Joint Surg., 50A:1171, 1968.
11. Littler, J.W.: Tendon transfers and arthrodeses in combined median and ulnar nerve paralysis. J. Bone Joint Surg., 31A:225, 1949.
12. Littler, J.W.: Personal communication, 1970.
13. Littler, J.W. and Burton, R.I.: Dynamics of finger extension, Part I and Part II. Sound-slide programs 467 and 468. American Academy of Orthopaedic Surgeons, 1976.
14. McKay, D., Pascarelli, E.F. and Eaton, R.G.: Infections and sloughs in the hands in drug addicts. J. Bone Joint Surg., 55A:741, 1973.

15. Micks, J.E. and Hager, D.L.: A method of accelerating fusion of small joints. (Abstract.) J. Bone Joint Surg., 50A:1269, 1968.
16. Moberg, E.: Arthrodesis of finger joints. Surg. Clin. North Am., 40:465, 1960.
17. Potenza, A.D.: A technique for arthrodesis of finger joints. J. Bone Joint Surg., 55A:1534, 1973.
18. Seewald, K.: Die arthrodese der fingergelinke mit gekreuzten bohrdrahten. Wien. Med. Wochenschr., 105:174, 1955.
19. Swanson, A.B.: Osteoarthritis of the hand. J. Bone Joint Surg., 55A:1769, 1973.
20. Swanson, A.B.: Flexible implant arthroplasty for arthritic finger joints. Rationale, technique, and results of treatment. J. Bone Joint Surg., 54A:435, 1972.
21. Swanson, A.B.: Disabling arthritis at the base of the thumb. Treatment by resection of the trapezium and flexible (silicone) implant arthroplasty. J. Bone Joint Surg., 54A:456, 1972.

14 Tendons

"The surgeon can fix it, God can heal it, but only the patient can make it work."

A tendon is, in essence, a cord which links a spring (the muscle, referred to as "the motor") to a bone. Like a fishing rod, it may require one or more guides (pulleys) to prevent bowstringing. For the muscle to recoil (contract) efficiently it must be stretched by the positioning of one or more joints (e.g. the wrist). The force of this recoil can make healthy tendons hypertrophy and injured ones separate or form hypertrophic callus and scar.

Tendon disorders are common. These are rarely neoplastic, seldom congenital, but commonly the result of inflammatory, degenerative or traumatic conditions. These may be isolated to one or more tendons, or may be generalized, involving all other tissues and structures. For practical purposes, the tendons affected by these disorders may be grouped anatomically and functionally as follows:

1. Disorders of the extrinsic digital flexors, the tendons with the greatest excursion (amplitude)
2. Disorders of the wrist extensors and flexors and forearm pronators and supinators, the "positioners"
3. Disorders of the extrinsic digital extensors, and
4. Disorders of the digital extrinsic-intrinsic "hood" mechanism.

Anatomy and Function

Tendons are the functional prolongations of muscles formed by the coalescence of muscle fibrils. They transmit the force of muscle contraction into joint movement. They are cords of condensed collagen having great tensile strength (approximately 10,000 lb to the square inch). To achieve their function of joint movement, tendons must be mobile and have a gliding mechanism.

Paratenon is a specialized areolar connective tissue sleeve and mesentery (mesotenon) of the tendons (Fig. 14-1). It is highly reactive and proliferative in the formation of pseudotendon and scar. It is found wherever there is no tendon sheath, namely, about the tendons of the forearm, dorsum of the hand, and in the midpalmar area. Paratenon provides a segmental blood supply by means of coiled elastic blood vessels so that tendon amplitude is not restricted.

Bowstringing across the concavity of joints is prevented by a retinacular sheath with periodic condensations in the form of pulleys where the greatest forces occur (Fig. 14-2). These pulleys are

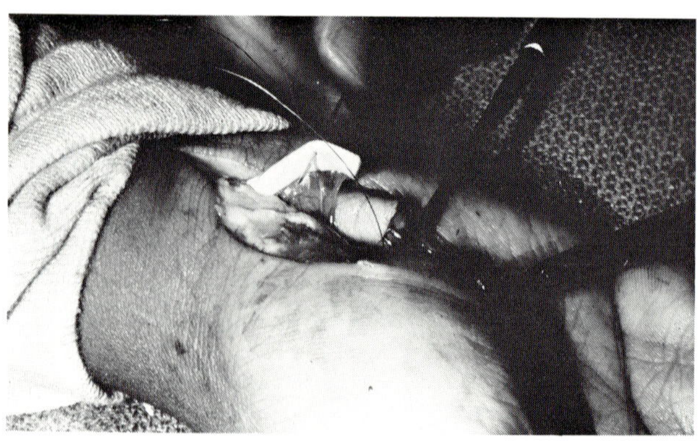

Figure 14-1. *Tendons have a mesentery (mesotenon) not unlike that of the intestine. Note the fine straight needle used to prevent retraction of the divided tendon.*

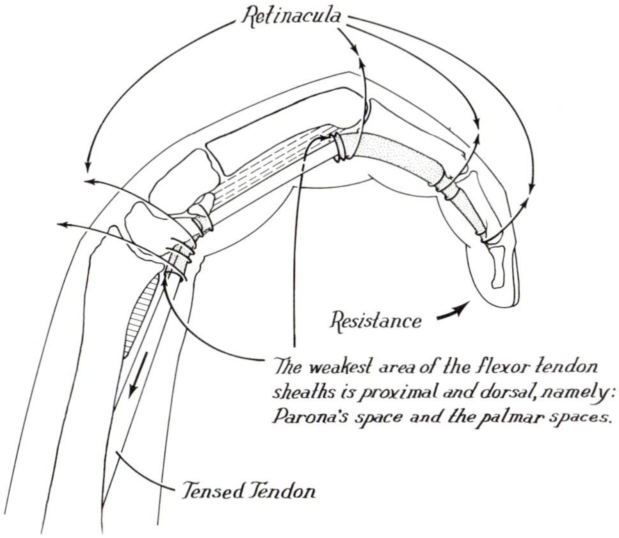

Figure 14-2. *Forces acting on the flexor pulley system during flexion.*

of indispensable importance for the long digital flexors. The most important pulley is that which is anchored to the proximal shaft volar plate of the proximal phalanx (Fig. 2-17). The second most important lies at the neck of the middle phalanx. The lubrication needed within these retinacular slings is provided by the synovial lining in the form of a bursa with visceral and parietal layers. These layers coalesce at the proximal and distal limits of the bursa, as well as along the deep surface of the tendon, forming a mesotenon. The major vessels are found in stalks called vincula. The short vincula are thick triangular membranes. They unite the terminal part of the superficial and deep flexor tendons to the dorsal wall of the tendon sheaths just proximal to the proximal and distal interphalangeal joints respectively. The long vincula are narrow translucent bands placed proximal to the short ones.

As tendons develop from cellular to relatively acellular structures, their blood supply diminishes. Circulation reaches tendons through the vascular arcades of the mesotenon and to a limited degree through the muscle proximally and the insertion distally. The intratendinous blood supply is not capable of nourishing more than one-quarter of the tendon length without collateral connections from the tendon bed.[11]

There are two major musculotendinous groups: (1) The extrinsic flexors and extensors (14 of each) arising in the arm and forearm, and (2) the 20 intrinsic muscles which lie exclusively within the body of the hand.

Crowding of the multiple tendons within a sheath-and-pulley system becomes a threat to excursion when the effects of injury lead to changes in volume of the tendon or its pulley. An isolated injury to the sheath or a single tendon within it may easily limit gliding of the companion tendons by the formation of short rigid adhesions and thick callus.

Amplitude, defined as the range of movement between maximal contraction and relaxation, can be critical for function. At the origin and insertion of the muscle-tendon unit, the amplitude of motion is zero. The maximal amplitude is usually at the center of the muscle-tendon unit. The average maximal amplitude of motion of the flexors and extensors of the wrist is 33 mm, extensors of the fingers 50 mm, flexor of the thumb 50 mm, and flexors of the fingers 70 mm.[1] It is difficult to measure the amplitude of motion of intrinsic muscles, but the adductor pollicis and the lumbricals have a range of approximately 20 mm. The gliding ranges of extrinsic tendons are shown in Table 14-1.

The multiarticulated architecture of the hand is maintained in delicate balance for movement by the interrelated actions of the extrinsic muscles, which provide power, and the intrinsic muscles, which provide dexterity. The thumb, index and long fingers are the principal digits of dexterity, and the long, ring and little fingers the principal digits for sustained grasp. Certain groups have common muscle bellies so that the tendon excursion of all must be free for any one to act adequately. That is, all of the tendon components to a common muscle must act at the same time (e.g. the extensor communis, or the flexor profundus to the long, ring and little fingers). Other musculotendinous units are totally independent. Anatomical variations to these generalizations occur.

The muscles must be stretched to contract effectively. Wrist movement, therefore, is the key to obtaining adequate tension for efficient function of the extrinsic muscles. To stretch the long digital flexors for power grasp, the extensor carpi radialis brevis, inserting centrally on the transverse arch, is the most important wrist extensor.[8] The synergistic relationships between wrist extension and digital flexion, and wrist flexion and digital extension, are therefore important. The normal amplitude of the extrinsic motors across the wrist ranges from 30 to 80 mm. However, wrist movement can compensate synergistically for deficiencies in the excursion of tendons to the digits.

The long and transverse arches of the hand, which must be assumed in cupping the palm and opposing the thumb and fingertips, are maintained

Table 14-1. *Tendon Excursions (modified from Boyes, J. H.*[1]*)*

	EXTENSOR PROPRIUS AND EXTENSOR COMMUNIS (in mm)	FLEXOR PROFUNDUS (in mm)	FLEXOR SUPERFICIALIS (in mm)
Index finger			
D.I.P. joint	0	5	—
P.I.P. joint	2	20	16
M.P. joint	15	15	16
Wrist joint	38	16	16
Full flexion (of all joints)	54	50	53
Middle finger			
D.I.P. joint	0	5	—
P.I.P. joint	3	17	16
M.P. joint	16	23	26
Wrist joint	41	38	46
Full flexion (of all joints)	55	85	88
Ring finger			
D.I.P. joint	0	5	—
P.I.P. joint	3	12	11
M.P. joint	11	15	21
Wrist joint	39	45	40
Full flexion (of all joints)	55	76	65
Little finger			
D.I.P. joint	0	3.5	—
P.I.P. joint	2	11	8
M.P. joint	12	15	17
Wrist joint	20	45	40
Full flexion (of all joints)	35	70	60

	EXTENSOR POLLICIS LONGUS (in mm)	EXTENSOR POLLICIS BREVIS (in mm)	ABDUCTOR POLLICIS (in mm)	LONG FLEXOR (in mm)
Thumb				
D.I.P. joint	8	—	—	12
M.P. joint	7	9	—	20
Carpometacarpal joint	6	7	5	8
Wrist joint	33	14	—	23
Totals	58	28	28	52

by the intrinsic muscles. These muscles also spread the hand and bring the fingers together and, through interweaving in the dorsal hood, share with the long digital extensors the action of interphalangeal joint extension. These two systems oppose one another in their actions on the metacarpophalangeal joint. In contrast to the digital flexors, the excursion of the extensor hood is minimal and deficits of 2 to 3 mm in any part of the hood may result in major deformities. The extensors of the digits generally cause more rapid but weaker motion than do the flexors.

Retinacular sheaths and pulleys lie across the wrist and along the volar aspect of the digits holding the tendons in place. Their synovial bursae provide the lubricant needed for tendon gliding, and also constitute avenues for the spread of infection. In disease and wound repair, tendon gliding is easily restricted by the constricting effect of these structures or by adherence of tendons to them.

Tendon Injury

Types of Injury

Tendon injuries are either open or closed, partial or complete. They are caused by direct or indirect violence, and any case may involve one or more tendons. Associated structures may be simultaneously injured.

Direct closed injury damages all tissues in the involved area. The tendons themselves undergo the same pathological changes as the surrounding soft tissue. In the wake of the initial traumatic edema and inflammation comes fibroblastic proliferation producing adhesions to tendons. A classic example of such injury occurs over the dorsum of the hand where peritendinous fibrosis (Secretan's disease)[12] results.

Tremendous forces are required to cause closed rupture of the normal flexor tendon. Such ruptures usually occur at either the origin or the insertion of a tendon. Occasionally the closed injury avulses the bone instead of, or in addition to, the tendon. This is frequently seen in the case of sudden forced hyperflexion or hyperextension at the distal interphalangeal joint, resulting in avulsion of the extensor or the flexor tendon at its distal insertion. Closed blunt trauma commonly causes attenuation and distortion of the extensor mechanism over the proximal interphalangeal joints of the fingers and the metacarpophalangeal joints of the digits.

Abnormal tendons may be easily ruptured with mild force. Such is the case in rheumatoid disease, in association with highly repetitive excursion of a tendon through a tight pulley (e.g. "drummer's thumb"*), in early postoperative tenorrhaphy, in the case of a poorly vascularized tendon graft and following partial division of a tendon.

The hope for recovery of function after open tendon injuries is governed to a large extent by whether the wound is tidy or untidy. However, the extension of even a tidy incisive wound to include the floor beneath the tendon or the sheath over it increases the chances of adverse adhesions and worsens the prognosis. Although an open wound may not specifically violate a tendon at the start, the function of a normal tendon can be curtailed by the reaction of injury in the tissues around it. All untidy tendon wounds are complicated problems, with a guarded prognosis for recovery even after the most skilled surgery. The most common open injuries are those to the extensor tendons in the hands and digits, where they lie close to the skin and are easily exposed to insult.

The anatomy of the vincula, the extensor hood and the juncturae tendina (conexus intertendineus) may easily mask a completely divided tendon from the unwary clinician. Likewise, partially divided tendons often pass unnoticed until further strain on the tendon insidiously or abruptly converts the partial injury into a complete one, days or even months later.

Reactions to Injury—Tendon Healing

The healing process following injury to a tendon and the tissues around it is the basis for principles governing tendon surgery. The cellular and biological events correspond to those that occur in the healing of other tissues.

The unique problem with tendons is the threat that wound healing poses to their gliding. In any wound, all the tissues are healed by a common coagulum that obliterates the tissue planes.[11] This coagulum matures into a scar as collagen is deposited. By the remodeling of collagen over a period of weeks and months, the tissue planes may become reestablished and the individual tissues anatomically distinct again. For this to occur, adhesions between planes must become soft, pliable and attenuated. The healed tendon may then glide actively if it has a functioning muscle, provided the joints are mobile and the tendon is not so bulky as to impinge on a tight tendon sheath.

A tendon heals almost entirely by the cellular response of its bed, leading to the penetration of capillaries into the tendon. This ingrowth results in adhesions which must modify in time to permit tendon excursion. Any trauma to the surface of the tendon, even touching it, incites adhesions. Traction on the tendon in the first three weeks of healing, the inducement of an inflammatory response by reactive sutures or infection and the impairment of circulation in the tendon bed lead to denser adhesions, which will restrict gliding. In certain individuals, even their own blood extravasated around the tendon provokes an extensive inflammatory response.

Separated tendon ends within a synovial sheath may fail to form any adhesions if there is no reaction to the blood in the sheath. However, retracted ends surrounded by paratenon invariably become fixed by the dense scar invoked by the cellular response of this tissue. In 3 to 6 weeks it may

*Trommelfinger (drummer's thumb) is the term coined for rupture of the extensor pollicis longus, which was an occupational injury among the elite of the Kaiser's drum corps.

surround the retracted tendon like a cocoon, precluding any elongation of the muscle-tendon unit. When the proximal and distal stumps are bridged by paratenon, this same reactivity may eventually transform the paratenon into a pseudotendon with longitudinally oriented fibroblasts, but without the glistening white fibrils of a normal tendon. Such a pseudotendon lacks the tensile strength needed for much stress, but it may function adequately where power is not needed, e.g. about the extensors on the dorsum of the hand.

Every effort must be made to bring a tendon wound into contact with soft areolar and fatty tissue. This provides a source of good vascularization and ultimately more yielding adhesions than are generally produced by the tougher tendon sheath. Resection of the tendon sheath in the area of tenorrhaphy, in the case of the flexors, or transfer of the tendon superficial to the retinaculum, in the case of the extensors, is often advisable. In cases where tendon is anchored to bone, as in tendon grafting or tendon advancement, the intramedullary canal should be exposed through a window so the tendon stump can be in contact with this rich blood supply.

The chronological pattern of tissue reactions after tenorrhaphy is as follows:

1. At three days the wound of the tendon is filled with granulation tissue, without any tensile strength. There is edema of the tendon ends and continuity is maintained only by the sutures. Each suture and needle tract is surrounded by an inflammatory response. There is appearance of fibroblasts in this proliferative phase, and the synthesis of new and lysis of old collagen begins.
2. At seven days, organization of the granulation tissue which has grown into and surrounds the tendon wound is beginning, but the tendon wound still lacks tensile strength. Fibroblasts continue to actively synthesize and secrete collagen and mucopolysaccharides. Tendon cells divide but contribute minimally to healing between tendon ends. Such healing is primarily dependent upon the migration and ingrowth of cells from the adjacent tissues. Thus, any substance used to surround or protect a tendon junction from forming adhesions with its bed will inevitably prevent the two essentials of healing (fibroblasts and new blood vessels) from gaining access to the tendon junction.
3. At fourteen days the tendon wound is filled with a bridge of fibroblasts and collagen but the tensile strength is still very limited. The great proliferative cellular reaction that has built up in and around the tendon is in continuity with that involving the surrounding injured tissues. All of this is referred to as the common coagulum.
4. At twenty-one days there is enough tensile strength to tolerate movement.
5. After three weeks, the time-consuming process of scar remodeling and maturation begins. The collagen and fibroblasts in the tendon union are eventually aligned in the direction of pull and adhesions may attenuate to permit gliding. Maximal remodeling may require more than six months. With adaptation of molecular structure to function, tendons become as strong as before the injury. Tendons surrounded by paratenon heal at a faster rate than tendons within synovial sheaths because the paratenon is a source of greater vascularity and accessibility of fibroblasts. The proliferative response it potentiates may be a disadvantage where maximal tendon amplitude is needed or where retinacular pulleys are essential.

A tendon graft or tendon transfer is revived by the ingrowth of capillaries and the formation of adhesions all along its length. As time passes, the collagen of the adhesions between the tendon and its bed must adapt biomechanically and become filmy, pliable and redundant enough to allow stretching if adequate tendon excursion is to occur. The degree of such adaptation can be influenced only in part by the skill and meticulous technique of the surgeon and the determined effort of the patient. The physical and chemical characteristics of the collagen in the scar about a tendon determine the degree of tendon function recovered.[11] The remodeling process in scar primarily aligns the fibroblasts and the bundles of collagen fibers to the direction of tensile force. Adhesions restricting glide are dense and have fewer blood vessels than non-restrictive adhesions. Restrictive adhesions resemble tendons, non-restrictive adhesions resemble normal paratenon.

All factors that influence wound healing in general affect tendon healing in particular. Paramount among these is the integrity of the circulation which, if impaired, delays healing, potentiates infection and favors adhesions. Immobilization hastens the resolution of the inflammatory stage, while appropriate mobilization aids remodeling and the gain in tensile strength of the scar. Tendon sutures promote the formation of scar through wounding and by the constriction of circulation. The size, character and placement of sutures are important considerations in tenorrhaphy.

Examination and Diagnosis of Injury

Accurate diagnosis of tendon injury is impossible without a knowledge of functional anatomy of the hand and the variable effects of different forms of injury on this function. With any history of injury to the hand, tendon involvement must be suspected, especially if the patient notices weakness or defective movement thereafter. The details of the history must clarify the exact moment of injury. If a flexor tendon injury occurs in the act of grasping while the tendon is drawn proximally, the distal tendon stump will lie well distal to the skin wound when the joints are extended. In contrast to this, if the hand is outstretched when the flexor tendon is divided, the distal stump will be found at the same level as the skin wound during extension.

Roentgenograms should be taken whenever there is a suspicion of associated fresh or preexisting bone or joint abnormality. They should also be taken when a retained foreign body is suspected (Fig. 14-3). In like fashion, appropriate laboratory tests must be performed to help determine the presence of relevant disease (e.g. rheumatoid disease or gout) which might predispose to or complicate a tendon injury.

Notes should be made immediately at the time of questioning and examination, and wherever applicable should be accompanied by a diagram of the site and nature of the injury. In addition to the chief complaints, the history must include a statement about the existence of any previous abnormality about the hand. Requestioning and reexamination are often necessary to reveal intentional or unintentional inconsistencies about the history and physical findings that are apt to mask the true diagnosis.

Following acute injury, examination of the hand is facilitated by having the patient recumbent and by adequately controlling his pain and apprehension. Elevation and gentle pressure on the wound will control most bleeding. The function of the entire hand and its comparison with the other

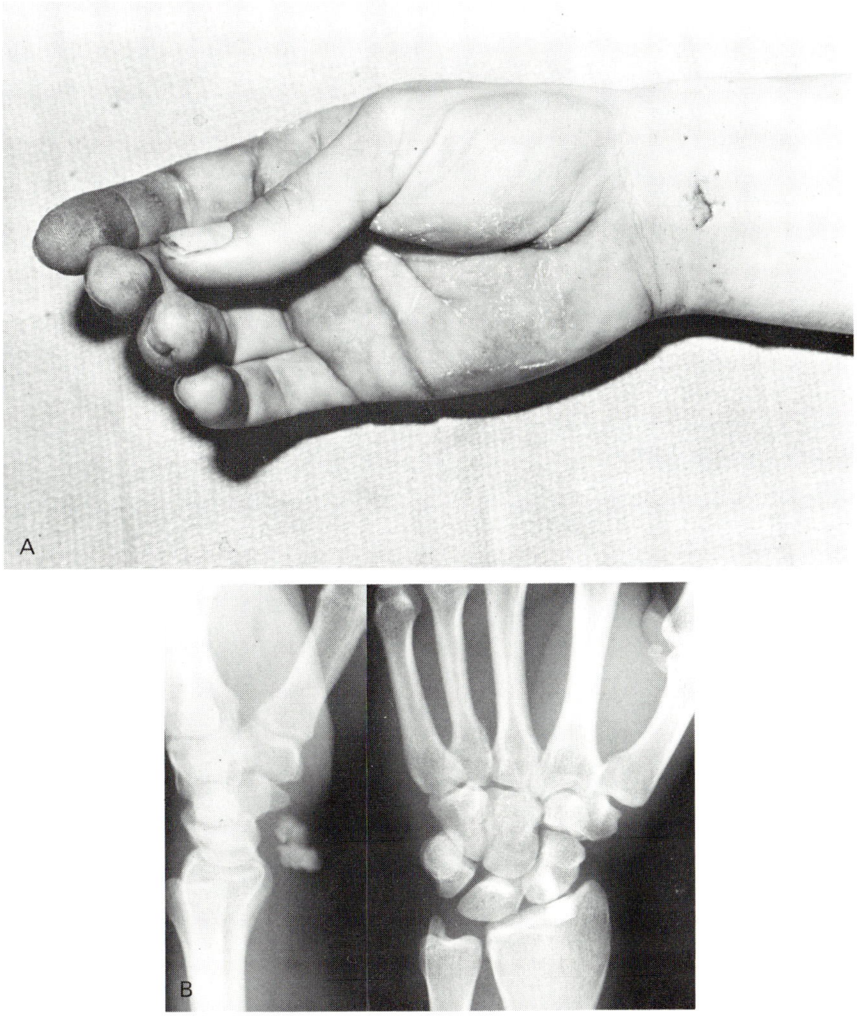

Figure 14-3. *A very minor skin wound at the wrist with complete severance of the flexor pollicis longus. The roentgenogram shows the radiopaque glass fragments which produced the injury.*

hand should be assessed as much as possible within limits of comfort before anesthesia is administered. Ideal facilities are needed for a detailed examination of the wound. A sphygmomanometer around the upper arm inflated to 250 to 300 mm Hg is indispensable for the evaluation and diagnosis of injury within a wound.

For evaluation of old injuries, the seated patient should have the neck and both upper extremities exposed for examination and comparison. He should have disrobed himself, allowing the physician the opportunity to observe the use of his extremities. At the beginning, he should hold both upper extremities high above his head and, while doing so, open and close his fists rapidly and repeatedly. Then he should spread and adduct his fingers; finally, he should sequentially oppose his thumbs to each fingertip. This provides at a glance the total upper extremity function and brings abnormalities to light much more readily than when the hands are held in the patient's lap.

The stance of both hands at rest must be observed and any abnormality of digital posture when the wrist is flexed or extended passively must be noted. Flexion of the fingers normally increases from the index to the little finger when the wrist is extended. Failure of a supple finger to flex under these circumstances indicates flexor tendon damage. When, however, the wrist is flexed, failure of supple digits to extend indicates extensor tendon damage.

Tendon tone should be tested at rest and during vigorous muscle contraction, and the cause of any weakness determined. The usual problems causing this are pain, paralysis, disruption, disuse or tenodesis. A tendon having undergone tenodesis is divorced from the elasticity of its muscle. When only one joint is crossed, the existence of a tenodesis cannot be distinguished from intrinsic stiffness of the joint without surgical exploration. When, however, the tenodesed tendon crosses two or more joints, and is tightened by the passive motion of just one of the joints, such tightening will force the remaining involved joints to move in the opposite direction. Thus, tenodesis of a digital flexor tendon in the forearm will draw the digit into flexion as the wrist is extended. Similarly, tenodesis of a digital extensor tendon at the same level results in digital extension as the wrist is flexed.

In closed injuries, a gap may be felt in the line of a tendon which, of course, can also be seen in the adequate examination of open injuries. In either closed or open injuries, the retracted proximal stump can occasionally be felt.

Although a tendon influences the movement of every joint is crosses, it primarily moves one joint. The flexor digitorum profundus, for instance, flexes all joints of the finger as well as the wrist, but its major role is flexion of the distal interphalangeal joint.

To test a muscle-tendon unit, the integrity of passive joint motion must first be established. Then the hand should be positioned to place the subject motor under the greatest passive stretch. Following this the patient should perform active movement with and without counter-resistance.

In the elective evaluation of old injury, three sets of hand measurements should be recorded and compared with the uninjured side (Chap. 28).

1. Goniometer measurements of wrist and digital joints in extremes of active and passive movement, including the abduction angle of the thumb. Normally the range of active movement will be equal to the range of passive movement.
2. The distance by which the fingertips fail to meet a straight line in extension, or to meet the proximal, mid- and distal palm in flexion, and the distance by which the tip of the thumb fails to meet the base of the little finger in flexion.
3. Grip meter and pinch meter readings.

The power of each muscle-tendon unit may be assessed and graded as follows:

Grade 0—complete paralysis
Grade 1—flicker of contraction
Grade 2—visible palpable contraction with gravity eliminated
Grade 3—contraction against gravity
Grade 4—contraction against gravity and some resistance
Grade 5—normal power

FLEXOR TENDON TESTING

Although these tendons lie deeper and are more difficult to visualize than extensors, testing their function is rather straightforward and less intricate than that for the extensors.

1. *Flexor digitorum profundus and flexor pollicis longus:* Keeping the more proximal joints extended, ask the patient to flex the distal interphalangeal joints.
2. *Flexor digitorum superficialis:* Eliminate the action of the flexor digitorum profundus by holding all other fingers of the patient's hand fully extended, and ask him to flex the finger with suspected tendon injury (Fig. 14-4). If the distal inter-

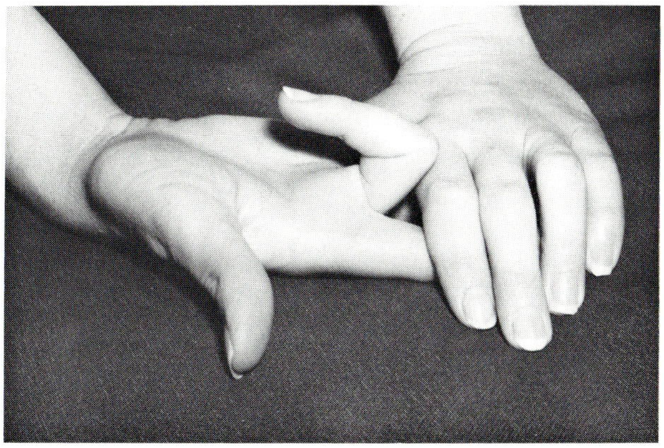

Figure 14-4. *The flexor digitorum superficialis is an independent digital flexor.*

phalangeal joint is flail, indicating absence of flexor digitorum profundus function, then flexion of the proximal interphalangeal joint will be by the independent flexor digitorum superficialis.

3. *Flexor carpi radialis:* Palpate this tendon radial to the midline when the wrist is flexed against resistance.
4. *Flexor carpi ulnaris:* Palpate this tendon under tension when the hand is forcibly spread. The flexor carpi ulnaris contracts synergistically to stabilize the wrist.
5. *Palmaris longus:* With the thumb opposed to the little finger and the wrist flexed forcefully, palpate this tendon in the midline. It is congenitally absent in about 20 per cent of cases.

EXTENSOR TENDON TESTING

Over the body of the hand and over the digits, the extensor tendons lie directly beneath the skin and injury to them is easier to visualize than in the case of the flexors. However, the intricacies of the intercommunications between components of the extensor hood mechanism of the digits, and between the components of the long extensors over the body of the hand, require that tests of function be painstaking.

1. *Extensor digitorum communis:* Keeping the interphalangeal joints flexed in a tight claw, the patient should perform active extension of the metacarpophalangeal joints. The extensor digitorum communis tendons can usually be seen and felt.
2. *Extensor indicis proprius* and *Extensor digiti quinti:* The patient should first make a fist and then independently extend the index and little fingers (as in finger-whistling) while the middle and ring fingers remain flexed (Fig. 14-5).
3. *Extensor pollicis longus:* The force and range of extension of the interphalangeal joint of the thumb must be tested. Only the extensor pollicis longus can forcibly extend or hyperextend this joint. However, the intrinsics can extend it weakly to a straight line.
4. *Extensor pollicis brevis:* When the patient's hand is spread forcefully, the examiner should palpate this tendon under tension over the dorsum of the thumb metacarpal. He must also note whether the metacarpophalangeal joint of the thumb is extended maximally by comparing it with the opposite normal thumb.
5. *Abductor pollicis longus:* The patient should spread the hand forcibly, and just distal to the radial styloid the examiner should palpate the abductor pollicis longus, which will be tensed deep to the extensor pollicis brevis as it synergistically extends the wrist.

INTRINSIC TENDON TESTING

The four tests for intrinsic tendon function are done against resistance and involve the following motions:

1. To test the dorsal interossei, spread the hand forcibly.
2. To test the volar interossei, ask the patient to resist the withdrawal of a piece of paper from between his extended fingers.
3. To test the thenar and hypothenar wads, cup the palm and pinch the thumb and little fingertips together forcibly. Feel the tone of the muscle wads and compare it with the normal side.

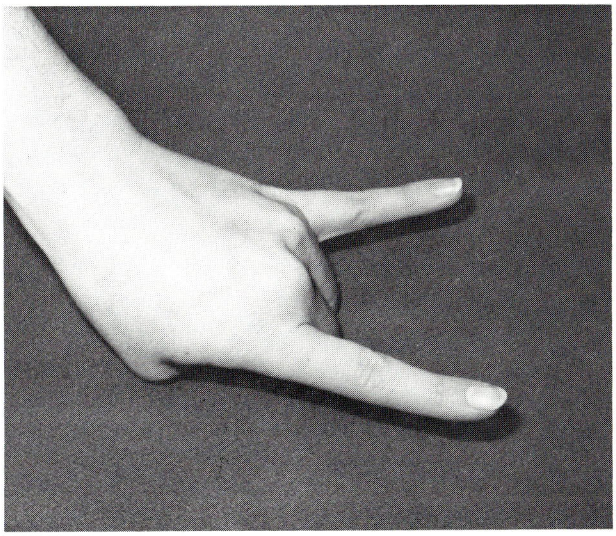

Figure 14-5. *The independent proprius extensors of the index and little fingers are tested as above.*

4. To test the intrinsic tendons, the wrist should be held in full extension and the fingers forcefully extended. If the intrinsics are working normally, it should take considerable passive force downward on the fingernail to flex the interphalangeal joints against this active extension.

ERRORS IN DIAGNOSIS

The misdiagnosis of tendon injuries is common for the following reasons:

1. Visualization in a wound is incomplete because of failure to use a tourniquet or extend the wound, or because of incomplete testing, faulty knowledge of anatomy, improper interpretation of the examination and inability or unwillingness of the patient to cooperate. The positive diagnosis of tendon severance can only be made by consistent absence of expected movement. False-positive diagnoses occur when the patient fails to move the tendon because of fear, pain or associated injuries to bones, joints, or nerves.
2. Even though a tendon has been completely divided, misleading movement of joints may occur by the presence of cross communications between normal and injured tendons (e.g. juncturae tendinum over the dorsum of the hand), or because of adhesions (pseudotendon) joining the two tendon ends, or because of an intact vinculum.
3. In open injuries, especially penetrating ones, there may be incomplete division of one or more tendons.
4. Blunt trauma to the dorsum of digital joints may result in extensive compromise of tendon integrity which may defy immediate diagnosis. An assortment of deformities develop insidiously as the injured extensor hood becomes attenuated. Successful prophylactic treatment entails an awareness of the potential changes that may occur after such injury.
5. Fresh lacerations over the proximal interphalangeal joint and metacarpophalangeal joint that involve only the middle extensor tendon may be missed because the hood mechanism has not yet decompensated by attenuation.

The diagnosis is not completed until the status of all other tissues is assayed. Open injuries involving the flexor tendons are commonly associated with serious nerve and arterial injury. Open injury to the flexor tendons in the fingers may also involve the flexor sheaths, the volar plates, joints, cartilage and bone, all of which have a bearing on the prognosis of good functional recovery. Similarly, extensor tendon injuries may involve the underlying joints or bones.

The recognition of normal and injured structures during an operation necessitates adequate light, assistance, instruments, exposure and tourniquet control of bleeding. If a definitive surgical correction is planned, the wound must be extended to identify and trace normal, unbloodied structures into the zone of injury.

SUMMARY OF TENDON DIAGNOSIS

1. Is there tendon injury? Look for any abnormal posture of the hand and digits. Test musculotendinous tone and individual tendon function precisely. Identify anatomical mechanisms that functionally mask the injury when it first occurs.
2. Where is the tendon injury in relation to the fibrous sheath and its pulleys? Where are the tendon ends in relation to the skin wound? Use a tourniquet and, if necessary, extend a wound to be certain about the injuries.
3. What is the type of tendon injury? Is it complete or incomplete? Is the wound tidy or untidy? Is there contamination? Is the tendon cut, crushed or torn? Are there associated injuries to other tissues? Is the muscle normal? Are there tendon adhesions? Are the joints supple?

Tendon Surgery

Tendon surgery is a special discipline with intricate and meticulous refinements and certain prerequisites to ensure success. These are:

1. The surgeon must have appropriate training, skill and technical facilities.
2. The tendon should be covered with healthy, padded and supple skin.
3. The joints over which the tendon acts must not be stiff or springy (Fig. 14-6).
4. The muscle acting on the tendon must have adequate contractability and be innervated or capable of being so.
5. The patient must be capable of rehabilitative effort by reasons of motivation or age.
6. The muscles to be restored should not be spastic and the area of their action not irrevocably anesthetic. This is subject to certain exceptions (Chap. 15).

Unfavorable circumstances for tendon repair exist when patients are over forty years of age, are poorly motivated, and have heavy inflexible hands with a tendency to excessive fibrosis (e.g. Dupuytren's fasciitis). In addition, the presence of

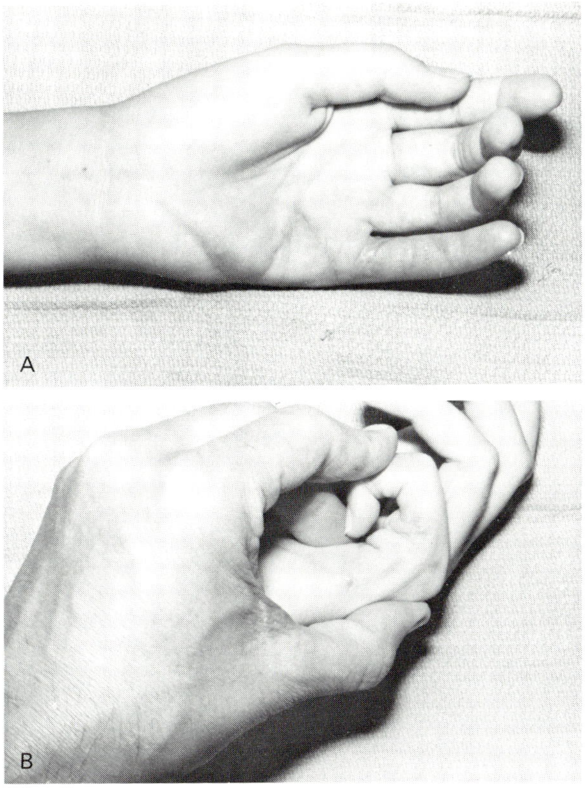

Figure 14-6. *The joints over which a repaired tendon will act must be supple prior to tenorrhaphy.*

an untidy wound, injury to neighboring tissues, trauma in and about the fibrous sheath or previous involvement of the subject tendon in injury, surgery, infection or other disease threatens the success of tendon reconstruction.

The Time of Tenorrhaphy

Surgical expertise markedly influences the results of tenorrhaphy and justifies, whenever possible, the referral of tendon surgery to the experienced surgeon. Definitive primary repair of injured tendons can be deferred up to 72 hours, provided the initial proper emergency wound care has been rendered. This includes a surgical skin preparation of the hand, temporary wound approximation by a few sutures or by dressing alone, immobilization, elevation and administration of anti-infective drugs (Chap. 4).

Primary repair of injured tendons is that which is done within 72 hours, while delayed primary repair is that done within the first two weeks. Secondary repair is done after there has been thorough resolution of edema and softening of scar, which may take 4 to 10 weeks or more.

PRIMARY TENORRHAPHY

A lengthy morbidity follows tendon injury and repair. All other things being equal, the earlier that tendon repair is done, the earlier function is restored and the less costly is the disability. Primary repair is preferable when the wound conditions are optimal (tidy) and the necessary surgical skill and facilities are available. Since a short delay is not at all deleterious to the outcome, the rushed repair of these injuries by an inexperienced or fatigued surgeon is not indicated.

DELAYED PRIMARY TENORRHAPHY

The delayed primary repair is chosen in special instances. It offers the surgeon time to evaluate and treat pressing problems exclusive of the hand. It also allows him time to observe the wound and ensure the absence of infection or undue swelling when they might be anticipated. If the wound remains soft, pliable, non-tender and free of heat, redness or pus, then tenorrhaphy may be done within 14 days.

SECONDARY TENORRHAPHY

If there are considerable associated injuries, or if wound complications have occurred, secondary repair is indicated. This often involves tendon grafting or transfers, and, at times, tenodesis. Adequate joint mobility is indispensable for these procedures. In order to use the original motor, the secondary repair must be done before elasticity (contractability) is lost; otherwise another motor will be necessary. After two months have elapsed, muscle contractability will probably be lost unless the musculotendinous unit has been tethered distally. Hence, secondary repair is done preferably within two months, providing all the prerequisites for reconstruction are met.

Secondary tenorrhaphy allows time for the replacement of skin and subcutaneous tissue when these have been lost or replaced by scar. It also permits time for the recovery from bone and joint injuries and the resolution of induration.

Preparation for Operation

The required surgical facilities consist of an adjustable operating table with an equally adjustable arm table, good light, appropriate magnification, specialized instruments, needles and sutures, buttons and felt padding, and adequate assistance. A tourniquet is indispensable. It must have been tested for its pneumatic competence and for the accuracy of its gauge before use. The patient must be comfortably supine with carefully placed padding under the tourniquet on the upper arm.

Barring pain, it may be advantageous to prepare and drape the extremity before the patient is anesthetized. He can then cooperate in the preparation, and it is possible to carry out last-minute retesting.

After suitable anesthesia is achieved, which requires total relaxation of the involved musculature, skin incisions are planned and marked with dye (Chap. 6). For primary tenorrhaphy, the extremity is simply elevated, but is *not* wrapped with an exsanguinating bandage before inflation of the tourniquet. Wrapping may cause freshly divided tendons to migrate far proximally from the zone of injury making them difficult to find. This problem does not exist with a secondary tenorrhaphy because adhesions have formed and migration is prevented. In the latter case the extremity should be exsanguinated by use of the Esmarch bandage before inflation of the tourniquet.

Tenorrhaphy requires the utmost in atraumatic technique to minimize the formation of adhesions to the tendon that will restrict its glide. Powder must be thoroughly washed off the surgical gloves and handling of the tendon and its bed must be reduced to an absolute minimum. Glistening surfaces of tendons and their beds must not be scratched or allowed to dry. The trauma of needles, sutures and forceps should be limited to the very ends of the tendon stump and its point or surface of attachment.

EXPLORATION OF THE FRESH, TIDY WOUND

After all loose clots have been removed, the need to extend the wound for adequate exposure must be assessed. The proximal and distal tendon stumps which are not readily found at the site of injury are traced and found in their sheaths or beds proximally or distally. Blood around retracted tendons signals their location. Finding the proximal stump is often hard, in contrast to finding the distal stump. The former may be drawn far proximally by the pull of its muscle, whereas the latter, if drawn away from the wound at all, is merely at the mercy of the joints which can be moved to readily bring the distal stump into view.

Three measures are helpful in advancing the proximal stump into the wound for retrieval: (1) squeezing the muscle wad to eject its tendon, (2) positioning the wrist so that the distance of the tendon end to the wound is reduced, and (3) putting traction on the muscle by the positioning of adjacent fingers whose tendons arise from it (e.g. profundus or extensor communis). (The insertion of a clamp into a tendon sheath to retrieve a proximal stump injures the bed and should be avoided.) If none of these techniques succeeds, the atraumatic retrieval of the stump requires a proximal counterincision for the recovery of the stump and its rethreading distally by suture to the tip of a polythylene catheter which is introduced along the sheath from the distal wound. Insufflation of the tendon sheath by lactated Ringer's solution via the catheter makes the advancement and retrieval of the catheter atraumatic (Fig. 14-27). Once the proximal and distal stumps have been identified, it may be helpful to tag them with nylon stay sutures, particularly when dealing with multiple tendon injuries. The proximal stump of the retrieved tendon may be secured in the wound for suture by a straight needle (Figs. 14-2 and 14-24).

Any injury to the tendon bed must be recognized, as it will influence the choice of the procedure. The resulting scar will fix the tendon in the bed. In certain instances the tendon can be separated from the injured part of the bed by the interposition of a thin silicone membrane, or the tendon can be totally transferred to a more favorable bed (e.g. out of a damaged fibro-osseous canal). An alternative method is the use of a silicone rod to develop a suitable pseudosynovial-lined bed where the original bed is extensively scarred. The lining usually takes 10 to 12 weeks to mature, after which a tendon graft or transfer is threaded through it.

When the site of a tendon juncture will lie within or glide through a fibrous sheath, enough of the sheath must be removed to prevent binding of the bulky tendon callus at this juncture during excursion of the tendon. Excision of the sheath must be done at its lateral margins with precision to avoid scarifying its shiny surface over the fibro-osseous floor, where the most unyielding adhesions form.

When multiple tendons are injured, the priority of repair is as described in the appropriate sections of this chapter. Primary or secondary tenorrhaphies in the case of complex tidy injuries (Chap. 16) must be chosen selectively on the basis of priority of tendon function and prognosis for recovery. The resection of dispensable musculotendinous units in multiple tendon injuries will often pave the way for better, albeit simplified, function.

This reduction of the aggregate mass of tendon and total wound callus improves the circulation available to the repaired tendons.

Lacerations of the wrist, palm and digits frequently divide nerves as well as tendons. The first priority is for the repair of tendons, although neurorrhaphy can often be done during the same operation. If so, the nerve repair should be done after the tendon repair. It must be remembered, however, that the surgical dissection needed to mobilize and repair a nerve may endanger the tenorrhaphy. When this seems likely, a secondary neurorrhaphy is preferred.

EXPLORATION OF THE FRESH, UNTIDY WOUND

The prime concern is achieving uncomplicated healing of the wound without infection. This entails appropriate debridement, the avoidance of unnecessary dissection, wound closure (primary or delayed) without tension, administration of antibiotics and the control of edema. Secondary tenorrhaphy is the rule for these wounds, but this does not preclude tacking together readily accessible tendon ends, or tethering a proximal stump so its muscle will not retract and lose its elasticity.

Where skin and subcutaneous tissue have been lost, wound closure is achieved by free grafts, rotation flaps and primary pedicle flaps (Chap. 6). If the fibro-osseous tendon canal is affected by an associated skeletal injury, tenorrhaphy is usually postponed until skeletal healing is complete. In the interim, the tendon sheath may be preserved by inserting a silicone rod (tendon prosthesis).

ELECTIVE EXPLORATION OF TENDON INJURIES

The problems are finding the tendon ends, developing the tendon bed and selecting the appropriate procedure. The tendon stumps may lie in the scar of the wound of injury, or they may be at a distance from it. If they are connected together by pseudotendon, this is identified by its somewhat grayish hue and the absence of white tendon fibrils when it is sectioned. Pertinent structures should be identified beyond the zone of injury proximally and distally, where they are normal, and then traced into the zone of injury. The bed of this zone need not even be entered if it seems best to bypass it in the course of reconstruction.

The degree of proximal retraction of divided tendon stumps depends upon the independence of function and force of contraction of their muscles and whether or not the tendons are tethered distally (e.g. lumbrical tethering of the profundus). Stumps of the totally independent flexor pollicis longus and extensor pollicis longus often recoil into the forearm. In the palm, the envelopment of the divided flexor tendons by a cocoon of paratenon and lumbrical may make their identification and dissection exceedingly difficult and preclude their repair.

DEVELOPING THE TENDON BED

A tendon or tendon graft will not glide through a bed of scar tissue or a snug sheath, nor will the callus of a tendon juncture pass through a pulley. The ideal bed for tenorrhaphies is one of healthy, fatty areolar tissue. A tendon graft threaded through a tendon sheath is more apt to glide if the synovial lining has not been injured and if the sheath lying between the pulleys has been resected. This will expose the graft to fatty-areolar tissue that will vascularize it with filmy and elastic, rather than rigid, adhesions. Tenorrhaphy by grafting places the sites of tendon suture (and subsequent tendon callus) strategically beyond the encroachment of pulleys. In tenorrhaphy without grafting, however, it is often mandatory to section or resect a pulley that will bind a tendon callus during tendon excursion, or else to relocate the tendon superficially and place the juncture on top of the pulley system.

For flexor tendons, an effort is made to preserve at least one pulley for the thumb and preferably two pulleys for the fingers to avoid bowstringing. These must freely accommodate the tendon.

If scarring or damage of the bed in which the tenorrhaphy lies is limited (less than 15 mm of its length), a 0.2-mm thick silicone membrane may be interposed between the bed and the tendon. This must not, however, surround the whole tendon. When there is more extensive injury and scarring to the bed, a new tendon canal may be reconstituted with a pseudosynovial lining by the insertion of a silicone rod. Eight to 12 weeks later this rod is replaced with a tendon graft.

At other times it is more expeditious to reroute the tendon, tendon graft or tendon transfer away from a scarred bed through healthy glide-facilitating fatty areolar tissue. Extensor tendons at the wrist level may be routed subcutaneously to override the extensor retinaculum. Similarly, a flexor pollicis longus may be routed directly through the thenar musculature from the forearm rather than through the carpal canal. Occasionally, a graft replacing the profundus tendon may be passed superficial to a scarred-down pulley to avoid adhesions inside it. When the tissue for a suitable tunnel is not otherwise available, it can be acquired from a local or distant pedicle flap of skin and fat.

SELECTION OF THE APPROPRIATE TENORRHAPHY (OR SUBSTITUTES THEREFOR)

The choices of tenorrhaphy or tenorrhaphy substitute, whether primary or secondary are:

1. No treatment
2. End-to-end tendon suture
3. Tendon advancement
4. Tendon transfer
5. Tendon graft
6. Fixation of joints by tenodesis or arthrodesis
7. Amputation

No treatment. When a tendon is partially divided (50 per cent) and its repair with immobilization would sufficiently risk normal function of companion tendons by the development of adhesions, no treatment may be necessary.

End-to-end tendon suture. When the ends are of comparable diameter and they can be satisfactorily approximated in a bed of tissue favorable to gliding the end-to-end suture is used. The juncture must be expected not to enter a fibro-osseous tunnel during its excursion.

Tendon advancement. When the proximal stump can be brought to the distal insertion of the tendon, beyond the tendon sheath, without overstretching the muscle and causing an adverse habitus and restriction of joint motion, this method is chosen. With these criteria, advancement is usually limited to not more than 1.0 to 1.5 cm, unless the tendon is lengthened near its musculotendinous junction.

Tendon transfers. Transfers are employed when the original muscle has lost its contractability or is paralyzed (Chap. 15).

Tendon grafts. Those hand surgeons who consider it essential that a tendon juncture and its suture line be kept outside of a tendon sheath favor tendon grafts. They are also used when additional tendon length is needed, or to thread a new pseudosynovial sheath (formed about a silicone rod) with a new tendon.

Tenodesis or arthrodesis. When the tenorrhaphy would markedly risk existing active joint motion (e.g. profundus graft through an intact superficialis), or when a supply of suitable musculotendinous units is not available, the reduction in number of acting units can be made functionally effective by appropriate tenodesis or arthrodesis. These procedures are most commonly considered for the distal interphalangeal joints, but in selected cases both the proximal and the distal interphalangeal joints of any given digit may be fixed in this manner.

Amputation. When 3 to 4 of the five essential tissues have been hopelessly injured, amputation is undertaken primarily. These essential tissues are: bone, tendon, nerve, vessels and skin. Amputation should be recommended when repairing an injury of similar magnitude will expose the patient to excessive physical, psychological and economic burdens. This is particularly germane in those cases where the overall loss of function is small compared to the existing function or where there will be marked risk to the patient's hand function or general state of health by initiating extensive reconstruction.

Aftercare

There are three phases of aftercare. Initially, for 3 to 4 weeks, is the phase of immobilization. Thereafter follows the phase of mobilization, which will vary in duration depending upon the extent and location of the tendon problem. The end-point of mobilization is objectively measured by goniometers and by grip and pinch meters. Most periods of convalescence involve several weeks or months of mobilization; it is not infrequent for this period to last a year or more after serious injuries. The final phase is that of adaptation and musculoskeletal accommodation to a fixed disability.

The patient has the prime responsibility for these three phases. However, even the best motivated and most intelligent patients need education, guidance and encouragement. This takes time and practice and must be custom tailored for each case. For the specifics of this postoperative management, see Chapter 4.

Flexor Tendons

The variation of anatomy along the course of the extrinsic flexor tendons, from the distal phalanges to the muscles in the forearm, affects the fate of their function after injury. To aid in understanding these variations and to establish sound principles of care, the anatomical zones are delineated along the length of each tendon (Fig. 14-7). The prime variation in these zones depends on: (1) the presence or absence of a snug flexor sheath and synovial-lined bursa (often referred to as the fibro-osseous tendon canal, with its fibrous condensations called pulleys), and (2) the number of tendons lying within the same canal and gliding simultaneously or independently. Tendons injured within a fibro-osseous tunnel may become adherent to the walls of the tunnel and fail to glide. When more than one tendon lies within the same tunnel, the tendons may stick to one another as well as to the wall. Where there is no snug tunnel to cause friction, there is no need for lubrication by a synovial bursa. Instead the tendon needs to be surrounded only by loose areolar tissue containing the blood supply (e.g. paratenon). In the middle third of the palm and proximal to the wrist the tendons are covered with paratenon rather than tendon sheath.

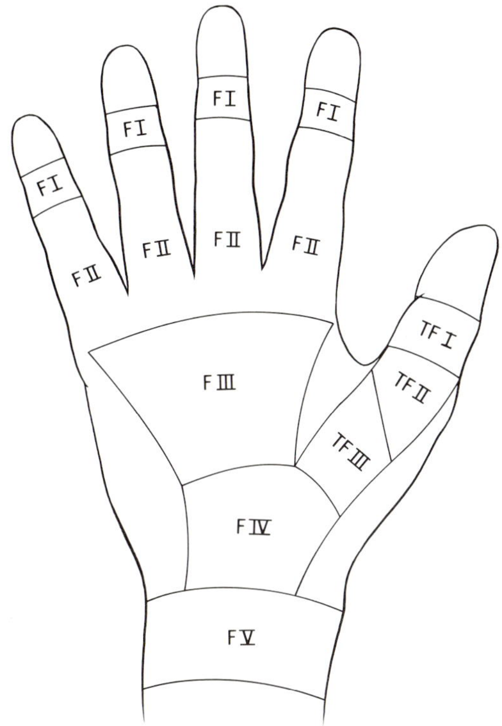

Figure 14-7. *Flexor tendon zones.*

Surgical Topography

From the distal phalanx of all fingers to the flexor muscles of the forearm, there are five zones. Since the thumb has only one interphalangeal joint, and, therefore, only one long flexor, its three distal zones are different from those of the fingers, but its two proximal zones, being the same, are shared with those of the fingers.

The flexor zones are designated as follows:

Zone *F-I of the fingers Zone **TF-I of the thumb	—Extends from the tendon insertion on the distal phalanx to the midshaft or near the base of the next proximal phalanx.
Zone F-II ("No-man's land") Zone TF-II	—Extends from Zone I to the proximal side of the most proximal digital pulley at the level of the metacarpal head.
Zone F-III Zone TF-III	—Extends from Zone II over the body of the metacarpals to the distal edge of the carpal canal.
Zone F-IV of the wrist	—Within the carpal canal.
Zone F-V of the forearm	—In the forearm proximal to the carpal canal.

*F—Flexor
**TF—Thumb flexor

Principles of Management

The condition of the wound and the complexity of the injury must be weighed in determining the timing and type of tenorrhaphy.

Primary tenorrhaphy with prophylactic antibiotic coverage can be done when the wound is tidy and not markedly contaminated. With irrigation of the wound and proper surgical preparation and dressing of the skin, primary tenorrhaphy can be delayed without detriment for 72 hours if necessary.

Tendon injuries in untidy and complex wounds are generally treated by secondary tenorrhaphy (weeks or months later) after the joints become mobile and the soft tissues pliable. This secondary approach does not preclude maintaining the muscle's length by tacking two readily accessible tendon ends together with fine nylon suture at the time of the injury.

When delayed primary or secondary tenorrhaphy is undertaken, 2 to 8 weeks after injury, the adhesions around the retracted proximal tendon stump are sometimes minimal and the muscle often sufficiently elastic to allow a direct tenorrhaphy. If, however, the injury caused loss of tendon substance, a tendon graft or transfer must be considered.

Eight to 10 weeks or more after injury, both the tendon and muscle are frequently so irreversibly retracted that direct repair would place too much tension on the junction or require too much flexion of the joints. In these cases, the choice of tendon graft, tendon transfer, tendon lengthening, distal tendon tenodesis or distal joint arthrodesis must be made.

Variation in treatment is necessary for particular fingers, particular patients and particular occupations. In general, the surgical procedure must *not* threaten the function of intact tendons. For example, a functioning flexor digitorum superficialis would never be removed to repair a flexor digitorum profundus in "no-man's-land." Furthermore, except in the youthful or totally pliable digit, normal flexor digitorum superficialis function should not be threatened by threading a flexor digitorum profundus graft through it.

In dealing with combined tendon and nerve injuries, the first thought should be the prevention of irreversible retraction of the musculotendinous unit. Tenorrhaphy, then, is the prime concern. Neurorrhaphy may be done at the time of tenorrhaphy if doing so will *not* entail surgical dissection prejudicial to the tenorrhaphy and thereby causing additional tendon-binding adhesions. When both tenorrhaphy and neurorrhaphy are done at the same sitting, the neurorrhaphy is always done last because it has a much more delicate suture line that will not tolerate the tension that might accidentally be placed on it during a tenorrhaphy.

Primary tenorrhaphy is contraindicated in fresh tendon injuries where the blood supply is also excessively compromised, if further surgical dissection will threaten the viability of the digit. Amputation of the severely damaged digit must be considered when its preservation will eventually compromise normal function of the rest of the hand, or unduly cripple the patient economically. In injuries of multiple digital flexor tendons, tenorrhaphy of any given tendon must be considered on its own merit. The proper selection of any tenorrhaphy requires a consideration of whether the tendon injury is within a fibro-osseous tunnel, or whether there is more than one tendon at the site of injury. Injury to the fibro-osseous floor of the tendon bed must also be recognized and considered in planning the treatment.

The presence of an injury to the floor of the fibro-osseous canal or the volar plate is often a contraindication to primary tendon repair.

The Treatment of Flexor Tendon Injury by Topographical Zone (*Fig. 14-7*)

The zone of injury influences the treatment.

FLEXOR ZONE F-I (FINGER)

This zone is traversed only by the flexor digitorum profundus which passes through the distal pulley and goes on to insert broadly on the distal phalanx. Its synovial sheath ends at the distal joint level, where the vincula brevia may tether the divided tendon enough to mask its injury. The maximum excursion of the tendon here is approximately 0.5 cm.

The relationship of the proximal and distal stumps of the divided flexor digitorum profundus to the wound depends upon whether or not the fist was open or closed at the moment of injury and whether or not the vincula brevia are still attached to the proximal stump, and also upon the vigor of muscular contraction which may pull the proximal tendon into the palm.

If the tendon is cut when the digit is fully extended, the distal stump will lie at the level of the wound. More often, the flexor digitorum profundus is cut during active flexion, and with extension the distal stump is pulled into the sheath beyond the wound.

Early and Late Treatment. Primary repair is done in tidy wounds if 50 per cent or more of the flexor digitorum profundus tendon has been divided. The zone of glide of the tenorrhaphy must be clear of the fibrous sheath and pulley system. If there is damage to either stump requiring trimming, a loss of 1.0 to 1.5 cm of length may be compatible with normal digital excursion. However, *any* shortening in one finger runs some risk of altering the fine balance of profundus action in adjacent fingers. This is usually expressed by a tendency of the affected finger to remain in a posture of some flexion and during active flexion, to flex ahead of the other fingers and, secondarily, limit the power with which they flex. Compensatory adjustment for such shortening must occur for normal function. This is much more apt to occur in the very young and is not likely in adults past 30 or 40 years of age.

Delayed primary treatment within two weeks may still allow direct repair. An alternative choice of primary or secondary treatment is a tenodesis of the distal stump of the flexor digitorum profundus or an arthrodesis of the distal joint (Chap. 13). A tendon graft should not be done unless the patient is willing to accept the potential loss of normal superficialis function by the formation of adhesions to the graft that is threaded through it.

FLEXOR ZONE F-II ("NO-MAN'S-LAND" OF THE FINGER)

This is that ensheathed zone of the finger from the middle phalangeal insertion of the flexor digitorum superficialis to the midpalm (proximal edge of the proximal pulley). The two long flexors lie within it, the profundus passing through the bifurcation of the superficialis. If the digit is in full flexion at the moment of injury in no-man's-land, the level of injury of the profundus and superficialis tendons will be staggered when the digit is extended, the distal stump of the flexor digitorum profundus being far more distal than that of the superficialis. The amplitude of glide of the flexor digitorum superficialis at the metacarpophalangeal joint is 2.5 to 4 cm and of the flexor digitorum profundus, 3 to 4.5 cm.

Treatment of injuries in Zone F-II requires the utmost skill and judgment to reduce the major threat of stiffness which, if sufficiently severe, may lead to the need for an amputation.

Injuries to Flexor Digitorum Profundus Only. The profundus tendon is *not* indispensable to useful finger function. Its repair or replacement when injured is of relative importance and certainly must be weighed against the risk of iatrogenic impairment to the excursion of a normal flexor digitorum superficialis by the formation of adhesions.

The combined action of the intrinsics and the flexor digitorum superficialis brings the distal finger fat pad firmly against the palm. Therefore, satisfactory finger function can easily be lost by indiscreet surgery designed to restore the normal action of the flexor digitorum profundus, but which leads to restrictive adhesions limiting not only the active flexion but also active and passive extension. Above all, an intact flexor digitorum superficialis must *not* be resected in an effort to restore the flexor digitorum profundus. If less than 50 per cent of the profundus tendon has been divided, it need not be sutured or immobilized. Doing so will unnecessarily beg for the formation of adhesions and the loss of tendon glide.

The choices of treatment of isolated flexor digitorum profundus injuries in Zone F-II are:

1. Primary and delayed primary definitive procedures:
   a. Tenodesis of the distal stump or arthrodesis of the distal joint is preferable if the wound is very untidy, the hand is not pliable or the patient is elderly. A tenodesis is apt to stretch, but it has a temporary disability time of only 3 to 4 weeks as compared to 6 to 12 weeks for an arthrodesis.
   b. If the wound is tidy and the hand supple, the preferred choice is to resect an adequate section of tendon sheath and pulley to clear the amplitude of the tendon juncture and to repair the flexor digitorum profundus. The tendon juncture must lie 1.0 to 1.5 cm distal to the bifurcation of the flexor digitorum superficialis. If the proximal stump is not in the wound of injury, it must be retrieved through a counterincision in the palm and rethreaded atraumatically back out the flexor sheath. A secondary tenolysis several months later is sometimes required.
   c. Primary tendon grafts should not be done.
2. Secondary definitive procedures (4 to 10 weeks or more after injury):
   a. Tenodesis of the distal tendon stump or arthrodesis of the distal joint is usually the best solution. The reasons for this are that the retracted flexor digitorum profundus stump is often hopelessly trapped in scar, the bifurcation of the superficialis and more distal pulley system obliterated and the elasticity of the profundus muscle markedly reduced.
   b. If, however, optimal conditions are present, the proximal flexor digitorum profundus stump may be joined to the distal stump or advanced. Upon the insistence of the thoroughly informed patient, a tendon graft may be elected.

Division of all the Flexor Digitorum Profundus and Half the Flexor Digitorum Superficialis. Such a diagnosis is possible only by surgical inspection of the wound. The divided limb of the flexor digitorum superficialis may be resected and the flexor digitorum profundus repaired. A 0.2-mm thick silicone film may be inserted as a barrier to adhesions between the two tendons. The other choices are distal stump tenodesis or distal joint arthrodesis. With the strictest selection of the patient, a tendon graft to the flexor digitorum profundus may be done as a secondary procedure. If such is the case, it might be necessary to first establish a pseudosheath with a silicone tendon prosthesis.

Division of both Flexor Digitorum Profundus and Flexor Superficialis. In tidy wounds, enough of the sheath must be resected to clear the excursion of the tendon juncture for primary repair of the flexor digitorum profundus (Fig. 14-8). The proximal stump of the flexor digitorum superficialis is usually resected by flexing the wrist and removing as much as possible. If its distal stump is shortened, the vincula brevia should be preserved. This will prevent bleeding and will leave a sufficiently long flexor digitorum superficialis stump to prevent a subsequent hyperextension deformity (recurvatum) of the proximal interphalangeal joint. A proximal removable tethering suture (Fig. 14-23) will take the strain off the tendon juncture, reducing adverse adhesions. Should the floor of the fibro-osseous canal be wounded, a 0.2-mm silicone film may be inserted to overlay this wound and bar adhesions between it and the tendon. All of this may be done primarily or delayed for as long as 1

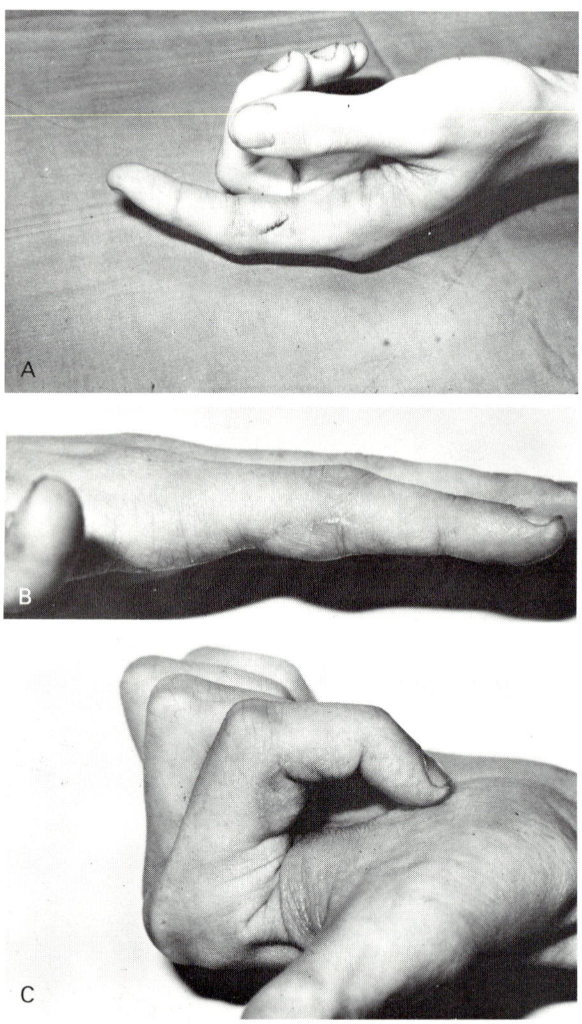

Figure 14-8. *Complete laceration of both flexor tendons in no-man's-land (Zone F-II). Primary repair of both tendons with resulting flexion and extension four months later. Usually only the profundus is repaired.*

to 2 weeks following the injury. Below the age of six years, primary tenorrhaphy is the procedure of choice. Thereafter, the surgeon may choose either a primary repair or a tendon graft.

When the flexor digitorum superficialis is divided distal to its decussation and is still tethered by the vinculum, and the flexor digitorum profundus tenorrhaphy will lie beyond the wound of the flexor digitorum superficialis, both may be repaired. A silicone membrane may be interposed between the two repairs.

Occasionally the surgeon who prefers grafting to primary repair may elect to do a primary tendon graft. However, most grafting is done as a late secondary procedure, 1 to 4 months after injury, when maximum pliability of joints and soft tissues has been reached. The stage for free tendon grafting may be set when the injury first occurs by inserting a short segment of silicone tendon rod to fill the tendon gap and keep the pulley system from collapsing and fibrosing.

An alternative to such preparation for free grafting is preparation for a form of pedicle grafting (Fig. 14-25). In the first stage of this procedure, when the injury is fresh, a silicone tendon prosthesis is placed in the digital sheath from the distal phalanx extending into the midpalm.[2] Distally it is anchored to the profundus stump, which is shortened to the level of the distal volar plate; proximally it is not anchored. The two proximal stumps of the flexor digitorum superficialis and flexor digitorum profundus are sutured end to end at the level of the lumbrical muscle, after resecting redundant parts of each. Eventually, when joints and the wound become thoroughly pliable (within 6 to 12 weeks) the flexor digitorum superficialis is divided in the forearm and drawn as a pedicle graft into the pseudosheath created by the silicone rod.

In any of these procedures the lumbrical plus state[10] must be avoided. This phenomenon results in paradoxical extension of the interphalangeal joints by dominance of the lumbrical over the action of the long flexors during forceful digital flexion. This can result from either recession of lumbrical origin or fibrosis and shrinkage of the muscle. The most common causes are too long a profundus tendon graft, an attenuated profundus tenorrhaphy with pseudotendon formation, or the use of a motor other than the profundus to flex the distal joint (e.g. superficialis). In each instance there is a condition favoring excessive tone or tightness of the lumbrical, usually by having its origin on the proximal profundus pulled too far proximally.[8] Lumbrical plus is particularly manifested during forceful flexion of all the fingertips to meet the distal palm. Instead of flexing, the affected digit extends forcibly at the interphalangeal joints (Fig. 14-9).

Paradoxical extension is prevented by: (1) at the time of tendon grafting, releasing a retracted profundus stump and lumbrical from cicatricial entrapment in a cocoon, and critical attention to the length of a tendon graft, (2) careful tenorrhaphy to prevent attenuation at the profundus-to-profundus or profundus-to-graft tendon juncture, (3) elective sectioning of the lumbrical tendon when employing a motor other than the profundus to flex the distal joint, so that the free proximal end of the profundus cannot pull excessively on the lumbrical by further proximal recession.

Treatment of the established lumbrical plus is to section the lumbrical muscle or tendon, divorcing it from the profundus. If possible, this should be done with local anesthesia so that the effectiveness of the treatment can be immediately tested.

In certain individuals it may be important to preserve the "holding" function of the ring and little fingers. This specialized function of furling around objects endlessly without fatigue is made possible by the independent action of the flexor digitorum superficialis. In considering the needs of selected artisans the flexor digitorum superficialis might be a more appropriate motor for the reconstructed flexor digitorum profundus in these two digits as long as the lumbrical is divided.

If any of these procedures in Zone F-II fail, tenolysis is considered 3 to 6 months later if tendon excursion is inadequate. There should, however, be good passive range of motion of joints and soft skin. Adherence of the tendon must be differentiated from "paradoxical extension" of the lumbrical plus state.

If both the radial and ulnar volar neurovascular bundles have been severed with the flexor tendons, the prognosis for recovery of function is guarded, particularly in the adult (Fig. 14-10). Primary amputation must be considered when injury to a finger is excessive (e.g. multiple tissues divided), especially if the rest of the hand is totally normal. A primary ray resection may be the most expedient answer to the patient's functional, cosmetic and economic needs.

Treatment when Zone F-II is Markedly Scarred. Several alternatives exist when Zone F-II is severely scarred: (1) arthrodesis of the interphalangeal joints (Chap. 13), (2) staged tendon reconstruction, and (3) amputation (Chap. 17). When the informed patient insists on tendon reconstruction in spite of the guarded prognosis, it is done in two stages. The first stage involves attention to the adequacy of skin cover and fat padding and the resection of scarred flexor sheath and tendon, followed by the insertion of a silicone rod to form a pseudosynovial sheath. In the second stage, 6 to 12 weeks later, a tendon graft is threaded through the new sheath and is motored by the flexor digitorum profundus or flexor digitorum superficialis of the affected finger or neighboring finger or by a transferred flexor digitorum superficialis. Barring that, the extensor carpi radialis longus can be transferred as a motor.

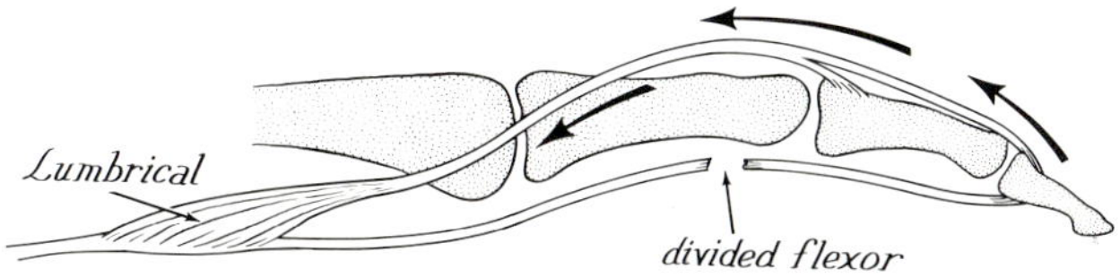

Figure 14-9. *Mechanics involved in the production of a lumbrical plus phenomenon (paradoxical interphalangeal joint extension due to overstretching the lumbrical during digital flexion).*

FLEXOR ZONE F-III (FINGER FLEXORS MIDPALM)

There are no sheaths or pulleys in this area. The synovial bursa of the little finger (the ulnar bursa) crosses it, but the flexors to the index, long and

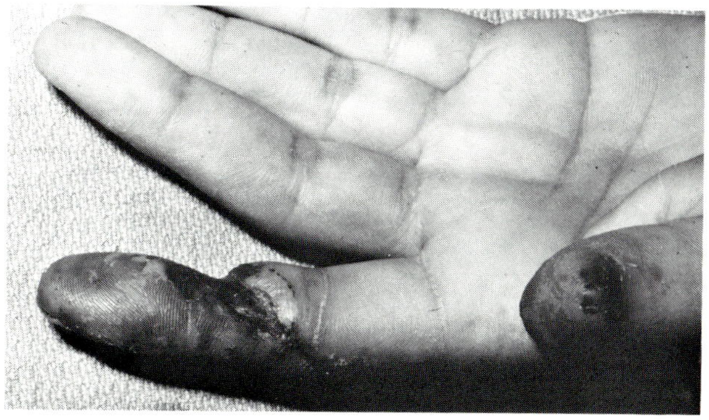
Figure 14-10. *Division of both neurovascular bundles and flexor tendons distal to the skin wound by an oblique laceration, eventually leading to digital amputation.*

ring fingers lose synovium here and are covered instead by paratenon. The flexor digitorum superficialis is superficial to the flexor digitorum profundus. The superficial arterial arch is immediately beneath the palmar fascia in the proximal part of this zone, and is in close relationship to the underlying nerves and adjacent tendons. The lumbrical muscles have their origin from the flexor digitorum profundus tendons in this area. As the tendons pass distally in this zone they become walled off from adjacent neurovascular bundles and lumbricals by the vertical septae of the palmar fascia. When these are dense and hypertrophied, as in Dupuytren's contracture, an injury may lead to excess fibrosis and tendon adherence.

When tendon lacerations occur with the fingers extended, the distal stumps will be found at the level of the wound when the fingers are extended for tenorrhaphy. If, however, the injury occurs during flexion (e.g. when the patient is gripping something), the distal tendon stumps lie far out in the flexor tendon sheaths when the digits are extended, producing, in effect, a Zone F-II injury. All possible combinations of injuries occur: complete and incomplete division of tendons, nerves and arteries. Hemorrhage is the worst when an artery has been only partly divided, and may severely obscure the anatomy and lead to excessive fibrosis.

Partial division of a tendon, particularly one slip of the superficialis, may, in time, be mistaken for a trigger finger (stenosing tenosynovitis) if it creates a "jog" during tendon excursion.

The treatment of tidy injury in Zone F-III depends on the level of the distal stump(s). When it lies well within the digit sheath the dictates for Zone F-II are followed. When the distal stump lies within Zone F-III, the specific factors to be attended are: (1) the resection of any dense palmar fascia, (2) interposition of the lumbrical or a thin sheet of silicone to separate the tenorrhaphies when both the superficialis and profundus are repaired, and (3) the deferment of neurorrhaphy until tenorrhaphy is complete.

If one or both tendons are divided less than 50 per cent, the tendon wounds are closed with 5-0 or 6-0 figure-of-eight nylon sutures and the digit is actively mobilized within 2 to 3 days under supervision.

When the wound is untidy, the potential for primary repair may be limited. Anticipating the probable need for a secondary procedure later on, the proximal and distal stumps (usually only the profundus), if easily accessible, may be tacked together, particularly for the purpose of maintaining muscle tone more than in expectation of a normally gliding tendon. Otherwise, they may be left apart and the tendon bed maintained with a silicone rod, pending delayed reconstruction with a graft. The motor for the graft is apt to become the adjacent superficialis. Conversion of the untidy wound into a tidy wound by debridement of injured tendons and lumbrical muscle may permit primary tenorrhaphy. To prevent a lumbrical plus phenomenon as the result of fibrosis of a macerated lumbrical or retraction of a proximal profundus stump, the lumbrical should be sectioned distally and a segment removed. Tenolysis may eventually become necessary to gain adequate tendon excursion, but is rarely undertaken less than 3 to 6 months after tenorrhaphy.

FLEXOR ZONE F-IV (CARPAL CANAL)

Zone F-IV is the fibro-osseous carpal canal, 25 to 35 mm long, containing the median nerve and the nine long digital flexors and their synovial bursae. It presents the same inherent problems as Zone F-II, aggravated by the presence of the median nerve which is often concomitantly injured. The nerve is the most superficial structure. It usually hugs the radial border of the canal and distally gives off the small (sometimes tiny) motor branch to the thenar muscles. In the next plane lie the superficialis tendons. In the floor of the canal are the tendons of the flexor pollicis longus and the profundi with their lumbricals. A median artery is present in 8 per cent of cases, and may be large and cause considerable hemorrhage.

Incisive injuries by broken glass or metal are often deceiving when tendons are incompletely divided or are anatomically tethered to one another. A careful surgical inspection of the wound is the only means of accurately determining the degree of injury. This usually requires extension of the wound, including complete division of the carpal ligament along the ulnar border. Untethered and independently acting musculotendinous units that are completely divided usually recoil into the forearm. The flexor pollicis longus and the flexor digitorum superficialis of the index and long fingers are the most likely to do this.

The flexors digitorum superficialis to the ring and little fingers are often tethered to one another and retract only when both are divided. The four flexors digitorum profundi, especially those of the ulnar three fingers, are tethered together and, accordingly, all have to be severed for any appreciable retraction of their stumps to occur. In many people, the flexor digitorum profundus to the index acts entirely independently of the other profundi, while in others it is tethered to the flexor pollicis longus.

The magnitude of tendon excursion in Zone F-IV may carry these tendon wounds into Zones F-III or V. This is a further reason to section the transverse carpal ligament (the pulley of the wrist) to give room for passage of callused tendon junctures and to reduce the likelihood of restrictive adhesions. To minimize the bulk of the common coagulum where multiple tendons are injured, the surgical principle of "reconstruction by simplification" should be followed, and, in the adult especially, tendons that are functionally dispensable should be resected. To this end, priority of repair is given to independence of flexion of the thumb and index and terminal flexion of all digits. Hence, the distal and proximal stumps of divided superficialis tendons may be resected. In children, all structures may be repaired in tidy injuries.

The lumbrical muscles are useful buffers against adherent scar between individual tenorrhaphies, if folded without tension about the repair. To separate the flexor pollicis longus tenorrhaphy from adherence to companion tendons or the median nerve, it is sometimes necessary to transfer it out of the carpal canal and thread it through the thenar muscles and subcutaneously across the radial aspect of the wrist. To achieve this a counterincision may be needed on the radial side of the thumb. The flexor digitorum superficialis of the index finger may be used as a motor if the flexor pollicis longus is hopelessly retracted. Tendon transfers and grafts are occasionally necessary in this zone when there has been loss of substance. Repair of the median nerve should be done last, after completion of the tenorrhaphies.

In postoperative immobilization the wrist should be sufficiently flexed to take tension off the repair and allow the digits to assume the position of rest (Fig. 14-11). This position is vital during the first three weeks of healing to facilitate subsequent mobilization. The wrist extensors are powerful and will, in time, force the remodeling of the adhesions allowing tendon excursion. They will also provide the desired stretch of the flexors that gives them power to augment this. Should the digits be immobilized in too much flexion, the extensors may be too weak to remodel the adhesions. Tenolysis is done in time whenever necessary.

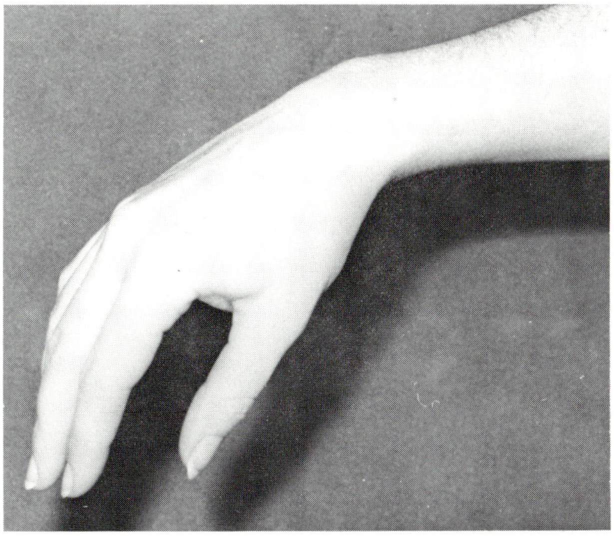

Figure 14-11. *Splinting of the hand in the position of rest to relieve any tension on flexor tenorrhaphies in the early postoperative period.*

FLEXOR ZONE F-V (FOREARM)

Within this zone, proximal to the carpal canal, the three wrist flexors (flexor carpi radialis, palmaris longus and flexor carpi ulnaris) are added to the nine digital flexors. The palmaris longus is an extremely variable structure and is absent in about 20 per cent of cases. If it is missing, the median nerve then lies as the most superficial central structure in the distal 2 to 4 cm of the forearm. More proximally, the nerve is beneath the superficialis muscles. This zone also contains the ulnar nerve and artery deep to the flexor carpi ulnaris. Occasionally there is a large median artery.

There is considerable variation in the length of flexor tendon substance and the breadth, thickness and length of the individual muscles to each tendon. The musculotendinous junction may be abrupt, long or tapered. In some instances it is possible to undertake a promising tenorrhaphy as far proximal as the middle third of the forearm.

Because of inhibition by the patient and the functional overlay of an intact muscle or tendon for an injured one, the existence and extent of injury to muscles, tendons, nerves and arteries cannot be defined without adequate exploration of the wound in ideal facilities. As in Zone F-IV, multiple structures may be simultaneously injured. The surgeon's dissection must first reach normal tissue in order to identify the structures properly and proceed from there into the zone of injury. A single surgical hook is helpful in identifying and testing the integrity of individual musculotendinous units (not nerves). Stumps of divided tendons must methodically be tagged with nylon stay sutures and matched in preparation for repair or resection.

In search for the proximal tendon stumps, it must be remembered that they can usually be retrieved by following the telltale trail of clotted blood within the parent muscle. Fasciotomy of the muscle compartment and an adequate extension of the skin wound will facilitate this, particularly in the presence of hemorrhea and hemopexis. The skin wound should be extended to offset the skin wound from the artery, tendons and nerves without creating poorly vascularized flaps.

As in Zone F-IV, the common coagulum is a problem to be resolved in time with the remodeling process. This can be minimized by reducing the number of muscle-tendon units repaired to those with the highest functional priority: (1) independent flexion of the thumb and index finger, (2) terminal flexion of the digits, and (3) the flexor carpi radialis for wrist flexion. If the ulnar nerve and the flexor carpi ulnaris are both injured at the same level, the nerve should be repaired and the proximal and distal tendon stumps of the flexor carpi ulnaris resected to reduce the amount of scar about the nerve juncture. In children, if the wound is tidy, all injured structures can be repaired. In adults, however, the dictum of "function by simplification" must be observed, as in Zone F-IV.

The most that can be done with injuries proximal to the musculotendinous junctions is to loosely approximate the muscle with its fascial envelope. The prognosis for effective recovery of function is then guarded.

In the early care of the tidy injury the priority in management is first to ensure the viability of the hand. When the radial and ulnar arteries are divided, the hand is cold and there is no capillary pulse, arterial repair is urgent and must be attended to first (Chap. 10). If, however, the hand is not cold and there is a good capillary pulse in all digits, then a thorough exploration of the wound and identification of structures to be repaired or resected can be undertaken under tourniquet control. After this the tourniquet can be released and the arteriorrhaphies pursued. Tenorrhaphy followed by neurorrhaphy can then be undertaken without the use of the tourniquet, with the hand and forearm modestly elevated.

In the care of untidy injuries and injuries with loss of substance, the prime considerations are viability, maintenance of sensibility, positioning for function, and restoring skin and fatty coverage with pedicle flaps if necessary. Extensive dissection and prolonged surgery are not warranted. Definitive reconstruction will follow in time when the wound softens. Eventually the amount of fibrosis governs whether tenolysis, tenotomy, resection of cicatrix, tendon graft or tendon transfer will be effective.

FLEXOR ZONE TF-I (THUMB)

This zone, extending from mid-distal to mid-proximal phalanx, has the terminal portion of the flexor pollicis longus, the only long flexor of the thumb, the muscle of which is the deepest and most radial digital flexor in the distal forearm. Its vinculum is a substantial structure on the deep side of the tendon over the interphalangeal joint. The synovial bursa starts at this joint and runs as the radial bursa to the distal forearm. The fibrous sheath begins just proximal to this joint. The radial and ulnar neurovascular bundles are just to the side of the sheath. The tendon excursion in this zone is about 1 cm.

Active interphalangeal joint flexion and tip-to-tip pinch are lost when the flexor pollicis longus has been totally divided in this zone, unless the intact vinculum tethers it; in this case flexion is weak and limited. The proximal tendon stump may be drawn far up the flexor sheath to the carpal canal or distal forearm. When the flexor pollicis longus and the flexor digitorum profundus of the index finger are anatomically joined, this juncture must be severed to permit retrieval of the proximal stump of the flexor pollicis longus in the forearm before rethreading it through the radial bursa. Partial division of the flexor pollicis longus can be diagnosed only by careful surgical inspection.

Inasmuch as the adductor pollicis is a powerful flexor of the metacarpophalangeal joint, the flexor pollicis longus can be considered a dispensable tendon. Consequently, when the flexor pollicis longus has been divided, good thumb function may be achieved by tenodesis of the distal stump or arthrodesis of the interphalangeal joint. These more predictable procedures are often preferable to that of trying to reconstruct the long flexor tendon mechanism, particularly if the injury is fresh and untidy, or old with a flexor sheath that is scarred and contracted.

Fresh tidy injuries of the thumb should be explored, and if more than 50 per cent of the flexor pollicis longus is divided it should be repaired. The sheath must be resected enough to make room for the excursion of the point of repair. If the distal stump is 1.0 to 1.5 cm or less in length, it may be resected and the proximal tendon stump advanced for insertion in the distal phalanx. If the distal stump is longer than 1.0 to 1.5 cm, advancement necessitates lengthening of the tendon in the forearm.

FLEXOR ZONE TF-II (THUMB)

Two anatomical points of importance in this zone, which extends from the middle of the proximal phalanx to the neck of the metacarpal, are the presence of a pulley on the proximal half of the proximal phalanx and the encroachment by the sesamoid bones at the metacarpophalangeal joint on the tendon tunnel. The amplitude of tendon gliding in this zone is 3 cm.

Marked retraction of the proximal stump of the flexor pollicis longus is the rule in injuries at this level. Retrieval usually requires a counterincision longitudinally in the distal forearm between the flexor carpi radialis and the radial styloid. The radial bursa may be difficult to thread with a catheter from distal to proximal, but it is easily accomplished from proximal to distal. A small window should be made in the bursa at the counterincision, which can be enlarged once the catheter emerges from the distal wound. Once the bursa is completely threaded, the syringe is shifted to the distal end of the catheter for the rest of the tendon-threading procedure.

If the thumb was tightly flexed at the moment of injury, the distal stump may be very short and far distal to the skin wound when the thumb is extended. In this zone there may be simultaneous injury to the adductor pollicis. If so, the reconstitution of the flexor pollicis longus is essential.

If the distal stump is short, the proximal end may be advanced distally with or without tendon lengthening in the distal forearm. When the distal stump is 2.5 cm or greater in length, a tendon graft should be utilized or the distal joint stabilized by a tenodesis or arthrodesis.

FLEXOR ZONE TF-III (THUMB)

In this zone, which extends from the neck of the metacarpal to the carpal canal, the flexor pollicis longus is very deep and surrounded by thenar musculature (Fig. 14-12). Its amplitude is 4 cm. The tiny thenar motor nerve and the digital nerves to the thumb traverse this area and are frequently injured along with thenar muscles and the flexor pollicis longus. Injuries at this level are often very bloody, obscuring the normal anatomy.

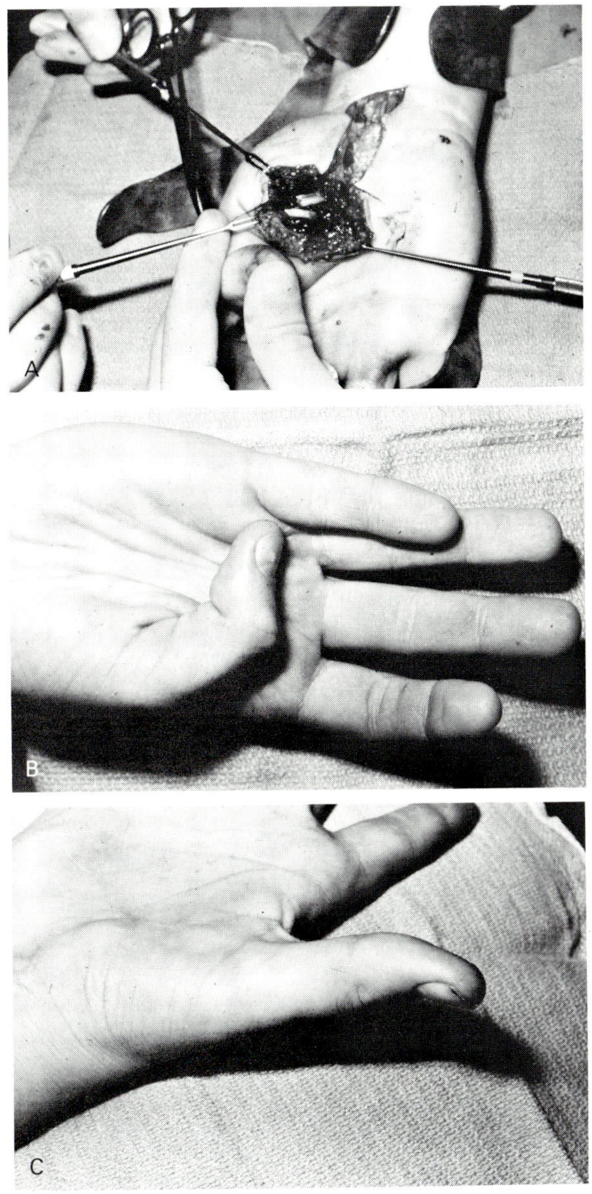

Figure 14-12. *Primary repair of the flexor pollicis longus in Zone TF-III. Note flexion of the distal phalanx to deliver the distal stump into the wound. Often only a tenodesis or arthrodesis is done for this type of injury.*

Whenever wounds at this level are untidy, secondary reconstructive procedures are generally indicated after blood has cleared from the tissues. This may consist of a tenodesis, arthrodesis or tendon graft. If a tendon graft is done, it may be routed as described in Zone F-IV on page 181.

The Treatment of Closed Injuries of Flexor Tendons

The most common effect of a closed injury to a flexor tendon consists of its entrapment within the flexor sheath by stenosis or adhesions. The injury is usually a contusion or crush with or without fracture. Swelling of either tendon sheath and tendon, or both, produces a trigger finger. Adhesions restricting excursion are especially common after a fracture of the proximal phalanx causing a tenodesis of the superficialis or the flexor pollicis longus.

Flexor tendon ruptures occur most often at the site of preexisting tendon abnormality. However, violent stress to a normal tendon may result in rupture at its insertion or its musculotendinous juncture. The patient usually experiences a sudden snap followed by loss of function. There may or may not be swelling or tenderness. A gap is sometimes palpable along the course of the tendon, and occasionally the retracted proximal stump can be felt.

When there is disease associated with the tendon or its bed, treatment should first be directed toward removing that disease (e.g. by synovectomy in rheumatoid disease), then, if the tendon is healthy, it should be repaired. However, if it is not healthy enough it should be replaced by a tendon graft or tendon transfer. Ruptured tendons are managed in the same way as open injuries, and the need for treatment is dictated by the patient's disability, his age and the prognosis for recovery of function after any surgery. Older people with minor disability often need only symptomatic treatment.

Most crushing injuries of the hand that cause sustained limitation of flexor tendon function do so through the formation of scar within the muscles and about the tendons. Volkmann's contracture is the most severe example of this phenomenon. Congestion of tissues with edema or blood is the forerunner of such scarring. The surgeon must be alert to the urgency of early preventive measures, such as widespread fasciotomy (Chaps. 9, 10, or 16).

Treatment of the established flexion contracture requires release or resection of the restraining scar, including tenotomy. Once the desired range of motion has been obtained and the tissues soften, secondary procedures may be planned consisting of: tendon transfer, tendon graft, tenodesis and, at times, arthrodesis. In the badly scarred but mobile digit the temporary placement of a silicone rod may provide a suitable sheath for a subsequent tendon graft. Amputation may be the most suitable treatment for a severely frozen digit or hand.

Extensor Tendons

The extensor system has intricacy and complexity apart from that of the flexor system, the specifics of which require detail in diagnosis and treatment.

Injuries may be closed or open and are often initially masked by the compensatory factors that maintain function even though it has been compromised and will deteriorate with time. Therefore, awareness of the impact of injury on function and the pathomechanics of the various deformities is imperative. Diagnosis must be precise to allow the timely prevention of these deformities through prompt splinting and surgery.

Treatment of open tendon injuries is dictated by the extent of tendon injury and the condition of the wound. In tidy incised wounds, primary tenorrhaphy is indicated. In untidy wounds and wounds with loss of substance, coverage has priority over reconstructive procedures.

In complex injuries where fractures and ligamentous damage coexist with the tendon injury, reduction and skeletal alignment and wound closure have priority over tenorrhaphy. However, elements of the separated extensor system may be approximated primarily when such is possible with ease.

Soft wet dressings, combined with internal and external fixation, are useful to maintain tissue integrity and functional position while evaluating viability and obtaining coverage in these severe cases.

The anatomical and functional features that make extensor tendon injuries quite different from flexor tendon injuries are the following:

1. Whereas flexor tendons are strong rounded cords with spiraling fibers, extensor tendons over the hand are thin and flat with longitudinal fibers which do not hold sutures well. At the wrist and in the forearm, their substance is more like that of flexor tendons.
2. Fibro-osseous tunnels are less prevalent and, therefore, less commonly a factor in generating restrictive adhesions. The adhesions that do occur generally cause less impairment of active joint motion because the normal extensor tendon amplitude is more limited than that of the flexors. Furthermore, the dorsal skin is not tethered as is the volar skin and can move with the tendon to which it is adherent rather than restrain the tendon's excursion.
3. Incomplete injuries of the extensor mechanism, particularly of the extensor hood, may be totally masked at first by the action of the still unaffected components of this mechanism. It is not only the

limited amplitude that makes this possible but also the abundance of interconnecting components of the extensor hood over the digit, and of the juncturae tendina over the body of the hand. Eventually, the unsplinted or unrepaired injury leads to the attenuation of the "normal" components in the longitudinal, lateral and volar directions so that deformities insidiously emerge.

4. The lever action of the digital extensor tendon system is much less powerful than that of the digital flexor tendon system. A flexor tendon passes over a joint at a greater distance (radius) from the joint axis and inserts farther beyond the joint than does the extensor tendon. Mechanically, this imparts greater power to the digital flexors than to the digital extensors. As a consequence, there is greater amplitude of the flexors per degree of joint motion than there is of the extensors, but the effect of the latter is more rapid motion. For this reason, tendon length is far more critical in repairs of the extensors over the digits than for repairs of the flexors. A millimeter or two in extra length in this area can result in failure of an extensor tendon graft or tenorrhaphy. Hence, the immobilization of joints in just the right amount of extension and the careful adjustment of tension of the extensor tenorrhaphy are crucial. If too loose, (e.g. too long) full active extension will not be achieved, and if too tight, stiffness due to limitation of flexion will result.
5. The absence of thick skin and a cushion of subcutaneous fat exposes the extensors to injury. Their vulnerability is increased by the tension created when the joints are flexed. Similarly, cutaneous trauma (e.g. burns) and infections easily involve these juxtaposed tendons.
6. The untethered loose dorsal skin is easily avulsed by a shearing force exposing the extensor tendons.
7. One nerve (the radial) innervates all of the extrinsic extensor muscles.
8. The proximity to the surface and limited retraction of the extensor tendons makes it feasible to repair many of their injuries with less elaborate facilities than are required for flexor tendons.
9. A finger with incomplete extension is generally far less a functional problem than a finger with incomplete flexion. The reverse is true of the wrist, where extension is indispensable for power grip.

Surgical Topography

The location of a tendon injury in relation to the joint or bone the tendon is traversing influences the development of functional impairment and deformity and thus the nature of treatment. Therefore, topographical zones are assigned for purposes of discussing the specific problems. The numerical order of the zones is from distal to proximal[13] (Fig. 14-13).

Extensor zones of the fingers, hand, wrist, forearm, and thumb are designated as follows:*

Finger, wrist, forearm:
- Zone E-I—Dorsum of the DIP joint
- Zone E-II—Dorsum of the middle phalanx
- Zone E-III—Dorsum of the PIP joint
- Zone E-IV—Dorsum of the proximal phalanx
- Zone E-V—Dorsum of the MP joint
- Zone E-VI—Dorsum of the metacarpal
- Zone E-VII—Dorsum of the wrist
- Zone E-VIII—Dorsum of the distal $\frac{1}{4}$ of the forearm

Thumb:
- Zone TE-I—Dorsum of the IP joint
- Zone TE-II—Dorsum of the proximal phalanx
- Zone TE-III—Dorsum of the MP joint
- Zone TE-IV—Dorsum of the metacarpal.

Principles of Management

Whenever possible, primary repair is favored over delayed repair. Without complicating factors there is no urgency and the repair can be delayed pending ideal circumstances for 72 hours to two weeks.

*DIP = Distal interphalangeal, PIP = proximal interphalangeal, and MP = metacarpophalangeal.

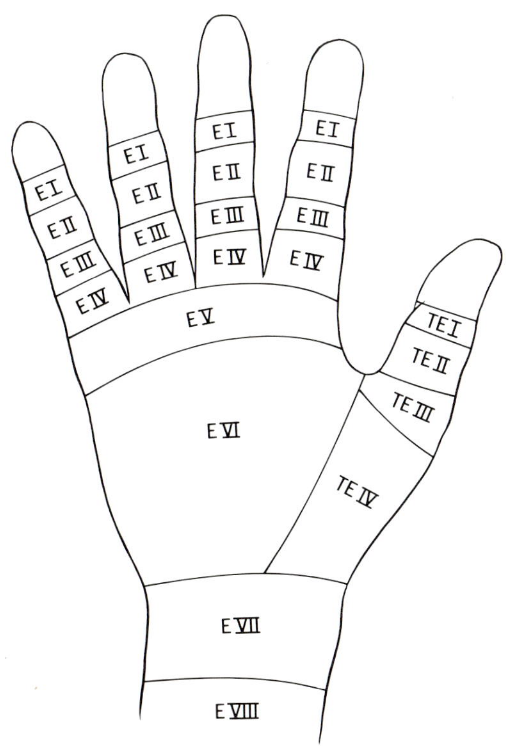

Figure 14-13. *Extensor tendon zones.*

Proximal to the metacarpals, retraction occurs after transection so that repairs are necessary as soon as possible (within 6 to 8 weeks) to keep the muscle from becoming irreversibly contracted. To prevent this problem when there is associated skin avulsion, the proximal stump may be tacked to the distal stump in anticipation of a formal tenorrhaphy later. The retrieval of retracted stumps may be accomplished through a proximal counterincision using a polyethylene catheter as described for flexor tendon retrieval (Fig. 14-27). The extensor retinacular pulley system can be circumvented by transferring the retrieved extensor tendon subcutaneously without impairing function.

The thin flat extensor tendons are repaired with a horizontal mattress or figure-of-eight suture for better purchase and less crowding than is achieved with the crisscross suture (Fig. 14-20).

The surgical procedures available for extensor tendon repair include:

1. Direct repair
2. Local tendon pedicle
3. Tendon transfer (e.g. extensor indicis proprius and digiti quinti to one of the other digital extensors)
4. Tendon graft
5. Tenodesis or arthrodesis

When there is no retraction of the tendon stumps, suturing may be contraindicated since favorable healing will follow splinting alone and adhesions, aggravated by the surgical handling of the tendon, will be reduced. When the tendon ends are approximately equal in an end-to-end repair, the horizontal mattress or figure-of-eight suture technique is generally used in Zone 1 through Zone 6 and a crisscross technique in Zone 7 and Zone 8. Tendons are usually joined by the weave technique when transfers or grafts are done. All restricting or constricting fascia should be excised, including the relevant portions of the extensor retinaculum.

The type of immobilization used for extensor tendon injury will vary greatly depending on the zone of injury and will be discussed under each one. In general, because of the limited forces of separation (retraction) of the cut ends, more freedom of motion of the uninjured segments of the extensor mechanism is allowed than in the case of immobilization following flexor tenorrhaphy. Once continous splinting has been stopped, intermittent protective splinting is employed at night and between periods of scheduled mobilization for a week or more. To overcome stiffness, dynamic splinting is sometimes necessary.

The Treatment of Extensor Tendon Injury by Topographical Zone

EXTENSOR ZONE E-I (OVER THE DISTAL INTERPHALANGEAL JOINT OF THE FINGER)

The distal interphalangeal joint is extended by two mechanisms: (1) the thin terminal extensor tendon, which is the terminal confluence of the tendon components of the extensor hood; its amplitude of movement is 5 mm or less, and (2) Landsmeer's oblique retinacular ligaments which are often of sufficient substance to act as static distal interphalangeal joint extensors when tightened by extension of the proximal interphalangeal joint.

The insertion of this tendon and the ligaments are into the epiphysis of the distal phalanx blending with the dorsal joint capsule just proximal to the nail bed. Operations on the nail can damage the extensor insertion and vice versa. The skin is thin, tight and adherent, making its separation from the underlying tendon difficult without the aid of magnification. Hyperextension of the distal interphalangeal joint must be avoided in splinting because this will impair the circulation in these tight tissues and jeopardize healing.

The injury may be confined to the extensor tendon or may involve skin, bone or joint. The impairment of extension may be complete or incomplete. Closed injuries ("baseball," "mallet," "drop finger" deformities) are more common than open ones. Sudden forceful flexion of the tensely extended distal joint ruptures the extensor or avulses its bony insertion causing loss of full active extension. Pain and tenderness are more prominent if there is a fracture and justify a roentgenogram for complete diagnosis.

The need for treatment is governed by pain and the impairment of "uplift" (active distal joint extension). Total impairment produces a flexion deformity of nearly 90° which may be a major functional and cosmetic disability. Partial impairment, with the loss of only 10 to 15° of extension, may require no treatment. The few millimeters of proximal migration of the hood following these injuries may produce an excessive pull of the central slip (medial extensor tendon) on the middle phalanx, resulting in hyperextension of the proximal interphalangeal joint (recurvatum). This, combined with flexion of the distal joint, produces a swan-neck deformity. Blunt trauma may weaken the tendon over the distal joint and insidiously lead to a flexion deformity by the process of attenuation.

There is minimal retraction of the proximal tendon stump following a laceration, but tenorrhaphy is difficult because of the adherence of the skin and the thin gauge of the tendon. Open injuries contaminate the distal interphalangeal joint and may injure the cartilage or ligaments.

Closed Injuries. Most closed injuries are treated non-operatively. No treatment is necessary if the informed patient so elects and the flexion deformity is no more than 15°. Deformities of greater than 15° should be treated for six weeks by splinting the distal joint in extension (*not hyperextension*). An accompanying fracture with a fragment larger than one-fourth the articular surface of the distal phalanx will require reduction or excision (Chap. 11).

Splinting is usually external. On occasion, internal fixation using an oblique or longitudinal Kirschner wire or hypodermic needle is preferred. The external splint must be padded with plastic or rubber foam and must cross the distal interphalangeal joint, obtaining as much contact with the middle and distal phalanges as possible and yet not blocking motion of the proximal interphalangeal joint. Barring adverse symptoms, the splint is not disturbed for six weeks. It is placed on the volar aspect when a dorsal wound or tenderness precludes direct pressure of the splint upon it. The flat dorsal surface of the aligned phalanges accommodates the splint better than the convexity of the volar fat pads (Fig. 14-14). Modifications of this type of splinting are used successfully. The splinted finger should be kept dry and checked regularly for position and skin irritation.

When it is imperative that the functional result is to be nearly normal, a greater degree of splinting is required. This is dictated by certain specific needs of individual patients, e.g. musicians. In these cases the digit and the hand, as well as the forearm, are immobilized in plaster, preventing any action on the entire flexor and extensor mechanisms for 3 to 4 weeks. The wrist is extended and the metacarpophalangeal and proximal interphalangeal joints are flexed, in addition to the specific splinting of the distal interphalangeal joint described above (which is maintained for the usual six weeks).

The sooner that splinting is instituted after injury, the better the chance for a good result. Splinting has been successful when started six weeks or longer after injury, but this is exceptional.

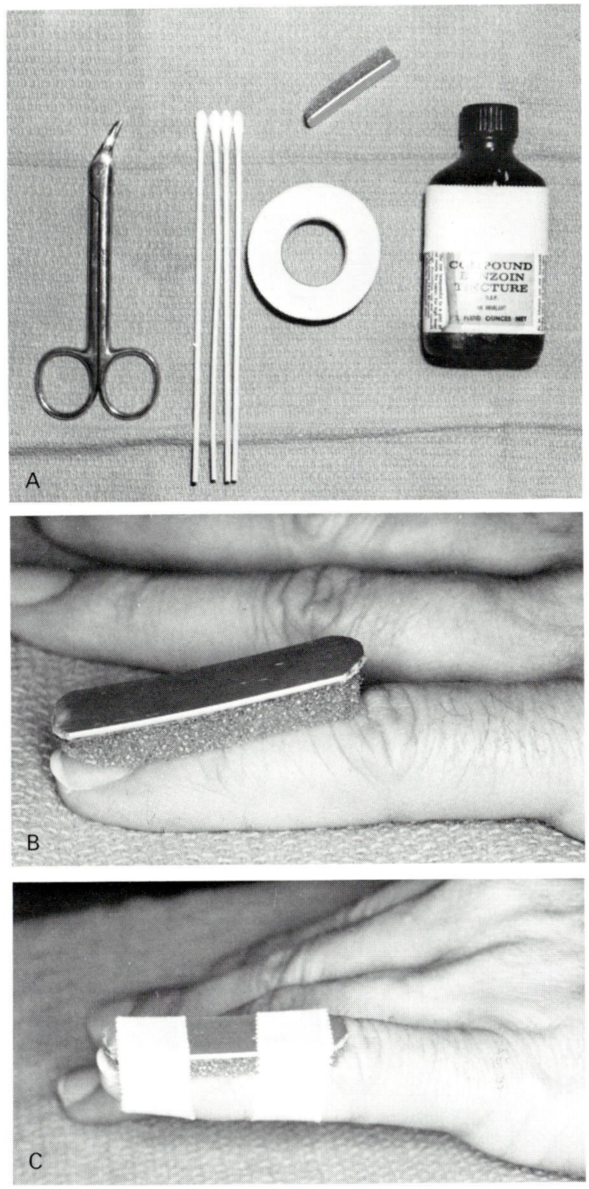

Figure 14-14. *Technique of splinting the mallet finger.* **A:** *The necessary materials for splinting.* **B:** *Application of a splint which will not limit proximal joint mobility.* **C:** *Securing the splint to the distal and middle phalanges with non-allergic tape.*

Treatment of these problems in children is just as important as it is in adults. One-third of patients will have some persistence of their deformity after six weeks of treatment. Splinting is discontinued at six weeks and joint motion is pursued to the patient's tolerance. A night splint may be used for an additional four weeks.

Open Injuries. The open mallet injury may be treated primarily or by delay for up to 72 hours.

The simultaneous repair of skin and tendon may be done immediately for tidy wounds. A horizontal mattress suture of 5-0 nylon is placed in the proximal stump. The distal joint is then pinned in a straight line with a longitudinal or oblique Kirschner wire. A Keith needle is passed through the distal stump of this tendon and obliquely through the bone and out at the fingertip. The suture ends are threaded through the eye of the needle and then withdrawn through the tip of the finger and tied over a pledget of dental roll. The skin wound is closed with 6-0 nylon. A forearm cast is applied for three weeks and the Kirschner wire left in place for six weeks. The pull-out nylon is removed at four weeks. Prophylactic antibiotics are administered.

Tendon advancement is generally unsuccessful and is apt to stiffen the joint in extension.

Untidy injuries may completely preclude the reapproximation of the extensor apparatus. The treatment of choice, then, is a primary arthrodesis (Chap. 13).

Chronic Mallet Deformity. Occasionally, an established mallet deformity of only 15 to 40° is cosmetically and functionally disturbing to the patient. When greater than 40°, it is often a major problem. Surgical treatment is justified only on demand by a well-informed patient who is willing to assume the risks of stiffness, adverse scar formation and possibly pain.

The surgical procedures to consider are: (1) section of the insertion of the central slip (medial extensor tendon), (2) arthrodesis of the distal joint, (3) excision of scar and advancement of the proximal stump of the terminal extensor tendon, (4) reconstruction of the oblique retinacular ligament, and (5) a tendon graft. Regardless of the type of surgical correction employed, transarticular fixation of the distal interphalangeal joint with a Kirschner wire for six weeks is advised. The patient must understand that arthrodesis has the highest predictability of success.

Section of the insertion of the middle extensor tendon on the middle phalanx (Fowler's procedure) releases the tethering effect of this structure against proximal migration of the distal components of the extensor hood. When the mallet deformity is between 15 to 40°, only 1 to 2 mm of migration is needed to produce normal extension of the distal interphalangeal joint. This much can be gained by Fowler's procedure. It is done with local anesthesia so that the patient can cooperate and its effectiveness can be immediately tested with forceful active motion. A proximal tourniquet is used to control hemorrhage. A midaxial incision is made along the proximal phalanx and the hood mechanism is elevated while the proximal interphalangeal joint is kept in hyperextension. Using small, short-bladed, pointed curved scissors, the insertion of the central slip is sectioned fiber by fiber without buttonholing the extensor hood. Postoperatively, mobilization is initiated under supervision within 24 to 48 hours.

An arthrodesis of the distal interphalangeal joint is indicated when the best chance for a painless joint is required (e.g. the patient is elderly or the joint is already stiff, painful and arthritic).

To excise the scar and advance the extensor tendon, a proximally or laterally based skin flap can be raised. Starting at the normal tendon proximally, the dissection proceeds into the zone of injury. The scar tissue is excised (not more than 1 to 2 mm) and the remainder of the procedure is performed as described for open injuries.

The oblique retinacular ligament is reconstructed by anchoring one end of a narrow tendon graft into the distal phalanx and the other into the flexor pulley of the proximal phalanx. For this graft to act effectively it must cross the middorsum of the distal interphalangeal joint. To satisfy both these demands and to avoid subluxation, the distal and proximal fixations are on opposite sides of the digit. Thus, the graft traverses obliquely across the dorsum. The length of the graft and its tension are critical. The distal fixation via a window in a bone is secured first after intramedullary fixation of the joint in full extension. Rather than opening the entire dorsum of the finger, a subcutaneous tunnel is created to a counterincision on the midaxial aspect of the proximal phalanx. The proximal end of the graft is threaded through a window in the flexor pulley along the midshaft of the proximal phalanx and sutured. With proper tension the proximal interphalangeal joint will lack 10° of full extension. During immobilization tension is taken off the graft by modest flexion of the proximal interphalangeal joint. The hand and wrist are splinted for three weeks. The transarticular wire is removed at six weeks.

Reconstruction of the extensor tendon is more difficult, but parallels the principles for reconstruction of the oblique retinacular ligament. More exposure is required distally and is gained by a proximally-based skin flap which is raised by incising across the apex of the eponychium and along the radial and ulnar borders of the digit. The distal half of the tendon graft is split into two tails and the apex of the split secured against further cleavage with a 5-0 nylon suture. The dorsal-lateral aspect of the distal phalanx is osteotomized by drilling on either side to receive the tails; alternatively, they are kept long and made to embrace the flexor side of the bone. The fixation of these tails follows the immobilization of the distal joint in full extension by a Kirschner wire.

Proximally, the graft is split also into two tails after having threaded it into a subcutaneous tunnel over the apex of the proximal interphalangeal joint and out of one or two radial and ulnar counterincisions near the base of the proximal phalanx. The proximal tails are threaded around the lateral bands while the proximal interphalangeal joint is held in full extension. The proximal interphalangeal joint is maintained in full extension with an oblique Kirschner wire after testing the tension of the graft. The tension is right if the proximal interphalangeal joint can be flexed 90° with simultaneous extension of the wrist and flexion of the metacarpophalangeal joint, and if full wrist flexion draws the metacarpophalangeal and proximal interphalangeal joints into full extension. Postoperative immobilization is for three weeks in a forearm cast with the wrist extended and the metacarpophalangeal joints flexed. At that time the fixation of the proximal interphalangeal joint is removed. The distal Kirschner wire remains for six weeks.

EXTENSOR ZONE E-II (OVER THE MIDDLE PHALANX OF THE FINGERS)

In this zone the lateral extensor tendons are fused distally to form the terminal extensor tendon and are connected proximally by the thin triangular ligament. The oblique retinacular ligaments fuse with the lateral aspect of the lateral extensor tendon and insert distally with the terminal extensor tendon. When there is injury to tendon, skin, bone or periosteum in this zone, disruption or fixation of the extensor mechanism may lead to a mallet deformity or loss of distal interphalangeal joint flexion.

Closed injuries rarely require primary treatment for the tendon injury. Later tenolysis or the resection of a bony callus or boss may be necessary. The latter procedure has a poor prognosis because of the tendency for recurrence. Tidy open injuries require splinting for four weeks. There may be no separation of the tendon as long as the distal joint is fully extended and the proximal joint partially extended. This obviates the need for tenorrhaphy. Tendon approximation is a secondary consideration when there is untidy skin and bony injury, but should not be deferred if it is easily accomplished. When there is good skin coverage, imminent fixation of tendon to bone may be arrested by interposing a thin sheet of silicone between tendon and bone. Late tendon reconstruction in this zone may require replacement of soft tissue cover, tenolysis or the procedures mentioned for Zone 1.

EXTENSOR ZONE E-III (OVER THE PROXIMAL INTERPHALANGEAL JOINT OF THE FINGER)

The central slip (medial extensor tendon) and the intrinsic tendons (lateral extensor tendons) combine through crisscrossing interconnections of the extensor hood to jointly extend the middle phalanx. The intrinsics contribute more to this action when they are stretched by extension of the metacarpophalangeal joint, and the central slip contributes more when it is stretched by flexion of the metacarpophalangeal joint. A transverse retinaculum tethers the extensor hood to the flexor sheath and holds the hood over the crest of the proximal interphalangeal joint. The amplitude of movement of the central slip is 5 to 8 mm.

The skin in this area is loose and redundant when the joint is fully extended but is stretched taut when the joint is fully flexed. In this stance, both skin and tendon are highly vulnerable.

Injuries in this region bring about joint deformities and stiffness. They may be open or closed, simple or complex. Dislocation of the proximal interphalangeal joint may cause a rupture of the transverse retinacular ligament and part of the collateral ligament on one side of the joint so that the extensor slips off the head of the proximal phalanx into the joint, requiring an open reduction because of locking (Chap. 12). A variant of this injury is a rent between the central slip and the lateral extensor tendon, resulting in volar displacement of the lateral extensor tendon and buttonholing of the subjacent phalangeal condyle between it and the central slip. Such displacement also creates a locked dislocation. An adherence of the central slip to the joint capsule causes stiffness in extension.

The buttonhole (boutonniere) deformity is the most common sequel of untreated injury to the extensor mechanism in this zone. Division or attenuation of the central slip is followed by a volar shift of the lateral extensor tendons as the head of the proximal phalanx "buttonholes" through the dorsal defect. The lateral tendons become flexors of the proximal interphalangeal joint as soon as they are volar to its axis, and the tension placed upon them by the flare of the condyles forces the distal interphalangeal joint into hyperextension.

Usually the buttonhole deformity does not develop immediately because all components of the extensor hood—the central extensor slip, the two lateral tendons and interconnections among the three—are not all simultaneously injured. Those that remain intact temporarily compensate for the injured ones. This accounts for the failure to recognize many of these injuries when they first occur. Without prompt treatment, the forces of "buttonholing" progress until the deformity is well established and active extension is lost. Following blunt trauma, the capsular thickening (traumatic synovitis) that occurs aggravates the attenuation of the hood and worsens the prognosis markedly when treatment is delayed.

Closed Injuries. A history of significant blunt trauma to the dorsum of the proximal interphalangeal joint, particularly at the moment it was fully flexed, demands scrutiny in the ensuing hours for the appearance of any soft tissue swelling and tenderness. Roentgenograms will demonstrate any coexisting injury to bone. As soon as swelling and tenderness appear, the proximal interphalangeal joint should be splinted alone in full extension, allowing the distal interphalangeal joint and metacarpophalangeal joints free. This splint should be applied in the same manner as that used for Zone I injuries (mallet deformity) and should be maintained for 4 to 6 weeks. If a Kirschner wire is used to immobilize the proximal interphalangeal joint, it should be placed obliquely, keeping it free of the extensor hood.

The treatment of associated fractures and ligamentous injuries must be integrated with the prophylactic treatment of a potential buttonhole deformity (Chap. 11). The usual dislocation of the proximal interphalangeal joint is a dorsal dislocation of the middle phalanx on the proximal phalanx, leaving the extensor hood intact. This does not predispose to the buttonhole deformity.

Unyielding adhesions between the central extensor slip and the dorsal joint capsule, producing an extensor habitus, may be unresponsive to dynamic splinting. If the roentgenogram of the joint is normal, a tenolysis may be done cautiously through a dorsolateral incision. The hood is elevated and the proximal interphalangeal joint hyperextended. Adhesions are divided without loss of integrity of the central slip so that a buttonhole deformity will not occur.

Functional disability and pain are indications for surgical correction of a buttonhole deformity if it persists after subsidence of the acute reaction to injury. The deformity may be incorrectly attributed to injury when, in fact, it is due to Dupuytren's contracture. At times, both etiologies for this deformity may coexist, making the prognosis for correction poor.

Once this deformity becomes established after trauma, it falls into two categories, one with supple joints and one with stiff joints. Those cases with supple joints that do not have thickening of the capsule and the extensor hood have a favorable prognosis for the recovery of extensor tendon function. Those with stiffness, however, often have so much thickening that there is little hope for the reconstruction of normal extensor function.

Preoperatively, the maximal mobility of stiffened joints must be obtained by active and passive exercise. Flexion of the distal interphalangeal joint helps to reduce the deformity by pulling the extensor mechanism distally, thereby reducing the volar shift of the lateral extensor tendons and the retraction of the medial extensor tendon.

The methods of tenorrhaphy are numerous (Fig. 14-15). For most instances one of the four following techniques will be suitable. Each requires transarticular fixation of the proximal interphalangeal joint by an oblique Kirschner wire for 3 to 4 weeks and a forearm cast for 2 to 3 weeks, followed by a digital splint across the proximal interphalangeal joint for 2 to 3 weeks.

1. The grayish central scar tissue of the extensor hood over the proximal interphalangeal joint is distinguished from normal white tendon tissue by magnification. It is excised in the form of a V-shaped specimen with the apex of the V distally. The specimen should not be more than 2 to 3 mm wide or overcorrection and stiffness will result. By hoisting the hood with fine hooks, thickened capsule over the cartilage may have to be carefully excised; sometimes the radial and ulnar transverse retinacular fibers have to be divided to release the lateral extensor tendons. The surgical defect in the hood is closed as a V into Y (Fig. 14-15**A**). In so doing, the medial extensor tendon (central slip) is advanced and the lateral extensor tendons (intrinsic bands) are repositioned dorsally into their normal relationship. Interrupted 5-0 or 6-0 nylon sutures are used in the repair, burying the knots.[5]
2. When shrinkage is more of a problem than capsular bulk (e.g. burns), dorsal reefing of the lateral bands as described by Littler is indicated[9] (Fig.

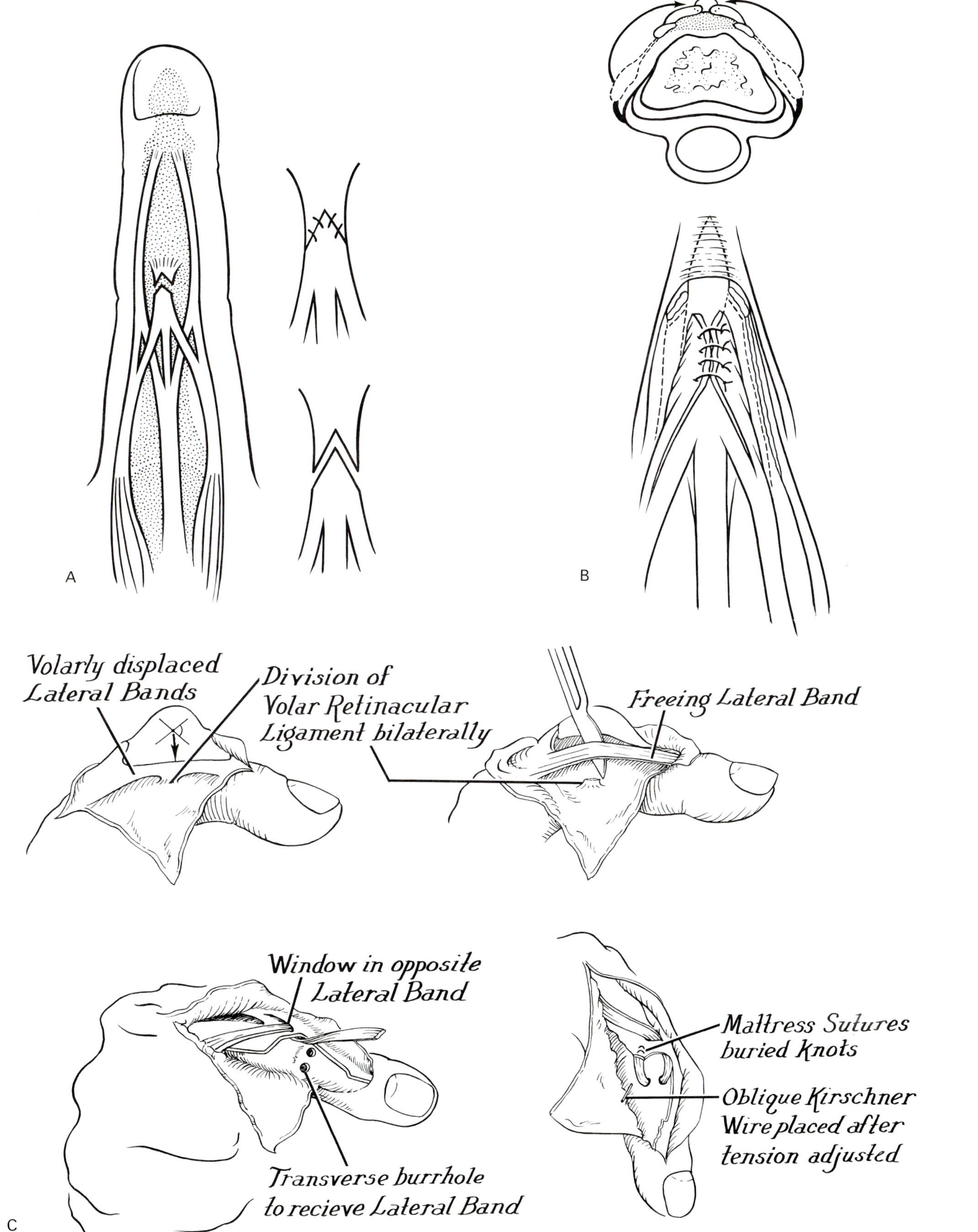

Figure 14-15. *Correction of boutonniere deformity.* **A:** *V-Y advancement.* **B:** *Reefing of the lateral extensor tendon.*[9] **C:** *Rerouting the ulnar lateral band.* (*Redrawn from Littler, J.W.*[8])

14-15**B**). The lateral extensor tendons are divorced from the terminal extensor tendon by sectioning them across the shaft of the middle phalanx, leaving enough of the terminal extensor tendon to provide continuity with the oblique retinacular ligaments. Continuity between the lumbrical and the terminal extensor tendon to reinforce extension of the distal interphalangeal joint may be maintained by longitudinal sectioning of half of the radial lateral extensor tendon. The midline approximation of the lateral extensor tendons over the proximal interphalangeal joint and the base of the middle phalanx restores extension of the proximal interphalangeal joint by the intrinsics. Arthrodesis of the distal interphalangeal joint may be undertaken if the function of the oblique retinacular ligament is inadequate to extend it.

3. A thin tendon graft is anchored at the base of the middle phalanx through a transverse hole. The redundant part is folded back proximally, spread out and sutured to the slightly advanced central slip. An alternative choice is to weave it through the central slip and at the same time around the lateral extensor tendons to elevate them.
4. Littler[8] has described an alternative method to using a free graft (Fig. 14-15**C**). The transverse retinacular fibers are freed and the lateral bands elevated. The ulnar lateral band is dissected free distally and rerouted across the dorsum through a window created in the radial lateral band and back to the hood after passing through a small burr hole in the middle phalanx. Postoperative treatment and splinting are the same as outlined for the free tendon graft.

In all of these procedures, the tenorrhaphy is completed prior to the transarticular joint fixation in order that the degree of tension can be tested.

With the wrist in extension and the metacarpophalangeal joint flexed, it should be possible to flex the proximal interphalangeal joint 90°, and with full wrist flexion the proximal interphalangeal joint should go into full extension. When the extensor mechanism is salvageable but the joint is destroyed, implant arthroplasty using a silicone spacer may be employed. Arthrodesis may be used to improve the angle of function when the deformity cannot be corrected by other means.

Open Injuries. These are tidy, untidy or complex with or without the loss of substance. In all open injuries with a functioning joint, adequate circulation and minimal potential for infection, tenorrhaphy and splinting are the rule. Even a partial separation of the central extensor slip requires tenorrhaphy. A good prognosis will follow this provided splinting is maintained by internal or external means for 4 to 6 weeks. A contaminated wound (e.g. inflicted by a tooth) is best treated as though already massively infected (Chap. 20, Bite Infections). In such circumstances, tendon repair, definitive closure of the wound and internal splinting are generally deferred 2 to 10 days until it is certain that infection is not developing.

The prognosis is always guarded in complex injuries when there is loss of substance or involvement of multiple tissues. Here the prime concerns are functional alignment and avoidance of infection by early closure of the wound. Tendon reconstruction is delayed until there is good soft tissue coverage and normal joint mobility. At times a short silicone tendon rod may be inserted primarily to form a pseudosheath in preparation for a tendon graft later. In carefully selected circumstances when the extensor hood and proximal interphalangeal joint have been destroyed but the flexor and volar sensory systems are intact, an implant arthroplasty together with a cutaneous pedicle flap may be done primarily. Subsequently, the extensor system may be reconstructed.

EXTENSOR ZONE E-IV (OVER THE PROXIMAL PHALANX OF THE FINGER)

There are no unique problems of repairing simple injuries within this area. Retraction is negligible, and when not present tendon sutures may not be needed. Splinting is maintained for 3 to 4 weeks. The complications here are similar to those about the middle phalanx (Zone E-II). A post-traumatic exostosis or boss under the lateral extensor tendon can tighten it enough to cause a state of intrinsic plus. This is relieved by section of the lateral band at the base of the digit in preference to resecting the boss, which is likely to recur.

EXTENSOR ZONE E-V (OVER THE METACARPOPHALANGEAL JOINT OF THE FINGER)

The extensor tendon with an amplitude of 15 to 18 mm is centrally anchored over the head of the metacarpal by the sagittal retinacular bands of the hood on either side, which limit retraction of the proximal stump. Incomplete division of the hood is often unrecognized at first by inexperienced examiners because the intact portion of the hood still compensates for the injured part. Just as in the case of injury to the proximal interphalangeal (Zone E-III), blunt and open trauma over the metacarpophalangeal joint may weaken the hood so that, with time, the force of flexion will attenuate the hood and bring about a loss of active extension.

Fixation by adhesions, tightening by shrinkage and capsular thickening are factors which can limit the excursion of the hood at the level and cause joint stiffness. Shortening of the subjacent collateral ligaments of the metacarpophalangeal joint often aggravates the stiffness following tendon injury and further prohibits flexion (Chap. 21). Injuries here may completely or incompletely divide the middle extensor tendon, and may be tidy, untidy or complex with or without the loss of substance. Penetrating injury of the joint is complicated by the shutter mechanism that exists between the extensor hood and the joint capsule, sealing in contamination.

Adherence to bone is rarely a problem. However, separations or attenuations of the radial sagittal band or contracture of the ulnar sagittal band will result in subluxation of the extensor tendon ulnarward when it is tensed during joint flexion. This is recognized as a snapping phenomenon. With progressive attenuation, chronic subluxation and ulnar drift occur.

Closed Injuries. Ulnar subluxation of the extensor tendon as a result of attenuation of the sagittal bands (lateral wings) following blunt trauma appears insidiously. Unlike that of the buttonhole deformity (Zone E-III), its onset cannot be readily enough anticipated to warrant splinting for the acute injury.

Ulnar subluxation of the extensor tendon usually requires relocation of the tendon by substitution for the incompetent radial sagittal band.[7] Repositioning of the middle extensor tendon over the apex of the metacarpophalangeal joint can be accomplished by tethering it in position with a distally based tendon pedicle (Fig. 14-16). The 3-mm wide pedicle is raised on the radial side of the long extensor, its base at the beginning of the extensor hood. This pedicle is looped around the radial collateral ligament. Tension is appropriately adjusted to allow full excursion of the joint passively and a normal habitus of the digit when the wrist is positioned in full flexion or extension. The pedicle is sutured with interrupted 4-0 or 5-0 nylon and the immobilization is maintained 3 to 4 weeks with the metacarpophalangeal joint in moderate flexion.

The "extensor plus" state may follow shrinkage and/or adherence of the extensor hood mechanism after injury in this zone.[6] As a consequence all three finger joints cannot be simultaneously flexed even though individually they move through a normal range of motion. This is corrected by release of the adhesions (tenolysis) or by prolongation of the medial extensor tendon and, if necessary, release of the sagittal band contracture. Local anesthesia is preferred, so that the adequacy of these procedures can be immediately gauged by having the patient's cooperation in active tendon and joint motion.

Exposure of the hood is gained through a dorsal lateral incision along the proximal phalanx and distal metacarpal. Then the central extensor tendon is elevated with a hook over the proximal phalanx and notched with a #11 scalpel. The notching is done alternately on the radial and ulnar sides in 2 to 3 locations at 1-cm intervals across the midline of the tendon so that no single tendon fiber remains intact the full length of any of the intervals (Fig. 14-17). The retinaculotomy is done on the ulnar sagittal band first. These notches must be precise and spare the lateral extensor tendons. The operation is followed by immediate and progressive mobilization.

Open Injuries. Tidy injuries may discretely divide the extensor tendon, the sagittal band or both. Although retraction is minimal, a repair of the divided portion of the hood is always indicated. The tendon should be elevated with hooks so that the joint capsule is not included in the sutures. If buried sutures are used, knots should be placed away from the apex of the knuckle when the joint is flexed or buried under the tendon; otherwise they will become symptomatic. There is a propensity for the development of a subdermal chronically draining bursa if great care is not taken to evert the skin, to avoid tight sutures and to leave skin sutures in long enough (e.g. usually three weeks).

External immobilization with a forearm cast to the proximal interphalangeal joints is employed for 3 to 4 weeks. To avoid stiffness, the metacarpal phalangeal joint must be in 40° flexion and the wrist in 30° extension. Local and systemic antibiotics are used before and after operation.

Complex injuries, and those in which tissue substance is lost, are treated as outlined for similar injuries in Zone E-III, except that internal fixation is used only if needed for fractures. In loss of substance injuries, once satisfactory skin cover has been replaced, an extensor tendon graft may be woven into the medial extensor tendon distally and the appropriate extensor tendon proximally. Ten-

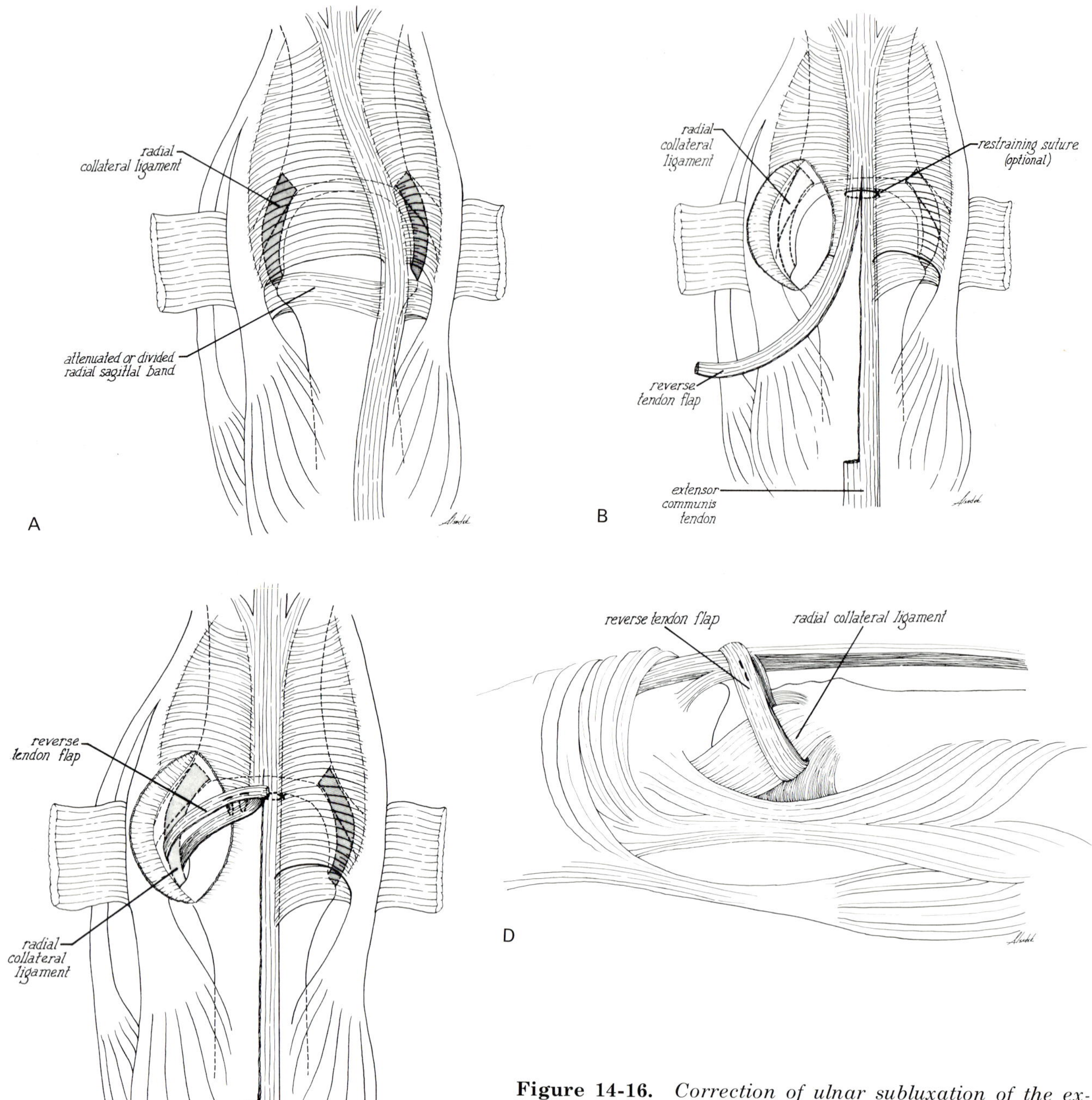

Figure 14-16. *Correction of ulnar subluxation of the extensor mechanism at the metacarpophalangeal joints by a reverse tendon flap.* (*Reproduced from Kilgore, et al.*[7] with *permission of the publisher.*)

sion is gauged by positioning the wrist. With full extension, the metacarpophalangeal joint should flex 45 to 60°, and with full flexion the metacarpophalangeal joint should fully extend. Immobilization of the wrist and metacarpophalangeal joint is required for four weeks.

EXTENSOR ZONE E-VI (DORSUM OF THE METACARPAL AND BODY OF THE HAND)

Within this zone are the four common extensors to the fingers, the two independent (proprius) extensors to the index and little fingers and the in-

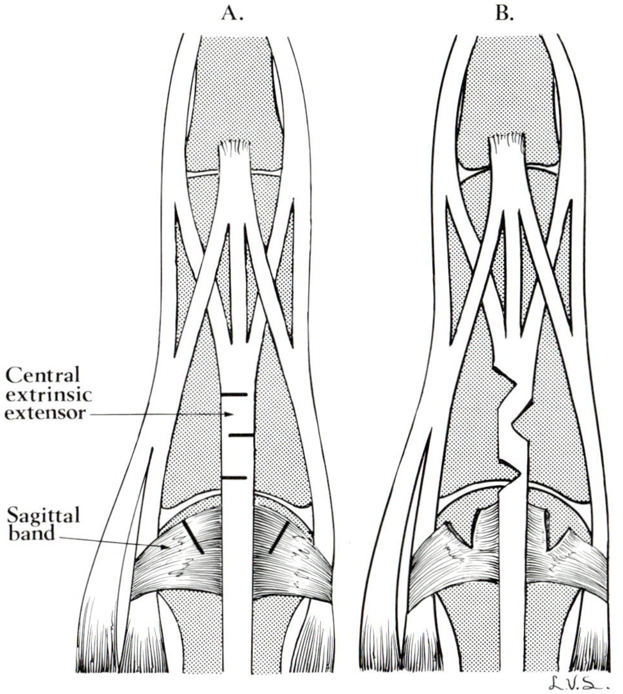

Figure 14-17. *Tenotomies for correction of extensor plus. (Reproduced from Kilgore, et al.[6] with permission of the publisher.)*

sertions of the three wrist extensors. Extensor tendon injuries to the index and little fingers can be masked if the injury is limited to just one of the two tendons of each finger. The juncturae tendina are also capable of masking injury to an adjacent tendon. With a divided proprius tendon, its companion extensor communis cannot fully extend the subject metacarpophalangeal joint if tethered by flexion of the other metacarpophalangeal joints.

Repair of these tendons is dictated by the functional requirements of the individual patient. A division of an extensor communis to the index or the little finger cannot be diagnosed without surgical exploration, whereas division of the extensor communis to the ring and long fingers may be diagnosed or suspected by failure of full and forceful metacarpophalangeal joint extension. A small mass developing after injury which moves with tendon excursion makes tendon injury suspect. Most often this mass represents tendon callus or cystic formation at the site of injury.

The vulnerability of the large veins on the dorsum of the hand readily complicates any injury or careless surgery. Adhesions between injured tendons and adjacent deep or superficial tissue (e.g. peritendinous fibrosis—Secretan's disease) are sequelae to trauma and may limit excursion.

Closed Injuries. Except for the uncommon problem of peritendinous fibrosis, it is unusual for closed injury to compromise the function of extensors in this area. Secretan's disease[12] is a brawny, persistent edema sometimes leading to massive (tumerous) peritendinous fibrosis. The blunt trauma preceding this process may appear insignificant and ecchymosis may be absent. There is nothing to be gained by use of local corticosteroids or massage. Surgery is ill advised and may aggravate and prolong the process. The patient should be warned to control edema and keep active, and told that the thickening of soft tissue on the dorsum of the hand may take months to improve. An elastic glove that is tailored to the hand helps to reduce the thickness of the scar.

Blunt trauma, fractures and infections can lead to adhesions that cause the extensor plus state discussed previously (Zone E-IV). This may require a tenolysis followed by immediate mobilization.

Open Injuries. Clean, tidy lacerations must be examined under tourniquet control of bleeding. Extension of the wound is often necessary. Divided tendons should be approximated with 4-0 or 6-0 nylon in the form of buried horizontal mattress, figure-of-eight, or crisscrossing sutures. If the juncture of the tenorrhaphy will pass into the fibro-osseous sheath at the wrist, enough of this should be resected to avoid blockage. Immobilization is carried out for 3 to 4 weeks with the wrist extended and the metacarpophalangeal joints in comfortable flexion. Prophylactic antibiotics are used locally and systemically.

Untidy wounds are treated according to the integrity of the soft tissue cover. Approximation of readily accessible tendon ends in the untidy wound may be done. Otherwise, tenorrhaphy should be postponed until the condition of the circulation, the skeleton and tendon bed can be made favorable.

Open injuries often result in adherence of the tendons to the overlying skin, producing puckering with motion. There may also be adhesions to the underlying bone, causing an extensor plus state. Tendon substance may be lost and, if skin is avulsed, the tendons may be widely exposed. Pedicle coverage is often necessary in order to prepare for tenorrhaphies or tenolysis. Tendon transfers and tenorrhaphies are done in the standard fashion.

Extensor tendon function that is compromised by full-thickness burns in this zone may spontaneously be replaced by scar tissue (pseudotendon) bridging the gap left by debrided eschar. When this is functionally satisfactory, no reconstruction is necessary. When unsatisfactory, tendon grafting is preceded by pedicle coverage to the dorsum of the hand.

Injuries of the Thumb Extensors and Abductor Pollicis Longus

The terminal extensor mechanism of the thumb is a conjoined one of the intrinsics and extensor pollicis longus. As in the finger, the dorsal hood of the thumb has lateral extensor tendons (intrinsic bands) fusing with the central extrinsic tendon (extensor pollicis longus). The intrinsics extend the interphalangeal joint to a straight line, but only the extensor pollicis longus can forcibly extend the joint or hyperextend it. The extensor pollicis longus, inserting at the base of the proximal phalanx, is the prime extensor of the metacarpophalangeal joint.

Injury to the terminal extensor causes a mallet thumb, which can secondarily lead to a hyperextension (recurvatum) of the metacarpophalangeal joint creating a swan-neck deformity, which is due to recession of the extensor hood and overpull of the extensor pollicis brevis. Injuries over the metacarpophalangeal joint lead to a buttonhole deformity with flexion of the metacarpophalangeal joint and hyperextension of the interphalangeal joint. The pathomechanics of this are similar to those described for Zone E-III of the finger.

The functional loss resulting from injuries proximal to the metacarpophalangeal joint depends upon the extrinsic tendons affected. In testing for the integrity of the abductor pollicis longus (a radial wrist deviator) the patient should be asked to spread his fingers forcefully to tense this tendon. This will also tense the overlying extensor pollicis brevis and deepen the anatomical snuffbox. Injuries in this area often involve the radial artery and nerve. Tenodesis of the thumb extensors following injury or surgery may be suspected by the limitation of active or passive flexion or active extension.

EXTENSOR ZONE TE-I (INTERPHALANGEAL JOINT LEVEL OF THE THUMB)

Closed Injuries. A mallet thumb without a fracture following trauma is uncommon. Its production requires great force, in contrast to a mallet finger. If it does occur it is apt to be complete and immediate. Treatment requires repair of the avulsed tendon or reduction of the associated fracture (see Zone E-I).

Open Injuries. The size of the tendon makes it easier to suture than the terminal extensors of the fingers. A 4-0 nylon suture is threaded as a crisscross or horizontal mattress suture which is buried or brought out and tied over a pledget of dental roll. The interphalangeal joint is immobilized in a straight line with an intramedullary wire for four weeks. In addition, the thumb, wrist and forearm are casted for three weeks.

In complex injuries with or without the loss of substance, attention is first given to wound closure and bone and joint alignment. Subsequently, a decision regarding arthrodesis or tendon grafting is made. If the latter is decided upon, the technique follows that described for mallet fingers (Zone E-I).

EXTENSOR ZONE TE-II (PROXIMAL PHALANX OF THE THUMB)

Closed injuries as a rule are not a major problem here. Open tidy injuries do not present problems with tendon retraction, but may develop late, restricted motion of the interphalangeal joint from adhesions. When there is loss of substance, a tendon graft bridging the proximal and distal ends of the divided tendon or interphalangeal joint fusion should be considered.

EXTENSOR ZONE TE-III (METACARPOPHALANGEAL JOINT OF THE THUMB)

Closed Injuries. A buttonhole deformity follows blunt injuries in this area, much as it does in Zone E-III of the fingers. It develops more insidiously because the forces creating the attenuation are not as severe. Injury to the extensor pollicis brevis, like that of the middle extensor tendon in the finger, is the key in the development of this problem. The extensor pollicis longus does not usually attenuate and, by remaining intact, is an important force causing the stretching of the extensor hood ulnarward. The apical defect is created by this ulnar pull countered by the radial pull of the thenar lateral extensor tendon. The proximal phalanx flexes with the force of the adductor pollicis augmented by the lateral extensor tendons which have shifted volar to the axis of the joint. The head of the metacarpal presents itself through the weakness which lies primarily in the extensor pollicis brevis and the radial sagittal band. A cross between the typical buttonhole deformity of the proximal interphalangeal joint and the ulnar drift deformity of the metacarpophalangeal joint results (Zone E-V).

There is a great difference in the normal range of flexion of the metacarpophalangeal joint. This deformity will be greatest in patients with maximum flexion of the joint. This aspect should guide the surgeon to use Kirschner wire fixation prophylactically for four weeks after a severe contusion. Lesser degrees of flexion may be adequately managed with external fixation of the wrist and thumb for 4 to 6 weeks. The metacarpophalangeal joint should be kept in full extension. The differential diagnoses immediately following injury, when there is marked swelling, are rupture of one of the collateral ligaments, dislocation or fractures. Once a buttonhole deformity develops, its treatment is surgical. A lateral incision should be made to develop a flap. The principles and techniques of repair parallel those described for treating this deformity in the finger. Scar and thickened capsule over the dome of the joint should be resected with magnification and healthy intrinsic and extrinsic tendon tissue should be elevated and advanced to close the gap. Often the extensor pollicis brevis must be specifically separated or dissected out of the extensor hood, advanced and imbricated in the hood or even drawn into a hole in the proximal phalanx (Fig. 14-18). In all instances, the joint must be stabilized with fixation by a Kirschner wire and the thumb and wrist immobilized in a cast for four weeks. In late cases, an alternate solution is fusion of the joint. When the buttonhole deformity accompanies an arthritic joint, an implant arthroplasty associated with the previously described tenoplasty should be considered.

Open Injuries. Tidy open injuries may divide all or part of the extensor hood. Retraction is usually minimal. The wound should be extended if necessary for adequate exposure of all intrinsic and extrinsic components of the hood. The repair with a figure-of-eight or mattress 4-0 or 5-0 nylon suture is usually sufficient. Fixation by a single oblique Kirschner wire is at times advisable to complement the plaster immobilization of the thumb and wrist for four weeks. Untidy wounds should be converted

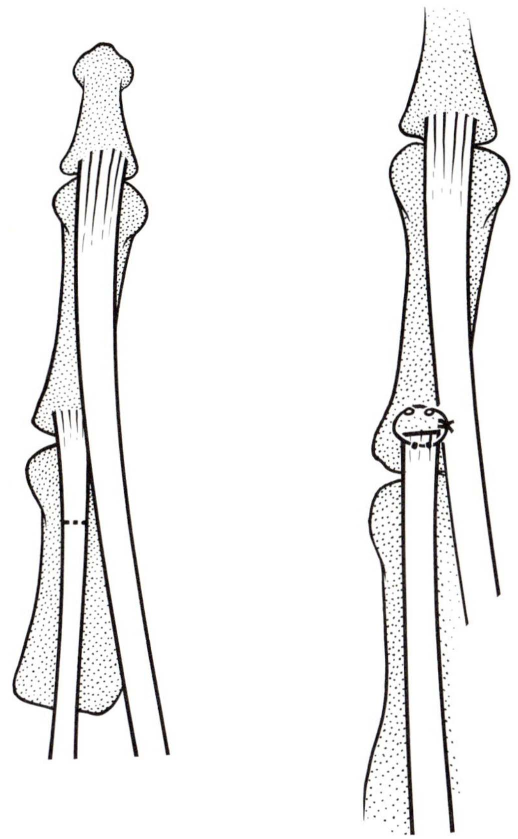

Figure 14-18. *Advancement of extensor pollicis brevis to correct a boutonniere deformity of the thumb.*

into tidy wounds if possible so that the treatment described above can be instituted. Reconstruction for complex injuries should be directed at maintaining active mobility of either or both the metacarpophalangeal or interphalangeal joint.

EXTENSOR ZONE TE-IV (OVER THE METACARPAL OF THE THUMB)

Closed Injuries. Blunt trauma rarely creates an isolated problem to the extensors in this region. They may adhere to a fracture site or become fixed in scarred skin and subcutaneous tissue from other causes (e.g. burns and infections).

Open Injuries. The two extensors of the thumb, especially the extensor pollicis longus, often retract into the forearm. The muscle of the extensor pollicis longus loses its elasticity rapidly so that an effort should be made to repair its tendon within two months. If the elasticity has been lost, then the extensor pollicis longus should be replaced by transferring the extensor indicis proprius (Fig. 15-

14). Should there be sufficient elasticity in the divided extensor pollicis longus, a tendon graft may be used to restore function.[3] Other considerations of injuries at this level parallel those described for open injuries on the dorsum of the hand (Zone E-VI).

EXTENSOR ZONE E-VII (UNDER THE EXTENSOR RETINACULUM OF THE WRIST)

In the six separate compartments of this zone, the long extensors of the wrist and digits lie in fibro-osseous tunnels surrounded by synovial bursae (Fig. 2-18). The particular points of anatomy to remember are: (1) the proximity of the radial nerve and artery to tendons as they cross the anatomical snuffbox, (2) the crowding of tendons in the first compartment (up to six components of the abductor pollicis longus), (3) the obliquity of the extensor pollicis longus crossing the radial wrist extensors and its sharp angulation around Lister's tubercle where it meets its muscle belly, (4) the breadth of the extensor retinaculum which blends proximally with the forearm fascia, (5) the location of dorsal sensory branches of the ulnar nerve, and (6) the abundance of dorsal veins.

Choking by the retinacular system or adherence within it is a common sequela to closed and open injuries at this level (Fig. 18-6). Unlike the flexor tendons, however, the transfer of tendons out of the tunnels and superficial to the retinaculum does not markedly detract from their effectiveness even though minor bowstringing occurs. Tenorrhaphy should be done so that the site of repair does not glide within the tunnel.

Closed Injuries. The prime problem of closed injuries relates to binding or adherence within the tendon tunnels, and occasionally a trigger phenomenon develops. This is most common with the abductor pollicis longus and extensor pollicis longus. The latter (extensor pollicis longus) occasionally ruptures at Lister's tubercle.

In industry, highly repetitive to-and-fro excursion of tendons creates frictional synovitis and sometimes crepitation (de Quervain's tenosynovitis) (Chap. 8). When rubor and calor are present, the possibility of rheumatoid synovitis must be considered in the differential diagnosis. The tendon ruptures that occur in this area commonly involve the extensors of the thumb, ring and little fingers as a result of rheumatoid arthritis and synovitis. Problems of synovitis are discussed in Chapters 24 and 25 (Fig. 14-19). Treatment consists of immobilization, administration of local steroids and surgical decompression of the fibro-osseous tunnels.

Wrist fractures, particularly of the distal radius, are apt to trap the extensors in the fracture site if there is improper reduction. Rough fracture margins may cut or fray the tendon. When this is properly anticipated, an open reduction to specifically transfer the tendons out of the fibro-osseous canal system may be justified. A fracture callus can also impinge on the tendons sufficiently to require such a procedure.

Open Injuries. Tidy open injuries present the same problems as those discussed for flexor tendon injuries in fibro-osseous canals. Tendons become adherent and, for this reason, tenorrhaphy requires that they be excluded from their sheaths.

This can be accomplished by resecting the sheath, by leaving it intact and displacing the tenorrhaphy superficially or by carefully elevating the retinaculum on a radially or ulnarly based pedicle and restoring it deep to the tendons.

Retraction of the proximal tendon stumps may be considerable, and retrieval often requires an extension of the wound or a counterincision in the distal one-third of the forearm. Operating under tourniquet control with magnification, the surgeon must protect the sensory branches of the radial and ulnar nerves as well as the radial artery. Multiple tendon injuries in this area create the problem of the common coagulum with adherence and loss of independent action. The concept of "function by simplication" must be invoked and the number of tendons repaired limited when all are

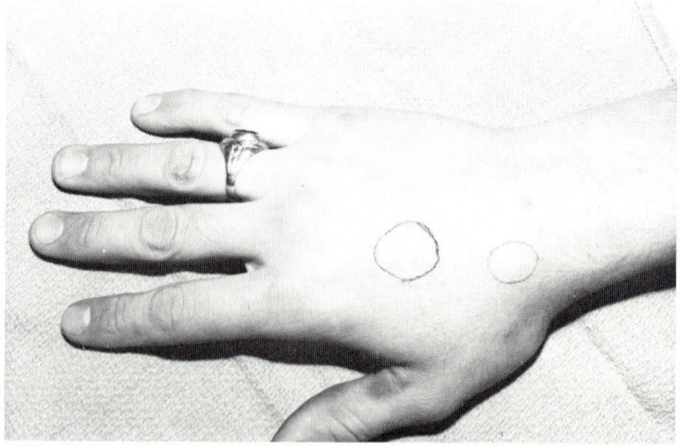

Figure 14-19. *Synovitis about the extensor retinaculum appearing as a dumbbell-shaped swelling which can be ballotted back and forth beneath the constricting retinaculum.*

divided. In choosing the tenorrhaphies the priorities for function are: (1) independent extension of the thumb, (2) mass extension of the fingers, (3) independent extension of the wrist, (4) radial wrist deviation.

In children and young adults, repair of all divided structures may be considered. Later in life, the usual tendons selected for repair are the extensor pollicis longus, the extensor communis, the extensor carpi radialis brevis and the abductor pollicis longus. These repairs are done with a crisscross weave suture of 4-0 nylon. Prophylactic antibiotics are used and the hand and forearm are immobilized from the proximal interphalangeal joints of the fingers and the tip of the thumb with the metacarpophalangeal joints in slight flexion and the wrist comfortably extended. Splinting is necessary for 3 to 4 weeks.

In complex injuries, alignment, wound closure, prevention of infection and resolution of edema are the targets of the initial treatment. Tendons that can be readily tacked together or tethered to maintain muscle tone are so treated. Primary or secondary coverage through pedicle flap transfer is necessary as a prelude to definitive tenorrhaphy. Subsequent tenolysis is often necessary.

EXTENSOR ZONE E-VIII (DISTAL FOREARM)

Thirteen tendons are in jeopardy in this area. The level at which tenorrhaphy can be done is limited by the length of the tendon with respect to its muscle. Those to the thumb have the shortest tendons. In contrast, repair of the extensor digitorum communis tendons is often feasible within the middle third of the forearm. The longest tendons are the wrist extensors. The sensory branch of the radial nerve is also subject to injury on the radial aspect of this zone where it emerges from beneath the cover of the brachioradialis. The nerve should be protected and, if necessary, transferred into a well-padded area to minimize the risk of symptoms from subsequent neuroma formation.

Closed Injuries. The prime impact of closed injuries on the function of the extensors comes from the sequelae of blunt trauma causing hemorrhea and congestion. Surgical decompression must be considered as an emergency before irreversible muscle ischemia develops. Unless this is appreciated, fibrosis and contracture, such as Volkmann's contracture, may follow. In anticipation of this need, the extremity must be evaluated hour by hour while it is immobilized and elevated. Intravenous low-molecular-weight dextran may be administered as an adjunct for its antisludging effect.

Myositis crepitans, which almost exclusively affects the abductor pollicis longus and extensor brevis of the thumb, is a stress myositis related to highly repetitive action of the muscles (Chap. 8).

Open Injuries. The identification of structures and the retraction of severed tendons within muscle bellies are the handicaps facing the surgeon in this area. Exposure is paramount and is accomplished by extension of the wound and the appropriate fasciotomy. The intramuscular blood clots invariably lead to the divided tendons which must be tagged and matched with their distal counterparts.

The tendons are repaired with 4-0 nylon in a crisscrossing or horizontal mattress fashion. The muscles are approximated loosely by fascial suture. Using the same priorities of repair cited in Zone E-VII, it is often necessary to reduce the bulk of callus in the wound. Splinting with a long-arm cast is employed for 3 to 4 weeks. Complex injuries of this area are managed similarly to those of Zone E-VII.

Techniques of Tendon Surgery

The objective of tendon surgery is to establish a secure bond at the end of a tendon (e.g. with another tendon, to bone or to ligamentous tissue) and to preserve the gliding properties of the tendon when such is needed. The point of fixation must be raw, whereas the gliding surface must be as free of any adhesions as possible. The former requires "freshening up" or abrading the point of attachment. The latter requires an immaculate "no-touch technique," avoiding injury to the epitenon. The surface of the tendon should never be compressed or squeezed and should be touched only by a rounded, smooth moistened instrument, not by the surgeon's gloves or forceps. At the end, where contact and bonding are desired, a stay suture, forceps or clamp can be used to hold the tendon. This traumatized area is then excised or used as the point of attachment. The tendon surface should not be unduly exposed to the air, but once exposed should be kept moist with lactated Ringer's solution and by closure of the wound around it as promptly as possible.

The surgeon's technique must also preserve the integrity of the circulation to the tissues comprising the bed in which the operated tendon will lie. When this bed is a tendon sheath, its surfaces must not be traumatized. The no-touch technique is essential.

Instruments must be carefully chosen for atraumatic and precise technique. Tourniquet ischemia and magnification are required, as is good assistance.

Table 14-2. *Prerequisites for Successful Tendon Surgery*

TISSUES
Good circulation
Adequate soft tissue cover
No infection
No edema
Minimal induration and scar
Mobile joints
Adequate motor function
PATIENT
Well motivated
Under 40 years of age
Pliable hands
SURGEON
Adequately trained
Access to adequate facilities

Mechanics of Tendon Suturing

Tendons are sutured for two purposes: (1) to hold the surfaces together, and (2) to resist separation.

The needs vary from one situation to another. The caliber of sutures and the method of securing the tissue must be adaptive. When there is no separation and spontaneous apposition by proper splinting, no sutures are necessary. Fine sutures* of 6-0 nylon will suffice when there is slight separation and no tension in the wound. These can be placed in an over-and-over figure-of-eight manner.

Stronger sutures are needed when there is considerable separation. This will be: 5-0 nylon for small tendons, 4-0 nylon for average adult tendons and 3-0 nylon when the force of retraction is excessive. The caliber of suture and its placement will be governed by the position of the tendon ends (stump-to-stump, side-to-side) and by whether a single suture or more will be used. The suture material must be wedged on a fine, atraumatic precision-honed cutting needle. The half-circle needle has advantages for use in confined areas.

The type of sutures used are: figure-of-eight, horizontal mattress and crisscrossing (Fig. 14-20).

The figure-of-eight sutures are used for stump-to-stump approximation where the objective is alignment and there is no tendency to separation. Several such sutures are used for side-to-side approximation and weaving at tendon junctures. The horizontal mattress suture is used when the tendon is flat and thin (e.g. extensor tendons) and the suture must prevent separation. This suture is generally placed 0.5 to 1.0 cm from the cut margin of the tendon.

The crisscross weaving suture of Bunnell[1] is used for resisting separation of tendons that are round and have adequate substance. A modification of this is a single over-and-over loop at the apex of the suture as it starts in the first stump. This loop is knotted in buried sutures and left open for withdrawal when the suture is to be pulled out (Fig. 14-20**C**). It helps to eliminate shearing and increases the hold on the retracting tendon.

The crisscross technique is performed with a 20-cm, double-armed atraumatic suture which starts on the tendon stump 1 cm or less from the end. It crisscrosses the tendon once, exiting on the face of the stump at opposite poles. Both needles must be placed within the tendon as crossed swords to avoid cutting the suture with the sharp needle. In entering the abutting tendon stump, the needles follow the same course as they did in the first stump. Holding the two ends of the suture taut, the second stump is advanced to meet the first one, coaxed with a moistened probe. The suture is then tied as maximal relaxation of the muscle tendon unit is achieved. The suture is tied with four knots, ensuring approximation of stumps of the tendon without telescoping of the tendon edges. This knot must not slip. To ensure against this the 3 to 4 knots must be placed flat upon the previous knots rather than slid down one limb of the suture.

Instead of the Bunnell suture, tethering the proximal tendon permits the placement of a 6-0 running suture or series of figure-of-eight sutures at the tendon juncture. The tethering suture of 4-0 nylon is placed in the tendon in the palm or fore-

*Any inert suture is satisfactory for tendon repair. Monofilament nylon is preferable to wire because: it does not kink, it is less prone to cut through tissue, and the knots are less likely to irritate.

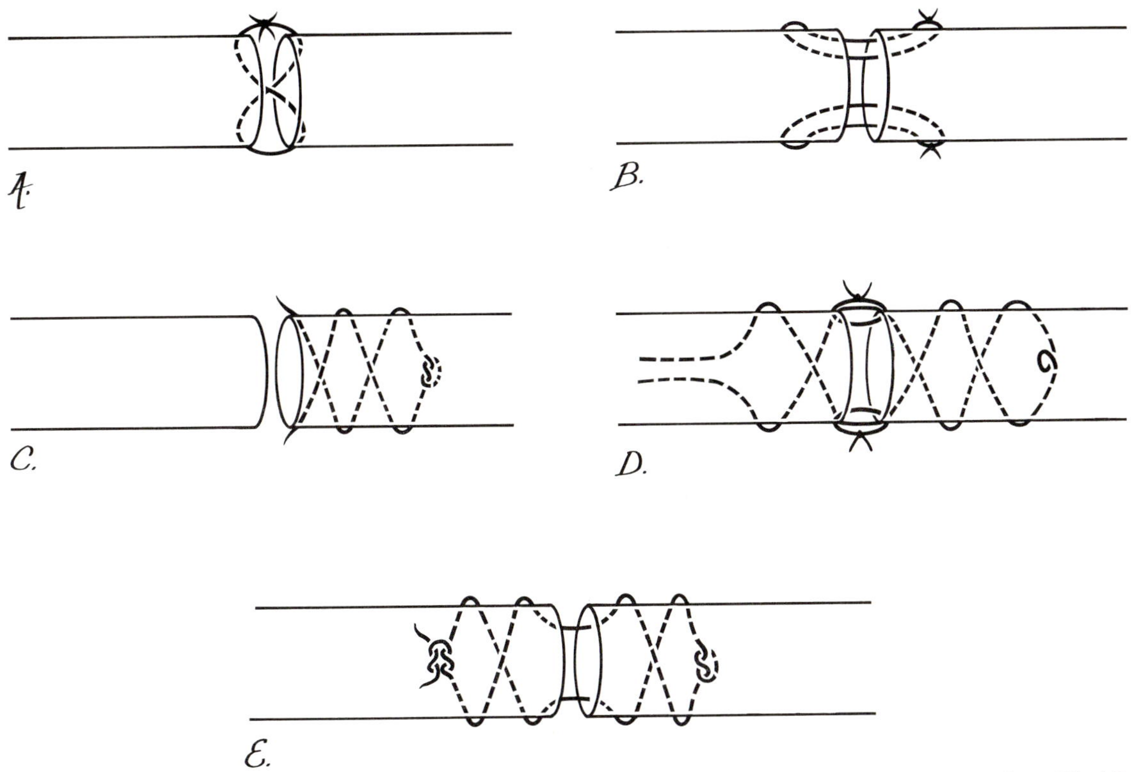

Figure 14-20. *Types of tendon suture.* **A:** *Figure-of-eight.* **B:** *Horizontal mattress.* **C–E:** *Crisscross (modified Bunnell).*

arm well proximal to the tenorrhaphy in the form of an over-and-over loop. Both ends of the suture are threaded on a long, straight needle which is passed parallel to the tendon and brought out through the volar aspect of the web or heel of the hand where it is tied over a dental roll (Fig. 14-21). It is withdrawn at three weeks. When this is used, it is imperative that no tension be placed on the distal tendon juncture by adverse positioning of the digit and wrist. The measure of adequate tethering is the laxity of the distal tendon juncture. This is, of course, judged before the skin wound is closed.

Pull-out sutures may be used anywhere, but generally are confined to anchoring a tendon or ligament into bone. After placing the Bunnell crisscross suture with nylon, the ends are threaded on a Keith needle which has previously been drilled in the desired direction through the bone or soft tissues, and the suture is withdrawn. The suture is then tied down over a pledget of dental roll with a surgeon's knot as the tendon (or ligament) is observed going into place. Three weeks later the one limb of the suture can be cut, the skin painted with iodine and traction placed on the other limb with a smooth-jawed needle holder to withdraw it.

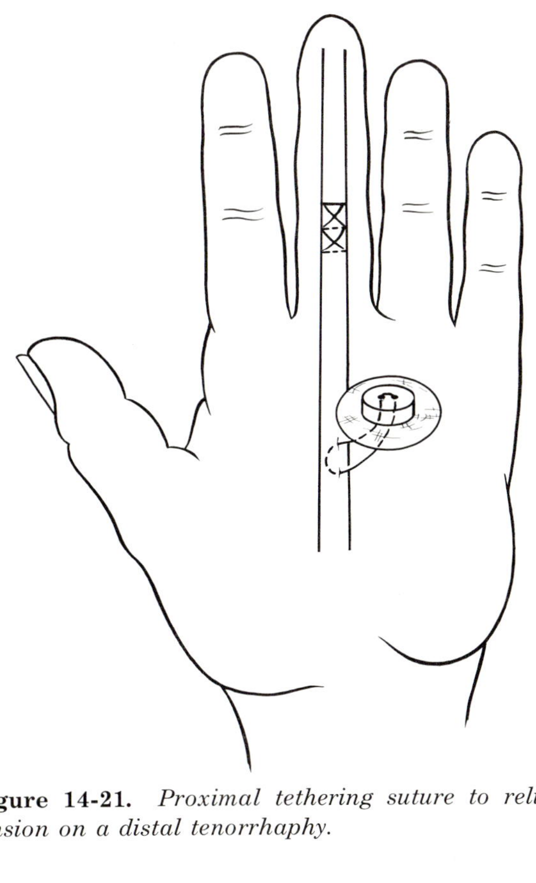

Figure 14-21. *Proximal tethering suture to relieve tension on a distal tenorrhaphy.*

When withdrawal is difficult, the suture will loosen with time, but if not it can be cut flush with the skin without any problem.

In certain instances, particularly ligamentous reconstruction using a tendon, a very tight fixation to bone may interdict the use of a button for fear of cutaneous necrosis. The suture (preferably wire) is tied against the bone by passing each limb separately through the bone on parallel needles to counterincision. This is a permanent suture.

The different types of tendon attachments are: tendon to tendon, tendon to bone, and tendon to ligament or pulley. In tendon-to-tendon junctures, there may be a partial or a complete separation. Subtotal separations are sutured as total divisions. The tendons being joined may be equal or unequal in caliber and may be flat or round. Partial separation (<50 per cent), if sutured, generally requires only a figure-of-eight suture. The risk of adhesions dictates against immobilization. The approximation of stumps for total and subtotal division requires a crisscross type of suture. Alternatively, a marginal continuous 6-0 nylon suture or figure-of-eight 5-0 or 6-0 nylon suture may be used if the proximal tendon is tethered.

In joining tendons of disproportionate diameters, a fish-mouth juncture, cocoon-type juncture or interweave may be used (Fig. 14-22). The fish-mouth technique involves slitting the larger stump longitudinally so that the smaller stump can be placed inside and sutured, after first scarifying the surface in contact with the other tendon. Appropriate calibered nylon sutures are used in figure-of-eight fashion. In lieu of this, a small tendon may be interwoven into the larger tendon as shown in the diagram (Fig. 14-22**B**). Interrupted sutures secure this juncture. Finally, if the palmaris longus or plantaris is being used as a graft, a cocoon-type juncture can be created as illustrated (Fig. 14-22**C**). The graft is threaded in a sigmoid fashion through a window in the recipient tendon, 1 cm from the end of the stump. Inasmuch as the graft can be splayed out, but the recipient tendon cannot, the entire cocoon is formed around the larger tendon by stretching out the graft between clamps. The graft envelops the recipient tendon in one direction proximal to the perforation and in the other direction distally. Interrupted 5-0 or 6-0 nylon sutures can be used.

Tendon is anchored to bone by creating a window in the bone to receive it. The bone is drilled with an oscillating burr or a small bone flap is raised with a narrow sharp osteotome. The tendon is held in the bone with a pull-out suture as previously described (Fig. 14-23).

When a tendon is anchored to a pulley or ligament, it is passed through a window and back on itself (Fig. 14-16**D**). An apical suture of 4-0 or 5-0 nylon is placed at the point of angulation and one or more sutures are placed between the two limbs of the tendon.

Tendon Advancement

Advancement of a tendon is done to overcome a gap, to stagger a tendon juncture from other injured tissue or to anchor a tendon beyond its sheath. This is commonly undertaken with repairs of the divided profundus tendon in Zones F-I, F-II, TF-I and TF-II. In undertaking this procedure, the advancement must not cause an imbalance through tethering of the parent muscle of adjacent tendons (e.g. profundus). The amount of advancement is generally limited to about 10 mm in an adult.

Tendon Lengthening

Tendon lengthening is done when the musculotendinous unit is too short. It is also necessary on occasion to achieve tendon advancement, in which case lengthening is usually done close to the muscle. In other instances, it is done to overcome stiffness when complete sectioning of the tendon is contraindicated. It can be done in one way to allow immediate mobilization (staggered incomplete tenotomies) (Fig. 14-17) and in another for immobilization (sliding complete tenotomy). In the staggered incomplete tenotomy, often done under local anesthesia for extensor tendons (extensor plus), the tendon is notched on alternate sides, 1 cm apart, at two or more levels. The notching must extend beyond the center of the tendon so that no single fiber of the tendon will remain in continuity. If the patient is awake, immediate active motion will determine the adequacy of the tenotomy. The surgeon will have to make this judgment after passive stretching of the involved digit if a general anesthesic or regional block is being used. Immediate postoperative mobilization must follow under guidance.

A complete tenotomy is done after first estimating the needed length with a gauge. This can be done preoperatively if desired. The length needed is deceptively more than would be guessed. As a rule, the deficiency should not be fully corrected because the muscle does not have its normal contractibility. The incision of the tendon can be long

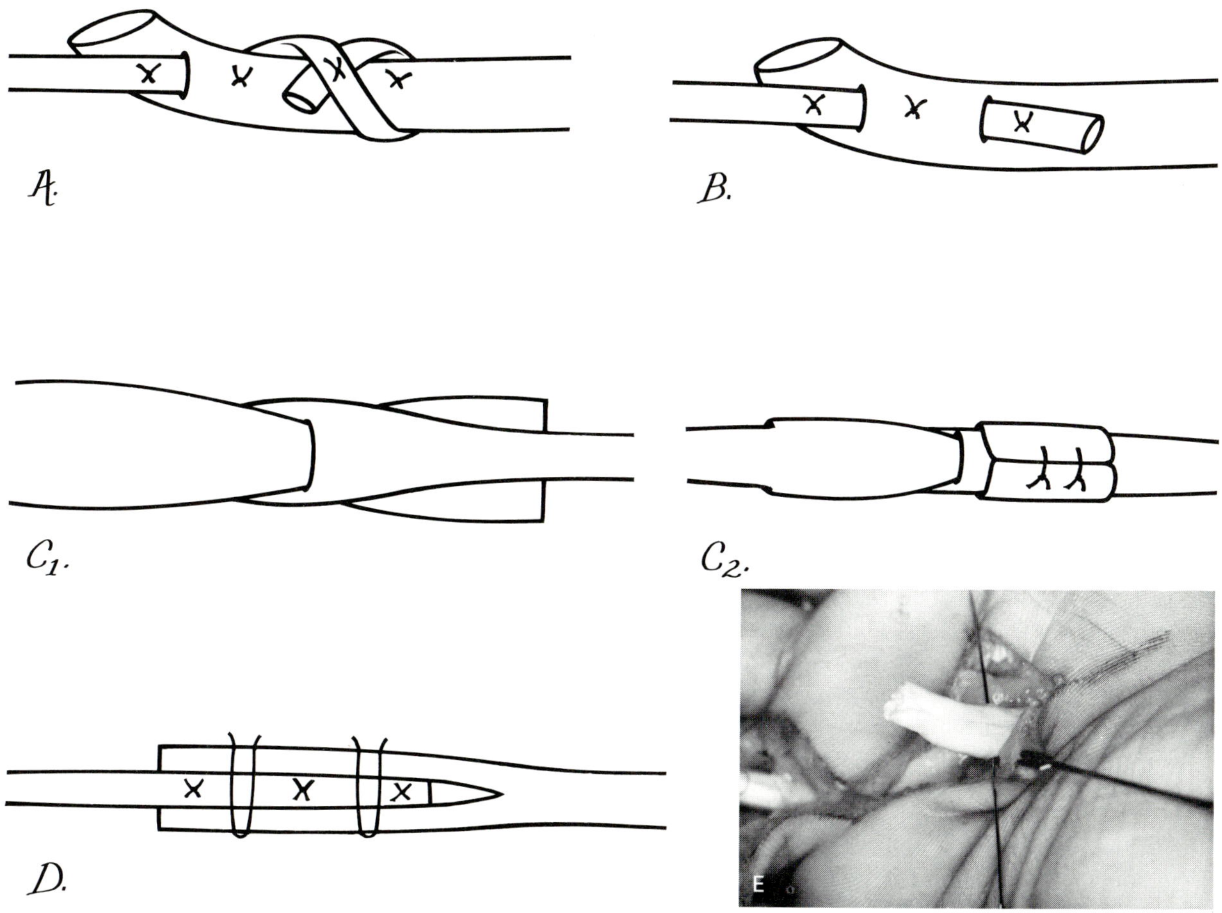

Figure 14-22. *Junctures for tendons of disproportionate size.* **A,B:** *Interweave.* **C_1,C_2:** *Cocoon.* **D:** *Fish-mouth.* **E:** *Needle through tendon.*

and oblique or bayonet in shape. In order to have adequate overlapping of the tendon ends for approximation once it is lengthened, the incision has to be twice as long as the gain desired. The side-to-side approximation is done with interrupted 4-0 or 5-0 nylon sutures. Immobilization is maintained for three weeks.

Tendon Grafting

The tendon bed to receive the graft is developed first. Once developed, it is protected by temporarily closing it and keeping it moist with lactated Ringer's solution. The tendon graft is then obtained from the same or opposite upper extremity or a lower extremity. A careful preoperative survey will generally enable the physician to anticipate the source of the graft and to prepare the patient for it (Table 14-3).

The removal of the palmaris longus (absent in 20 per cent of patients) is done through two transverse incisions (Fig. 14-24). The one at the flexor crease of the wrist is made first with caution to protect the median nerve, to avoid bleeding from the multiple veins in the area and to maintain the surface integrity of the graft. It is delivered as a glistening tendon completely free of any drag by peritendinous tissue. A stout clamp is placed on it as far distally as possible and the tendon is transected beyond the clamp. Slight traction is placed on the clamp and the proximal limit of the tensed tendon is palpated in the midforearm. A transverse counterincision, 2 cm long, is made at this level. With retraction, pointed curved scissors are used to spread the fascia longitudinally over the tendon. It is undermined and moistened blunt-nosed scissors are passed beneath it. A soaking wet gauze is placed proximal to the scissors to receive the tendon which is forcefully flipped out after release of the distal clamp. The tendon is again clamped at its cut end and elevated under tension. Any remaining muscle belly is shaved off with a scalpel and the tendon is clamped as far proximally as possible and divided. If temporary storage is necessary, it is placed in a bowl by itself with lactated

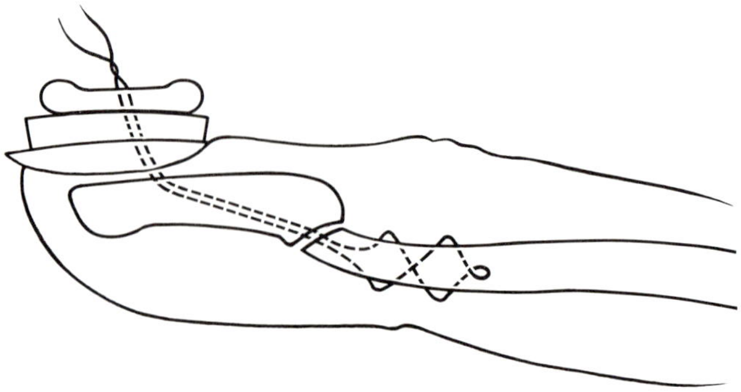

Figure 14-23. *Tendon juncture to bone.*

Ringer's solution. When it is time to thread it into place one end is suture-ligated with nylon for a stay suture. Throughout, immaculate no-touch technique is maintained except for the very ends of the graft.

In the absence of a palmaris longus, the plantaris is the second graft of choice. It may be the preferred source for many-tailed grafts to correct the clawhand. Like the palmaris longus, it is absent in 20 per cent of cases, and may be present on only one side. It is found medially and deep to the Achilles tendon through a 3- to 5-cm longitudinal incision. A proximal thigh tourniquet should be used to control bleeding. The tendon is freed from its bed, clamped as far distally as possible and divided. A long tendon stripper (e.g. Brand stripper) is passed over the tendon and directed proximally with the tendon held under marked tension. When the stripper has reached the proximal third of the calf, it is twisted to shred the muscle fibers attached to the tendon, which will suddenly come free.

The proprius extensor tendons to the index and little fingers make suitable grafts and are removed

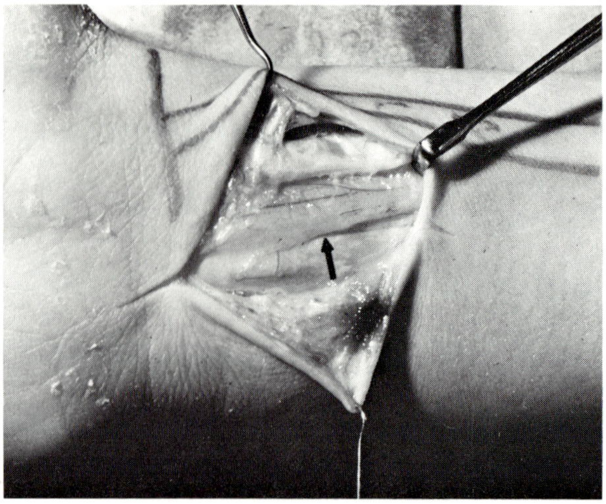

Figure 14-24. *Median nerve immediately beneath the skin in the midline of the wrist with absence of palmaris. This vital nerve has been mistakenly removed by the inexperienced surgeon while seeking a tendon graft.*

through a small initial transverse incision over the head of the metacarpal. These tendons are found on the ulnar side of their respective extensor communis tendons. A longitudinal counterincision is made in the middle of the forearm and the graft is tensed alternately to make its musculotendinous junction move. This facilitates its identification there. It is undermined and removed in the same fashion as described for the palmaris longus.

The flexor superficialis is recommended as a graft only when it has been traumatically severed and it would otherwise be removed, or, if intact, its function can be justifiably sacrificed for more important function elsewhere. Its caliber is usually larger than the other grafts. This can be a favorable or an unfavorable feature. This tendon is used

Table 14-3. *Tendon Grafts: Their Source, Procurement, and Suitability*

SOURCE OF TENDON	SUITABLE SIZE	AVAILABILITY	ACCESSIBILITY	RESULTANT DISABILITY	PARATENON	RATING OF CHOICE
Palmaris longus	Yes	Local	Yes	None	Yes	First*
Plantaris	Yes	Remote	Yes	None	Yes	Second
Extensor proprius (Index or little finger)	Yes	Local	Yes	Slight	Yes	Third
Extensor digitorum longus (foot)	Yes	Remote	No	Slight	Yes	Fourth and Fifth
* Flexor digitorum superficialis	Too big	Local	Yes	Variable	No	Fifth

* The flexor digitorum superficialis is often the first choice for a tendon graft if it has already been divided and it is not going to be repaired.

in the two-stage "pedicle" grafting of the superficialis tendon to the profundus motor via a pseudosheath formed about a previously placed silicone rod. In this instance its proximal musculotendinous attachment is maintained until the second stage (Figs. 14-25, 14-26, 14-28).

The extensor digitorum communis of the toe is used as a last source of tendon grafts when the more commonly used ones are not available. If the extensors of the second, third, and fourth toes are used, they are removed from the dorsum of the foot through serial transverse incisions. Care must be taken to divide the juncturae tendina and not to injure the dorsal vessels. As many as five incisions might be required to remove the tendons which cannot be handled as gently during the dissection as is ideally desirable to protect their epitenon. The incisions are begun at the base of the toes and the proximal limit of dissection is at the distal edge of the superior extensor retinaculum where they fuse into a single tendon. Thus, the graft consists of a single base with three or four distal tails (a many-tailed graft) which is useful when several grafts are connected to a single motor.

RETRIEVAL AND THREADING OF TENDONS

The retracted tendon that has been freshly divided may recess far into the sheath or remain close to the wound. In the former instance, a counterincision will be needed to find it. In the latter it may be presented in the wound by simply positioning the wrist and fingers and squeezing the muscle belly in the proximal forearm.

Before performing a proximal counterincision, the following retrieval measures should be taken without injuring the lining of the tendon synovial sheath:

1. In trying to present the proximal stump of an independently acting tendon, position the wrist in flexion for flexors and in extension for extensors and squeeze the forearm musculature. At the same time look for the bloody tendon stump to appear within view or easy reach in the wound. It will be there if it has been tethered by the vascular stalk of its mesentery (vinculum).
2. In trying to present a retracted tendon that is interconnected with others to a parent muscle (profundus or extensor communis), do exactly the same as in (1) above, but, in addition, place the

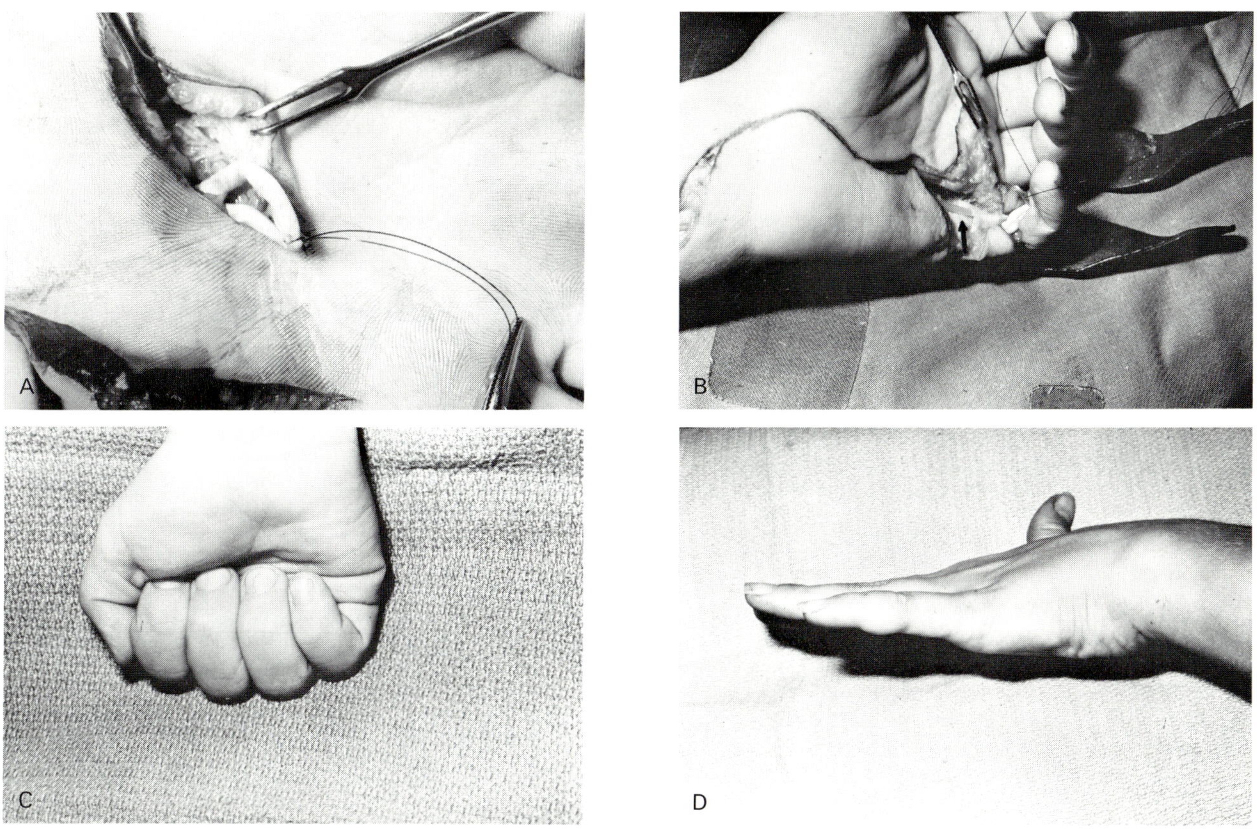

Figure 14-25. *Two-stage tenoplasty.* **A:** *End-to-end suturing of profundus and superficialis with distal insertion of a silicone rod.* **B:** *Proximal division of the superficialis and its distal transfer by attaching to the end of the silicone rod.* **C:** *Full flexion six months postoperatively.* **D:** *Full extension six months postoperatively.*

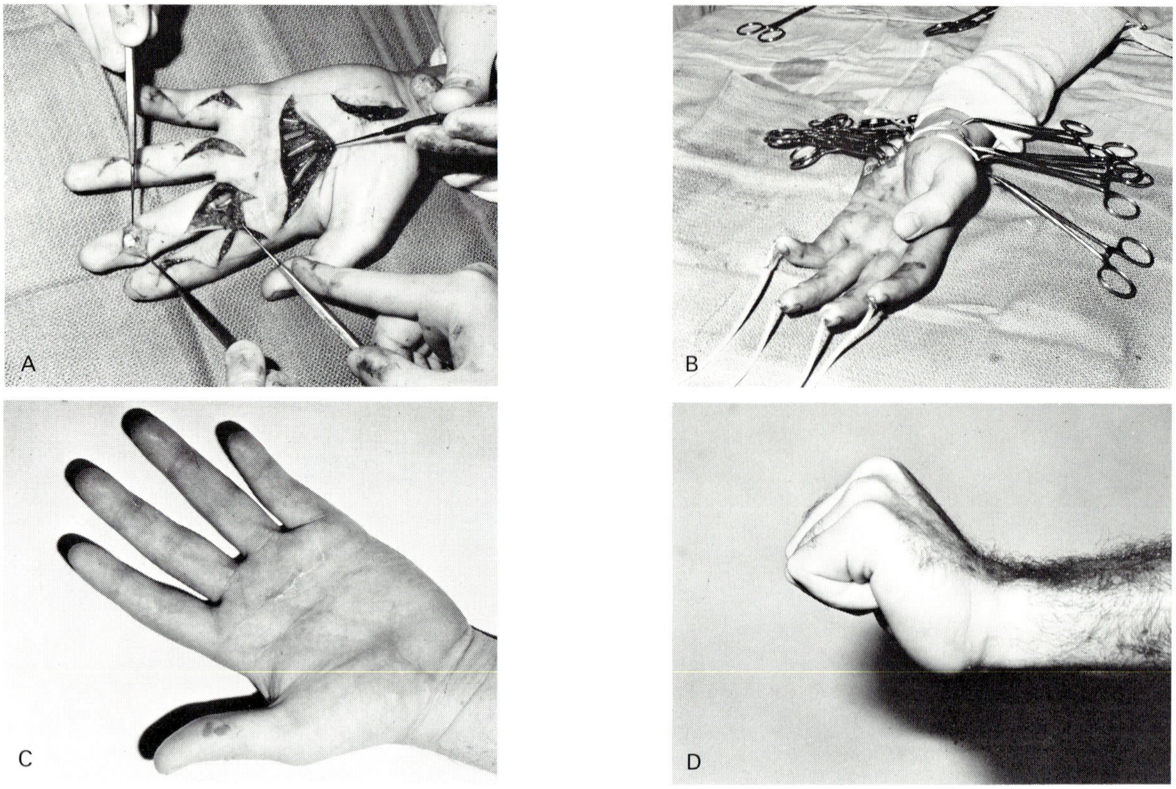

Figure 14-26. *Two-stage tenoplasty (alternate technique).* **A:** *Distal tendons resected and silicone rods in place.* **B:** *Tendon grafts advanced by suturing them to the silicone rods and drawing them through the new pseudosheaths.* **C:** *Extension six months after the second stage.* **D:** *Flexion six months after the second stage.*

fingers in the opposite direction to the wrist to stretch the parent muscle and propel the injured tendon into the wound. As soon as the stump presents itself, it should be secured transversely with a stay suture at its tip.

When the retracted stump is beyond reach, a counterincision is needed in the palm or forearm. The search is made for the sign of blood in the path of the retracted tendon, and when it is found an opening is made and the tendon flipped out, held with a stay suture through the tip and kept moist with lactated Ringer's solution. The next step is to thread a retrieval catheter from the distal wound along the tendon pathway and out the counterincision, or vice versa (Fig. 14-27). The catheter (a sterile infant feeding tube) is attached to a syringe filled with lactated Ringer's solution. This solution is flushed into the tendon pathway, distending it and permitting the catheter to be advanced without force.

The end of the catheter is flipped out of the counterincision with a moistened blunt-nosed instrument and is sutured tip to tip to the tendon stump. With further flushing, the catheter is withdrawn, pulling the tendon stump behind it into the distal wound. The catheter then serves as a tractor on the tendon stump while the definitive tenorrhaphy suture is placed. Once that suture is complete, the traction suture and catheter are removed. An alternative method of holding a retrieved proximal stump from retracting is to skewer it with a small Keith needle, placed trans-

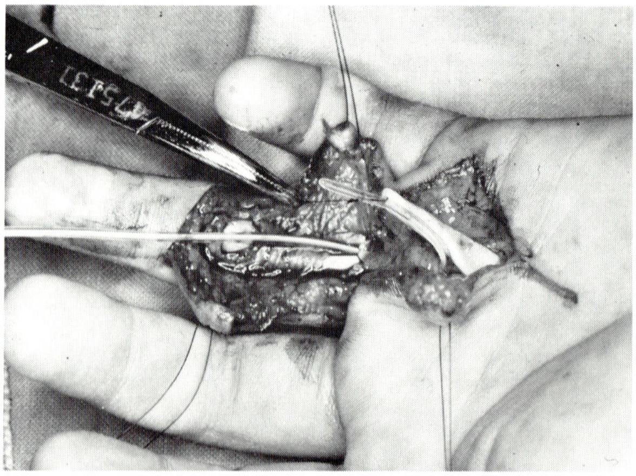

Figure 14-27. *Atraumatic retrieval of a proximal tendon stump or tendon graft facilitated by the passage of a pediatric feeding tube irrigated with lactated Ringer's solution to distend the collapsed sheath.*

versely 1 cm proximal to the stump. This needle is withdrawn when tenorrhaphy is complete (Fig. 14-22**E**).

A tendon graft is threaded into place with the same technique if the tendon canal has not been unroofed. In threading a tendon transfer or graft through a new path, the bed is made through fat, soft areolar tissue or muscle. This is done by forcing moistened blunt-nosed scissors with a hole at the tip (Littler scissors) along the desired pathway from one incision to another. The traction suture from the tendon is then treaded through the hole in the scissors and the scissors is withdrawn. With the wound properly moistened and exposed, the tendon stump is pulled out to the new location.

In threading a graft through a pseudosheath created by a silicone rod, the tip of the graft should be sutured to the rod so that the graft will be pulled into place behind the rod as it is removed. A clamp is then placed on either end of the graft to prevent its accidental removal prior to the completion of the tenorrhaphy.

GRAFTING

The first suture of the graft is the distal crisscross one anchoring it into the bone or to the distal tendon stump. Once this is secure the proximal end is united to the recipient motor by whatever technique is best for the circumstance (stump-to-stump, tendon weave, fish-mouth, or cocoon). After placing one or two sutures, the adequacy of tension is tested by positioning the wrist. *The grafted digit should assume a stance that is slightly exaggerated in the direction of the repair when the wrist is moved.* If the tension is satisfactory, whatever additional sutures are needed can be placed and the redundant portions of the graft removed. In the absence of flexor tendon pulleys, bowstringing of the graft will occur, making it more difficult to judge the proper length and tension. Placing the distal fixation of a flexor graft first will permit the closure of the digital skin without the awkwardness of having to suture later when the finger is flexed. The digit can then be flexed while the proximal juncture is made and the proximal wound readily closed.

IMMOBILIZATION

Immobilization is directed at relaxation of the repaired muscle-tendon unit for 3 to 4 weeks. Mass action and the synergistic movement of muscles of the flexor and extensor group make it impossible to limit the immobilization to just the repaired motor unit. Splinting must always include the wrist, which is positioned to relieve tension on the suture line without having the digit in a position of extreme flexion or extension. The cast is extended around the thumb alone after repair of any of its motors, and is extended in boxing-glove fashion around all the fingers after repair of any of the long flexors. It includes the metacarpophalangeal joints for repair of any of the finger extensors in Zones E-IV and E-V, but extends in partial boxing-glove fashion for repairs in Zone E-I to E-III. In Zones E-I to E-III, there is often internal fixation (see Extensor Tendons), and, in addition, the injured finger and at least one adjacent finger are splinted together. It must be stressed to the patient, however, that the cast is only a relative, not an absolute, splint. He must understand that all motion of unsplinted joints of the upper extremity must be *without* force during the three-week period if synergistic tension on the tendon suture is to be avoided.

Pulley Reconstruction

Pulley reconstruction has the same inherent difficulties as reconstruction of a collateral ligament. To be normal it must have no slack and a precise snugness. This is difficult to achieve without compromising the circulation of the pulley and the tendon and without creating adhesions. As a rule, only one flexor pulley is reconstructed. This is done along the proximal shaft of the proximal phalanx. A tendon graft is used, threading the two ends through a transverse hole in the phalanx to encircle the flexor tendon or a silicone rod. Fine wire should be used to thread the stumps of the graft into the hole on either side of the phalanx. The tails of the wire are threaded on separate Keith needles which pass in opposite directions through the bony window of the phalanx. To tie the suture, one of the Keith needles reverses its direction and traverses the bone again through a parallel, but separate, path. The two suture ends then lie on the same side of the phalanx and can be tied.

The surgical approach for this may be either a volar zigzag or both radial and ulnar midaxial incisions. It should not be done at the same time as a tendon graft or transfer. A functioning flexor tendon should be made to move actively, under the surgeon's direct supervision in the immediate postoperative period, protecting the pulley by full extension of the metacarpophalangeal joint and volar counterpressure by the surgeon over the head of the proximal phalanx. This should be done daily. The digit is protected against indiscriminate flexion by splinting for four weeks.

Two-stage Tenoplasty (Figs. 14-25, 14-26)

In complex flexor tendon injuries, the resultant scar tissue may be such that the flexor system can be salvaged only by a two-stage tenoplasty. A silicone rod (3 or 4 mm) is inserted for about 12 weeks to permit the formation and maturation of a pseudosynovial sheath about it. The digit should have sensibility or the rod may erode through the skin without warning. The scarred flexor tendons and sheaths are removed, saving, if possible, at least one pulley, and, if not possible, reconstructing one.

The rod is anchored to the distal phalanx (or to a 10- to 15-mm distal stump of the profundus) and its proximal end is brought out through the carpal canal into the forearm where it is free to move. The digital joints are kept supple by passive motion postoperatively. Six to 12 weeks later, incisions are made at the proximal and distal limits of the rod and a tendon graft is threaded into the pseudosheath behind the rod as it is removed. This graft is anchored distally and proximally as previously described.

A modification of this procedure is uniting the proximal stump of the divided profundus and superficialis tendons end to end at the level of the lumbrical muscle, at the time of placement of the silicone rod. In this case the proximal limit of the rod is to the lumbrical, not in the forearm. When the rod is removed, the superficialis tendon is divided in the forearm and becomes the tendon graft (Fig. 14-28). This provides a graft with a previously healed proximal juncture. It may be necessary to free some adhesions about this previous tenorrhaphy in the palm. This procedure is sometimes chosen as a primary procedure when an excessive scarring is anticipated in the digit.

Tenodesis

Tenodesis is a technique of establishing a static force to act across one or more joints. If it acts across a single joint it will restrict the motion of that joint in one direction. Thus, a profundus tenodesis across the distal joint, or a superficialis tenodesis across the middle joint, of the finger restricts extension of the joint. When a tenodesis acts across more than one joint it will become an agent of motion if tensed. Thus, flexor tendons to the digits having undergone tenodesis in the forearm will flex the digits when the wrist is extended, whereas extensor tenodesis will extend the fingers when the wrist is flexed. The tendon must be anchored to bone or ligamentous tissue, and each must be roughened to promote an adequate fibrous bond (Fig. 14-23). Immobilization is for 3 to 4 weeks, and if internal fixation is used it may be left for 4 to 6 weeks.

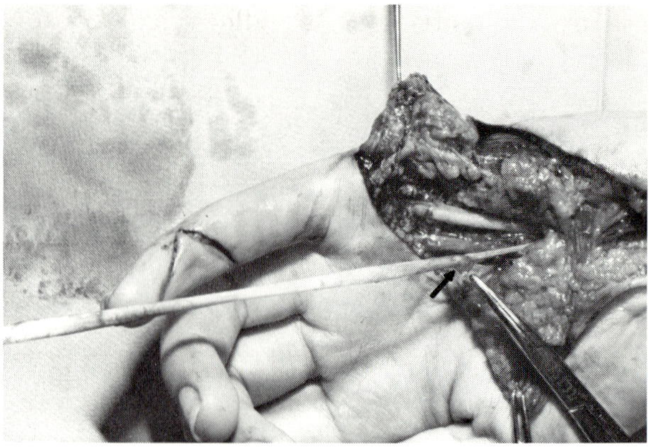

Figure 14-28. *Superficialis tendon used as a pedicle graft prior to attaching to the previously inserted silicone tendon prosthesis. The arrow indicates the profundus-superficialis juncture.*

Tenolysis

Tenolysis is undertaken to overcome adhesions that are restricting excursion of the tendon (Fig. 14-29). It is also undertaken to liberate one tendon from another to reestablish independent amplitude. The inherent risks are rupture and readherence. These are minimized by careful dissection and carefully supervised but persistent postoperative active motion. This is started within 24 hours. Its only limitations are those imposed by the needs for healing of the skin wound.

The incision should be chosen to give effective exposure, but at the same time placed so that immediate postoperative motion will not jeopardize its healing. Part of a tenolysis may be blind if the surgeon is meticulous. Tissues must be kept under tension, particularly the tendon being freed. At the conclusion, the surgeon must be able to

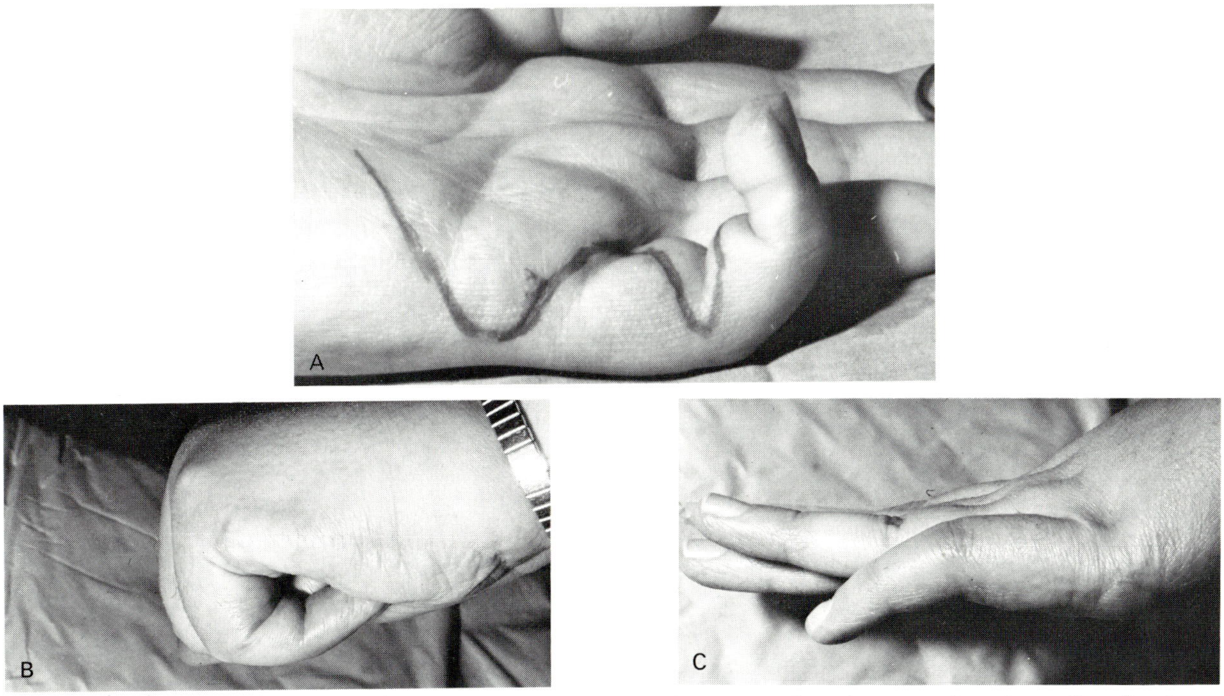

Figure 14-29. *Tenolysis may be necessary if improvement in the range of motion stops 3 to 4 months after tenorrhaphy* **(A).** **B** *and* **C** *illustrate the improved flexion and extension six weeks after tenolysis.*

establish a full excursion of the tendon and joints. The more the excursion has been liberated, the better the prognosis. Because of the limited tendon amplitude and therefore ease of readherence, the most difficult lysis to achieve is that of the extensor hood over the dorsum of the proximal and middle phalanges.

The most common sources of failure for tenolysis are: (1) to immobilize the tendon for longer than 24 hours after lysis, (2) for the patient to fail in the hard work of repeated active contraction of the musculotendinous units, (3) for the tendon to be divided, and (4) for a concomitant procedure requiring immobilization to be done (e.g. neurorrhaphy).

Tenolysis which requires immediate mobilization is incompatible with simultaneous procedures that require immobilization.

Reverse Tendon Flaps

A reverse tendon flap is used to tether a joint or tendon against specific motion or subluxation without compromising the basic motion and function expected of that tendon. It involves the development of a flap of tendon with a distal base. This flap sometimes has to be relocated. It usually consists of one-third to one-half of the width of the parent tendon.

The technique is useful in many circumstances, such as:

1. Restriction of hyperextension of the distal interphalangeal joint by a pedicle of the profundus fixed to the pulley of the middle phalanx
2. Restriction of hyperextension of the proximal interphalangeal joint by a pedicle of the superficialis into the pulley of the proximal phalanx
3. Restriction of the swan-neck (recurvatum) deformity by the lateral extensor tendon routed volar to Cleland's ligament and the axis of the proximal interphalangeal joint to the pulley of the proximal phalanx[8] (Fig. 14-30)
4. Restriction of subluxation of the extensor tendon over the metacarpophalangeal joint by an extensor pedicle around the radial collateral ligament
5. Creation of a pulley for the profundus or a collateral ligament of the proximal interphalangeal joint by a superficialis pedicle
6. Creation of a pulley for the abductor pollicis longus by an extensor carpi radialis pedicle
7. Creation of a pulley for all the extensor communis tendons from the extensor carpi radialis
8. Creation of a pulley for an opponensplasty by the flexor carpi ulnaris
9. Correction of subluxation of the extensor carpi ulnaris by a restraining ligament from its radial border.

Immobilization is for 3 to 4 weeks, but guarded motion in the direction of action of the parent

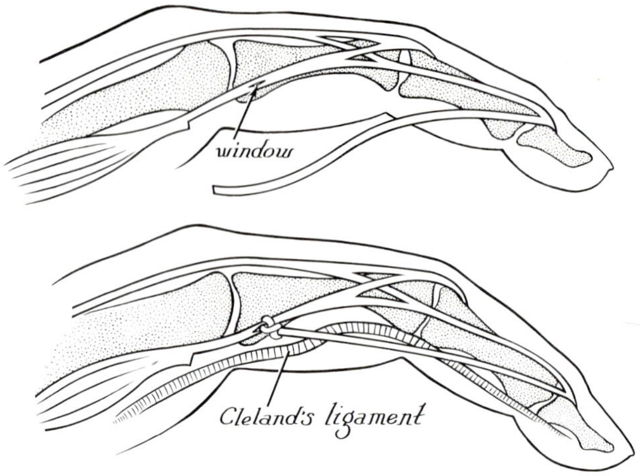

Figure 14-30. *A strip of lateral band freed from its volar edge, tunneled under Cleland's ligament and reattached to create a dynamic tenodesis in correcting the swan-neck deformity.* (*Redrawn from Kilgore and Graham.*[4])

tendon may be allowed under supervision beginning 24 to 48 hours postoperatively.

References

1. Boyes, J.H.: *Bunnell's Surgery of the Hand,* 4th ed. J.B. Lippincott, Philadelphia, 1964.
2. Chong, J.K., Cramer, L.M. and Culf, N.K.: Combined two-stage tenoplasty with silicone rods for multiple flexor tendon injuries in "no man's land." J. Trauma, 12:104, 1972.
3. Hamlin, C. and Littler, J.W.: Segmental tendon graft restoration of extensor pollicis longus disruption. Presented at 30th Annual Meeting of American Society for Surgery of the Hand, San Francisco, February 28, 1975.
4. Kilgore, E.S. and Graham, W.P.: Operative treatment of swan-neck deformity. Plast. Reconstr. Surg., 39:138, 1967.
5. Kilgore, E.S. and Graham, W.P.: Operative correction of boutonniere deformity. Surgery, 64:999, 1968.
6. Kilgore, E.S., Graham, W.P., Newmeyer, W.L. and Brown, L.: The extensor plus. Hand, 7:159, 1975.
7. Kilgore, E.S., Graham, W.P., Newmeyer, W.L. and Brown, L.: Correction of ulnar subluxation of the extensor communis. Hand, 7:3:272, 1975.
8. Littler, J.W.: In: *Reconstructive Plastic Surgery* (Converse, J.M., Ed.). W.B. Saunders, Philadelphia, 1964.
9. Littler, J.W. and Eaton, R.G.: Redistribution of forces in correction of boutonniere deformity. J. Bone Joint Surg., 49A:1267, 1967.
10. Parkes, A.R.: The lumbrical plus finger. Hand, 2:164, 1970.
11. Peacock, E. and VanWinkle, W.: *Surgery and Biology of Wound Repair.* W.B. Saunders, Philadelphia, 1970.
12. Secretan, H.: Hard edema and traumatic hyperplasia of the dorsum of the metacarpus. Rev. Med. Suisse Romande, 21:409, 1901.
13. Verdan, C.E.: Primary and secondary flexor and extensor tendon injuries. In: *Hand Surgery* (Flynn, J.E., Ed.). Williams and Wilkins, Baltimore, 1966.

15 Nerves

Injury causes the most common nerve disorders affecting the hand. Three different types are recognized: (1) *neurotmesis,* in which all nerve continuity is lost, (2) *axonotmesis,* in which there is only partial loss of continuity and (3) *neuropraxia,* in which there is no loss of continuity.

In neurotemesis spontaneous regeneration is unlikely. The condition results from injury which may be tidy (incisive) or untidy (mangled with possible loss of substance). In axonotmesis the sheath is intact but some of the axons are physically interrupted. This usually results from compression, stretching or concussion. Spontaneous recovery occurs but is less complete and less frequent than in neuropraxia. Neuropraxia usually is a result of compression or ischemia. All axons remain in physical continuity but are functionless. Recovery may be spontaneous or the damage may be permanent, depending upon the duration of compression or the extent of the ischemia.

Neurotmesis invariably requires a surgical repair, whereas neuropraxia and axonotmesis are expectant problems for which neurolysis may become necessary after 3 to 6 months. All these phenomena have the same functional impact on the extremity as the disruption of the telephone or electrical system would have on a city.

Central nervous system afflictions often affect the function of the upper extremity. There are spastic states and different degrees of motor paralysis, with or without sensory disorders, or there may be sensory paralysis without motor disturbances (e.g. tumor and syringomelia). Significant alterations in function are also produced by peripheral neuropathies. There are millions of lepers in the world with sensory and motor deficits of the median and ulnar nerves. In many instances this disease has caused severe sensory and motor palsy with secondary clawing of the hand and trophic ulcerations. In our own western civilization, nutritional deficiencies caused by alcoholism have produced a host of neurological disturbances.

One of the least understood disorders mediated by the peripheral nerves is pain. The complex interrelationship of the psyche and the soma is usually at fault in the problem of chronic pain, and is often extremely perplexing, even defying solution. Relief of pain is a prime obligation of the doctor, but the patient must share in the responsibility for this relief. Persistent pain arising in the extremity is usually the consequence of inflammatory, chemical or physical processes acting on peripheral nerves. The most common physical causes of acute pain are stretching, compression and ischemia. The most common physical causes of chronic pain are fibrosis, entrapment and neuroma formation.

Regeneration of a sensory nerve is invariably associated with chronic dysesthesia which may last for weeks or months with disabling results. Similar dysesthesia (probably mediated through the sympathetic fibers that coexist with somatic peripheral nerves) is frequently seen in the aftermath of any major injury, or surgery to any part of the upper extremity. Inflammation of the tissues generates pain by its biological effect on nerve endings. The magnitude of this effect is undoubtedly related to the extent of neurotoxicity. One of the most prominent pain-provoking neurotoxic states is that produced by the herpes virus, in which the pain is out of all proportion to the magnitude of swelling, inflammation and tension.

Each peripheral nerve contains a great number

of nerve fibers (axons), individually enclosed within an endoneurial sheath. These units are in turn bound together into bundles or funiculi by adjacent connective tissue, the perineurium. The bundles are held together by a loose areolar connective tissue framework called the epineurium, which serves as a definitive external sheath that separates the nerve from the surrounding tissues. The collagen and elastic fibers of these sheaths have good tensile strength and hold sutures well. Thus the endoneurium, perineurium and epineurium constitute the connective tissue framework of a peripheral nerve needed for the support, isolation and insulation of its various components. Each of these has specific architectural or structural characteristics which should be understood.

In his study of the comparative amounts of connective tissue in cross-sectional areas of nerves, Sunderland[39] found the smallest amount to be about 22 per cent and the greatest 88 per cent. In general, anywhere from 30 to 75 per cent of a peripheral nerve is made up of connective tissue, depending upon the nerve and the specific level in question. There is more connective tissue when the neural components are small and numerous and less when the bundles are few or of a larger size. There is also more at those sites where peripheral nerves pass across joints.

The endoneurium, which surrounds each complex made up of axons and Schwann cells, is mostly composed of collagenous tissue. This supporting connective tissue forms the fine, intrafunicular septae that separate nerve fibers inside a funiculus. These septae contain the interfunicular blood supply.

The perineurium invests each bundle or funiculus with a relatively thin but dense and distinctive sheath of fibrous tissue. It contains elastic and collagen fibers which intermesh by passing circularly, obliquely and longitudinally. These fibrils form from 7 to 17 concentric lamellae or tubes, the number varying depending upon the size of the funiculus. When the funiculi at the end of a freshly cut nerve are carefully examined, it will be seen that they have the ability to move back and forth independently within the perineurium. The epineurium, the outer sleeve, also moves somewhat independently in relation to its contents, the funiculi making the entire unit an unstable composite of slippery tubes like fine-cooked spaghetti.

Injection studies demonstrate that the microcirculation of each funiculus runs in the perineurium. The internal circulation of the nerve is piped to it segmentally through the mesoneurium in a relationship similar to that of the intestine and its mesentery. All the nutrient vessels enter the nerve along the line where the mesoneurium attaches to the nerve and not around the remainder of its circumference. Blood is supplied in a segmental fashion, being both dispersed and collected through a series of arcades within the mesoneurium. The grouping of arcades seems to change from one area to another to meet needs and requirements imposed by local anatomical variations. In areas such as the shoulder, elbow, and wrist, where great degrees of mobility are required of the nerve, the mesoneurium is longer, more complex and contains more vessels. When there is little or no tension on these vessels, they telescope in an accordion-like arrangement. As tension increases with movement, the vessels within the mesoneurium stretch out to accommodate for the changing position of the nerve. The nutrient vessels entering a given portion of nerve through the mesoneurium will, therefore, appear to vary in number depending upon the position of the limb and the degree to which they are stretched. Peripheral nerves possess considerable strength and elasticity. Though it is not possible to isolate and separate the mechanical properties of each component part of a peripheral nerve, there is evidence to show that a great deal of the tensile strength and elasticity of nerve trunks is derived from the perineurium. It plays a major role in maintaining the integrity of the nerve trunk under tension.

Rupture of endoneurial and perineurial tubes leads to axonal escape from the endoneurial tube that is formed by the Schwann cells. These cells then proliferate to repair the rupture and, if successful, will contain the regenerating axon. Otherwise, the uncontained axons will become entangled with the proliferating fibroblasts arising from the connective tissue of the nerve. Thus neuromas can occur, even when there is continuity of the nerve, if the endoneurium and perineurium are ruptured.

Evaluation of Nerve Function and Diagnosis of Disorder

A knowledge of the usual functional anatomy and its variations is a prerequisite to the assessment of any disorder of peripheral nerves. Dysfunction peripheral to the brachial plexus usually results in anatomically "pure" sensory and/or motor deficits, as distinguished from more proximal injuries which produce effects that overlap the distribution of several peripheral nerves.

Painful stimuli originating peripherally often

radiate to the shoulder and thorax, making diagnosis difficult for the unwary physician. One of the most common examples of this is the carpal tunnel syndrome, in which the presenting complaint can be pain over the upper chest and shoulder girdle as well as in the upper extremity (Chap. 8).

Spasticity is prima facie evidence of a central nervous system disorder. Hyperreflexia or an asymmetrical areflexia, in the absence of peripheral nerve or muscle injury, also reflects a central nervous system disturbance.

Most afflictions originating peripheral to the brachial plexus can be diagnosed by testing the muscle and sensory function appropriately. The habitus of the extremity often signals the involvement. Thus a wristdrop with profoundly weakened grip is telltale of a "Saturday-night paralysis" from lying on the upper arm and compressing the radial nerve as it crosses the distal third of the humerus.

Division of the median and ulnar nerves distally at the wrist leaves the digits at the mercy of the tone of the extrinsic muscles and a clawhand results. This consists of hyperextension of the metacarpophalangeal joints, supination of the thumb and furling of interphalangeal joints into flexion. The palm is flattened with total loss of effective pinch. Eventually there is profound atrophy of intrinsic muscles. In addition, there is corresponding anesthesia.

In isolated injury of the ulnar nerve in the distal half of the forearm, clawing is confined to the ring and little fingers and is more pronounced than the clawing of the index and long fingers following isolated injury of the median nerve in the distal forearm. Clawing signifies that the extrinsic muscles are innervated. Thus median and ulnar nerve injury about the elbow will not produce clawing. Since clawing requires hyperextension of the metacarpophalangeal joints, tightness of the collateral ligaments, volar plate or joint capsule may reduce or prevent clawing.

Proximal injuries of the median and ulnar nerves have other characteristic stigmata added to the peripheral sensory and intrinsic muscle palsies in the hand. A high median palsy results in loss of forearm pronation (except by gravity), loss of action of the flexor pollicis longus, all the superficialis muscles, the profundi to the index and long fingers, and the flexor carpi radialis. A high ulnar palsy will paralyze the profundi to the ring and little fingers as well as the flexor carpi ulnaris. The latter is most easily tested by having the patient spread the flattened hand forcefully to tense this tendon (Fig. 15-1).

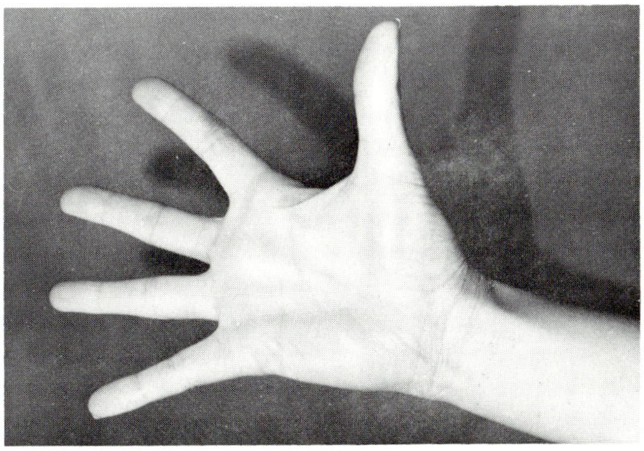

Figure 15-1. *Tensing the flattened hand demonstrates both the flexor carpi radialis and carpi ulnaris.*

The technique of testing for integrity of profundus and superficialis tendons is described in Chapter 14.

Occasionally the deep volar interosseous branch of the median nerve is compromised. This produces an isolated paralysis of the flexor pollicis longus, the profundus to the index finger, and the pronator quadratus, without any sensory loss. The pronator quadratus can be differentially tested from the pronator teres by determining the power of pronation when the elbow is fully flexed, reducing the effectiveness of the pronator teres by relaxing it.

High radial nerve palsy produces a wristdrop with paralysis of all the long extensors including the brachioradialis. In contrast, paralysis of the deep dorsal interosseous branch affects the more peripheral extensors, the abductor pollicis longus and both long thumb extensors, but does not weaken wrist extension. Testing for the muscles innervated by this branch is done by having the patient spread the flattened hand and extend the distal joint of his thumb with force. The superficial radial nerve (pure sensory) is highly vulnerable in the distal third of the forearm and readily produces a painful neuroma in any of its 3 to 5 terminal branches.

Fresh injuries often perplex the surgeon because false-negative tests of nerve function are common. Intact motor action may be withheld because of pain and apprehension, not paralysis. In testing sensibility, transient physiological anesthesia ("protective" neuropraxia) may occur; therefore, repeated testing of function is mandatory. An accurate diagnosis is ensured when the results of repeated evaluation are consistent and anatomically compatible. This is particularly true in the case of incomplete nerve damage.

Muscle palsy is evidenced by weakness or total failure to act and the concomitant loss of contractile tone (Fig. 15-2); however, wasting (mus-

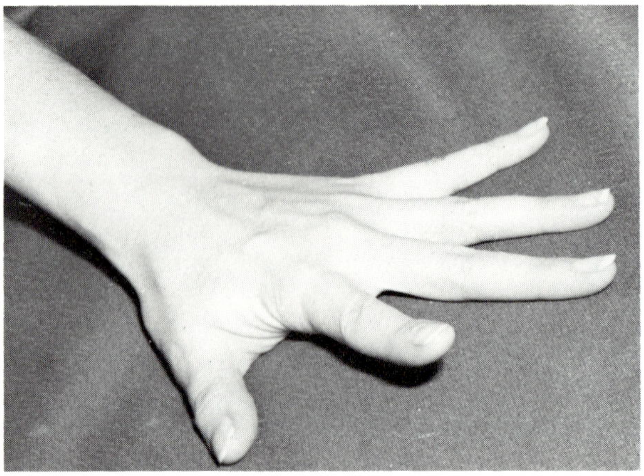

Figure 15-2. *The integrity of the first dorsal interosseous is demonstrated by spreading the fingers and extending the thumb, then abducting the index finger.*

cle atrophy) due to paralysis takes several weeks or months to become readily apparent. It is distinguished from disuse atrophy by its confinement to specific patterns of innervation. Electromyographic testing may be valuable where clinical weakness or atrophy is not yet diagnostic.

The infinite variations in neuroanatomy give rise to considerable overlap in sensory and motor innervations of the hand. In addition, there are many overlapping functions of different muscles (muscle for muscle and muscle group for muscle group), so that loss of action can be masked by compensatory function. This, indeed, is a fortunate circumstance for function, but it is often the basis of unjustified credit taken by the surgeon for the results of neurorrhaphy. A true assessment of such overlapping functions is the result of a detailed and time-consuming motor and sensory evaluation after differential blocks of peripheral nerves. On practical grounds, neither the patient nor the surgeon takes time for this somewhat academic exercise.

The presence of sweat signifies that the sensory innervation is intact. Dryness is the telltale evidence of sensory impairment if it is limited to the distribution of an injured nerve, and the patient has not had a sympathetic block. Examination of the skin of the palm and digital fat pads with a magnifying glass will usually demonstrate glistening beads of sweat. If the skin is dry, fine particles of tissue paper and cotton will not adhere to it as they do if sweat is present.

A more sophisticated test for sweating is the ninhydrin fingerprinting test.[21] Other functional tests of sensibility which correlate with the epicritic modalities are the following blindfold tests: (1) the identification of various standard coins and small objects, (2) the identification of five different grades of sandpaper by lightly touching or rubbing them, and (3) the Weber test of two-point discrimination.[19] Normally, the two ends of a paper clip on the digital fat pad should be identifiable when they are 4 mm or less apart. Sensory nerve conduction studies can also be made. However, these do not always correlate with the clinical findings. In all this testing the clinician must compare the abnormal limb with the normal one.

The return of motor function after nerve regeneration is assessed by the appearance of active contraction and by the strength regained. The initial testings may be falsely negative if they are made against resistance (gravity). Thus, in testing the early recovery from a wristdrop, the forearm should be neither pronated or supinated. A thorough examination necessitates an evaluation of the independence of action of individual muscles, their excursion, speed and power of action and the overall coordination and control of the hand. Once motor function has begun to appear, progression may be very rapid.

Electromyographic testing may demonstrate early muscular reinnervation prior to the objective clinical findings. The first changes are the decrease of fibrillation and the appearance of slow polyphasic discharges produced by attempts at voluntary movement. Early fatigability of the recently reinnervated muscle fibers is reflected by the late peak following the initial spike of the action potential, referred to as the slow polyphasic unit of regeneration.

The final assessment of muscle function is, of course, performance and endurance. Grip meter readings are used in chronological sequence as an index of progress, as cited by Zachary.[42] Highet[42] has a useful calibrated scale for testing muscle strength:

0—no contraction
1—a flicker
2—contraction
3—contraction against gravity
4—contraction against resistance
greater than gravity
5—normal

In evaluating regeneration of a sensory nerve, Tinel's sign (the electric shock noted with discrete percussion over the nerve) is useful. It corresponds to the level of peripheral migration of Wallerian regeneration. The failure of any progression of the Tinel's sign past 4 to 6 months signifies arrest of regeneration. Tinel's sign does not imply the quality or extent of function of the regenerated nerve.

The rate of regeneration varies, depending on the age of the patient, the blood supply and the location of the injury. It is most rapid in preadolescents.[26] In the forearm it may progress up to 100 mm/month but distal to the wrist it advances at the rate of 1 mm/day. The order of appearance of sensory modalities in regeneration is: (1) Tinel's sign, (2) deep pain, (3) tingling, (4) light touch and temperature, (5) position sense and (6) sudomotor activity (sweat and epicritic sensibility).

The Tinel phenomenon (electric shock reaction to touch) is the basis for Paul Brand's concept of the "inhibited hand" introduced in contrast to the "uninhibited hand." All sensory nerve regeneration imparts hypersensitivity over its geographical distribution during the phase of regeneration. This may last for months, and unfortunately sometimes is permanent. As a result of this sensory experiment, it is only natural that the patient withdraw from using the hand—hence the term "inhibited hand." When the hand is "blind" by failure of any sensory regeneration, the insensitive part is traumatized by overuse and the absence of pain (Figs. 15-3, 20-12). Thus, lepers with combined ulnar and median nerve palsy have trophic digital ulcers as a consequence of the "blind" hand gripping with extreme force to compensate for what they cannot feel. Proprioception of the unaffected forearm muscles is their only clue to the hand's performance. This typifies the "uninhibited hand."

Through education and guidance, the patients with the inhibited hand will usually tolerate the period of disturbed sensibility and overcome the dysesthesia. Those with the uninhibited hand often need more guidance and education to avoid injuring the anesthetic part. A maximally developed proprioceptive feedback can do much to compensate for skin blindness. This requires a tailored program of activity involving proprioceptive correlation of objects calibrated by size and weight which the patient may pinch, grip and hold alternately under direct vision and when blindfolded. Thus the continued use and protection of this uninhibited extremity is the direct responsibility of the patient.

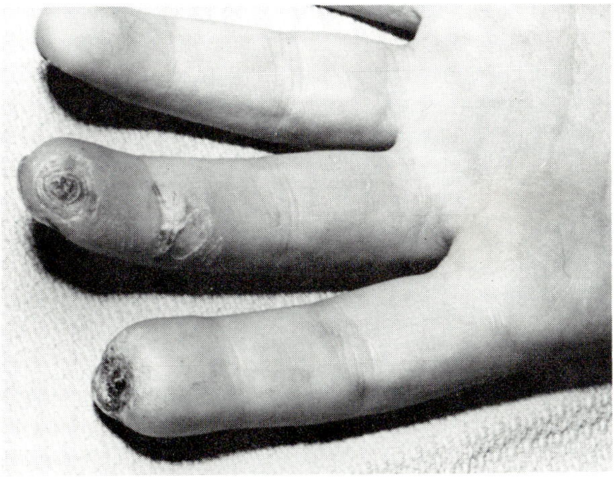

Figure 15-3. *Ulceration of the fingertips of a boy with an "uninhibited" hand due to complete division of the median nerve.*

Inhibition or lack of inhibition may be geographically broad or narrow. If it involves the dominant side of a digit (e.g. the radial side of the distal phalanx of the index), a careful study of boundaries by the patient, coupled with the protective coating of the involved area with moleskin, felt, or sponge padding, is helpful.

As a general rule, the changes in the nerve distal to the site of injury become fixed and relatively irreversible after a year. However, motor end-plates atrophy beyond recovery far sooner. These degenerative changes are most difficult to offset in the intrinsic muscles. Delay in the repair of the divided median or ulnar nerve beyond two months leaves little chance for appreciable intrinsic muscle recovery despite reasonable sensory regeneration.

It is impossible to recover all function lost by division of a peripheral nerve. The reasons for this are mechanical and biological (Fig. 15-4). A nerve in cross section consists of thousands of microscopic axons in bundles called funiculi. The stroma supporting these axons is connective tissue. Fifty per cent or more of the cross-sectional surface area of a peripheral nerve may be stromal and not axonal. Hence, the impossibility of matching all axons becomes clear. It would be like precisely matching all the straws of two brooms. Complicating this is the fact that the major nerves are mixed and sensory and motor axons will not function if they are mismatched. Furthermore, their geographical relationship is constantly shifting axon for axon, funiculus for funiculus, millimeter to millimeter along the nerve (Fig. 15-5). Add to this the inescapable swelling that occurs in wound healing and some hemorrhage (at times a sizable clot from an endoneurial vessel) and ultimate fibrosis, and the impact of distortion on matching axons becomes evident.

Notwithstanding these problems, useful function can be recovered by neurorrhaphy. Of the three major nerves in the arm, the median is the

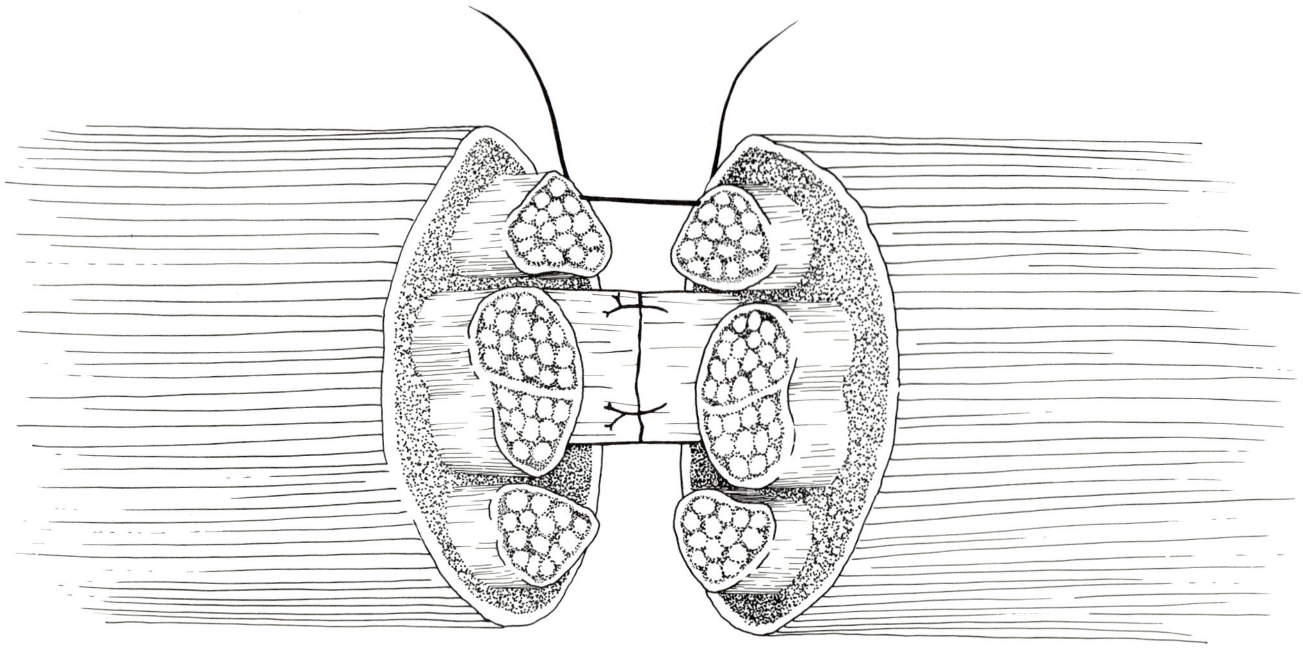

Figure 15-4. *Schematic representation of the technique of the funicular repair of peripheral nerves. (Redrawn from Grabb, W.C.: Management of nerve injuries in the forearm and hand. Orthop. Clin. North Am., 1:419, 1970.)*

most important to repair for reasons of its sensory distribution. The radial nerve, which is predominantly motor, generally recovers better after repair than either the median or ulnar nerve.

Time of Repair

There is still controversy about the value of primary versus secondary neurorrhaphy of divided peripheral nerves in tidy wounds. The consensus among hand surgeons favors primary repair, particularly when the injury is in the forearm or hand. The reason for this is that the nerve and its funicular components are more easily identified and matched then than at the time of secondary repair when perineurial scar may obscure the anatomy. In addition, considerable time and expense are saved by preventing disability and repeated treatment. There are those[30] who prefer secondary neurorrhaphy, claiming that the added thickness of the connective tissue sleeves (epineurium and perineurium) facilitates suturing. However, surgeons of that sentiment are invariably faced with the need to resect more proximal and distal nerve stump at the time of repair. This increases the

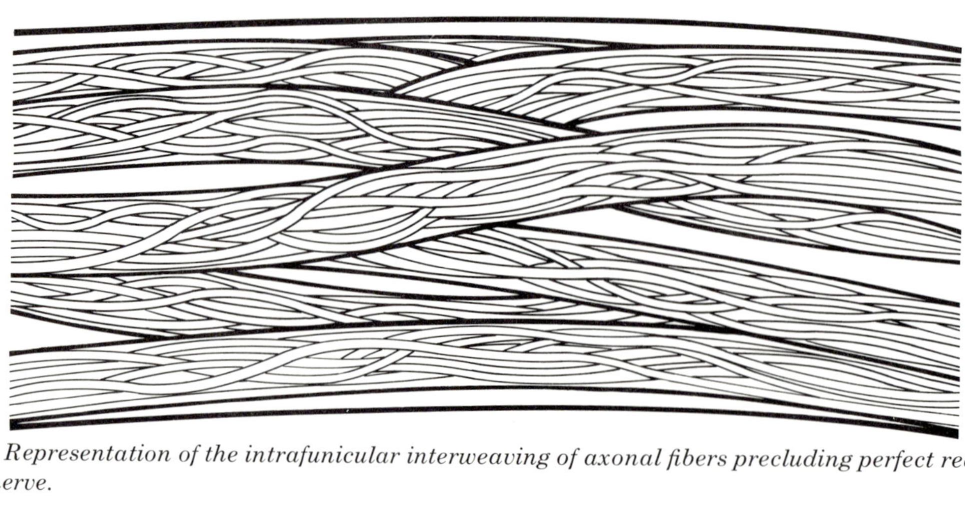

Figure 15-5. *Representation of the intrafunicular interweaving of axonal fibers precluding perfect reapproximation of a divided nerve.*

amount of tension on the suture line and the need for adverse positioning of joints to reduce this tension is introduced unless a nerve graft is employed.

All surgeons agree that tension is inimical to a favorable result from neurorrhaphy. Prejudicial tension is produced not only by stretch but also by congestion within the epineurial and perineurial sheaths themselves. In recognition of the deleterious effect of tension, many surgeons[27] today no longer do epineurial repairs of the major nerves and avoid the need for extensive mobilization of nerves and adverse positioning of joints. The epineurium is slit and even resected, liberating the funiculi which are then matched for size and geography proximally and distally. Nerve grafts are used liberally to overcome any gaps so that joints do not have to be positioned unnaturally.[27]

When tidy nerve injury occurs near the nerve cell body, the disturbance of cellular metabolism is sufficiently greater that there is less unanimity of opinion about the benefits or primary neurorrhaphy[13] (Fig. 15-6). A delay of 3 to 4 weeks is advocated by many experienced surgeons to allow the cell body to recover and enter the phase of neuronal regeneration.

Nerve Injury

Fresh injury to peripheral nerves may be open or closed. If closed, the mechanism of injury is usually stretching, contusion, compression or transient crushing. If there has been a fracture with a sharp edge, there may be division of the nerve (the radial nerve in humeral fractures, the ulnar nerve in elbow fractures and the motor branch of the ulnar nerve in fractures of the base of the fifth metacarpal). Barring such fractures, the treatment of closed nerve injuries is usually expectant for as long as six months.

During or after this period experience will direct the surgeon to consider nerve decompression. Such a procedure becomes an emergency in the face of mounting congestion or signs of motor and sensory

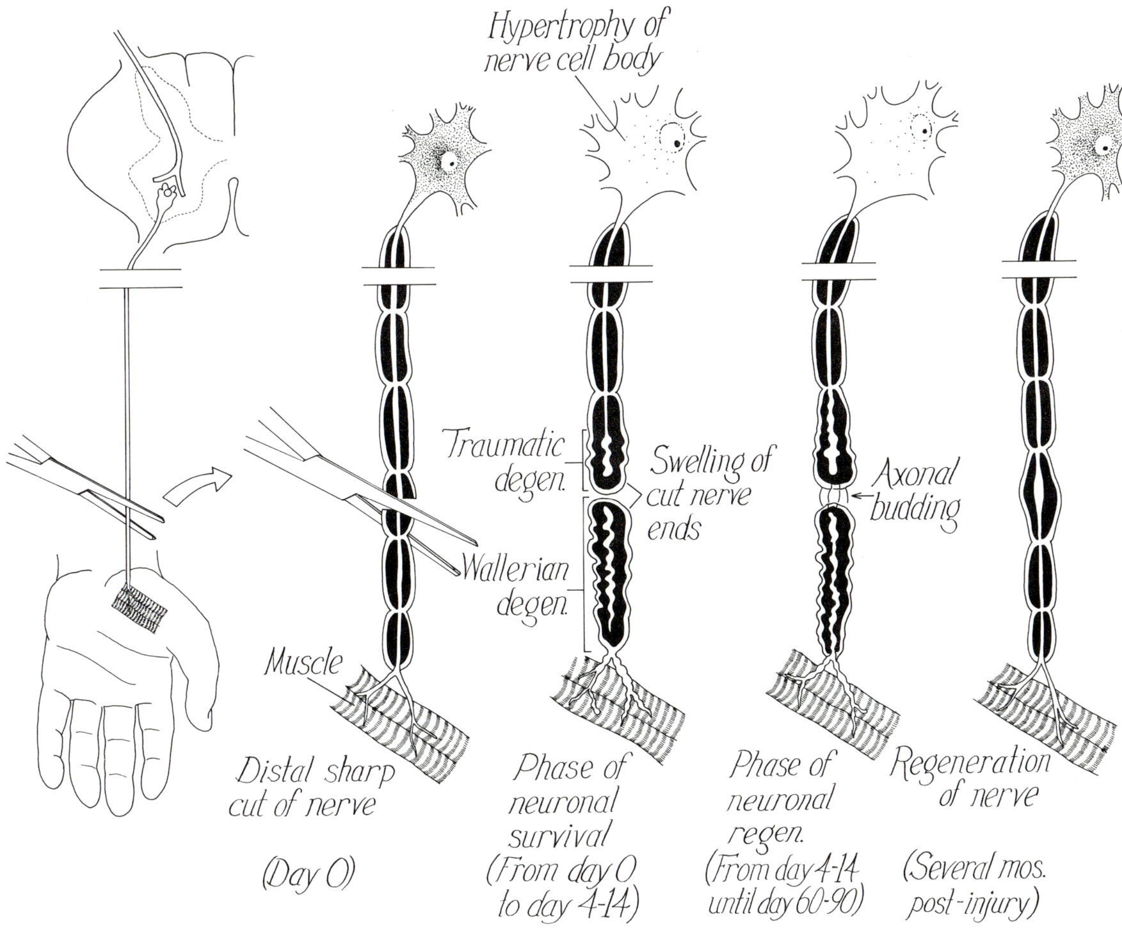

Figure 15-6. *Injury to any peripheral nerve fiber induces changes in the cell body. These changes are greater the closer to the cell body the injury occurs. (Redrawn from Grabb, W.C.: Management of nerve injuries in the forearm and hand. Orthop. Clin. North Am., 1:419, 1970.)*

paralysis (Fig. 15-7). Any severe swelling of the extremity, whether inflammatory or traumatic, may present this crisis. Treatment requires slitting not only the skin and fascia but any structure constricting the nerve, e.g. the pronator teres choking the median nerve. Although an attempt is ordinarily made to cover the decompressed nerve with some soft tissue that has good blood supply, the closure of the skin wound is less urgent and may require grafting. While awaiting recovery, joints must be kept limber and sometimes splints (particularly night splints) are needed to prevent overstretching of paralyzed muscles and to preserve the functional habitus of the hand. The patient must learn to avoid injury to anesthetic skin and denervated joints.

At times, nerve decompression necessitates an endoneurolysis, slitting the epineurium in one or more planes. This may be facilitated by the injection of saline beneath the epineurium and requires magnification to identify and protect crisscrossing funiculi. Endoneurolysis is essential when there is

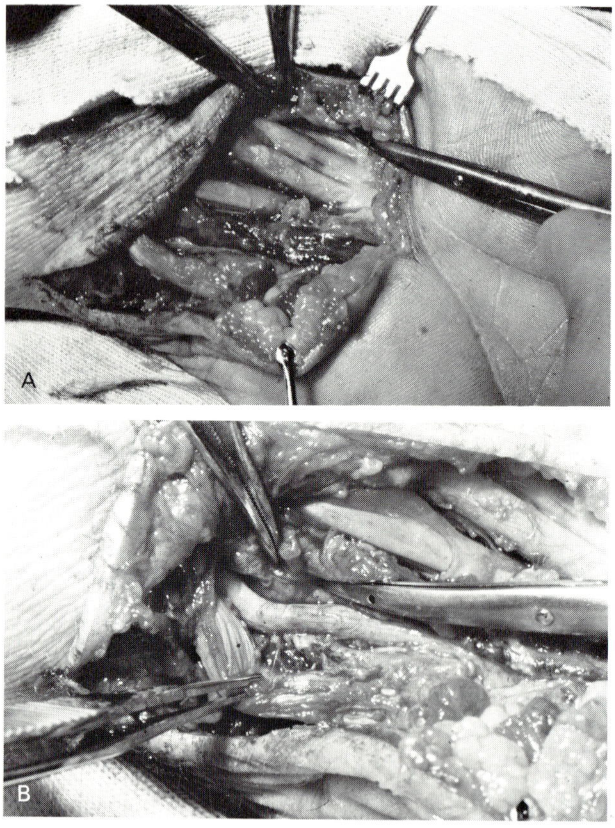

Figure 15-7. *An acute median and ulnar nerve entrapment at the wrist occurring after a Colles' fracture. Removal of the thrombosed veins* **(A)** *and decompression of both nerves immediately relieved the symptoms. (Courtesy of Dr. Alexander Kalenak.)*

any hourglass constriction of the nerve, or if its consistency is firmer than normal.

When neurotmesis is suspected, then the treatment must be surgical under the most ideal conditions of experience and facilities (magnifying equipment, instruments and sutures).

In open injuries, the emergency treatment of the wound must spare all nerves from iatrogenic crushing by the avoidance of indiscriminate clamping of bleeding vessels (Figs. 15-8, 9-8). The placement of a tourniquet (sphygmomanometer) is mandatory. It should be inflated rapidly to 300 mm Hg in order to discretely identify the bleeding vessels within the wound. Manual compression of the surrounding tissues will extrude blood from the vessels, permitting their identification.

Whether or not a primary or secondary nerve repair is done is largely a matter of surgical judgment. Tidy wounds, or wounds which can be easily tidied, favor primary neurorrhaphy. With proper emergency surgical preparation, wound approximation, splinting, elevation and administration of prophylactic antibiotics, the primary nerve repair may be delayed for hours or several days.

In the interests of the best prognosis, secondary neurorrhaphy is advisable when the structures in a tidy wound are so stained with blood that small nerves cannot be identified without excessive dissection, leading to a greater amount of scarring. Secondary repair is essential when the wound is untidy and adequate cover is not available for the nerve.

In the untidy wound, attention should be directed at the viability of tissues, the prevention of infection, debridement, alignment and the restoration of acceptable cover to the zone of injury. During debridement, the astute hand surgeon will cap-

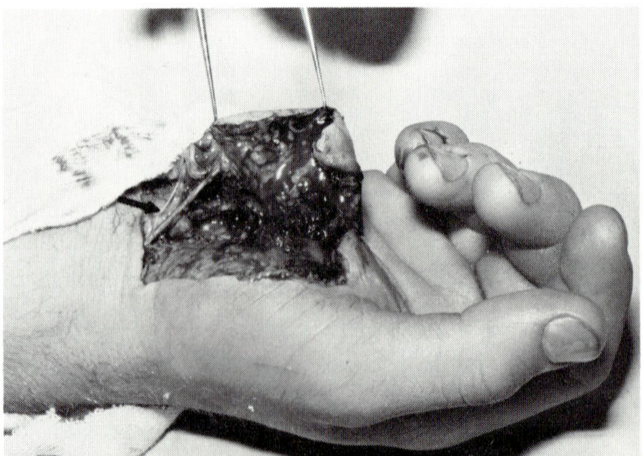

Figure 15-8. *The palmar cutaneous nerve is still intact after avulsion injury of the palm.*

italize on an opportunity to salvage nerve tissue which can be used for grafts where needed elsewhere in the same hand.

Neurorrhaphy

Neurorrhaphy is intended to correctly align as many axons as possible by matching the funiculi and epineurial vessels of the proximal and distal stumps. This meticulous surgery requires magnification by at least a 2- to 4-power loupe and often an operating microscope with 12- to 20-power magnification. A microscope cannot be used, however, when the wrist and elbow joints have to be flexed to bring the nerve ends together.

The proximal and distal stumps of the nerve being repaired need not be trimmed if the injury is fresh and the stumps are tidy. Untidy stumps of a freshly injured nerve and stumps in secondary neurorrhaphy must be trimmed back and made tidy. However, for the sake of axonal alignment, the amount resected should be kept to a minimum. A tidy stump is obtained by transverse sectioning with a new razor blade pressed down upon the nerve as it lies on a wet tongue blade (Fig. 15-9). Another technique for sectioning is to hold the nerve by a piece of plastic sheeting which is wrapped around it and secured by a mosquito hemostat placed parallel to the nerve.

Small nerves, such as digital nerves, are repaired with interrupted 10-0 to 12-0 atraumatic nylon sutures placed through the epineurial cuff at points 180° apart. There must be no telescoping or overlapping of neural elements, no projection of any unmatched and angulated funiculi from the margin of the nerve juncture. As a rule two such sutures will suffice, but at the most four are placed, the nerve being mobilized from its bed and rotated to place a suture on the deep side. When the funiculi are easily identifiable, they should be specifically matched and secured with one perineurial suture. In this case the epineurium is slit. At the conclusion of neurorrhaphy, 2 to 3 mg of triamcinolone may be placed in the soft tissue about the nerve to lessen the local inflammatory reaction.[31]

Larger caliber nerves such as the median, ulnar and radial are repaired by funicular approximation.[27] This requires a microsurgical dissection of the major nerve funiculi out of the proximal and distal stumps and careful matching by size and location. There will be up to 4 or 5 major funiculi for each large nerve. The epineurial sleeve is slit and may be resected. One or two 10-0 to 12-0 nylon perineurial sutures are placed for each funiculus and tied loosely (Fig. 15-4). The technique must be

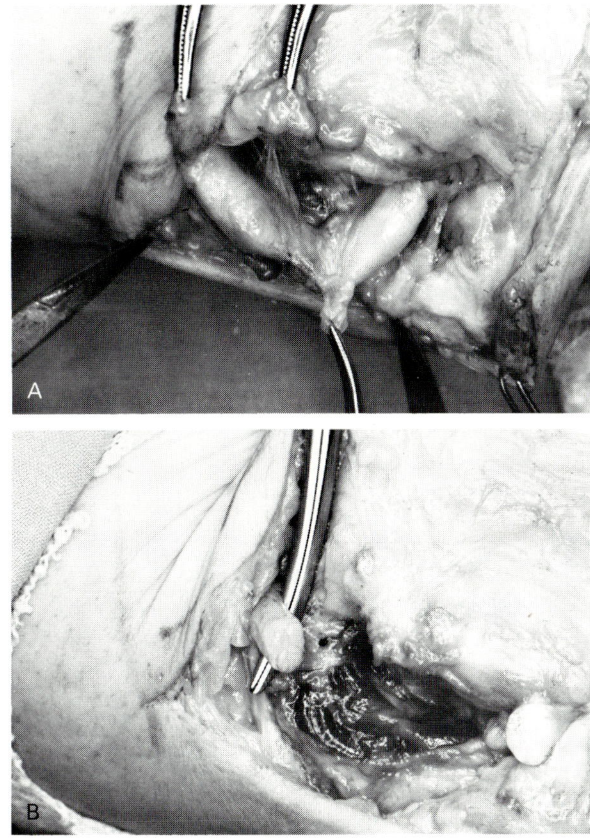

Figure 15-9. *A neuroma in continuity of the ulnar nerve resected prior to neurorrhaphy. (From Graham, W.P., et al.: Treating the injured hand.* Contemp. Surg., 4:67, 1974.)

totally devoid of any tension on the suture line.

A gap in the nerve is overcome by mobilization of the nerve proximally and distally, positioning the joints to approximate the stumps, or insertion of a graft (Fig. 15-10**A**). A graft avoids any tension; however, it creates a new (albeit acceptable) disability in the donor site and it must be revascularized by its new bed. The preferred donor nerves are the sural nerve (35 cm), the superficial radial nerve (20 cm) and the medial antebrachial cutaneous nerve of the forearm (12 cm). In placing the graft, the various-sized funiculi of the proximal and distal stumps must be carefully mapped and joined by an appropriate-sized funiculus of the graft.[27] To reduce the amount of scar at the junctures of the graft and the stump, the levels of the repair of the various funiculi may be staggered by shortening some of them (Fig. 15-10**B**).

Mobilization of nerves to overcome gaps often requires extensive dissection. This decreases the blood supply to the nerve, and may result in denervation of some structures. It invariably involves positioning of the joints so that it is difficult to do a meticulous microsurgical repair and to avoid ten-

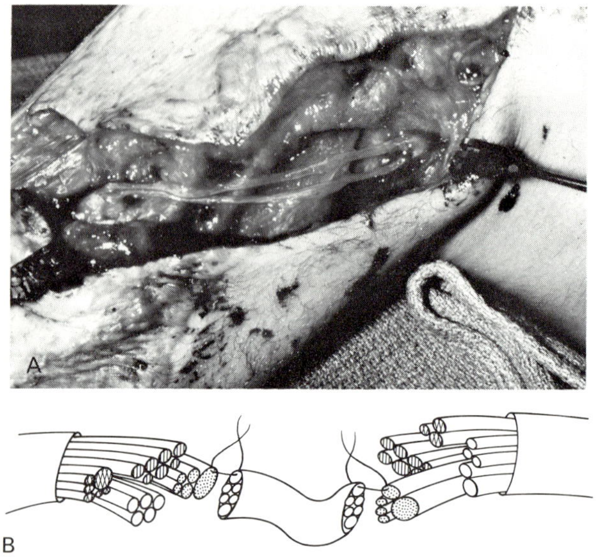

Figure 15-10. *Interfunicular nerve graft replacing an avulsed neural segment. Interfunicular grafting is facilitated by staggering the levels of neurorrhaphy and allowing the individual grafts to be as free as possible to ensure their approximation to the bed for revascularization.*

sion on the suture line. A limited amount of mobilization and joint flexion is, however, acceptable in lieu of a graft when there is *no tension.* Under such circumstances, the segmental blood supply of the nerve will not be jeopardized. Many surgeons are utilizing interfasicular grafting in preference to extensive proximal and distal mobilization and extreme joint positioning.[27]

If no alternatives exist, a gap of 5 cm may be overcome in the median, ulnar or radial nerves by extensive mobilization, combined with flexion of the joints. To gain maximum length requires mobilization from the arm to the forearm. The easiest nerve to free is the ulnar, which has few branches and a relatively superficial location between the arm and forearm. It usually has to be transposed anterior to the medial epicondyle after opening the cubital tunnel by slitting the flexor carpi ulnaris. If necessary, the branches to the profundi and the flexor carpi ulnaris are divided. Length is gained for the median nerve by liberating it from its deep position in the distal arm, antecubital area and forearm so that it can come to rest subcutaneously. As a rule concomitant elbow flexion is needed more to gain length with the median nerve than is the case with the ulnar nerve. To gain length in the radial nerve, it is mobilized from its spiral groove in a tunneling fashion, brought out on the medial aspect of the upper arm through a counterincision and rerouted straight across the antecubital fossa.[28]

In certain circumstances a nerve pedicle is the only available technique for overcoming a gap. This is commonly the case in the surgery of Volkmann's ischemic contracture. This technique is also resorted to in loss-of-substance injury of the forearm. The existing problem is the totally anesthetic hand, and the objective is restoration of sensibility over the distribution of the median nerve. The proximal remaining ulnar nerve becomes the donor pedicle (Fig. 15-11).

Theoretically, the advantage of a pedicle over a free graft is that the pedicle, even when transferred, retains some inherent circulation. Transecting and shifting the proximal ulnar nerve to join the proximal stump of the median nerve maintains the natural direction of axoplasmic flow (Fig. 15-11**D–F**). Furthermore it allows for tracing regeneration and timing the second stage. When

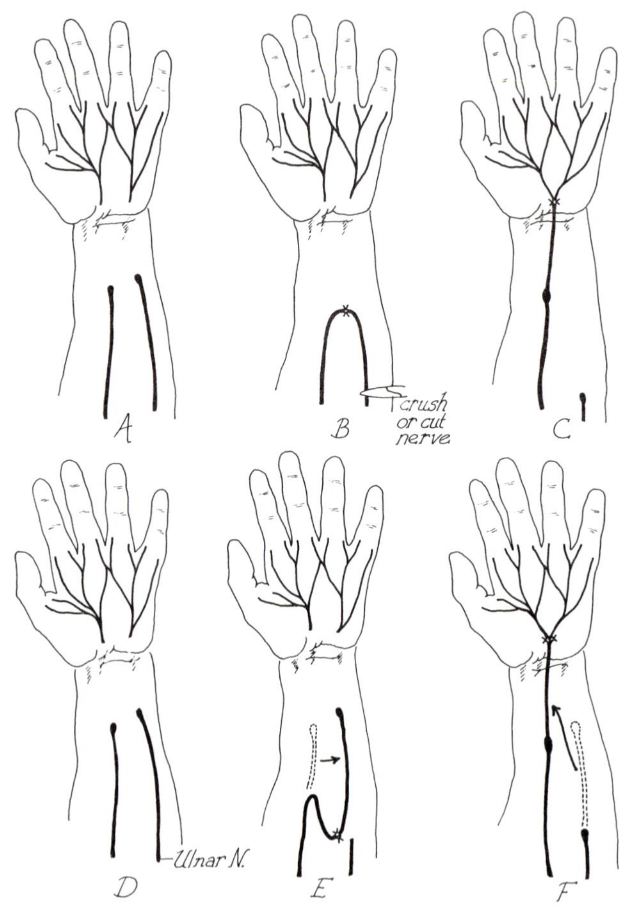

Figure 15-11. *Restoring a missing segment of median nerve by use of the adjacent damaged ulnar nerve. If the procedure can be performed as illustrated in* **D–F,** *the second stage is done when the Tinel's sign reaches the end of the median nerve segment. (Redrawn from Chase, R.A.:* Atlas of Hand Surgery. *W.B. Saunders, Philadelphia, 1973.)*

Tinel's sign reaches the distal stump the pedicle is advanced and joined to the distal stump of the median nerve.

In a partial nerve injury, the surgeon is guided by whether or not the injury is fresh or old, tidy or untidy. He must decide whether to simply do an epineurial approximation or to resect epineurium proximally and distally and perform a funicular repair with perineurial sutures. Furthermore, he has to decide how much, if any, of the proximal and distal funicular stumps need to be resected on the basis of existing maceration in fresh injuries and scar in old injuries. As a rule, with some mobilization of the funiculi proximally and distally an approximation is possible without tension on the perineurial sutures and without undue kinking of the adjacent intact nerve.

The amount of postoperative joint flexion to avoid tension at the nerve juncture must be determined before closing the skin. If there is no tension, postoperative immobilization is necessary only until the skin heals. When splinting is needed to prevent tension on the nerve juncture, it must be maintained for 3 to 4 weeks. If a sizable gap has been overcome by positioning, this period will be prolonged for several weeks while the flexed joints are gradually extended.

When there is total anesthesia the patient will lack any awareness of discomfort from a congested portion of the hand or from a pressure point of a splint. Accordingly, great care must be taken in applying the dressing and cast in these circumstances.

The indications for reexploration of a neurorrhaphy are:

1. The failure of any sign of regeneration at 3 to 4 months for a sensory nerve and at 4 to 6 months for a motor nerve.
2. The arrest of regeneration distal to the neurorrhaphy as detected by Tinel's sign. This most frequently occurs at the distal end of a nerve graft. Occasionally it occurs at some point of compression distal to the neurorrhaphy where it can be treated by a neurolysis. If bipolar nerve-stimulating electrodes are available, proof of regeneration is possible and obviates the need for repeating the neurorrhaphy. The neurolysis itself will offer the maximum chance for improvement.
3. The existence of a disabling neuroma that is intractable to non-operative treatment.

POSTOPERATIVE CARE FOLLOWING NEURORRHAPHY

At the start the patient must be made aware of the factor of time involved in the recovery of function after any neurorrhaphy. This involves months and occasionally years. The patient must realize that his adaptation to the paralysis and perseverance in pursuing the disciplines of rehabilitation are the keys to successful recovery. The surgeon must see the patient frequently enough in the immediate postoperative period to help him understand the natural history of recovery and the various signs and symptoms he can expect.

During the first month the patient must guard his hand against congestion by adequate elevation and the avoidance of constricting forces. At all times he must protect the anesthetic skin and joints. When the cast and dressing are removed the joints must be kept limber and the strength of intact muscles maintained. Splints may be applied to counteract marked muscle imbalances. This is particularly applicable to a radial nerve palsy.

Once the patient has gained some recovery of nerve function, he must train and educate his motor and sensory systems to achieve a full measure of rehabilitation. This embodies not only the strengthening of returning function but also the development of compensatory and dormant functions to the maximum.[12] When a vocational readjustment seems inevitable, this should be started as soon after injury as possible. At all costs the patient should avoid the rut of daily inactivity and despair.

Loss of Sensibility

RADIAL NERVE

The sensory loss resulting from division of the radial nerve has limited functional importance. The distribution of sensory innervation is on the dorsal radial aspect of the hand. Cross-innervation from the ulnar nerve frequently compensates to give protective sensibility. The greatest clinical problem along the sensory distribution of this nerve is the formation of a disabling neuroma in the distal third of the forearm. This propensity exists in any one of the several terminal branches, and is the reason that they are generally not repaired when divided. Lying in a vulnerable site, the distal radial nerve is frequently injured. Surgery in this area, most commonly in ganglionectomy and tenovaginotomy for de Quervain's tenosynovitis, has created some disabling neuromas (Fig. 8-7).

At times the skin innervated by this nerve is used for transfer of sensibility to the thumb as a neurovascular island[1] (Fig. 15-12).

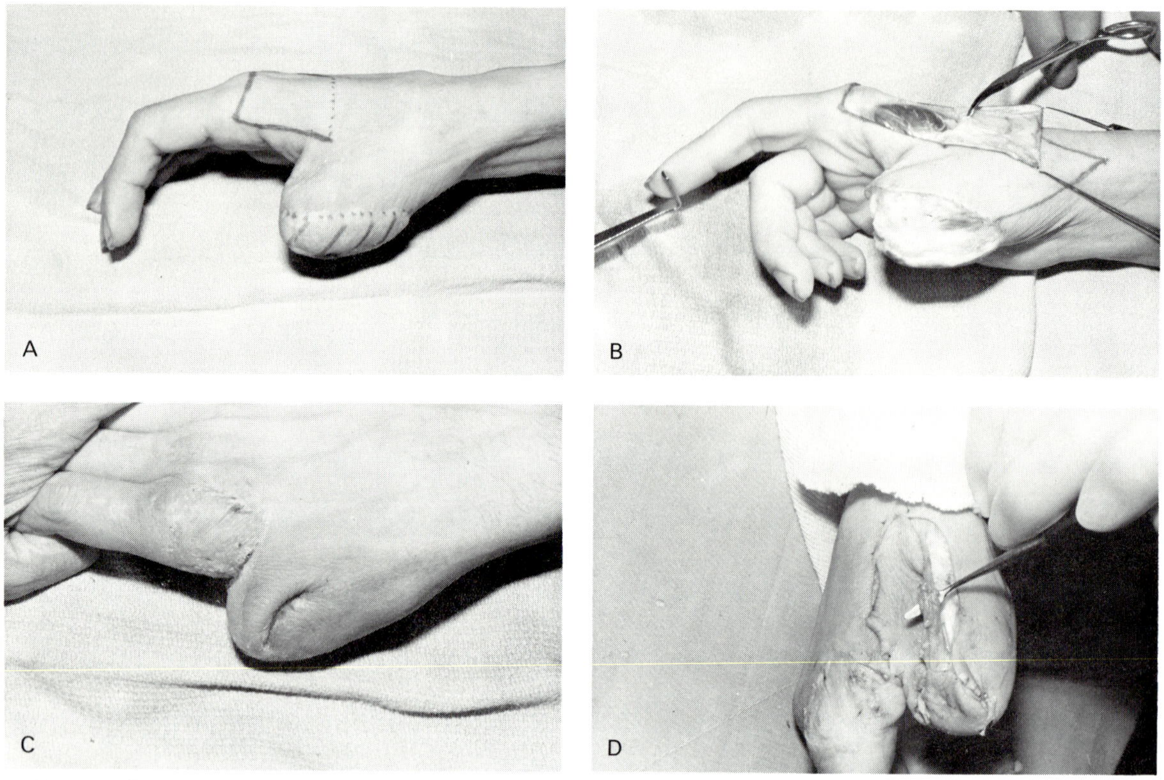

Figure 15-12. *Two-stage transfer of radially innervated pedicle from dorsum of index finger to tip of thumb. After the cutaneous flap is vascularized, the nerve is dissected proximally and transferred to a subcutaneous position on the thumb. The skin of the flap is divided and inset.*

When additional sources of nerve grafts are needed, this sensory nerve may be employed.

MUSCULOCUTANEOUS NERVE

The division of this nerve results in no appreciable functional loss of sensibility. It rarely, if ever, gives rise to a symptomatic neuroma. Its sensory component, the lateral antebrachial cutaneous nerve of the elbow and forearm, is a potential source of nerve grafts.

MEDIAN NERVE

The most important sensory distribution of the hand is vested in this nerve. The importance of its sensibility generally demands surgical repair. When paralyzed there is "blindness" of the radial two-thirds of the palm and the working surfaces of the thumb, index and long fingers. The distal two phalanges of the index and long fingers are invariably deprived of all sensibility. As such, they are frequently traumatized by daily use (Fig. 15-3). Burns from cigarettes held between them are exceedingly common. The fingertips of lepers lacking sensibility succumb to trophic ulcers.

All levels of this nerve have a propensity for developing symptomatic and disabling neuromata. When they occur at the level of the wrist, palm and digits, they may cause permanent disability. The palmar cutaneous branch is the cause of a disabling neuroma equal in magnitude to the radial nerve mentioned above (Fig. 15-8). This often tiny nerve falls prey to accident and intraoperative trauma in the region of the tubercle of the navicular. It is the reason why incisions crossing the wrist should zigzag to the ulnar rather than to the radial side.

ULNAR NERVE

The sensory importance of this nerve is its innervation of the ulnar side of the hand. Its dorsal branch presents some of the same types of problems described for the radial nerve but to a much lesser degree. More often, the most troublesome neuromata are found about the elbow and the volar-ulnar digital nerve to the little finger.

Transfer of Sensibility by a Neurovascular Island Pedicle

When there is no other means of restoring sensibility to a digit such as the thumb or index that critically requires it, a neurovascular island pedicle may be undertaken. This technique makes it possible to transfer a patch of padded skin on a neurovascular pedicle from an area of lesser functional importance. Thus, nearly normal sensibility and sweat can be restored to a "blind" thumb or index. The source of the pedicle may be a digit requiring amputation (Fig. 17-11), or the least functional side of a normal finger, such as the ulnar side of the ring or long finger. These pedicles are usually transferred at the time of secondary reconstructive surgery, but have been used at times for resurfacing at the time of injury.

The technique depends upon the surgeon's ability to elevate the digital artery, nerve and vena comitantes into a sufficiently long stalk to permit the transfer without tension or kinking. An anomaly limiting the length of the artery must be anticipated. Hence, the dissection of the pedicle should always begin in the palm to ascertain that an adequate artery reaches the superficial arch. The commitment to complete the rest of the dissection is made only after assurance of adequate length. Preoperative arteriography may be helpful in determining the feasibility of this procedure (Fig. 15-13).

Exposure of the pedicle is through a zigzag incision in the palm in continuity with a midaxial incision in the digit. Under tourniquet control and magnification, the dissection starts in the palm at the level of the superficial arterial arch and proceeds retrograde. All of the tiny branches of the vascular stalk are coagulated or ligated with 8-0 nylon except at the yoke of the common volar digital artery. Here great care is exercised to ligate the limb of the yoke upon the adjacent digit using 6-0 nylon without encroachment upon the neurovascular stalk of the island. The epineurium of the common volar digital nerve may have to be split. This is done with great precision back to the level of the superficial arch.

After the stalk has been developed in the palm, the size of the island needed is mapped out. First, the recipient site is outlined and denuded. The excised skin is defatted and used as a template to outline the donor island. If this template is of satisfactory quality, it may be used subsequently as a full-thickness skin graft to the donor site. The decision must then be made whether or not to release the tourniquet for 10 to 15 minutes before proceeding with the dissection of the island. It is a distinct advantage to have tourniquet control from the moment of elevation of the island until it is sutured in place and the dressing has been applied. Release of the tourniquet before this point invariably results in congestion of the graft, making it progressively more difficult to seat and to close the wound around it.

The island is raised by incising the skin with a #15 scalpel. Holding the margin with stay sutures, it is dissected out, dividing the fascia with fine scissors. The full thickness of the digital fat pad should be freed from its bed with the skin and should not be traumatized by the dissection. Once the pedicle is raised, it is transferred to the recipient site.

The recipient digit may be opened in the same way as the donor digit and the two incisions joined in the palm. If possible, however, it is preferred to separate these incisions with a bridge of palmar skin which is tunneled beneath to accommodate the island pedicle. The passage of the pedicle through the tunnel must be accomplished without any compression, tension or twisting. This is facilitated by moistening the wound and the pedicle, by controlling the island with proximal and distal stay sutures and, in some instances, by carrying out the transfer within a moistened silicone or rubber drain.

The island is sutured in place with a minimum number of nylon sutures. This allows the egress of blood and serum from the wound into the wet dressing which is then applied.

The wound of the donor finger is covered with a thick split-thickness skin graft or the defatted skin previously used as a template from the recipient finger. A moistened, tied-down dressing (Stent) is applied to immobilize the graft. The digits are gently compressed against a soft roll of wet gauze for 3 to 5 minutes after the tourniquet is released and prior to application of the cast. Immobilization is maintained for at least a week, but the pedicle should be inspected within 2 to 4 hours and daily for the first 2 or 3 days.

With attention to these details, there is assurance of functional success with good sweating and two-point discrimination of about 4 mm. Lesser

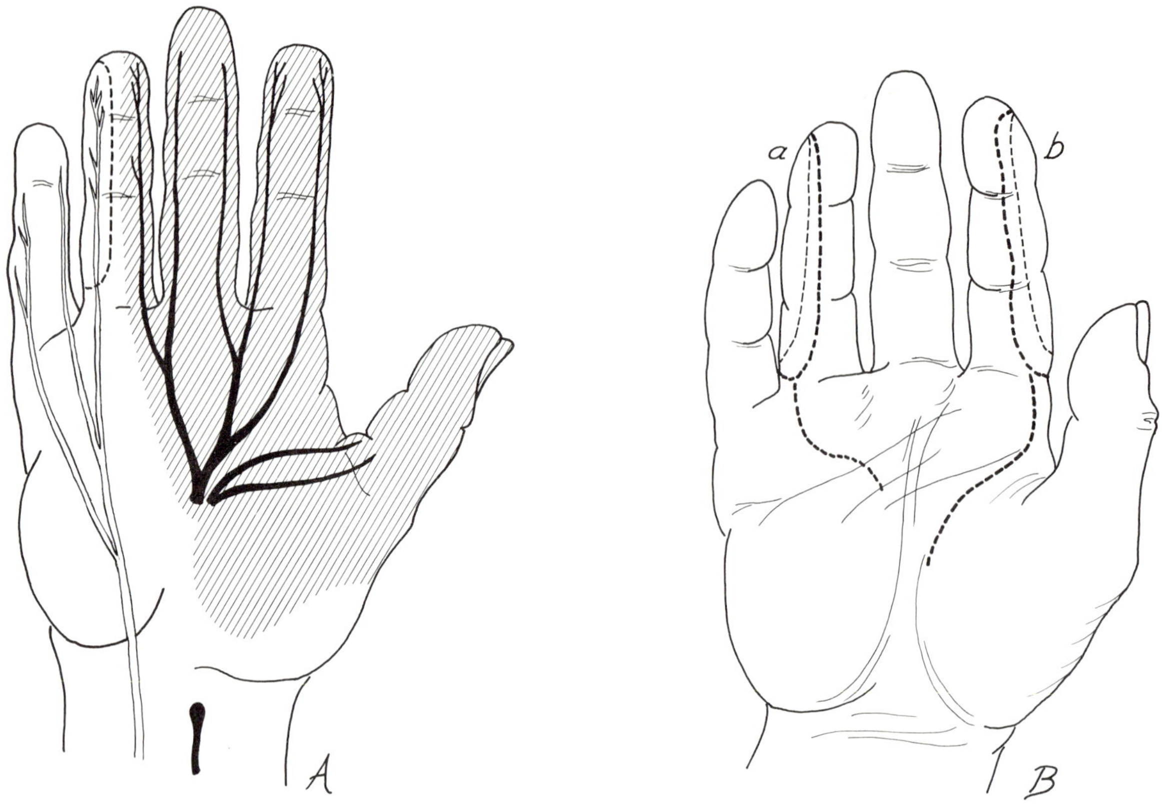

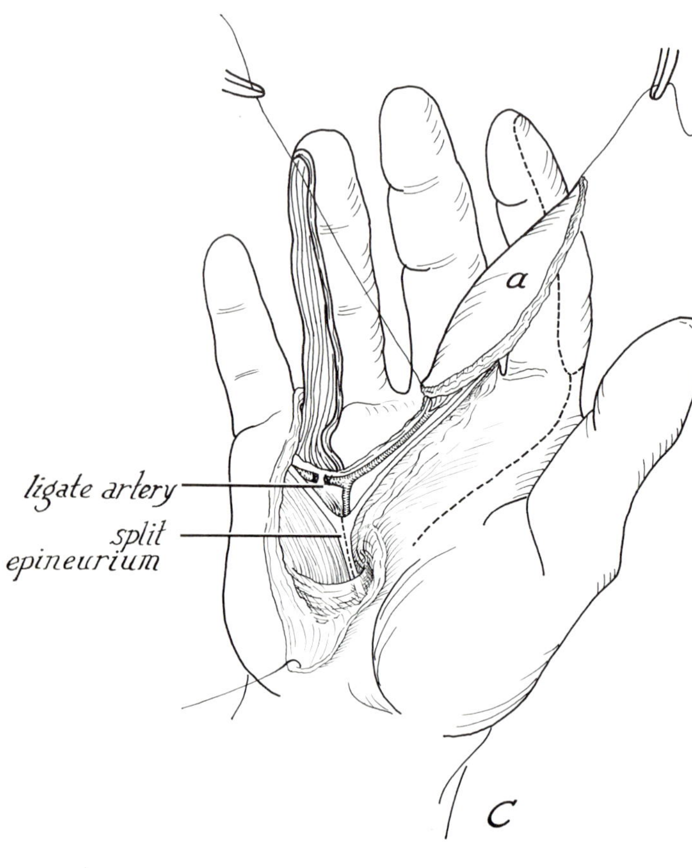

Figure 15-13. *An example of restoring sensation to the index finger (prime manipulating digit) by an island pedicle flap to treat irreversible median nerve loss. (Redrawn from Chase, R.A.:* Atlas of Hand Surgery. *W. B. Saunders, Philadelphia, 1973.)*

epicritic sensibility can be transferred by a pedicle flap, e.g. flag flap from the skin innervated by the radial nerve. Such transfers are usually made to the thumb (Fig. 15-12). Even though the cortical registration of these sensory islands never completely shifts to their new geographical location, the functional value of the transfer remains.

Neuromas

Neuromas result from nerve injury and may occur within an intact nerve (neuroma in continuity) or at the proximal end of a divided nerve (stump neuroma). A neuroma consists of disorganized axons interwoven with scar of variable quantity and quality. This scar can virtually "choke" the nerve and close off the avenues for axonal regeneration. The neuroma of a sensory nerve may be the source of painful stimuli regardless of its size or location. The neuromas that cause disabling pain are usually at pressure points, or are subjected to tension within dense immobile scar. Sometimes neuromas enlarge insidiously with or without symptoms. At times symptoms do not develop until years after injury. This is particularly true of the median nerve at the wrist.

The meticulous surgeon does his best to minimize neuromas by strict adherence to the following principles:

1. Preservation of the integrity of a well-vascularized soft tissue bed around the site of injury to a nerve.
2. Utilization of the techniques of neurorrhaphy previously described.
3. Proper placement of the proximal stump of a divided nerve. This must always be free of edema, and in a bed of healthy fat or muscle, and never overlying a prominence where it can be compressed.

A nerve stump should never be cut flush with the end of the bone in amputations. Keeping the nerve long will facilitate the transfer of its stump into a protecting bed. A good example of this is the transfer of digital nerves of the index finger into the substance of the first dorsal interosseous muscle during an index ray resection. If transfer of the stump is not feasible, an alternative solution is placement of the stump inside the marrow cavity of the adjacent bone. This requires a sufficiently large hole in the bone to prevent any constriction or tension on the nerve. A terminal neuroma that is symptomatic need not always be resected when the nerve is transferred. If the nerve is sectioned, the end should be ligated with 5-0 nylon.

When the nerve stump in question is too close to the parent nerve to allow relocation, capping the nerve with a silicone sleeve should be considered. An alternative or adjunctive method which may help reduce the amount of scar and neuroma formation is the local injection of 2 to 5 mg of triamcinolone around the nerve stump at the time of nerve ligation.[31] An injection of absolute alcohol within the nerve sheath after its ligation has brought relief of pain in some intractable cases. Very small amounts should be used to avoid the flow proximally into the normal parent nerve.

Before deciding to operate on a painful neuroma the physician must be sure that the patient has conscientiously tried to reduce his misery by percussing the neuroma. This is a "toughening up" phenomenon which works empirically. Prior to operative intervention 5 mg of triamcinolone may be injected around the site of the neuroma after establishing an effective nerve block. This may be repeated up to three times at 1- to 3-week intervals. The patient should be warned of the occasional depigmentation of the skin and atrophy of the subcutaneous fat that may be produced.

Repeated surgery by qualified surgeons for painful neuromata is contraindicated and serves to reinforce the patient's psychological fixation on his pain. One procedure well done must be considered adequate surgical therapy for the relief of his pain. If the pain continues, it must be made clear to him that the control of pain is beyond the providence of surgical treatment, and the patient must learn to live with it. If disability settlement is an issue, it must be promptly rated. Activity in the form of work does more to distract the patient from his awareness of pain and reduce his anxiety over it than any form of treatment or medical compassion.

A neuroma of the sensory branch of the radial nerve about the distal third of the forearm and the wrist is one of the most common and symptomatically intractable. It often develops following trivial trauma and surgery by inexperienced operators. It usually is most symptomatic in the forearm but has been sensitive enough to require surgical treatment at the level of the proximal phalanx of the digits it innervates.

Other locations of particularly troublesome symptomatic neuromata are: (1) the main median nerve and the palmar cutaneous branch at the wrist, (2) the main ulnar nerve and its dorsal sensory branch at the wrist, (3) the branches of the median and ulnar nerves in the palm and digits and (4) the ulnar nerve at the elbow.

Injuries to Pure Motor Nerves

The pure motor nerves are the posterior interosseous nerve of the radial, the volar interosseous nerve of the median nerve, the deep motor branch of the ulnar nerve and the recurrent motor branch of the median nerve. Any of these may be specifically injured by discrete penetrating wounds. All are difficult to repair primarily because of their anatomical depth, the frequent coexistence of marked bleeding, and, in the case of the nerves to the intrinsic muscles, their small size.

The deep motor branch of the ulnar nerve can be considered the most important to repair since it is the most difficult for which to compensate. The alternative to motor nerve repair is tendon transfer.

Tendon Transfers

Tendon transfer means to take a musculotendinous unit and alter its natural function by adding to that function or shifting that function to a new role. The latter often requires a geographical displacement of the unit. Transfer achieves the following: (1) restores voluntary movement to one or more joints, (2) stabilizes one or more joints by rendering an antagonist to existing muscle power, (3) adds power in the face of weakness, (4) restores basic prehensile function and (5) restores manipulative function and dexterity.

The conditions that may be improved by transfers are:

1. Nerve palsy. Most transfers are undertaken to compensate for the functional loss imposed by partial or complete paralysis of one or more of the major peripheral nerves.
2. Muscle deficits. The second most common need for transfers is to replace the loss of function incurred by the physical or functional absence of one or more musculotendinous units. Physical absence is seen congenitally and as a result of surgical resection or avulsion injuries. Deficits can also result from irreversible retraction of divided musculotendinous units, e.g. old rupture of the extensor pollicis longus.
3. Spastic states. These problems of imbalance are caused by central nervous system disorders.

The prerequisites for a successful transfer are:

1. The patient has a functional need for the intended reconstruction, understands the problem, and is willing to make the effort to achieve success.
2. The joints to be acted upon have a satisfactory range of motion.
3. The soft tissue bed and the skin cover over it are adequate. There is a minimum of scar and a reasonable potential that the transfer will glide through the bed.
4. The transfer is expendable. Thus, the function lost because of the transfer is dispensable and the potential gain by it is worthy of any risk of failure.
5. It is capable of its new function. It will span the distance required with adequate amplitude (Table 15-1), power and, if need be, act independently.
6. It is chosen for its synergistic action. Whenever possible, transfers should be selected from among the following synergistic groups:
   a. wrist extensors, digital flexors and adductors
   b. wrist flexors, digital extensors and digital abductors.
7. The direction of its pull should be as much as possible in a straight line from muscle origin to tendon insertion in order to retain its efficiency and power. Accordingly, angles and pulleys should be avoided as much as possible.
8. The joints moved by the transfer and the skin over them should have enough sensibility to register motion.

Table 15-1. *Tendon Amplitude (effective range of muscle contraction)*

FLEXION	MILLIMETERS
Profundus and superficialis	60–70
Flexor pollicis longus	52
Flexor carpi radialis	40
Flexor carpi ulnaris	33
EXTENSION	
Extensor pollicis longus	58
Extensor communis and extensor indicis propius	55
Extensor carpi radialis longus and brevis	37
Extensor digiti quinti	35
Extensor pollicis brevis	28
Abductor pollicis longus	28
Extensor carpi ulnaris	37

Technical Considerations Relating to Tendon Transfers

Incisions must be planned to preserve the circulation and minimize scarring as well as to provide an adequate bed. Wherever possible flaps should be used, rather than incisions placed directly over the tendons, so that the skin wounds will be offset from the tendons. Whenever the transfer crosses the wrist, the ability to position this joint tests the effectiveness of the transfer and relieves tension on the transfer postoperatively. For this reason, if wrist fusion is indicated, it should be postponed until all tendon transfers have been completed and are working.

Pulleys are essential for the effective function of certain transfers. They direct the line of pull of a tendon and distribute the mechanical advantage of this pull if the transfer crosses more than one joint. Too many pulleys, however, increase the risk of tendon adherence. When a natural anatomical pulley is not available, an unyielding fascial band, tendon or bone may serve as a pulley. Adherence between the tendon and pulley will occur if: (1) the pulley is too tight, (2) raw surfaces are present and synovium is lacking and (3) tension on the transfer causes a point of pressure between the pulley and the tendon during healing.

The size of the tendon can cause difficulty. If it is too small and delicate for the demands upon it, rupture may result. If it is too large, it may be awkward to anchor because of its bulk and may become adherent in the sheath and pulley system.

Bone is the ideal anchoring point. Fixation to bone eliminates a tendon callus and adhesions along the body of the tendon where a smooth surface is needed for gliding. However, of necessity, many transfers involve stump-to-stump approximation or the interweaving of tendons. Under these circumstances, a satisfactory bed of fatty and areolar tissue free from constricting pulleys and fascia and raw periosteum is essential.

The ideal sources of tendon grafts for the prolongation of transfers are the palmaris longus or plantaris. However, any other dispensable tendon may be used.

Tendon transfers in spastic hands have excessive tension acting on the tendon wounds by virtue of the hyperactive muscles. The tendons must be anchored more securely than usual, but without compromising the surrounding circulation. The involuntary spasticity makes it difficult, and often impossible, to remove strain on the suture line by positioning the wrist.

Arthrodesis and tenodesis are used to complement tendon transfers, and may be substituted if suitable transfers are not available.

TIMING OF TRANSFERS

Transfers are considered under two circumstances: (1) a primary transfer at the time of injury when the likelihood of recovery from the loss seems very limited, and (2) after the passage of time when the irreversibility of the loss is unquestioned (Table 15-2). If the motor loss has a minimal impact on function or the potential tendon transfers can offer very little improvement in function, these procedures are not indicated. Transfers can be done immediately when there is a motor deficit through a loss of substance injury. However, in the case of nerve palsies, they are generally delayed until there is no reasonable hope of overcoming the paralysis by regeneration of the nerve.

To justify the transfer there has to be a reasonable hope of marked improvement in function. In the case of a low median nerve injury opponensplasty is often unnecessary (40 per cent or more of cases) because of innervation of sufficient pronating thenar muscles by the ulnar nerve. In the case of low ulnar nerve palsy, tightness of ligaments about the metacarpophalangeal joints of the ring and little fingers often prevents hyperextension. Clawing, therefore, is negligible, and there is no need for transfers.

Table 15-2. *Timing of Transfers in Nerve Palsy Following Neurorrhaphy (based on failure to show any evidence of recovery)*

Brachial plexus	6–12 months
Musculocutaneous	6 months
Radial	
High	6 months
Posterior interosseous	4 months
Median	
High	6 months
Anterior interosseous	4 months
Low	4 months
Ulnar	
High	6 months
Low	4 months

Before tendon transfers are undertaken, there must be satisfactory skeletal alignment, mobility of joints, adequate skin cover and sensibility, and muscle power of the intended transfer. To achieve this may require considerable time. Finally, the construction of tendon transfers must precede an intended fusion of the wrist.

Specific Transfers

HIGH RADIAL NERVE INJURY

To achieve elbow extension, the latissimus dorsi is mobilized from its insertion on the humerus and transferred down the arm to be inserted into the triceps. In lieu of this, the biceps tendon may be transferred posteriorly, provided there is an intact brachialis. Successful function with these transfers is difficult to achieve. Fortunately, gravity is frequently adequate for the needs of extension, although the elbow is flail when the arm is raised overhead.

The weakness of supination needs no correction as long as the biceps is intact. For wrist extension, the pronator teres is exposed through a longitudinal incision in the middle third of the radial aspect of the forearm and shaved off the radius. It is passed superficial to the brachioradialis and joined end to side to the extensor carpi radialis longus or brevis. The surfaces of the two tendons are scarified before they are joined.

For finger extension the flexor carpi ulnaris is transferred. A skin flap with an ulnar base is raised on the distal forearm. A short longitudinal incision exposes the tendon of the flexor carpi ulnaris, which is mobilized over a distance of 8 to 10 cm, avoiding injury to the ulnar nerve and artery. It is then transferred subcutaneously around the ulna and joined with the extensor communis proximal to the extensor retinaculum. Tension and the line of pull of this junction are critical. The four tendons of the extensor communis are held with a straight needle placed transversely as the flexor carpi ulnaris is threaded through them. The extensor digiti quinti is excluded from this transfer to avoid excessive extension and abduction of the little finger.

Thumb extension is achieved by transfer of the extensor pollicis longus radialward to join it with the palmaris longus. The latter is mobilized through two transverse incisions, one at the wrist and the other proximally at its musculotendinous junction. It is passed subcutaneously to join the extensor pollicis longus. If the palmaris longus is absent, thumb extension can be achieved by including the extensor pollicis longus in the common transfer to the flexor carpi ulnaris, leaving the flexor carpi radialis for wrist flexion. Immobilization with a long arm cast is required for four weeks. Isolated loss of the extensor pollicis longus can be corrected by transferring the extensor indicis proprius (Fig. 15-14).

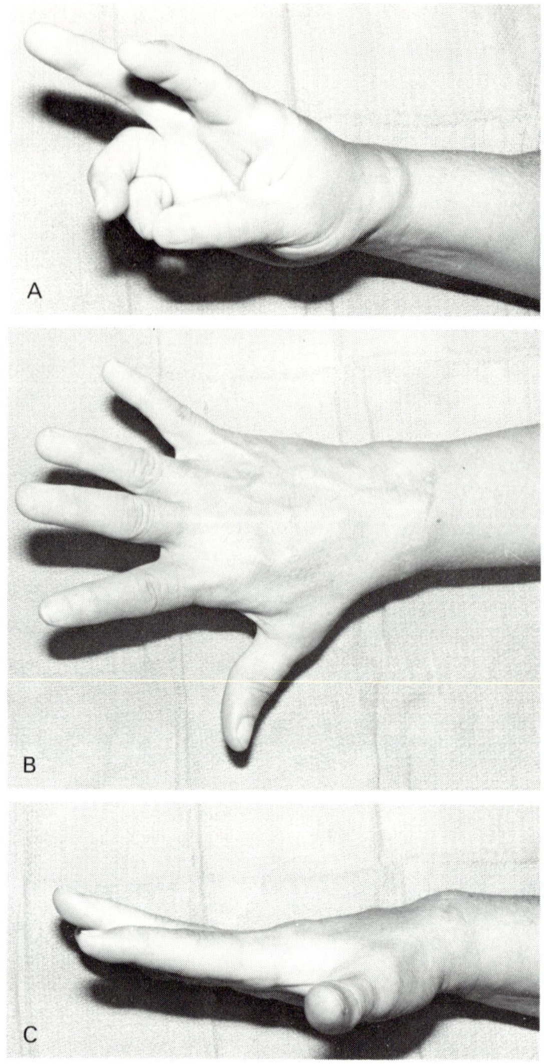

Figure 15-14. *Reconstruction of avulsed extensor pollicis longus by transfer of the extensor indicis proprius. Note three months after injury there is still a slight extensor lag of the index finger.*

LOW RADIAL NERVE INJURIES (POSTERIOR INTEROSSEOUS)[3,41]

Deficits	*Needs*	*Transfers*
Finger extension	Finger extension	Flexor carpi ulnaris to extensor communis
Thumb extension	Thumb extension	Palmaris longus to extensor pollicis longus
Radial wrist deviation	Radial wrist deviation	Pronator teres to abductor pollicis longus

Injury to the posterior interosseous nerve does not paralyze the extensor carpi radialis longus. Consequently, the pronator teres is available and can be transferred into the abductor pollicis longus for radial wrist deviation. The other transfers are the same as indicated previously for high radial nerve injuries.

The hand and arm are immobilized in a long-arm cast with the elbow flexed to 90°, the forearm pronated, the wrist fully extended and the fingers and thumb in the functional position in a boxing-glove splint. Splinting is discontinued and exercise begun at four weeks. This is generally a very successful transfer.

MUSCULOCUTANEOUS NERVE INJURIES

Deficits	*Needs*	*Transfers*
Elbow flexion	Elbow flexion	Steindler flexorplasty
Weak supination	None	None

To restore elbow flexion, the medial epicondyle with its forearm flexor muscle attachments is moved proximally on the humerus (Steindler flexorplasty).[24] A laterally based antecubital skin flap is used to expose the medial epicondyle and the ulnar nerve is liberated from the ulnar groove and the cubital tunnel. Then the median nerve is exposed. Both nerves are protected and retracted. A shaving of the medial epicondyle is removed with a knife in children and a chisel in adults. The flexor wad is mobilized distally off the elbow joint and ulna. The preservation of the branches of ulnar and median nerves limits this mobilization. The distal 5 to 7 cm of the humerus is bared laterally by splitting the fibers of the brachialis. With the elbow flexed to 45°, the highest point on the anterolateral aspect of the humerus that can be reached by the epicondylar bone plug is marked. A cortical hole is made to match it. The plug is secured in this hole with wire sutures into the humerus as the median nerve is retracted medially.

Immobilization is maintained for four weeks with a long-arm boxing-glove cast with the elbow flexed to 60° and the forearm fully supinated.

If preoperatively the patient can weakly flex the elbow with the shoulder abducted and the force of gravity neutralized, the prognosis for function from this procedure is good. Alternatives are transfers of the pectoralis major[10] or the sternocleidomastoid.[8]

HIGH MEDIAN NERVE INJURIES

Deficits	*Needs*	*Transfers*
Weak pronation	None	None
Weak wrist flexion	None	None
Partial loss of thumb flexion	Thumb flexion	Brachioradialis to flexor pollicis longus
Independent finger flexion	None	None
Index and long fingertip flexion	Finger flexion	Profundus II and III to profundus IV and V
Thumb pronation (opposition)	Opponensplasty	Extensor carpi ulnaris to rerouted extensor pollicis brevis or extensor carpi radialis longus to rerouted extensor pollicis brevis.

The anesthesia produced by this injury will have some bearing on the rate and quality of recovery. Forearm pronation, wrist flexion and thumb pronation (opposition) may all be possible despite the severity of this palsy. Forearm pronation is aided by gravity and the action of the brachioradialis. The flexor carpi ulnaris flexes the wrist and the thenar muscles, innervated by the ulnar nerve, pronate the thumb (40 per cent of cases).

The transfers available for opponensplasty after high median nerve injury are: (1) extensor carpi ulnaris or extensor carpi radialis longus to the abductor pollicis brevis,[32] (2) extensor indicis proprius, plus adductor pollicis transfer, and (3) the abductor digit quinti.[23]

The opponensplasty requires that the mean pull on the thumb ray corresponds to the direction of the fibers of the abductor pollicis brevis. Stripping the extensor pollicis brevis tendon out of its muscle belly in retrograde fashion to its insertion obviates the need for attaching a tendon transfer onto the thumb. Two incisions are necessary for this, one over the muscle belly in the forearm and one on the radial side of the metacarpophalangeal joint of the thumb. Injury to the radial nerve must be avoided and the full length of the tendon must be obtained. Before stripping it out, however, the extensor carpi radialis longus is dissected out and transferred. Its insertion is exposed through a short longitudinal incision and, with the stump in a clamp, it is divided and placed under alternating tension as its musculotendinous junction is palpated and exposed in a proximal counterincision. Another incision is made as a skin flap with a volar base over the ulnar styloid. The extensor carpi radialis longus is then withdrawn and transferred to this incision across the dorsum of the forearm. The extensor pollicis brevis is also stripped out and transferred subcutaneously over the thenar wad to join and be interwoven with the extensor carpi radialis longus. Passive wrist extension should fully pronate the thumb. Although its amplitude is only half that of the extensor carpi radialis longus, the extensor carpi ulnaris, divided at its insertion at the base of the fifth metacarpal and stripped out, is a useful substitute transfer for the extensor carpi radialis longus.

The extensor indicis proprius routed around the ulnar side of the wrist and across the thenar wad is another effective choice for opponensplasty. Its effectiveness is augmented by shifting the insertion of the adductor from the ulnar to the radial base of the proximal phalanx of the thumb.[7]

Opponensplasty with the abductor digiti quinti is technically the most intricate of the three procedures listed. Extreme care must be taken to identify and avoid injury to the neurovascular stalk of the muscle in dissecting it from its bed and off the pisiform bone. This stalk lies on the deep side of the muscle toward the heel of the hand. Properly done, the muscle is turned 170° like the page of a book so that as it overlies the thenar wad the neurovascular stalk is seen now on its superficial rather than deep aspect. Its two heads are interwoven with the tendon of the abductor pollicis brevis and its base remains attached to the flexor carpi ulnaris.[23]

The limitation of flexion of the thumb is only a loss of interphalangeal flexion and may be a relatively insignificant loss as long as the interphalangeal joint does not hyperextend. The adductor remains as a forceful flexor of the metacarpophalangeal joint. Hence, the choice is: doing nothing, activating the flexor pollicis longus with the brachioradialis, or fusing or tenodesing the interphalangeal joint in 15 to 20° of flexion. If the second choice is preferred, the incision should be longitudinal on the volar-radial aspect of the distal forearm. With due regard for the radial artery and nerve, the brachioradialis tendon is mobilized from the distal radius and transferred over the flexor pollicis longus. The two are scarified and sutured together. There should be adequate flexion of the interphalangeal joint upon passive wrist extension.

Paralysis of the long flexors of the index and long fingers is amenable to correction by the following means:

1. Attachment of the radial profundi to the ulnar profundi. The tendons to the long and index fingers should be separated from the parent muscle and from each other to allow adequate adjustment of tension during the transfer. In the case of the long finger an advancement of about 10 mm may be necessary.
2. Transfer of the brachioradialis into the profundus of the index and long fingers. An alternative is transfer of the brachioradialis into the profundus of the index to give it independent action. This use of the brachioradialis may necessitate stabilization of the distal joint of the thumb. Postoperative immobilization in a boxing-glove cast is required for 3 to 4 weeks. This should be a long-arm cast if the brachioradialis or long wrist extensors are transferred; otherwise only a forearm cast is needed.

MIDMEDIAN NERVE INJURIES (ANTERIOR OR VOLAR INTEROSSEOUS NERVE)

Deficits	*Needs*	*Transfers*
Thumb flexion (partial)	Distal joint stabilization	Tenodesis, arthrodesis
Index and long fingertip flexion	Digital flexion or distal joint stabilization	Profundi II and III to profundi IV and V. Tenodesis or arthrodesis

Most individuals will not be sufficiently disabled to want any reconstruction done with an isolated paralysis of the anterior interosseous nerve, which results in paralysis of the pronator quadratus, flexor pollicis longus, and profundus of the index and long fingers. If needs dictate, the following choices are available: (1) tenodesis or arthrodesis of the distal joint of the thumb, index and long fingers, (2) joining the radial two profundus tendons with the ulnar pair as described above, and (3) activating the flexor pollicis longus with the extensor carpi radialis longus.

LOW MEDIAN NERVE INJURY

Deficits	*Needs*	*Transfers*
Thumb pronation (opposition)	Opponensplasty	Extensor carpi radialis longus or extensor carpi ulnaris to rerouted extensor pollicis brevis Extensor indicis proprius with transfer of adductor Superficialis of ring[34] Abductor digiti quinti

The superficialis tendon is exposed through a lateral incision along the proximal phalanx and divided proximal to the vinculum longum at the point at which it is pierced by the profundus. This leaves a distal stump which is tethered proximally to the vinculum longum, preventing the development of a swan-neck deformity (recurvatum). It also prevents bleeding which follows sectioning of the vascular pedicles, the vincula. In order to withdraw the superficialis into the forearm, its decussation in the digit must be divided.

The forearm is entered through an incision which raises an ulnar-based skin flap. The superficialis tendon is withdrawn and transferred around the flexor carpi ulnaris near the pisiform, while the ulnar nerve and artery are protected. A third incision is made on the dorsal radial border of the thumb, exposing the extensor hood. The superficialis tendon is threaded subcutaneously on top of the abductor pollicis brevis and split into two tails. The ulnar tail is anchored on the dorsal ulnar aspect of the extensor hood over the metacarpophalangeal joint and the radial tail is threaded into the hood just distal to the joint. The length of this radial tail is fashioned so that it will extend the metacarpophalangeal joint fully before both tails begin to pronate the thumb.[5]

The disadvantages of opponensplasty using the superficialis tendon of the ring finger are: (1) loss of independent flexion of the ring finger with impairment in holding tools that require the thumb and index fingers to be free (a bitter postoperative complaint of some craftsmen, dentists, etc.), (2) secondary swan-neck deformity of the ring finger, and (3) secondary stiffness with limitation of extension of the ring finger.

Postoperative care is the same as has been described for reconstructive procedures after high median nerve injury.

HIGH ULNAR NERVE INJURY

Deficits	*Needs*	*Transfers*
Weak ulnar wrist deviation	None	None
Ring and little fingertip flexion	Fingertip flexion or stabilization	Profundi IV and V to profundus III. Tenodesis or arthrodesis
Adduction of fingers	Adduction of little	Extensor digiti quinti to radial lateral band of little finger
Abduction of fingers	Abduction of index	Extensor indicis proprius to radial lateral band of index finger
Adduction of thumb	Adduction of thumb	Extensor indicis proprius (or brachioradialis) for thumb adduction

Since clawing may not occur with high ulnar nerve paralysis, there may be no need for any transfers. The basis for reconstruction is to correct the imbalance of the thumb created by the adductor paralysis and to correct the abduction stance of the little finger. In addition the index finger may need a transfer to replace the first dorsal interosseous, thereby improving the dynamics of pinch.

The suitable transfers for these problems are:

1. The extensor indicis proprius is routed around the ulnar side of the index metacarpal and attached to the adductor tendon of the thumb. This is done through two small incisions. The first is on the dorsum of the head of the index metacarpal where the extensor indicis proprius is divided as it joins the extensor hood. The second is a zigzag incision on the dorsum of the thumb web, giving access to the extensor indicis proprius and the adductor pollicis tendon. The former is threaded between the index and long metacarpals and over the surface of the adductor to its tendon, where it is anchored.

2. In substituting for the first dorsal interosseous the extensor indicis proprius is shifted from the ulnar side of the hood to the radial side. When this is the case, adductorplasty of the thumb must be done in another way. Two procedures have merit:
   a. The Boyes transfer of the brachioradialis lengthened by a tendon graft.[4] This is routed in the same fashion as the extensor indicis proprius tendon using either the index or long metacarpal as the pulley.
   b. The Royle-Thompson transfer using the superficialis to the ring finger.[36] In this procedure the superficialis tendon is mobilized in the ring finger as described for opponensplasty but instead of bringing it out in the forearm it is brought out in the palm and tunneled over the thenar muscles. The two tails are anchored to the thumb in the same fashion as with the Brand opponensplasty technique.[5]

The abduction stance of the little finger can be corrected by transfer of the extensor digiti quinti. Through a longitudinal incision over the dorsum of the space between the little and ring metacarpals the extensor digiti quinti is severed from the extensor hood. It is transferred volar to the intervolar plate ligament. This ligament becomes the pulley as the extensor digiti quinti acts on the radial intrinsic band of the little finger to which it is attached.

Whenever the proprius tendons are used for transfers, all possible length must be achieved by splitting the dorsal aponeurosis to free the tendon. The aponeurosis is then repaired. Postoperative management is routine as described for the previous transfers. If the loss of tip flexion of the ring and little fingers is troublesome, this can be treated by joining the profundus tendons of these digits to that of the adjacent long and index fingers in the distal forearm.

LOW ULNAR NERVE INJURY

Deficits	*Needs*	*Transfers*
Clawing of ring and little fingers	Correct clawing	Extensor carpi radialis longus via carpal tunnel prolonged through lumbrical canal to lateral bands
Adduction of fingers	Correct clawing	Extensor carpi radialis longus via carpal tunnel prolonged through lumbrical canal to lateral bands
Abduction of fingers	Abduction of index	Extensor indicis proprius to radial lateral band
Adduction of thumb	Adduction of thumb	Extensor indicis proprius or brachioradialis

The problems and treatments remain the same as those for the high ulnar nerve lesion except that clawing is more apt to occur. The correction of clawing may be done in one of two ways:

1. The extensor digiti quinti is transferred as described for high ulnar palsy. The difference here is that the tendon is split and one tail goes to the radial lateral band of the little finger and the other to the radial lateral band of the ring finger. Both pass through separate tunnels in their respective intermetacarpal spaces and the intervolar plate ligaments serve as pulleys.
2. The extensor carpi radialis longus is divided at its insertion, retracted into the forearm and transferred subcutaneously around the radial side of the forearm toward the carpal tunnel. After it is lengthened by a palmaris graft split into two tails, it is passed through the carpal tunnel deep to all the tendons. The tails are threaded along the lumbrical canals to the lateral bands of the little and ring fingers to which they are secured. By positioning the wrist in 45° of passive extension, the metacarpophalangeal joints should be drawn into 50 to 70° of flexion if the tension of this transfer has been correctly adjusted. Postoperative care is the same as that for other similar transfers.

COMBINED HIGH MEDIAN AND ULNAR NERVE INJURY

Deficits	*Needs*	*Transfers*
Weak pronation	None	None
Wrist flexion	None	None
Digital flexion	Digital flexion	Extensor carpi radialis longus to thumb. Extensor carpi ulnaris to fingers

Deficits	*Needs*	*Transfers*
Thumb pronation	Opponensplasty	Extensor indicis proprius for adduction. Extensor pollicis brevis anterior to abduct thumb
Clawing	Correction of clawing	Brachioradialis with many-tailed graft

The massive functional sensory and motor loss imposed by this injury requires a careful study of the patient's adaptability and the results of staged procedures before performing further surgery. It is impossible to do more than restore basic function in most instances. The success of functional restoration depends upon the simplicity of the plan for it and the proper timing of the procedures. What is hoped for is the restoration of at least a "key" pinch and basic grasp. Arthrodeses may help to simplify the hand. However, this is rarely necessary or advisable for the wrist, the function of which is indispensable in most instances to augment the effectiveness of transfers.

The long extensors are available for transfer. The centrally placed extensor carpi radialis brevis, however, should be spared for wrist stabilization and extension. Standard transfers consist of the extensor carpi ulnaris routed around the ulnar side of the distal forearm to join the profundi and flex the fingertips. The extensor carpi radialis longus is routed radially around the forearm to the flexor pollicis longus. Pronation of the thumb can be achieved by routing the extensor pollicis brevis volarly through a midwrist pulley (palmaris longus).[6]

The extensor indicis proprius is used for adductorplasty as previously described. The brachioradialis, together with a tendon graft split into four tails, is passed through the carpal tunnel and along the lumbrical canals to the radial intrinsic bands of the long, ring and little fingers and to the ulnar lateral band of the index finger. This overcomes clawing.

The hyperextension of the metacarpophalangeal joints of the fingers that leads to the claw deformity can be corrected in a static way by tethering the joints in some flexion. The method of Zancolli of excising part of the volar plate and advancing the remainder to bring the metacarpophalangeal joint into 30° of flexion has had limited success.[43]

Another technique is to tether the superficialis at two levels, one to the pulley system of the proximal phalanx and the other to the transverse carpal ligament so that the metacarpophalangeal joints are slightly flexed. If further stabilization and control are needed, the metacarpophalangeal joint of the thumb and the distal joints of the fingers may be arthrodesed or tenodesed at the best angle to achieve the desired improvement in function.

LOW COMBINED MEDIAN AND ULNAR NERVE PALSY

Deficit	*Needs*	*Transfers*
Clawing	Correct clawing	Extensor carpi radialis longus
Thumb adduction	Adductorplasty	Extensor indicis proprius
Thumb pronation	Opponensplasty	Extensor pollicis brevis
Weak thumb flexion	Stabilize	Arthrodesis of interphalangeal joint

The imbalance of the thumb is correctable by: an adductorplasty using the extensor indicis proprius and the index metacarpal as its pulley, an opponensplasty by transferring the extensor pollicis brevis around a midwrist pulley (palmaris longus), and active metacarpophalangeal joint flexion of the thumb via the flexor pollicis longus by fusing the interphalangeal joint.

The clawing of the fingers is corrected with a four-tailed graft to the extensor carpi radialis longus via the carpal tunnel, with each tail going to an intrinsic band volar to the intervolar plate ligament. This should be the radial lateral band for the long, ring and little fingers but the ulnar lateral band of the index finger so that the fingers will adduct as well as flex at the metacarpophalangeal joint.

COMBINED RADIAL AND MEDIAN NERVE INJURY

Deficits	*Needs*	*Transfers*
Wrist and digital extension	Wrist and digital extension	Flexor carpi ulnaris
Index and long finger flexion	Index and long flexion	Profundus II and III to profundus IV and V
Thumb pronation	Opponensplasty	Abductor digiti quinti
Instability thumb tip	Stabilize	Tenodesis or arthrodesis

In combined radial and median nerve palsy, if the lesions are high, the only motors left are the two ulnar profundi, the flexor carpi ulnaris and 15 intrinsic muscles. With transfer of the flexor carpi ulnaris dorsally, all the digital extensors may be activated. Thumb flexion and possibly some pronation exist by virtue of the adductor acting on the metacarpophalangeal joint and action of some of the thenar muscles innervated by the ulnar nerve. If an opponensplasty is needed, the abductor digiti quinti is available. When needed, tenodesis or arthrodesis can stabilize the distal joint of the thumb. Finger flexion can be achieved by joining the radial profundi to the ulnar profundi. If necessary, the wrist can be stabilized with an external splint.

If the radial nerve palsy is combined with a low median nerve palsy, the flexor pronator system is intact and available for dispensable motors to correct the radial palsy.

COMBINED RADIAL AND ULNAR NERVE INJURY

Deficits	*Needs*	*Transfers*
Wrist extension	Wrist extension	Pronator teres to extensor carpi radialis brevis
Digital extension	Digital extension	Flexor carpi radialis
Ulnar clawing	Correct clawing	Zancolli capsulodesis and middle joint arthrodesis
Thumb adduction	None	None

If there is a combined radial and ulnar nerve palsy, the pronator teres may be transferred for wrist extension and the flexor carpi radialis for thumb and finger extension. The interphalangeal joint of the thumb can be fused, allowing the flexor pollicis longus to act as a metacarpophalangeal joint flexor and adductor. The clawing of the ring and little finger may need to be corrected by static measures (Zancolli capsulodesis, proximal interphalangeal joint arthrodesis).

In cases of overwhelming paralytic involvement of two or more major nerves, it has been possible to restore basic prehension with a combination of functional tenodesis, digital joint fusions and appropriate reassignment of function to available musculotendinous units. The mobility of the wrist is of the greatest importance under these circumstances. It is possible, therefore, to have gravity flex the wrist so that extensor tenodesis in the forearm will open the hand. A single wrist extensor combined with appropriate functional fusion of interphalangeal joints and tenodesis of the long flexors in the forearm can bring about a useful degree of grasp.

Nowhere in the surgery of the hand are the ingenuity of the surgeon and his ability to program treatment adaptively more crucial to function than in these cases of paralysis (Fig. 15-15).

Compression States of Nerves

All the major nerves of the upper extremity are subject to the effects of compression, given the appropriate circumstances. This state has been variously referred to as constriction or entrapment. The process is mechanical and may be acute or chronic and intermittent or progressive. The clinical manifestations depend on the acuteness and the severity of the compression. The rapid progression of symptoms and signs must be treated as an urgent problem. Chronic states should be mechanically relieved before the changes in the nerve become irreversible.

The mechanical aspects involve, for the most part, a disproportion between the size of the nerve and the space around it. Such disproportion can result from congenital anatomical factors, conges-

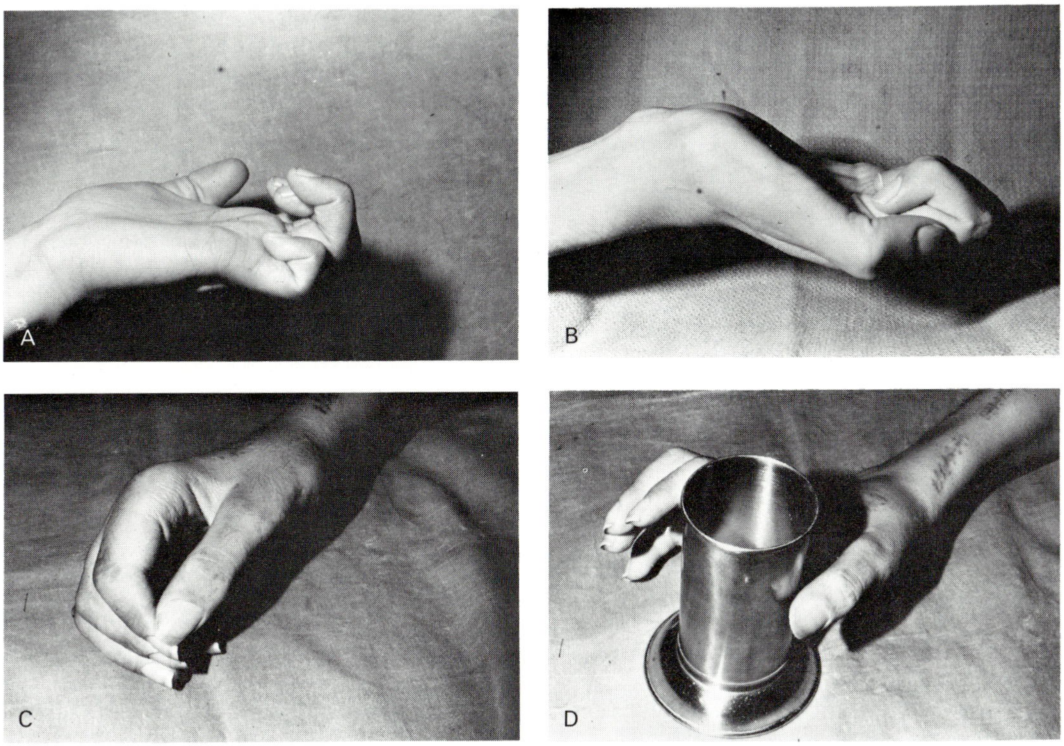

Figure 15-15. *Reconstruction of long-established claw deformity by distal and proximal interphalangeal joint arthrodesis and transfer of extensor carpi radialis longus into the transposed extensor pollicis brevis for opposition—"restoration of function by simplification."*

tive changes in the extremity, traumatic deformities (dislocation and angulation), cicatrix, secondary changes of aging often referred to as "rheumatic changes" and space-occupying lesions.

The pathological state in the nerve is initially one of neuropraxia, which unattended may steadily increase and result in intractable axonotmesis.

Median Nerve Compression

The most common entrapment of the median nerve occurs in the carpal canal, causing the carpal tunnel syndrome. Elsewhere the nerve can be trapped as it traverses the pronator teres muscle in the proximal forearm or beneath the ligament of Struthers in the distal arm. Its deep volar interosseous branch can be trapped by the superficialis sling in the midforearm. Individual branches in the hand and digits can also be compressed.

CARPAL TUNNEL SYNDROME

The median nerve, the softest and most volar structure in the carpal canal, is brought against the transverse carpal ligament, especially when there is forceful digital flexion with simultaneous wrist flexion. The nine long flexor tendons, when tensed, compress the median nerve against this ligament.

Typically, the patient notes paresthesias and numbness over the distribution of the nerve. These subjective complaints spare the little finger. Pain may radiate to the shoulder, neck or chest. The patient is often awakened from a sound sleep. The same symptoms may develop after repetitive vigorous gripping or after acute wrist flexion (Phalen's test[33]). There may or may not be weakness, softness or atrophy of the thenar musculature. The clinical test for this is forceful tip-to-tip pinch between the thumb and ring finger which should produce a "golf-ball hard" contraction of the abductor pollicis brevis (Fig. 15-16). Roentgenograms of the wrist should be taken whenever there is the slightest question of a skeletal derangement which might precipitate this condition. This often requires that the wrists be compared and that the projection include "carpal tunnel views."

Two-point discrimination and blindfold pick-up testing may be impaired. Judicious employment of well-executed sensory and motor nerve conduction and electromyographic studies may be used to

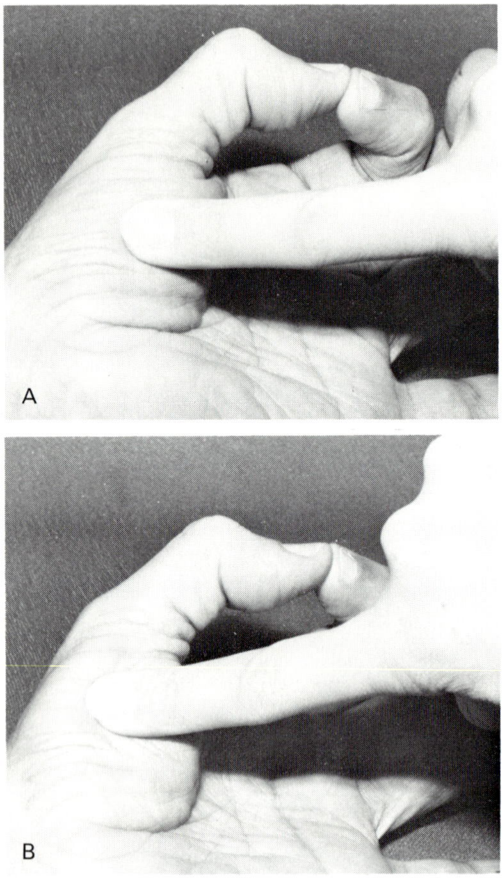

Figure 15-16. *Demonstration of the normal "golf-ball hard" thenar wad* **(A)** *in comparison to the soft indentable denervated musculature following median nerve injury* **(B).**

confirm the existence or non-existence of this condition when the clinical impression is in question.

Water retention plays a prime physiological role in the precipitation of symptoms.[29] This distends the transverse carpal ligament and swells the tendons and median nerve beneath it. Hence, the classic symptomatology that wakens the patient at night is due to the stagnation and accumulation of tissue fluid. Relief comes from elevation and exercise, which milk away the offending fluid.

The condition is most commonly idiopathic in postmenopausal women. It concomitantly exists with other manifestations of aging in the musculoskeletal system. It must be anticipated as a sequel to wrist fracture, dislocations and crushing injuries as well as any condition causing massive forearm and hand swelling (burns, drug abuse, etc.). Other causes are musculoskeletal hypertrophy, repetitive effort, rheumatoid arthritis and synovitis and tumorous conditions within the canal (ganglion, lipoma, etc.). The most common developmental anomalies associated with this are a persistent median artery and anomalous intrinsic or extrinsic muscle bellies.

Treatment of Carpal Tunnel Syndrome. The treatment of the carpal tunnel syndrome is both operative and non-operative. The non-operative treatment is reserved for all cases in which there is no emergency and in which the sensory and motor impairment is not objectively demonstrable. The operative treatment is indicated whenever there is acute injury with rapidly progressing impairment of nerve function, chronic symptomatology with objective evidence of motor paresis and space-occupying lesions encroaching on the canal.

The modalities of non-operative treatment consist of cessation of the aggravating activity, splinting to prevent wrist flexion, elevation and the injection of the canal with triamcinolone. The operative treatment is section of the transverse carpal ligament with or without endoneurolysis and with or without reconstruction of the carpal ligament.

The injection of the carpal canal is done with the patient supine. The triamcinolone mixture is injected deep to the nerve, entering the carpal tunnel on the ulnar side of the palmaris longus tendon. Frequent aspiration ensures that vessels are not entered. The injection is given slowly and disseminated afterward by active digital movement while the surgeon compresses the wrist. *The nerve must not be injected.* The patient is also advised that a transient reactive "flare" of increased pain may occur after the effect of the lidocaine has worn off. Nearly all patients will obtain temporary relief of pain from the initial injection and about 40 to 50 per cent may be sufficiently improved by 2 or 3 injections so as to preclude the need for surgery. When symptomatology is limited to the sleeping period, a splint of the wrist should be worn during that time.

In considering operative treatment, the following points should be appreciated: (1) The usual temporary disability is one month and a bulky dressing will be required for 10 to 14 days. (2) There is postoperative wound pain of variable duration. (3) The tiny palmar cutaneous branch of the median nerve may give rise to a very painful postoperative neuroma if it has been injured. (4) Recovery of normal grip strength may be delayed for weeks, even months. In this regard, preoperative gripmeter readings should be recorded.

The essence of successful surgical technique is adequate visualization and adequate decompression. Blind surgery (through a transverse incision) leads to overriding and incomplete division of the ligament with persistence of the symptoms. It also risks the chance of cutting the median nerve or its branches.

The exposure requires an incision beginning at the midpalm along the ulnar side of the thenar crease (the linea vitalis) and in the distal 4 cm of the forearm (Fig. 6-8). When treating idiopathic carpal tunnel syndrome without thenar palsy, a 2.5-cm skin-fat bridge across the heel of the hand is left for its protective and cosmetic value. In all other cases, the proximal and distal wounds should be joined with a zigzag to the ulnar side at the wrist flexion crease, sparing the palmar cutaneous branch of the median nerve. This small sensory nerve leaves the radial side of the median nerve at varying distances proximal to the wrist flexion crease. Its detection is aided by the use of a magnifying loupe (Fig. 15-8).

Once the superficial tissues and palmar fascia are divided, the extremely tough transverse carpal ligament is sectioned on its ulnar aspect with heavy, blunt-nosed scissors or a knife if a groove director is placed to protect the median nerve. These instruments should be moistened and introduced in the canal with ease and without force. Division of the carpal ligament is complete when the nerve and tendons can be seen throughout their course in the canal. The portion of the ligament most commonly overridden and left intact is its distal limit. After complete division of the ligament, the surgeon's little finger should freely pass through the canal.

The recurrent motor branch of the median nerve must not be injured, and at the discretion of the surgeon may be specifically identified and decompressed. There are considerable variations in its size, point of origin and course after leaving the median nerve. At times it may even be a dual nerve[17] (Fig. 15-17).

The clear-cut indication for endoneurolysis is clinical evidence of palsy of the thenar musculature (abductor pollicis brevis). The muscle most often involved hugs the thumb metacarpal and during forceful thumb pronation is soft and hollow when it should be hard and full. This is inevitably accompanied by an hourglass deformity of the nerve and requires total exposure of the nerve (Fig. 15-18). Endoneurolysis is also indicated if the epineurium is thick, its vessel obliterated and the funiculi obscured, or if a zone of induration is discovered by palpation.[14]

The Technique of Endoneurolysis. Magnification is essential to the conduct of this meticulous procedure. Subepineurial Ringer's solution may be helpful in separating nerve bundles from connective tissue. This should be introduced with a 30-gauge needle slowly and without force. The epineurium should be tensed with microforceps while undermining and splitting it with fine-pointed microscissors. Neural vessels should be spared. The epineurial incision should not spiral about the nerve because of the possibility of injuring funiculi or vessels. The incision need only extend the length of the constriction. At the surgeon's discretion, epineurial stay sutures may be used, more than one slit made in the epineurium and triamcinolone instilled in the wound prior to closure. At the conclusion, the funiculi should be exposed like spaghetti. Other salient abnormalities are dealt with as the need arises. Space-consuming lesions should be removed e.g. boggy synovium, ganglion, tumor or displaced bones.

The ligament need not be biopsied, and may be reconstructed. This is done by developing reciprocal flaps with a distal base on one side and a proximal base on the other. These are sutured side by side across the tunnel with 5-0 nylon sutures. The product is a new ligament approximately 2 cm in width with adequate clearance for the contents of the tunnel (Fig. 15-19). This restores to some measure one of the stoutest ligaments of the body, the function of which is the maintenance of the transverse carpal arch and protection of the median nerve, as well as serving as a pulley for the flexor tendons.

Wound closure is done in a single layer. Postoperative splinting is done with a well-padded plaster forearm cylinder with the wrist in extension. The fingers are left free for immediate guarded motion. Some dressing is continued for 10 to 14 days.

Successful surgery is followed by immediate relief of the patient's subjective complaints, including the shoulder, neck, and chest pain that has been referred proximally.[9] Often these patients had mistakenly attributed their shoulder pain to bursitis. In the presence of an hourglass deformity of the nerve, a reversal of the muscle paralysis and return of normal sensibility cannot be expected. However, pain is invariably relieved.

The prognosis is guarded and the diagnosis may be in doubt in those patients who have not had some measure of immediate postoperative relief. Carpal tunnel decompression conducted according to the principles indicated above offers the maximal potential for surgical relief. Unless some new disorder develops there should be no grounds for further surgery if symptoms continue.

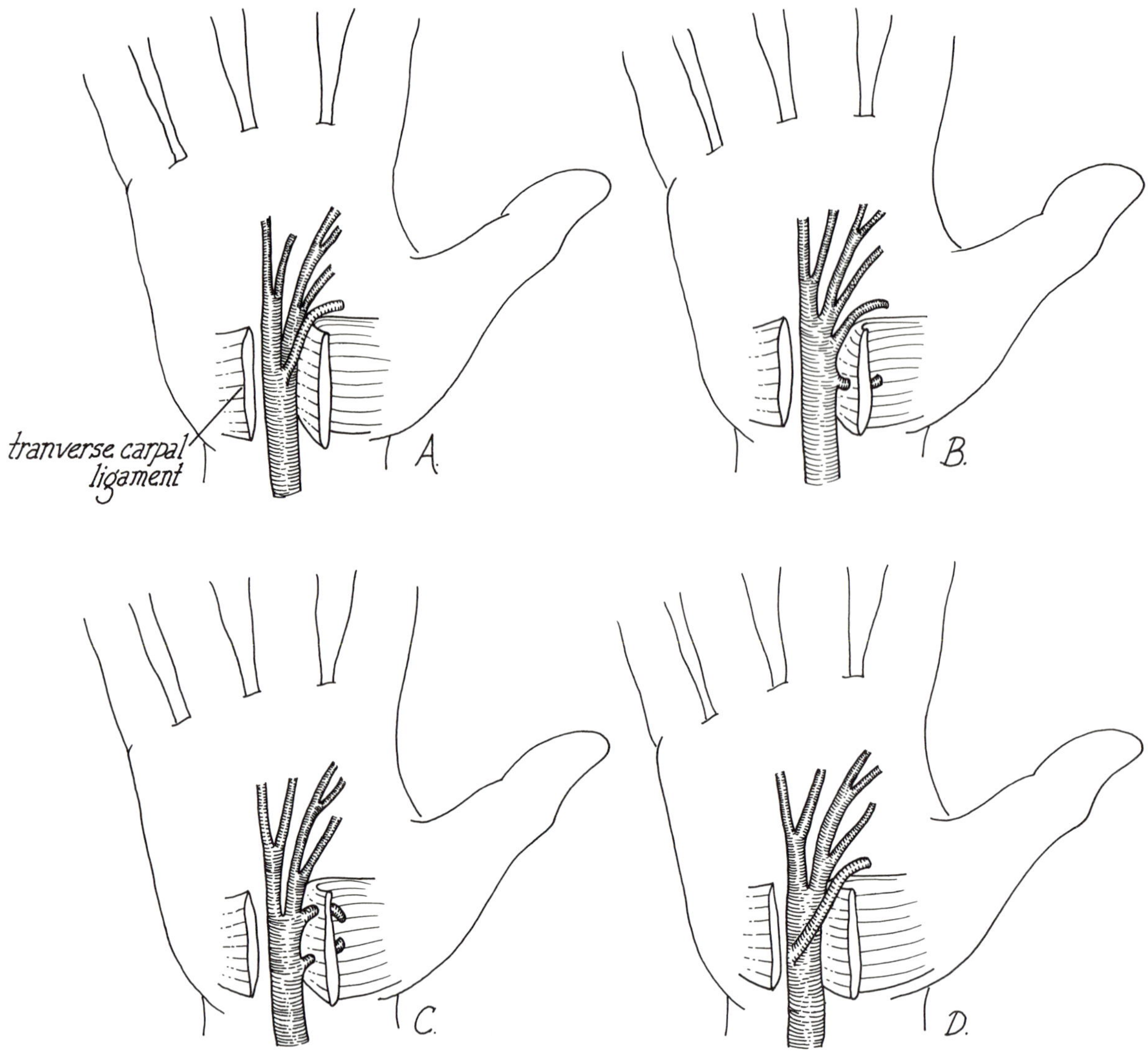

Figure 15-17. *Wide variations in the origins and path of the motor branch of the median nerve (dual, or arising from the ulnar side of the main nerve within the canal).* (*Redrawn from Graham, W.P.*[17])

The carpal tunnel syndrome that accompanies acute swelling and induration must be treated as an emergency (Fig. 15-7). The most common iatrogenic basis for this problem is inappropriate treatment of fractures and dislocations of the wrist: (1) overzealous mashing of tissues in achieving reduction, (2) inadequate reduction and (3) immobilization in the flexed position (Cotton-Loder position).

OTHER ENTRAPMENTS OF THE MEDIAN NERVE

Entrapment in the proximal forearm occurs where the median nerve passes through the substance of the pronator teres. Compression at this site results from marked congestion caused by severe trauma, cellulitis, compression by the body of a comotose patient, muscle hypertrophy and a congenital aponeurotic ring between the two heads of the muscle. Compression at this level probably has a greater incidence than is frequently recognized. It may be indistinguishable from the compression caused by the aponeurotic ring between the radial and ulnar heads of the superficialis muscle which lies just distal to the pronator tunnel and is the site of the anterior interosseous nerve syndrome. However, the entire median nerve will be involved at the level of the pronator.

The clinical manifestations of the pronator syndrome lacks the clear definition characteristic of the carpal tunnel syndrome. There is usually pain which may be poorly localized and may radiate

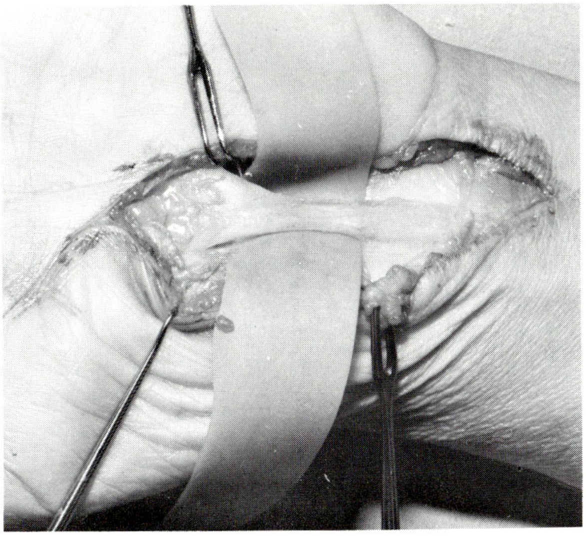

Figure 15-18. *Classic hourglass deformity of the median nerve in long-standing carpal tunnel compression.*

proximally and distally along the nerve. This may be accentuated by deep pressure on the pronator, which may feel tighter than normal. Tensing the pronator teres against resistance may precipitate and aggravate symptoms. There may or may not be dysesthesia and intrinsic weakness similar to the carpal tunnel syndrome, as well as paresis of the extrinsic muscles (the radial two profundi, the flexor pollicis longus and the superficialis). Electromyographic abnormalities with a sensory and motor conduction delay may be found.

Constriction at this level must be differentiated from constriction above the elbow in the rare instance of entrapment of the nerve beneath the ligament of Struthers. This ligament bridges the hollow between the supracondylar process and the medial condyle of the humerus.[22] Compression here will add paralysis of the pronator teres to the previously mentioned signs. The lacertus fibrosis must be divided and attention given to securing adequate hemostasis in dissecting under the pronator teres and the superficialis.

Entrapment of the volar (anterior) interosseous nerve occurs at the level of the aponeurotic bridge joining the humeral and radial heads of origin of the superficialis muscle. Entrapment here may spare the rest of the median nerve in which case the clinical findings are limited to motor palsy *without* any sensory disturbance. The muscles affected are the profundus to the index and long fingers, the flexor pollicis longus and the pronator quadratus. The pronator quadratus is tested by evaluating the strength of pronation with the elbow fully flexed. This is an uncommon compression syndrome for which the etiology is the same as that discussed under the pronator tunnel syndrome. Treatment is the same for both.

Cervical Nerve Root Compression and Scalenus Anticus Syndrome

These entities are discussed here because their manifestations are frequently allied to the carpal tunnel syndrome and other entrapments of the median nerve. Twenty-five years ago it was fashionable to diagnose the scalenus anticus syndrome (thoracic outlet syndrome) and to treat it by scalenotomy. The carpal tunnel syndrome was scarcely recognized. Today's experience has proven beyond a doubt the reversal of incidences.

Cervical nerve root compression is relatively common and is caused by trauma and degenerative changes about the cervical spine, the latter predominant as an etiological factor. The prime clinical findings are pain and associated muscle spasm, both of which cause limitation of motion of the head and neck. The pain and dysesthesias are apt to be poorly localized and are often accentuated by extension of the neck and simultaneous rotation to the contralateral side. With progression there will be objective muscle weakness and reflex changes. This may include winging of the scapula if the long thoracic nerve is paralyzed by a C-5, C-6 involvement.

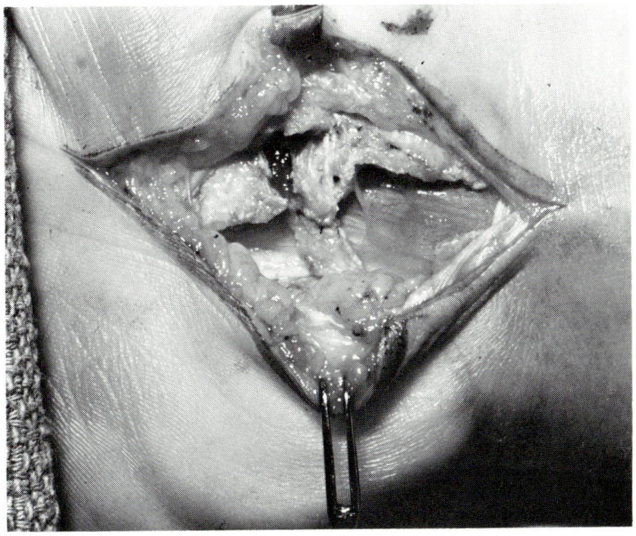

Figure 15-19. *The interdigitation of two portions of the carpal ligament to reestablish a loose sling in this area.*

Standard cervical roentgenograms may show narrowing of the disc space and other changes in the contour and relationships of the vertebral bodies. In addition, oblique views may show hypertrophic bone encroaching on the foramina. Intractable cases deserve a myelographic study.

A wryneck occurs when pain and spasm are marked. This however, more often than not, is simply a desmitis rather than a radiculitis or nerve compression problem.

Initial treatment for cases exclusive of fracture, dislocation and tumors is always conservative. It consists of the immobilization of the head and neck with a cervical collar. Severe and intractable cases are subjected to continuous or intermittent cervical traction which must be adapted to the patient's comfort. Concomitant antispasmotics, analgesics and anti-inflammatory agents are administered. If there is not adequate improvement in 1 to 2 weeks, a myelogram is considered. When this shows nerve root compression, surgery is undertaken before there is evidence of permanent paralysis.

The scalenus anticus syndrome—variably called the thoracic outlet, cervical rib, costoclavicular and hyperabduction syndrome—refers to symptomatology created by a variety of compression phenomenon on neurovascular structures deep to the clavicle. Pain, paresthesias or numbness occur through compression of the brachial plexus. The involvement is primarily over the distribution of the ulnar nerve, however; peripheral sensory or motor loss is rare. Roentgenograms should be taken to determine the presence of a cervical rib or elongated transverse process at C-5 or C-6. Arterial and venous compression are not considered prominent features of this entity. Poor posture is the most common basis for this problem and frequently responds to corrective exercises.

Failure to improve after 3 to 6 months of conservative effort justifies resection of the first rib for relief. The transaxillary approach is preferred.[35]

Ulnar Nerve Compression

Ulnar nerve entrapment is less common than that of the median nerve. It occurs at three sites: the ulnar groove behind the medial epicondyle, the cubital tunnel through the aponeurosis of the flexor carpi ulnaris and at the wrist and heel of the hand (loge de Guyon). Etiological factors contributing to ulnar nerve palsy are primarily traumatic, but may also be developmental and secondary to degenerative or metabolic changes and tumorous conditions. In the case of the ulnar groove and cubital tunnel, sustained body pressure is the most common reason for palsy in contrast to true entrapment.

The level of compression is determined by the muscles involved in the paralysis. Compression in the ulnar groove affects the flexor carpi ulnaris and the profundus to the ring and little fingers as well as the 15 intrinsic muscles innervated by the ulnar nerve. Compression in the cubital tunnel does not paralyze the flexor carpi ulnaris. Compression at the wrist can be distal or proximal. When it is distal there is paralysis of the interossei, the adductor pollicis, and the ulnar two lumbricals without sensory loss, since only the deep motor branch is affected. When it is proximal in the wrist, there is paralysis of all of the 15 intrinsic muscles and sensory loss that spares the dorsal branch of the ulnar nerve.

The subjective complaints in ulnar nerve compression are inclined to be more of numbness and dysesthesia than of deep miserable pain. Loss of dexterity and loss of grip and pinch strength are prominent complaints. As with median nerve compression, electromyographic and nerve conduction studies may be diagnostically useful.

ULNAR GROOVE COMPRESSION

The bony groove between the olecranon and the medial epicondyle is of variable depth. When shallow, it gives poor protection to the ulnar nerve, which can be traumatized by repeated subluxations out of it. This groove is bridged by a fascial sling which varies somewhat in its thickness and laxity. As a consequence of trauma the canal can be encroached upon by either bone or fascia and the nerve compressed. The diameter of the canal is markedly reduced with flexion of the elbow.[2] Routine roentgenograms of the elbow and tangential views of the groove are essential.

The immediate or rapid onset of paralysis arising at the level of the ulnar groove follows sustained pressure in the unconscious patient or is a consequence of direct violence or severe injury with intense swelling.

"Tardy ulnar palsy"[20] originates in the ulnar groove and follows trauma by several years. Cubitus valgus and post-traumatic deformities of the ulnar groove play a role in the causation of tension or friction on the nerve to bring about this palsy. Repetitive occupational stresses, including extension-flexion elbow motion and local percussive forces during certain activities, have been incriminated. Direct local trauma can lead to fibrosis and fixation of the nerve in the groove. At times an hourglass constriction with a pseudoneuromatous enlargement proximal to the groove is found. Laxity of the fascial sling over this groove permits subluxation of the nerve. The resulting trauma caused by snapping and friction on the nerve causes edema and fibrosis of the nerve. Osteoarthritic exostoses, rheumatoid synovitis, ganglia and other masses are occasionally sources of compression.

CUBITAL TUNNEL COMPRESSION

The nerve enters the cubital tunnel as it leaves the ulnar groove. This tunnel is formed by the epicondylar and olecranon heads of the flexor carpi ulnaris. The aponeurotic ring may be tight enough to indent the nerve, with the formation of a proximal pseudoneuroma and an hourglass deformity. Developmental factors and hypertrophy of use contribute to the role of trauma in the production of compression in this area.

THE TREATMENT OF COMPRESSIONS IN THE ULNAR GROOVE AND CUBITAL TUNNEL

In view of the juxtaposition of these two areas and the difficulty in incriminating entrapment at one or the other site, any treatment should be delivered simultaneously to both areas. Acute paralysis resulting from simple direct pressure on the elbow (e.g. in sleep, leaning on the elbow as with driving, etc.) is treated expectantly for 3 to 4 months if the tissues are soft and pliable. Triamcinolone may be initially injected around the nerve. If there is no sign of recovery, the nerve should be explored and decompressed. Emergency decompression is done whenever the paralysis develops rapidly, or is associated with a fracture or established congestion and brawny edema.

The surgery is done with loupe magnification and tourniquet ischemia. A 15-cm median longitudinal incision is made anterior to the crest of the epicondyle. The normal nerve is identified proximally and is traced into the ulnar groove. The fascial sling across the groove is divided superficial to the nerve. The nerve should be elevated from its bed. This may require division of some of the tiny articular branches and ligation of a host of veins. The nerve is then traced to the cubital tunnel, which is divided with scissors with the nerve in sight at all times.

If there is no tension about the ulnar nerve lying in its normal bed with the elbow flexed and the problem is not one of repeated subluxation of the nerve, it does not have to be transferred. If the nerve is tight when the elbow is flexed or recurrent subluxation has occurred, it should be transferred anteriorly. In doing so, the muscular branches to the flexor carpi ulnaris and profundus muscles must be preserved as much as possible. The nerve is held in its new bed without any kinking by a very loosely fitting fascial sling constructed from the aponeurosis of the flexor musculature. In lieu of transferring the nerve anteriorly, the medial epicondyle may be resected subperiosteally[15] (Fig. 15-20). This removes the fulcrum that causes tension during flexion. In the case of tardy palsy, it may be necessary to do an endoneurolysis using the same technique described for the median nerve in the carpal canal. The operation must concomitantly deal with any associated problems (ganglion, etc.).

The elbow is immobilized at a right angle in a well-padded cylinder long-arm cast for a week to 10 days. The duration of disability for the procedure itself is 3 to 4 weeks.

COMPRESSION AT THE WRIST (LOGE DE GUYON)

Here the nerve runs deep and radial to the pisiform bone and gives off the hypothenar motor branch, the volar sensory branches to the ring and little fingers and the deep motor branch. The latter passes through a discrete aponeurotic sling of the origin of the hypothenar musculature and then disappears around the ulnar side of the hook of hamate into the depth of the palm (Fig. 2-18).

The causes for compression in this canal are: direct trauma, brawny swelling and induration about the wrist, arthritis, tumors and simple compression (against the handle of a crutch). At times the condition coexists with carpal tunnel syndrome.

The treatment of ulnar nerve compression in Guyon's canal is non-operative, emergency operative, and elective operative. Very few cases fall into the non-operative and emergency operative categories. The non-operative treatment is initiated when there are no local bone or soft tissue changes about the canal and the problem is one of acute simple compression (leaning on the handle of crutches). The source of compression must be rec-

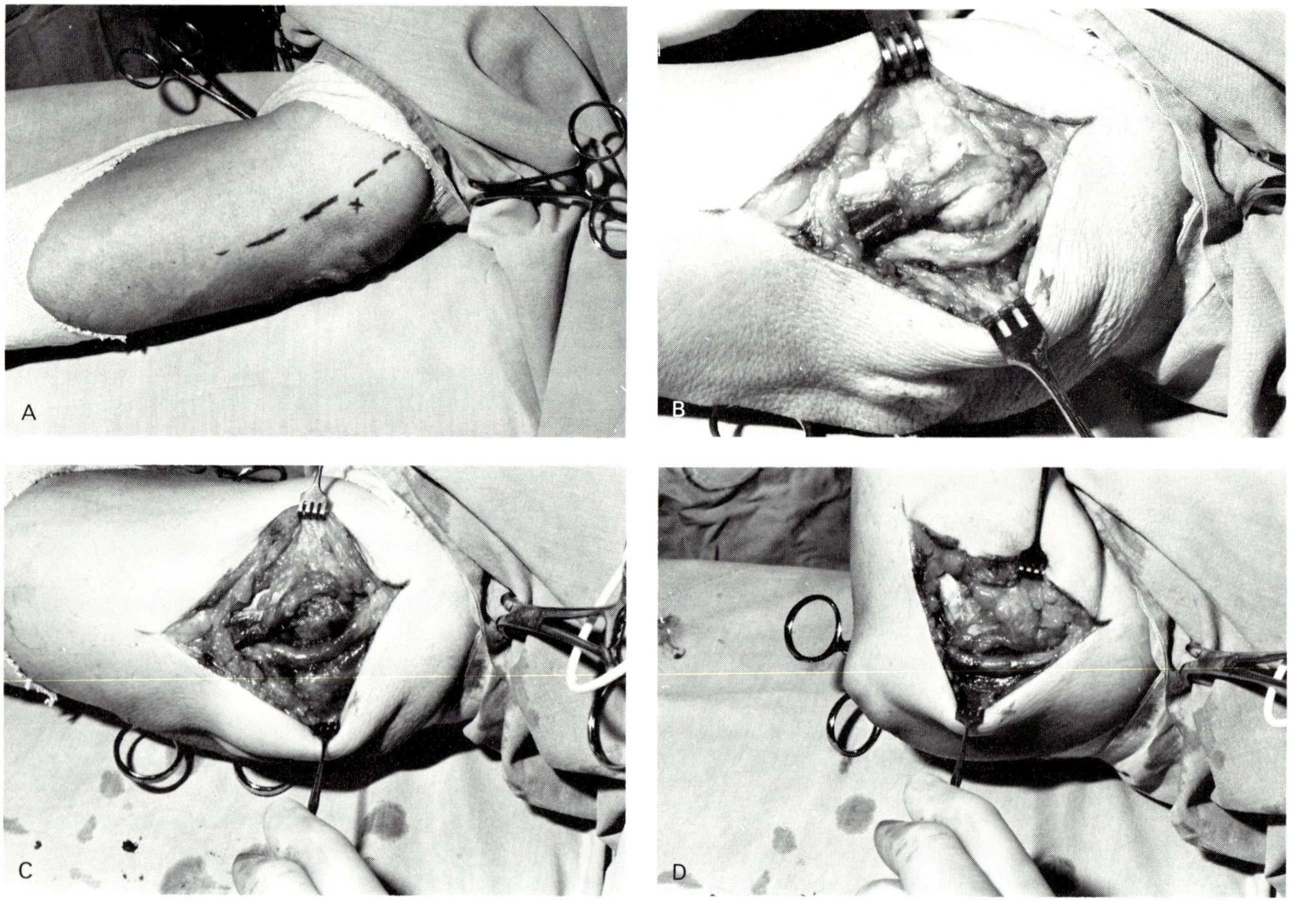

Figure 15-20. *Technique of ulnar nerve release and medial epicondylectomy for entrapment of the nerve in the ulnar groove. After the epicondyle has been excised, the nerve should no longer be tensed with flexion and extension* **(C,D).**

ognized and eliminated. One to 3 injections of 2 to 5 mg of triamcinolone can be placed about the nerve over a period of 3 to 6 weeks. Recovery is monitored by testing the strength of the first dorsal interosseous muscle (Fig. 15-21). Emergency surgery is done for acute progressive paralysis and established paralysis in the face of indurated congestion of the wrist. Elective surgery is done in all other cases of ulnar palsy in the loge de Guyon, including those which failed to respond to nonoperative measures.

The incision for decompression is slightly ulnar to that for decompression of the carpal tunnel. One incision can be used to decompress both median and ulnar nerves. The ulnar artery must be recognized and preserved. All constrictive fascial elements around the nerve in Guyon's canal, including the fibrous hypothenar aponeurosis around the deep motor branch, are sectioned. The nerve and its branches are thus totally liberated. Small arterioles and veins crossing over it must be divided for adequate exposure. This is especially important in order to identify and avoid injury to the deep motor branch, which is well hidden. Any induration along the nerve is reason for an endoneurolysis as described for the median nerve in carpal tunnel release. Postoperatively, the hand is dressed for 10 to 14 days. The duration of temporary disability is usually four weeks or more. Failure to respond to these conservative measures may necessitate tendon transfers to correct the deformities of intrinsic paralysis.

Compression of the Radial Nerve

The most common compression state of the radial nerve is that referred to as the "Saturday-night paralysis." This results from the narcotized patient (usually alcoholic) going to sleep with his arm resting over the back of a chair with his head upon the arm. The radial nerve is compressed against the humerus in the spiral groove. Most of the time this paralysis clears spontaneously, but

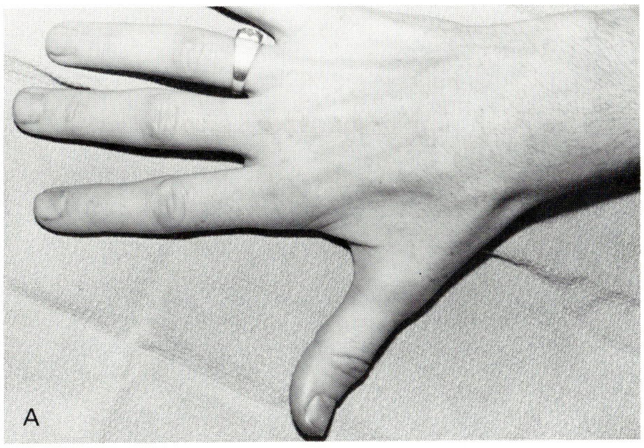

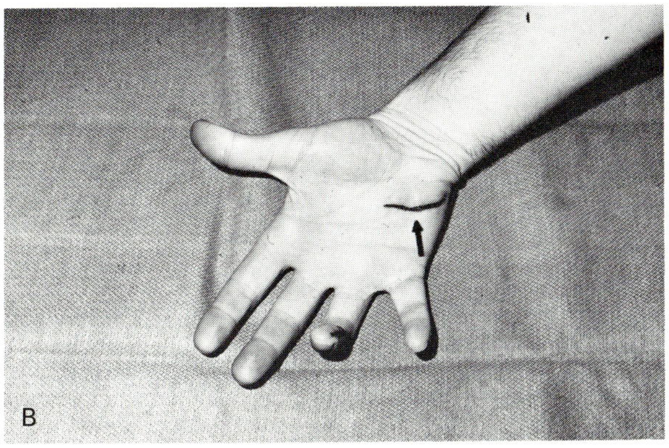

Figure 15-21.A: *Atrophy of first dorsal interosseous muscle in classic ulnar palsy.* **B:** *Clawing resulting from division of the deep motor branch of the ulnar nerve (arrow). Note the ulceration of the ulnar aspect of the distal phalanx of the ring finger.*

occasionally it is permanent. Treatment is expectant. A cock-up splint may be worn to correct the wristdrop. Tendon transfers must be considered if there is no sign of recovery in 4 to 6 months.

This is also the site of entrapment of the nerve by a fracture of the humerus. Here the problem may arise acutely or insidiously. When it is acute, it is difficult to know if the nerve is divided, kinked or crushed at the fracture line. Emergency exploration should be considered. When the onset is insidious, cicatrical entrapment or incorporation in the fracture callus must be considered. Here too the treatment is surgical.

Compression of the Dorsal Interosseous Nerve

The site of entrapment of this nerve is at the aponeurotic window of the supinator[38] (Fig. 15-22) or within the substance of the supinator muscle as it winds around the lateral aspect of the radius. Here it may be choked following direct trauma, compressed by hypertrophy of the muscle, by congestion or tumor within the forearm or by synovitis about the elbow. Paralysis causes a classical pattern. There is no sensory deficit, but there is motor weakness. This involves the abductor pollicis longus, the extensor pollicis longus and brevis and the extrinsic extensors of the fingers.

The treatment is expectant when there is no gross evidence of disease and the cause has been direct pressure. The wrist extensors are intact and therefore a cock-up splint is not needed. Triamcinolone may be injected around the nerve. Emergency decompression is undertaken when the paralysis is acute and progresses rapidly. Elective decompression is undertaken in all other cases.

Exposure is through a dorsal lateral longitudinal incision of the elbow and proximal forearm. The normal radial nerve is identified between the brachioradialis and the brachialis and traced to where it branches into the superficial sensory nerve and the dorsal interosseous. The latter is traced to its entry into the arcade of Frohse, which is divided to liberate the nerve. The extremity is mobilized as soon as the skin wound is healed.

Miscellaneous Neurological Entities Affecting Hand Function

There are a host of neurological afflictions which have their impact on the function of the hand. These may affect the sensory or motor systems singularly or in combination and may be grouped accordingly. Some of them vary in onset from acute to insidious. When insidious, they may take a considerable period of time to diagnose. The predominant features that help to distinguish these from a peripheral process is that the distribution of symptoms and signs is diffuse, may occur in both extremities, or is not limited to a specific peripheral nerve. Some of these conditions are relapsing, some progressive, and some intractable to any known treatment.

Conditions involving the motor and sensory systems are hysteria, multiple sclerosis and Charcot-Marie-Tooth disease. Hysteria, particularly the chronic form, primarily affects women. When seen in the male, it is almost always a compensation neurosis directed at obvious material gain. The foundation is usually anxiety and the manifestation is in the form of motor or sensory paralysis. It typically has a stocking-glove distribution. Treatment necessitates psychiatric expertise.

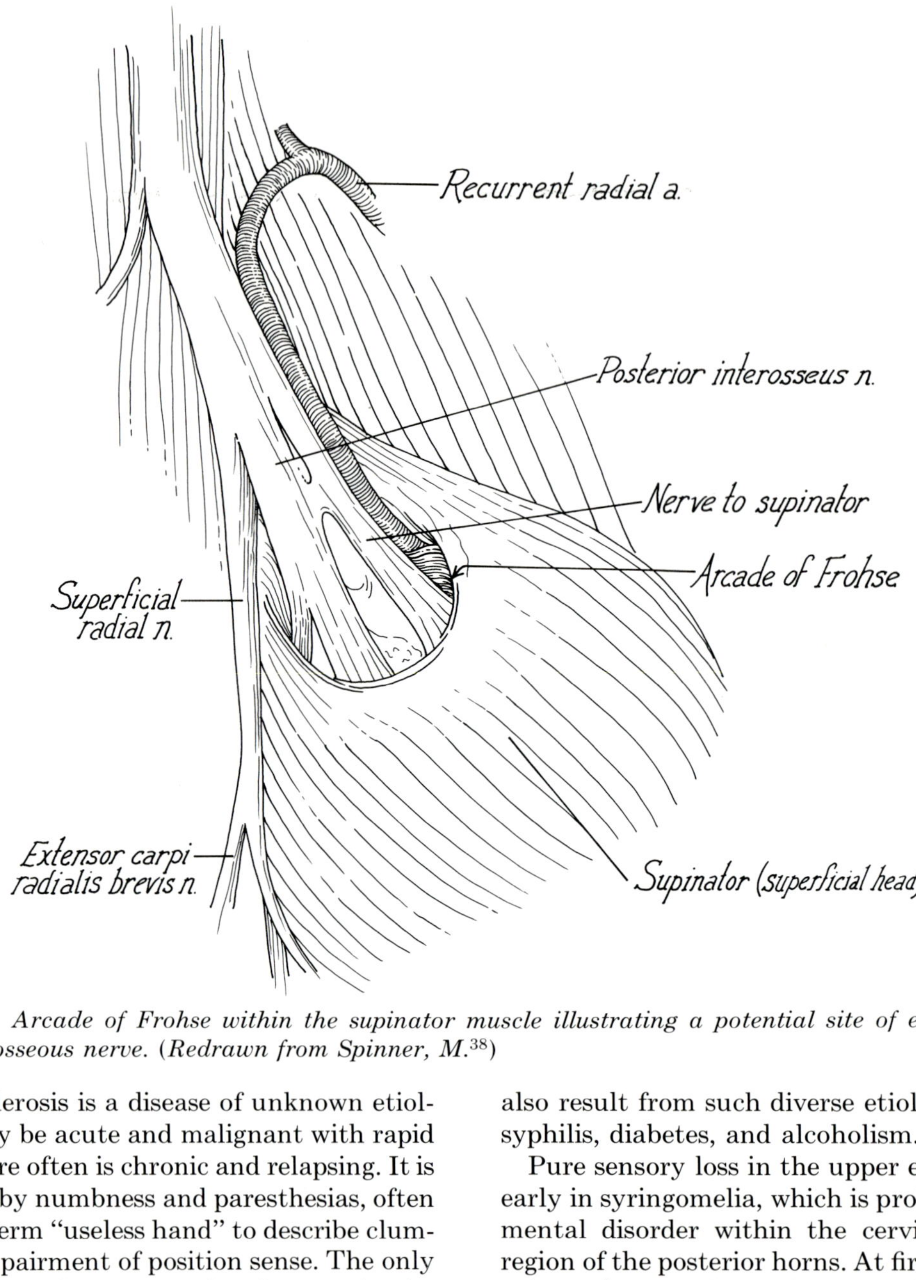

Figure 15-22. *Arcade of Frohse within the supinator muscle illustrating a potential site of entrapment of the posterior interosseous nerve.* (*Redrawn from Spinner, M.*[38])

Multiple sclerosis is a disease of unknown etiology which may be acute and malignant with rapid death, but more often is chronic and relapsing. It is characterized by numbness and paresthesias, often invoking the term "useless hand" to describe clumsiness from impairment of position sense. The only laboratory tests of note are the changes in the colloidal gold curve of the cerebrospinal fluid, which are not diagnostic. There is no specific therapy.

Charcot-Marie-Tooth disease is a hereditary chronic degeneration of peripheral nerves. The symptoms are weakness and muscular wasting with paresthesias and other rather slight sensory changes. This condition may be arrested at any stage. As a rule, the lower extremities are primarily affected but eventually there may be extensive atrophy of hand and forearm musculature which requires reconstructive surgery.

Combined sensory and motor neuropathy can also result from such diverse etiologies as leprosy, syphilis, diabetes, and alcoholism.

Pure sensory loss in the upper extremity is seen early in syringomelia, which is probably a developmental disorder within the cervical cord in the region of the posterior horns. At first there is loss of pain and temperature in a cape-like distribution over the shoulders, arms and hands. Trophic changes follow, including Charcot joints. Later on, there are motor changes. Neurosurgical treatment is generally unsatisfactory.

Afflictions primarily influencing the motor functions are seen in lead neuropathy, poliomyelitis, amyotrophic lateral sclerosis, parkinsonism and cerebral palsy. Chronic exposure to lead leads to paresis of the upper extremities predominantly affecting the radial nerve. Clinically the paralyzed muscles are those which are most used. A wrist- and finger drop eventually develops. Laboratory assay of lead in the urine and stippling of the erythrocytes are diagnostic. The source of exposure must be eliminated and chelating agents given to facilitate excretion of the lead.

Poliomyelitis no longer seriously threatens hand function now that immunization is commonplace. For the unfortunate few who have contracted it, its impact on motor function of the hand can be lessened by appropriate musculotendinous transfer procedures, tenodesis and joint fusion.

In amyotrophic lateral sclerosis weakness and atrophy combined with spasticity and hyperreflexia result from the gradual degeneration of motor neurons. There is no effective treatment. Progression of the disease is relatively rapid with death from aspiration pneumonia.

Parkinsonism frequently develops asymmetrically and may start as a slight tremor in the fingers of one hand. With progression, the typical cogwheel phenomenon develops. Rigidity and tremor are markedly aggravated by emotional tension. There is no specific treatment insofar as the hand itself is concerned.

Spastic dysfunction of the hand is seen commonly in cerebral palsy, postencephalitis, cerebral trauma and cerebral vascular accidents. Since the abnormality is cortical, the possibility of restoring peripheral function by surgery is limited. The persistent cortical stimulation may be the undoing of an otherwise well-conceived tendon transfer, musculotendinous lengthening or arthrodesis.

Successful surgery requires a well-motivated patient who has volitional grasp and release and reasonable sensibility in the hand. The common deformities are pronation of the forearm, flexion of the wrist, thumb-in-palm, and flexion of the fingers with or without swan-neck configuration.

Spasticity will be of variable magnitude within any group of muscles and will be altered by the emotional state and consciousness of the patient. It is these unpredictable and often uncontrollable issues that make the prognosis for treatment guarded. Many patients are helped by an effective program of splinting designed to correct deformities, to prevent their progression, to overcome the spasm of the predominant group of muscles and to stabilize the hand in a functional habitus. In addition, through positioning and stabilizing the hand, the splint helps the surgeon evaluate the potential of corrective surgical procedures. When splinting overstretches spastic muscles, hyperactivity of the stretch reflex is accentuated.

Swanson describes some specific procedures to overcome the various spastic states.[40] To correct the pronation deformity of the forearm, the flexor carpi ulnaris may be transferred to the radius or the radial wrist extensors, the pronator teres may be sectioned or transferred, or the radius may be osteotomized distal to the insertion of the pronator teres.

Wrist flexion is corrected by transfer of the flexor carpi ulnaris around the ulnar border of the forearm to its distal dorsum to interweave with the extensor carpi radialis brevis.[18] The tension must be carefully gauged not to preclude wrist flexion and finger extension.

Excessive coexisting spasticity of finger flexors may be relieved by release of the flexor muscle wad with preservation of the origin of the flexor carpi ulnaris. Six weeks of immobilization in a long-arm cast with forearm supination and wrist dorsiflexion follows surgery.

The procedure of choice for a flexion deformity of the fingers is a release of the flexor muscle wad from the medial epicondyle, the ulna and the interosseous membrane, sparing injury or traction to either the median or ulnar nerves. If wrist flexion is to be corrected, the origin of the flexor carpi ulnaris is spared and its tendon is transferred dorsally as described above. As a consequence, a new resting length is attained which breaks the cycle of excessive stretch-induced spasticity without unduly weakening the flexor efficiency of the muscles released from their epicondylar origin.

The muscles are exposed through a longitudinal incision on the ulnar aspect of the proximal forearm and elbow. If the flexor pollicis longus needs to be released, a separate radial border incision is necessary. The merits of this procedure can be assessed preoperatively by a local block of the flexor muscle group. Inability to gain digital extension with the wrist in more than 40° flexion favors this release.

Because the wrist is the key joint for moderating extensor-flexor muscle force on the digits, its elimination by arthrodesis may be regretted in these conditions. If it is done, it requires overwhelming attention to immobilization (usually with Steinmann pins) to counteract the constant force of spastic muscles.

To correct the thumb-in-palm deformity, the aim is to release the spastic intrinsics and reinforce the extensor pollicis longus. The former is accomplished through a palmar incision on the ulnar side of the thenar crease. With due care to avoid injuring the ulnar and median motor nerves, the adductor pollicis and the thenar muscles are freed and raised from their origin and allowed to shift distally as the thumb is positioned in full abduction

(Fig. 15-23). The brachioradialis is mobilized a sufficient distance through a forearm incision to facilitate its transfer into either the short or long thumb extensors. The metacarpophalangeal joint is stabilized against hyperextension by fusion or a Zancolli type of capsulodesis.

The swan-neck deformity is an imbalance consisting of hyperextension of the middle joint with flexion of the distal and proximal joints. The middle phalanx may be locked in the hyperextension. Treatment is the prevention of hyperextension. This can be effectively accomplished by tenodesis of one slip of the superficialis tendon to the pulley or bone of the proximal phalanx holding the proximal interphalangeal joint in 20 to 40° of flexion with a Kirschner wire for 8 to 10 weeks.

Occasionally a pure hygienic problem of maceration and odor deserves release, without the intention of restoring function. Here the choice is between multiple tenotomies followed by prolonged postoperative casting or denervation of the extrinsic and intrinsic muscles. The latter is a more extensive operation but far more predictable and immediate in accomplishing its goal and does not require immobilization beyond the period of skin healing.

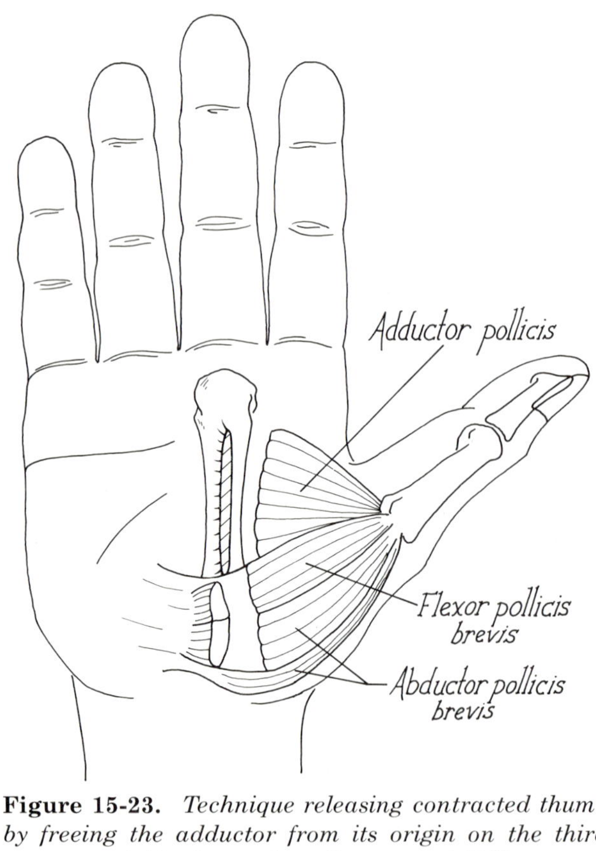

Figure 15-23. *Technique releasing contracted thumb by freeing the adductor from its origin on the third metacarpal.* (*Redrawn from Swanson, A.B.*[40])

Disorders of the Sympathetic Nervous System

These are problems manifested most often by pain and vascular disturbances, e.g. sympathetic dystrophies and vasospastic disorders. These conditions are discussed in detail in the chapters on pain and vascular disorders respectively. The upper extremity lacks parasympathetic innervation. The sympathetic nervous system functions in a dual capacity to create both adrenergic and cholinergic effects.

Hyperhidrosis of the palms or axillae is sometimes severe enough to be a functional and social handicap. When it is unresponsive to antiperspirants and anticholinergic drugs, the only recourse is a bilateral sympathectomy to treat the problem in the palms. Preoperative blocks must be administered to demonstrate the sequelae of the operation to the patient.

Axillary hyperhidrosis may be treated by resection of the hair-bearing skin and underlying subcutaneous fat. Closure of the vertical wound is done with multiple Z-plasties.[11] An alternative method, resecting only the subdermal glandular-bearing fat, has been described by Skoog.[37]

References

1. Adamson, J., Horton, C. and Crawford, H.: Sensory rehabilitation of the injured thumb. Plast. Reconstr. Surg., 40:53, 1967.
2. Apfelberg, D.B. and Larson, S.J.: Dynamic anatomy of the ulnar nerve at the elbow. Plast. Reconstr. Surg., 51:76, 1973.
3. Beasley, R.W.: Tendon transfers for radial nerve palsy. Orthop. Clin. North Am., 1:479, 1970.
4. Boyes, H.H., Ed.: *Surgery of the Hand.* 4th ed. J.B. Lippincott, Philadelphia, 1964.
5. Brand, P.W.: Reconstruction of the hand in leprosy. Ann. R. Coll. Surg. Engl., 11:350, 1953.
6. Brand, P.W: Tendon transfers for median and ulnar nerve palsies. Orthop. Clin. North Am., 1:447, 1970.
7. Burkhalter, W., Christensen, R.C. and Brown, P.: Extensor indicis proprius opponensplasty. J. Bone Joint Surg., 55A:725, 1973.
8. Carroll, R.E. and Gartland, J.J.: Flexor plasty of the elbow; an evaluation of a method. J. Bone Joint Surg., 35A:706, 1953.
9. Cherington, M.: Proximal pain in carpal tunnel syndrome. Arch. Surg., 108:69, 1974.

10. Clark, J.M.P.: Reconstruction of the biceps brachii by pectoral muscle transfer. Br. J. Surg., 34:180, 1946.
11. Davis, P.K.B.: Surgical treatment of axillary hyperhidrosis. Br. J. Plast. Surg., 24:99, 1971.
12. Dellon, A.L., Curtis, R.M. and Edgerton, M.T.: Reeducation of sensation in the hand after nerve injury and repair. Plast. Reconstr. Surg., 53:297. 1974.
13. Ducker, T.S., Kempe, L.G. and Hayes, G.J.: The metabolic background for peripheral nerve surgery. J. Neurosurg., 30:270, 1969.
14. Eversmann, W.W. and Curtis, R.M.: Internal neurolysis, an adjunct to the treatment of the carpal tunnel syndrome. J. Bone Joint Surg., 54A:897, 1972.
15. Gore, D. and Larson, S.: Median condylectomy for subluxing ulnar nerve. Am. J. Surg., 111:851, 1966.
16. Grabb, W.C., Bement, S.L., Keopke, G.H. and Green, R.A.: Comparison of methods of peripheral nerve suturing in monkeys. Plast. Reconstr. Surg., 46:31, 1970.
17. Graham, W.P.: Variations of the motor branch of the median nerve at the wrist. Plast. Reconstr. Surg., 51:90, 1973.
18. Green, W.T. and Banks, H.H.: Flexor carpi ulnaris transplant and its use in cerebral palsy. J. Bone Joint Surg., 44A:1343, 1962.
19. Guyton, A.C.: *Structure and Function of the Nervous System.* W.B. Saunders, Philadelphia, 1972.
20. Hunt, J.R.: Tardy or late paralysis of the ulnar nerve. A form of chronic progressive neuritis developing many years after fracture dislocation of the elbow. J.A.M.A., 66:10, 1916.
21. Klhuner, K.G., Edshage, S. and Wiehelm, A.: Ninhydrin test—an objective method for testing local anesthetic drugs. Acta Anaesthiol., Scand., 4:189, 1960.
22. Kopell, H.P. and Thompson, W.H.: The pronator syndrome. N. Engl. J. Med., 259:713, 1958.
23. Littler, J.W. and Cooley, S.G.E.: Opposition of the thumb and its restoration by abductor digiti quinti transfer. J. Bone Joint Surg., 45A:1389, 1963.
24. Mayer, L. and Green, W.: Experiences with Steindler flexorplasty at the elbow. J. Bone Joint. Surg., 34:180, 1946.
25. Mayer, L.: Tendon transfers in the arm. In *Hand Surgery* (Flynn, J.E., Ed.). Williams and Wilkins, Baltimore, 1966.
26. McEwan, L.: Median and ulnar nerve injuries. Aust. N.Z. J. Surg., 32:89, 1962.
27. Millesi, H.: The interfascicular nerve graft. J. Bone Joint Surg., 53A:813, 1971.
28. Mutz, S.: Anterior transposition and neurorrhaphy of the radial nerve. Presented at the 29th Annual Meeting of the American Society for Surgery of the Hand. Dallas, January, 1974.
29. Nicholas, G.G., Noone, R.B. and Graham, W.P.: Carpal tunnel syndrome in pregnancy. Hand, 3:80, 1971.
30. Nicholson, O.R. and Seddon, H.J.: Nerve repair in civilian practice: results of treatment of median and ulnar nerve lesions. Br. Med. J., 2:1065, 1957.
31. Pataky, P., Graham, W.P. and Munger, B.L.: Terminal neuromas treated with triamcinolone acetonide. J. Surg. Res., 14:36, 1973.
32. Phalen, G.S. and Miller, R.C.: The transfer of wrist extensor muscles to restore or reinforce flexion power of the fingers and opposition of the thumb. J. Bone Joint Surg., 29A:993, 1947.
33. Phalen, G.S.: Reflections on 21 years experience with the carpal tunnel syndrome. J.A.M.A., 212:1365, 1970.
34. Riordan, D.C.: Tendon transplantations in median nerve and ulnar nerve paralysis. J. Bone Joint Surg., 35A:312, 1953.
35. Roos, D.B.: Transaxillary approach for first rib resection to relieve thoracic outlet syndrome. Ann. Surg., 163:354, 1966.
36. Royle, N.D.: An operation for paralysis of the intrinsic muscles of the thumb. J.A.M.A., 111:612, 1938.
37. Skoog, T.: *Plastic Surgery.* W.B. Saunders, Philadelphia, 1974.
38. Spinner, M.: The arcade of Frohse and its relationship to posterior interosseous nerve paralysis. J. Bone Joint Surg., 50B:809, 1968.
39. Sunderland, S.: The connective tissues of peripheral nerves. Brain, 88:841, 1965.
40. Swanson, A.B.: Surgery of the hand in cerebral palsy and muscle origin release procedures. Surg. Clin. North Am., 48:1129, 1968.
41. White, W.W.: Restoration of function and balance of the hand by tendon transfer. Surg. Clin. North Am., 40:427, 1960.
42. Zachary, R.B.: Results of nerve suture. In *Peripheral Nerve Injuries* (Seddon, J., Ed.). Medical Research Council Special Report, Series #282. Her Majesty's Stationery Office, London, 1954.
43. Zancolli, E.A.: Clawhand caused by paralysis of the intrinsic muscles. A simple surgical procedure for its correction. J. Bone Joint Surg., 39A:1076, 1957.

16 Complex Injuries

Complex injuries of the hand are either open or closed and involve multiple or all structures. Invariably the venous and lymphatic circulation is jeopardized and often the arterial supply as well. Hence treatment is primarily directed at preservation and recovery of circulation.

The extent of the injured tissues is the determinant of the efforts at salvage. Since the sickle surrendered to the mechanical cornpicker and the smithy gave way to lines of punch presses, the hazards to workers' hands of compound and complex injuries continue to increase. V-belts and pulleys, unyielding steel rollers, shredding instruments and presses which close with tremendous force all produce damage to several or all of the tissues which comprise the hand. The term "cornpicker hand" has become a well-known synonym for such mutilation.[13] When multiple tissues are seriously damaged the additive effect threatens the integrity of the entire hand as an anatomically functional unit.

The possibilities for subsequent reconstructive procedures are determined, to a great extent, by the initial management of the injury. The hand surgeon must exercise a high order of surgical judgment, drawing from his knowledge of infection and wound healing, orthopedic principles, muscle and nerve pathophysiology, techniques of skin coverage, functional dynamics and priorities in the hand.

Salvage and reconstruction must be governed by the functional needs and economic restrictions of the patient, which are influenced by his age, occupation and motivation.

The conditions which influence complex injuries are listed below:

Closed wound
Open wound
Tissue destruction
Loss of substance
Ischemia
Inflammation (chemical)
Contamination

Examination

An accurate examination of a mangled hand is difficult to carry out in the emergency room. Pain and apprehension, bleeding and hematoma, inadequate lighting and deficient instrumentation all pose handicaps to a good evaluation. The complex injury must be handled in the operating room under adequate anesthesia and conditions suitable for performing major surgical procedures. A general survey in the emergency room—an evaluation of the circulation, x-ray examination, gross neurological assessment and an assessment of skin deficits—is adequate for planning. Probing the wound and manipulating the injured tissues at this time give little additional information and may add significantly to contamination and tissue damage.

The emergency management of the wound is discussed in Chapters 3 and 4. Briefly the injury should be cleansed, covered with a sterile dressing and immobilized as soon as possible.

The two emergencies requiring immediate transfer to the operating room are external hemorrhage or rapid progression of swelling from internal hemorrhage. Where such transfer is not feasible, the emergency treatment for persistent hemorrhage is: (1) direct pressure on the site of external hemorrhage rather than blind clamping or ligature, (2) removal of all constricting garments and jewelry which serve as venous tourniquets and elevation of the injured part, (3) the application of a sphygmomanometer proximal to the zone of injury. This must be inflated and maintained at 100 mm Hg above the systolic blood pressure. It can usually be tolerated for 20 to 30 minutes without anesthesia. Tetanus prophylaxis in the appropriate form and broad-spectrum antibiotics are initiated early.

Triage

The principles of problem sorting learned in management of mass casualties and in wartime medical logistics are of great aid in planning the surgical repair. A surgical triage is performed at the time of first examination. All tissues retaining reasonable health should be preserved for use in immediate repair or banked as parts for future reconstruction. The sequence of repair is: (1) skeletal alignment and stabilization, (2) the restoration of circulation, (3) soft tissue coverage and (4) tenorrhaphy and neurorrhaphy.

Judgment regarding the potential use and function of an injured part is difficult to make at this time since the surgeon does not know the injured's specific job requirements, motivation and adaptability. The function which can be coaxed from a mangled part by a determined and persistent patient after good surgical care is often amazing.

However, an overly sanguine approach may lead to disaster. A surgical judgment difficult to master is a clear assessment of what can realistically be accomplished versus what might hypothetically be accomplished for the patient. The "what-have-we-got-to-lose" approach may lead to disaster if the surgeon assumes unreasonable risks. A patient may be subjected to prolonged disability with physical and economic hardships, and the opportunity for a cleanly healed wound may be lost by accepting a high risk of tissue survival (Fig. 16-1).

It is helpful, for purposes of assessment and planning, to reduce the hand to its component tissues: vessels, bone and joint, skin, tendon and nerve.

VESSELS

Viability is the first concern on the care of injury. The only absolute indication for amputation is irreversible loss of blood supply.[15] This is the baseline from which planning should start. An accurate assessment of the circulation can best be made under operating room conditions after a thorough surgical toilet.

Collateral arterial supply is generally excellent in the proximal hand and will usually ensure survival if one major source remains. Preoperative or intraoperative arteriography is helpful in examining the larger vessels which may be amenable to repair. End-vessels such as digital arteries are difficult to repair and to maintain patent, even with microsurgical technique. Venous channels which are primarily on the dorsum of the hand are extremely important to preserve and are easily compromised. Injury to this drainage complex produces acute and chronic edema as well as hemorrhea, destroying existing and potential function.

BONE AND JOINT

The mechanical functions of the hand are dependent on certain spatial relationships of a group of multijointed lever arms. Further, the circulatory pattern and the soft tissue components of the hand are developed to conform to the bony scaffold. The health and function of these elements are aided by preservation of the form of the hand (e.g. the proper alignment of rays and the restoration of longitudinal and transverse arches, the pronation of the thumb and extension of the wrist). These features aid not only the function but the resting of injured tissues. These immediate gains, with the difficult problems in secondary realignment of malpositioning, place skeletal restoration in the high priority group of tissues. Similarly, circulatory restoration may be impossible until skeletal stabilization has been achieved.

SKIN

The soft tissue covering of the hand bears much of the brunt of the trauma in complex injuries. Avulsion, shredding, tearing, crushing and friction are among the forces which physically remove or devitalize areas of skin. Restoration of the skin-fat cover assumes a high priority. Its protective cover is essential to control infection and maintain the

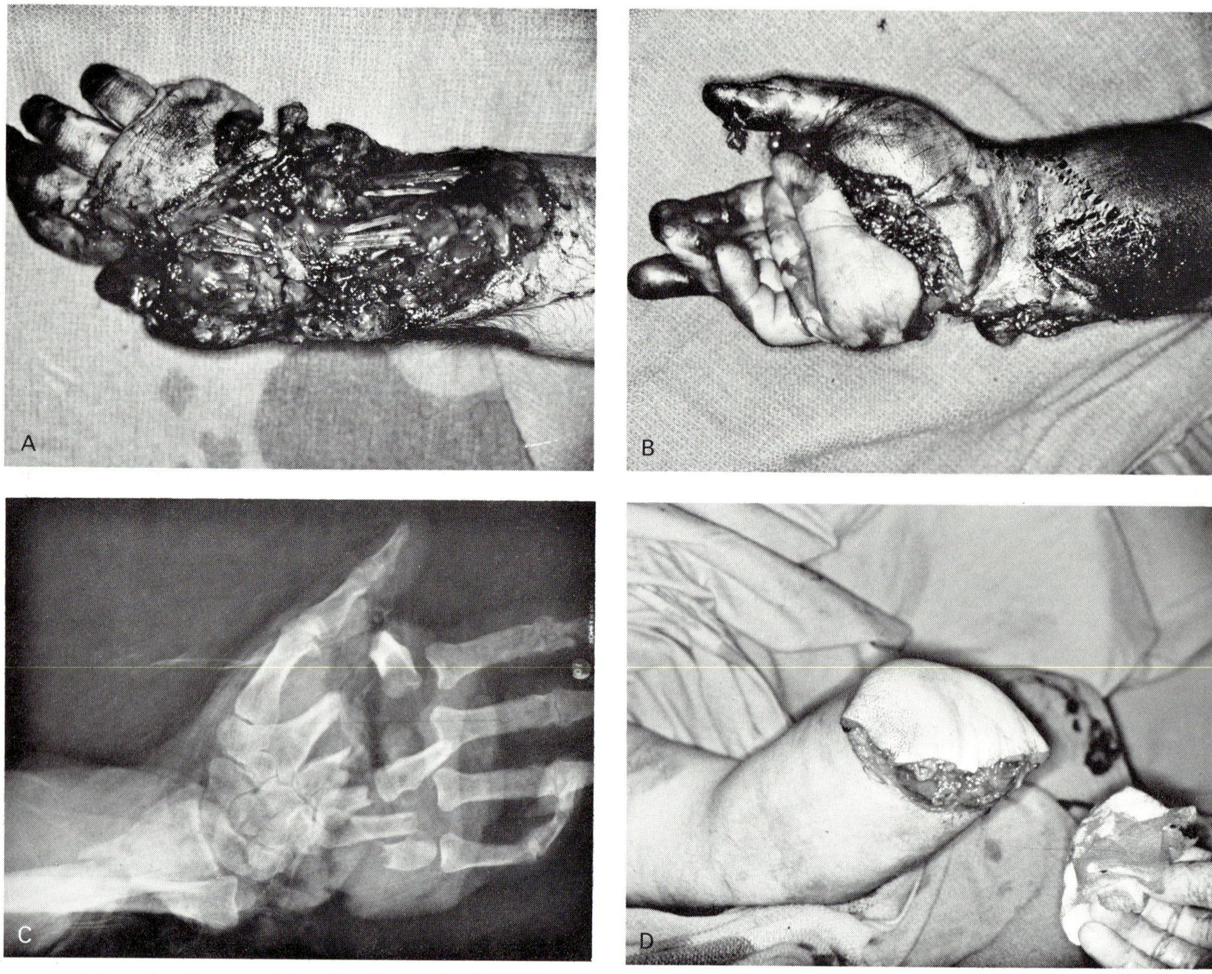

Figure 16-1. *A 49-year-old printer crushed his hand between the rollers of a press* **(A,B)**. *Multiple compound fractures* **(C)** *and extensive soft tissue loss and loss of circulation and nerve supply made a midforearm amputation necessary* **(D)**. *He returned to his job as a printer using a hook prosthesis within three months.*

function of nerve, tendon, bones and joints. A general plan for soft tissue coverage must be in mind before entering the operating room. A need for a flap or graft influences choice of anesthetic, positioning and draping and instrumentation.

Equally important, an appropriate explanation of the general plan of the surgery and the possible involvement of other uninjured anatomical areas as donor sites should be made to the patient beforehand. He should not awaken from anesthesia to find his hand unexpectedly bound to the abdomen in a pedicle.

TENDON AND NERVE

The considerations for disrupted tendons and nerves in this category of injuries are parallel. Their blood supply and protective beds are often compromised even if continuity is retained. When the continuity is interrupted, the proximal and distal portions may be widely separated by loss of substance or so altered by injury as to be unsalvageable or unrecognizable. Additional dissection may threaten already embarrassed circulation and is generally contraindicated. However, easily approximated grossly intact stumps of either tendons or nerves may be brought together. This may be done definitively if feasible without unduly prolonging the initial operating time and if satisfactory skin coverage is available. Otherwise proximal and distal stumps may be tacked together by very fine sutures merely to prevent their retraction.[3]

In the absence of tenorrhaphy the space beneath important pulleys may be temporarily maintained by silicone rods, providing skin cover is satisfactory and bacterial contamination has been insignificant.

A denuded tendon or nerve is prognostically deceptive of its future function in these injuries. Internal microscopic and physiological disruption, particularly of nerves, often compounds the grossly recognized problem of circulatory impairment. This leads to dysfunction through fibrosis or neuropraxia and axonotmesis.

Definitive Care

Reconstructive surgery begins immediately and is synonymous with initial repair.[4]

The basic operative management has three major goals:

1. To preserve existing function and viable tissue and to comprehensively debride non-viable tissue or tissue which will predispose to excessive scar.
2. To ensure the form and stability of the hand by reduction and stabilization of the skeleton.
3. To gain primary wound closure.

Both experimental studies and clinical observations incriminate retained foreign material, clots and ischemic tissue as the principal causes of healing failure and wound infection. The persistence of dead space predisposes to infection and fibrosis. Debridement must not further injure the hand or compromise its blood supply and should proceed in an orderly progression from the surface to the depths of the wound. The degree of tissue reactivity to foreign materials varies with the substance. The surgeon should not add noxious agents in preparing skin or in efforts to sterilize the wound. Irrigation with isotonic solutions may aid the gentle removal of clots as well as foreign material and loose tissue.

Judgment is necessary in appreciating when the retention of minute particles will not jeopardize hand function more than the act of their debridement. An example of this is the tattooing of the extensor hood in the hand of a lithograph pressman who has a wringer injury. This ink staining is minimally reactive and need not be totally eliminated at the expense of extensor function.

The salvage and recovery of function rest heavily on the surgeon's judgment and skill in debriding. Redundant tissue which might be prejudicial to healing and future function should be excised, e.g. the volar plate and collateral ligaments about amputated digital joints.[14] However, all healthy tissue must be preserved although there may be no immediate use for it.[17] Skin from filleted fingers may be extremely valuable in future surgery if properly banked in vivo at the time of initial repair (Fig. 16-2).

The determinants of viability are the color and bleeding of tissues.[15] Pink skin with prompt capillary filling and bright red bleeding from open wounds confirm viability. Dark and viscid blood is ominous. Microvascular sludging and thrombosis may render initially viable tissue ischemic. Such progressive retrograde thrombosis is most common as a result of venous impairment.[18] Crushing shearing forces, reverse avulsion flaps and upper extremity congestion commonly cause this.

When bleeding obscures meticulous debride-

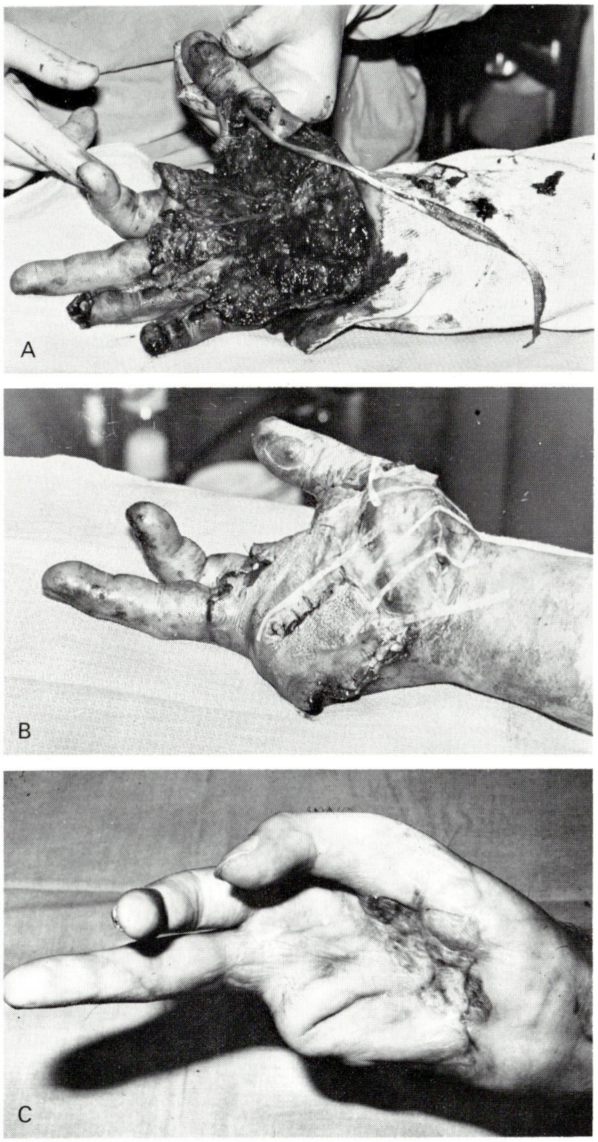

Figure 16-2. *This 25-year-old man was injured when the Civil War cannon he was loading inadvertently discharged. The palmar and ulnar aspects of the hand were torn away* **(A).** *The filletted skin sleeves of the ring and little fingers were used to help close the palmar defect* **(B,C).** *Later tendon grafts and thumb web expansion improved his grasp.*

ment, the tourniquet should be used judiciously. Reactive hyperemia will follow its release and is useful in the determination of tissue viability.

Skeletal Restoration

Skeletal distortion by dislocation and fracture causes tension of tissues, impairing circulation. The mechanics of the hand are also seriously disturbed or impossible without intact bones and joints. Reduction of fractures and dislocations should be conducted as a primary procedure within the limits of good circulation. Secondary correction of these distortions is often difficult and may further threaten mobility.

Although anatomical reduction implies the restoration of both arches of the hand, the axial alignment of the digital rays and the opposition of the thumb, it should not be accomplished by further damaging the hand.[9] Ideal alignment must sometimes be compromised to maintain an adequate blood supply.

Reduction and alignment may require internal fixation (Chaps. 11, 12) (Fig. 16-3). Unstable joints may be pinned in the position of function. At times the simple molding of the hand about a soaking wet gauze is a better choice for aligning extensively comminuted fractures and preserving blood supply. Well-padded external fixation ensures the immobilization needed for healing.

Avascular bone will not heal unless the bed has good circulation. This consideration should dictate the debridement of free comminuted fragments and the secondary use of bone grafts. It is often necessary to maintain the length of metacarpals. An alloplastic spacer may be used for this purpose, pending restoration of skin-fat coverage and an ultimate bone graft (Chap. 11).

Hopeless disruption of joints may require primary arthrodesis or even a primary silicone prosthetic arthroplasty.

Wound Closure

Wound closure should never be at the expense of good circulation. Tension must be avoided at all costs and drainage of serum and blood must be facilitated. Sometimes these objectives may be served only by leaving the wound open. If necessary a drain can be inserted. At times wound approximation may be accomplished by porous paper tape strips, fine mesh gauze or the positioning of the hand, rather than further injuring the skin

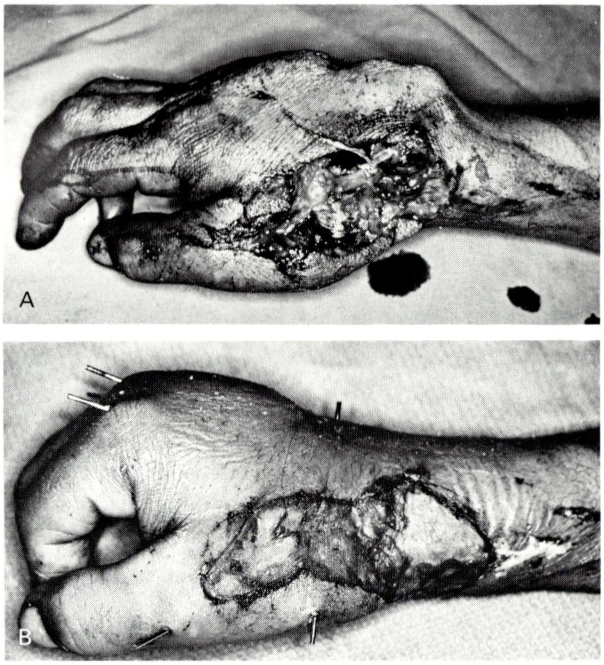

Figure 16-3. *A 42-year-old machinist caught his right hand in his lathe, sustaining multiple soft tissue avulsions* **(A)** *and compound comminuted fractures of the carpals and metacarpals. Open reductions with Kirschner wire fixation were carried out to restore architecture. The apparent skin defect was lessened after fracture reduction and split-thickness grafts were used for wound closure* **(B).**

edges and circulation by suturing. As long as there is no compromise with adequate tissue coverage, the simplest method which will meet the requirements will usually be the most satisfactory.[10]

Skin flaps with precarious circulation (distally based flaps) should sometimes be detached, defatted and reapplied as full-thickness skin grafts. If the bed is healthy there is a reasonably good chance of survival. Thin split-thickness skin grafts are most predictable to take on a poorly vascularized bed (Fig. 16-4). These should be applied as postage stamp or meshed grafts only when the circumstances are most unfavorable for their survival.

Primary definitive cover (pedicle flaps and thick free grafts) should not be used when there is a high threat to survival by factors of poor circulation, contamination or the patient's adverse health or psychology.[5] Closure by secondary intention should be avoided if it risks stiffness and excessive scar.[12] Wounds 1 cm or greater in diameter should be considered for split-thickness grafting in order to minimize local scarring and delayed healing.

Primary neurovascular island pedicle grafts can be used in only selected and unique circumstances by the expert surgeon. These will restore sensibil-

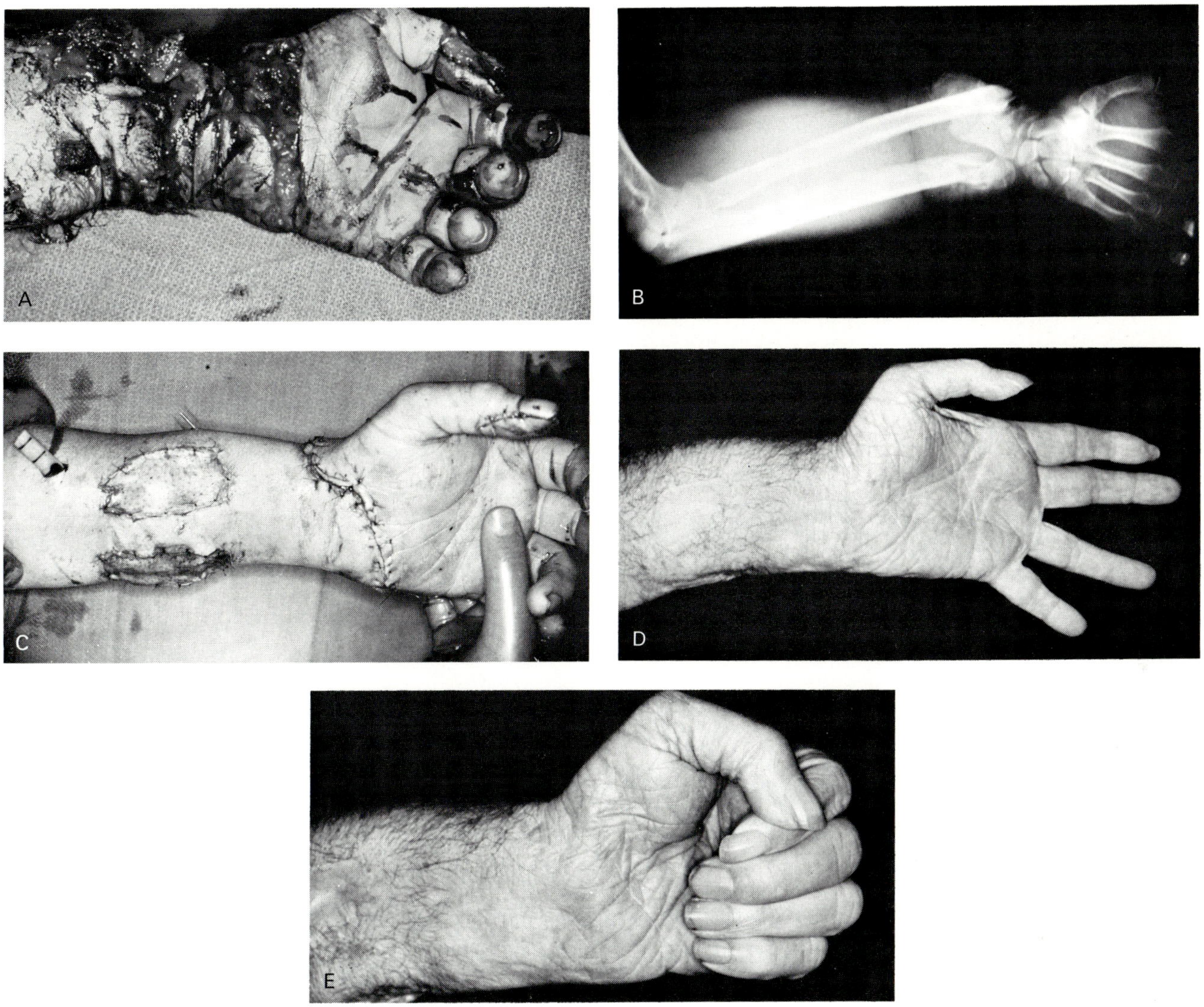

Figure 16-4. *A hay baler crushed this older man's only remaining hand (the other had been lost in a cornpicker several years earlier), resulting in extensive soft tissue avulsion* **(A)** *and compound fractures* **(B).** *Following wound toilet, split-thickness skin grafts were used to resurface the defects* **(C)** *with primary healing and good recovery of function* **(D,E).** *The patient has not needed further surgery.*

ity and circulation after the avulsion of a functionally critical surface of a digit.[6]

Pedicle flaps are primarily used to cover denuded bone, tendons or nerves (Chap. 9). Local tissue shifts are useful where deficits are relatively small and the circulation could be jeopardized by further dissection. Distant pedicle flaps are required for larger surface losses and to transfer better fat padding and enhance the blood supply (Fig. 16-5).

Priorities in Planning Secondary Reconstruction

Every effort is made to overcome edema. This requires elevation and as much active motion as possible. Customized elastic gauntlets and the intermittent wearing of a surgeon's rubber glove may expedite the resolution of swelling.

Mobility of all joints of the upper extremity must be sought by progressive active and passive exercises until the existence of cicatrix or bony blockade becomes insurmountable. At that point surgical intervention may be elected if a reasonable improvement in function can be expected. This may consist of: (1) replacement of skin cover, (2) tenolysis and (3) joint procedures, i.e. arthrolysis, arthroplasty or arthrodesis. Functional passive mobility may convert to active motion by appropriate musculotendinous procedures. Appropriate skeletal alignment and stability are sought by suitable procedures such as rotation and wedge osteotomy and bone grafting.

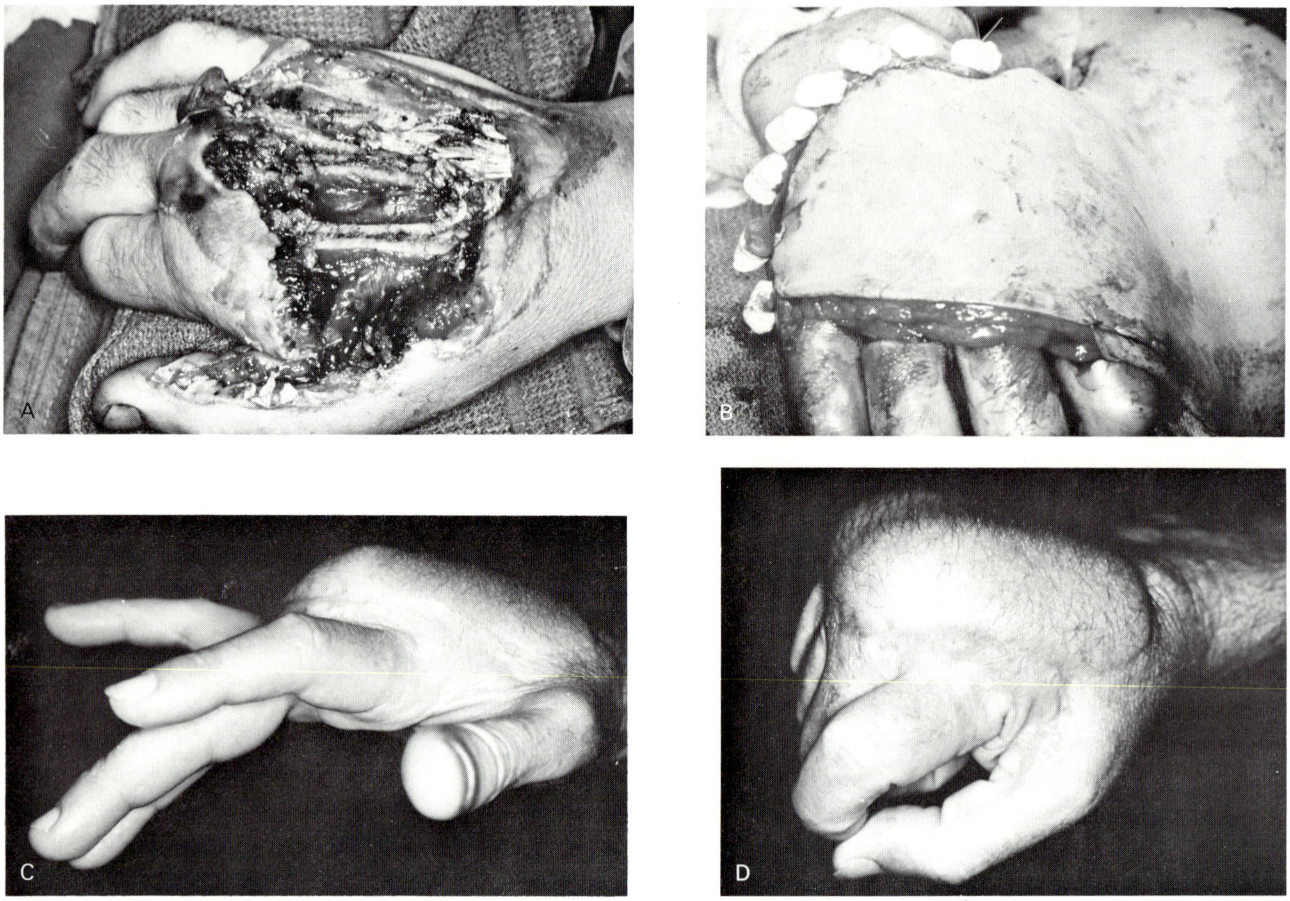

Figure 16-5. *An extensive dorsal wound destroying skin, extensor tendons and cortices of the metacarpals occurred in this young workman* **(A).** *The only complete fracture was through the distal index metacarpal. After a thorough debridement including all marginally viable tissue, flap coverage from the abdominal wall was used* **(B)** *as the best means of preserving the underlying structures. A partial loss of active extension* **(C,D)** *is the only functional deformity following the initial repair.*

Pain can be the undoing of all efforts at reconstruction and rehabilitation. It must be prevented. Pain which is caused by impaired circulation, scar tissue and direct trauma to nerves should be surgically prevented or relieved whenever possible. The patient must be physically and psychologically active to make progress and develop confidence in his recovery. Patients lacking initiative may be helped by extended daily physiotherapy and occupational therapy (Chap. 27).

Impaired sensibility may be overcome by suitable procedures which include neurolysis, neurorrhaphy with or without resection of a neuroma, nerve graft or neurovascular island pedicle transfers (Chap. 15).

Specific Injuries

Specific complex injuries to the hand are listed below. All injuries require a detailed specific history for a proper diagnosis, intelligent selection of treatment, and prognosis.

- Concussion, explosion and high velocity
  - Gunshot
  - Firecracker
  - Grenade
  - Staple gun
  - Cement gun
- Digital degloving
- Compression, crushing, ischemic
  - Wringer with and without avulsion
  - Press injuries
- Mangling
  - Power drive
  - Cornpicker
  - Lawnmower
  - Lithograph
  - Power press
  - Animal bites

Injection and puncture (gas, liquids, plastics, drugs, aniline dyes)
- Inert foreign body
- Reactive foreign body
- Aerosol bomb
- Mace
- Thermal foreign body

Electrical injuries

Concussion

In this group of injuries the effect may be less apparent on the surface than it is beneath by virtue of the wave of concussion and the nature and path of the foreign body. There may be a latent period before the impact of the concussion upon circulation becomes evident.

A roentgenogram may be helpful in demonstrating retained foreign bodies and concomitant skeletal injury. These foreign bodies do not necessarily require removal if their presence does not impair function. The common fear of intravascular migration of such foreign bodies from the hand is generally unfounded. The placement of a small drain to the depths of the wound aids against infection when augmented with systemic antibiotics (Chap. 9).

The mangling that results from blast injuries of firecrackers and bombs is treated according to the discussion under mangling injuries.

Digital Degloving ("ring" injury)

A digit bearing a ring may be degloved by a strong centrifugal force. As a rule this involves the ring finger and classically occurs during a fall when the victim hooks his ring in an attempt to restrain his descent. Part or all of a digit may be torn off.

There are three gradations of this injury.

SKIN ELEVATION ONLY

The distal circulation may be intact albeit precarious. The repositioning of the skin with or without sutures, the administration of low-molecular-weight dextran or heparin along with elevation and immobilization may permit salvage of the skin sleeve. An axial decompressing incision distal to the point of injury may further aid in supporting the local circulation.

COMPLETE AVULSION OF THE CUTANEOUS SLEEVE

Loss of the cutaneous sleeve leaves the digital skeleton with intact tendons and ligaments but devoid of nerves and vessels. Occasionally these soft tissues still remain attached to the distal phalanx.

If the thumb is involved, a tube pedicle should be applied from the contralateral deltopectoral area and later augmented by a neurovascular island transfer. An alternative to this would be amputation of the thumb and pollicization of the index finger.

Any other digit so affected should be treated with a ray resection (Fig. 16-6). In a youthful patient a ray transfer may be considered to compensate for the long or ring fingers. Such transfers take 8 to 12 weeks for the metacarpal to heal and risk the occurrence of joint stiffness and non-union because of the need to strip the periosteum. In this instance ray II is transferred to ray III and ray V to ray IV (Chap. 17).

AMPUTATION

The cutaneous sleeve is avulsed with one or more phalanges which may or may not tear flexor or extensor tendons from their musculotendinous junction. The treatment here should follow the precepts of Chapter 17 on amputations or those enumerated in the foregoing paragraph.

Compression, Crushing and Ischemic Injuries

These injuries result from compression of the extremity between rollers, which are usually motor driven at variable rates of speed. At times only one roller is powered. The clearance between the rollers is highly variable and may be either fixed or spring loaded. At times only the friction between the rollers and the skin advances the extremity to cause injury. However, all too often it is the workman's glove that is suddenly seized, pulling the extremity after it. Classically the first injuries so described were those caused by the home laundry washing machine wringer (still sold today in this era of automatic equipment).

Certain specific injuries result depending upon the speed of the rollers, their compressive force, the anatomical point of arrest (thumb web, elbow or

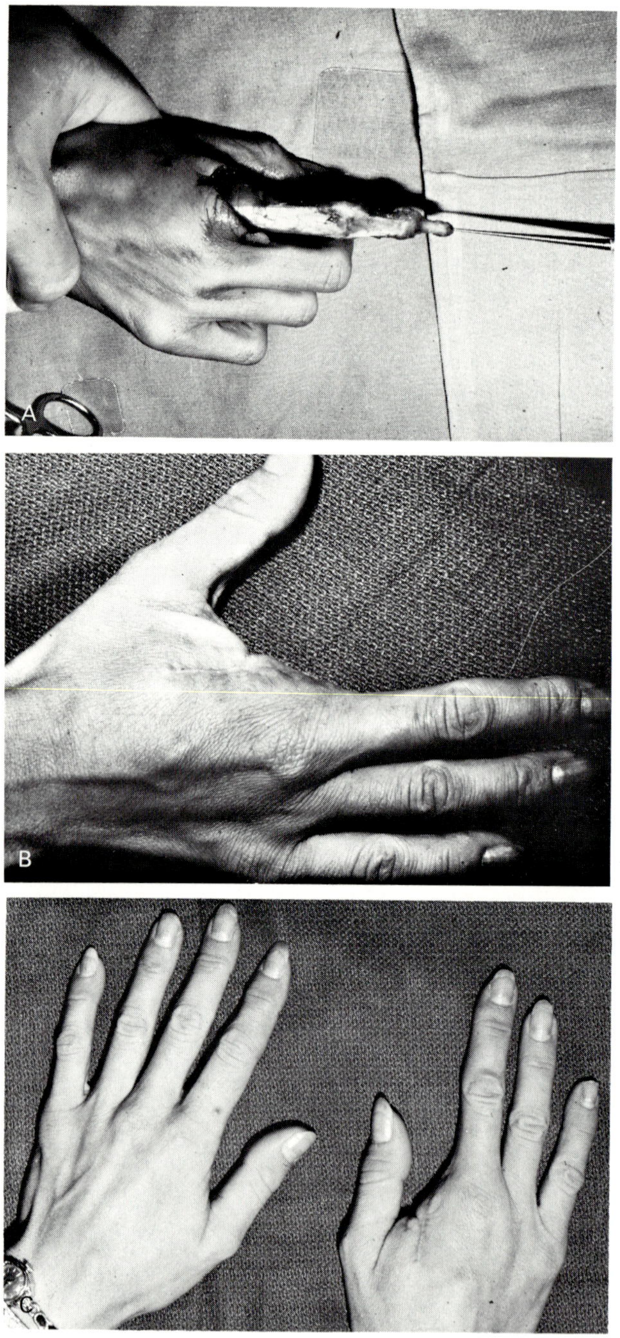

Figure 16-6. *This 30-year-old seamstress suffered a degloving injury of her major index finger when she caught it in a power lawnmower* **(A).** *An immediate ray amputation with transfer of the first dorsal interosseous muscle into the long finger was done. An excellent functional and cosmetic result was obtained* **(B,C).**

axilla) and the patient's withdrawal reaction. Low-speed rollers with limited compressive force may do little more than frighten the patient. High-speed rollers with marked compressive force and a violent withdrawal reaction by the patient may severely disrupt circulation, produce fractures or dislocations and avulse soft tissues. Even traction injuries of the brachial plexus can result.

These injuries are emergencies and because they may thoroughly threaten the circulatory dynamics of the extremity (venous return) they must be attended to promptly and observed frequently in a responsible environment (hospital). The initial outward appearance may belie the extent of deep injury resulting from simple compression with or without a shearing force. Either factor can cause injury to vessels, resulting in hemorrhea and thrombosis. The shearing force can produce extensive separation of skin and subcutaneous tissue from the underlying fascia, leading to a dead space which often requires drainage.

Roentgenograms are imperative in most of these injuries. For proper scrutiny of the fresh injury the patient should be kept supine and the extremity elevated on a pillow or in a stockinette sling. Under these circumstances progressive brawny edema monitored by circumferential measurements and progressive nerve palsy require prompt decompression of skin and fascia (Chap. 10). Decompression may be needed even in the presence of a good peripheral pulse. Unrelenting throbbing pain urgently signals the need for decompression.

Specific skin injuries consist of avulsions and friction burns.[16] The avulsions may be closed or opened, limited or extensive, but usually spare the palm which is tethered by its fascia. Distally based flaps are the rule and their circulatory embarrassment is so common that the physician must consider replacing them primarily as a free graft or secondarily by grafts from other areas.

At the point of arrest of the power-driven rollers friction burns, often third and even fourth degree, result. Primary debridement and early secondary grafting should follow. Thick split-thickness grafts should be used in the thumb web, while elsewhere the grafts should be tailored to the surface and the circumstances. The graft should not be applied until hemostasis and the circulatory integrity of the bed are assured. Fractures and dislocations should be promptly reduced and appropriately splinted. As with all injuries, it is desirable to reinstitute active physical effort of all parts as soon as possible to forestall stiffness and contractures. Open injuries demand the administration of antibiotics. Low-molecular-weight dextran may be useful in the presence of circulatory embarrassment.

In addition to friction and compression, a laundry mangle produces thermal trauma from the steam or heat emitted (Fig. 16-7); this may constitute the only injury sustained. Depending on the

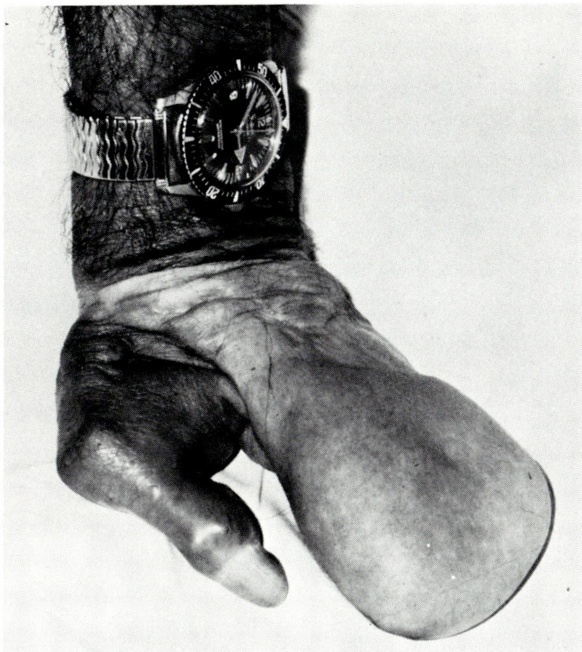

Figure 16-7. *This middle-aged man caught his hand in a hot mangle, suffering both crushing and thermal injuries. After amputation of the fingers his hand was covered with two abdominal flaps for the palm and dorsum.*

nature of the mangle, one or both surfaces of the hand may be burned.

A host of either closed or open crushing injuries result from a vast array of other circumstances. The history is of paramount importance in these injuries, predicting the threat to functional integrity. It should be a guide to appropriate treatment in the same manner as that cited for wringer injuries.

Mangling Injuries

All of these injuries are open, with disruption of multiple tissues and skeletal distortion. These injuries are the greatest challenge to the surgeon in estimating salvageability of function and viability, especially when more than a single digit is involved. The magnitude of the salvage effort should be governed by the magnitude of the involvement and the likelihood of restoring basic useful function. If only one or two fingers are involved amputation may spare hopeless reconstructive efforts and costly time. When the injury is greater the decision to amputate or not may be difficult, even for the most experienced hand surgeon. The key to success lies in adequate debridement, maintenance of circulation, prevention of infection and aiming for simple rather than complex function.

The bulk of these injuries result from power-driven machines: in industry and construction, in farming (cornpicker) and in the home (lawnmower). Bites of a frightened or infuriated animal have been known to mangle single or multiple parts of the upper extremity by their fury and force. The additional factor of contamination here makes the need for the preservation of circulation and the administration of systemic antibiotics imperative.

Injection Injuries (*punctures*)

Through no more than a puncture wound, animal toxins, pathogenic organisms or foreign materials are inoculated. The result is influenced by the toxicity of the substance injected, the amount of the inflammatory response and the magnitude of the dead space created. The temperature of the injection may produce a thermal or cryogenic injury. When the substance is not inert the local reaction may result in chemical necrosis. The injection can consist of gas, liquids, semisolids or solids. Without experience, the patient and the doctor can be tragically misled by the frequently innocuous appearance of the hand in the first few hours after injury (Figs. 16-8**A**,16-9**A**). The hand may appear and function normally. Hence the history is critically important to the immediate institution of proper treatment.

SIMPLE PUNCTURE

If the injury is a simple contaminated puncture with the injection limited to bacterial contamination, then the treatment may be confined to elevation, immobilization and administration of antibiotics. Examples of such injuries are bites, stings and nail or needle punctures.

When a toxic substance (e.g. aniline dye from an indelible pencil) is introduced, local chemical necrosis will occur. Immediate local excision of the exposed tissue and foreign material must be considered to avoid extension of the cellulitis and secondary cicatrix.[11]

GAS INJECTION

Gas under pressure may cause serious systemic effects, even death if injected directly into the systemic circulation. However, if injected into the tissue spaces, it may dissect widely even into the trunk without creating any systemic effect. If subcutaneous crepitation is not evident the diagnosis

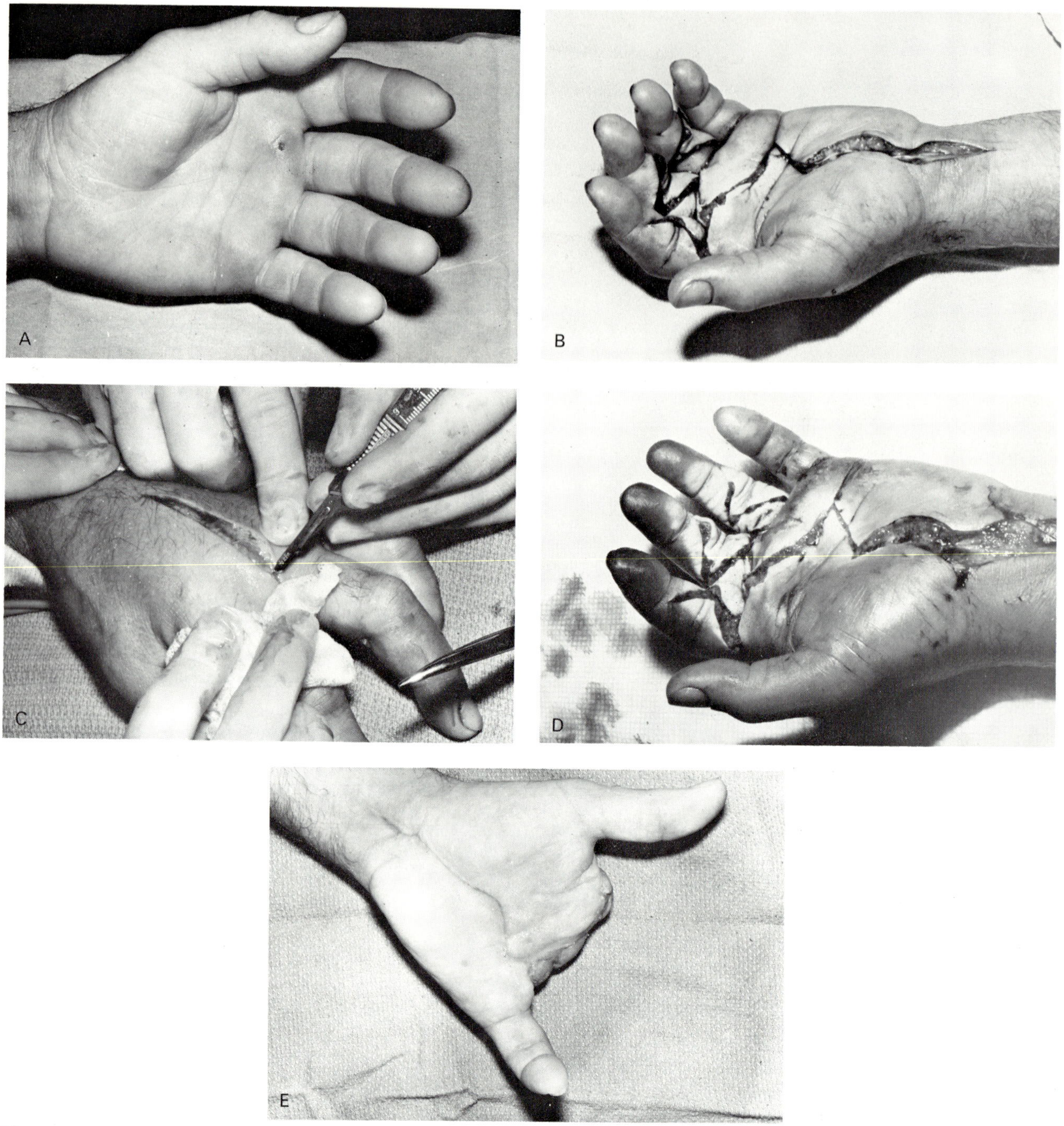

Figure 16-8. *This middle-aged painter sustained an injection injury of his minor hand on the volar aspect of the index metacarpal head with paint thinner* **(A).** *Despite decompression of the digits, dorsum of the hand and palm within six hours of his injury, he suffered loss of three fingers* **(B,C,D).** *A rotation osteotomy of the little finger and deepening of the first web are planned.*

can be confirmed by roentgenography. The problems generated are those of tissue tension with circulatory embarrassment, dead space in the presence of bacterial inoculation and chemical toxicity if the gas in not inert.

Expectant treatment with immobilization, elevation and systemic antibiotics usually suffices for these injuries.

LIQUID INJECTION

A liquid, like a gas, may spread widely through tissue planes, and when it is under high pressure may immediately diffuse without distending tissue spaces.[8] Subjectively the patient describes only a sudden hot feeling at the moment of injection. The injection may block nerve impulses, delaying the

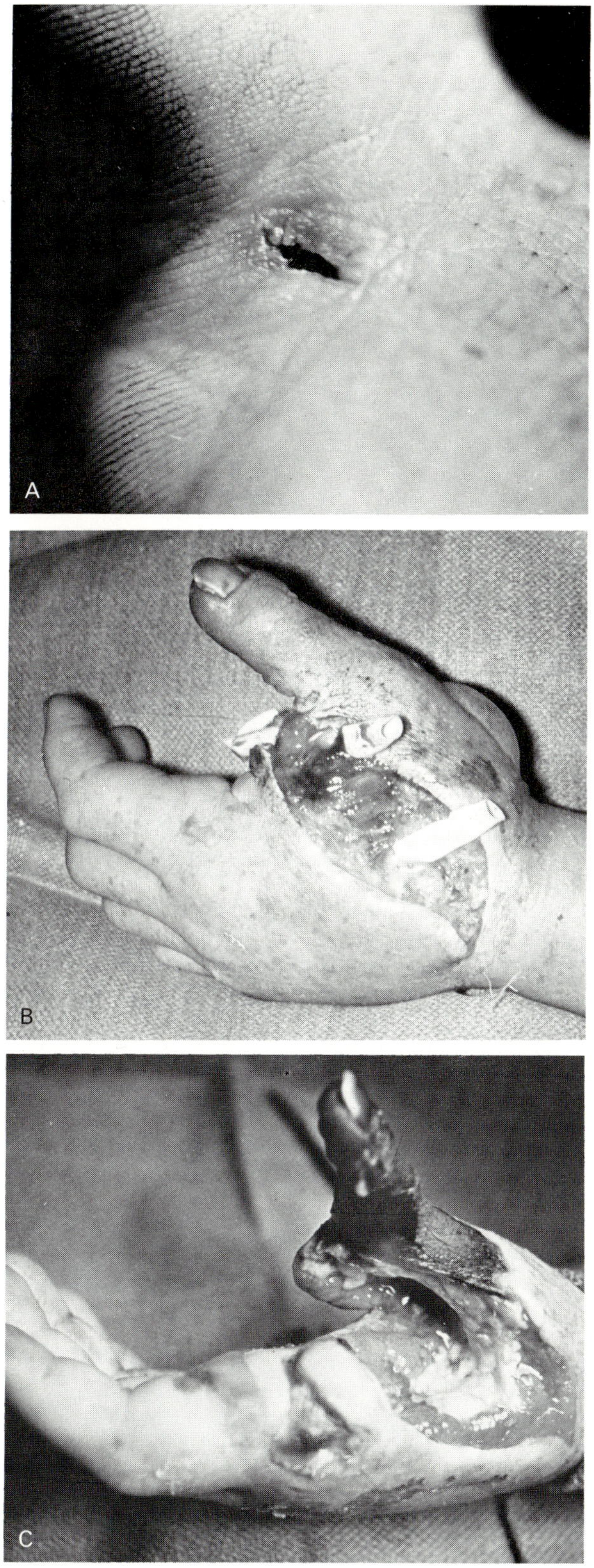

Figure 16-9. *The only obvious injury was a small puncture wound in the thenar web at one hour after an injection injury from a grease gun* **(A).** *In spite of immediate and wide decompression, drainage and irrigation* **(B),** *signs of ischemia were present at 48 hours* **(C)** *and frank necrosis of the thumb by 5 days.*

onset of pain for an indefinite period. The lack of pain must not delude the surgeon into inaction. Ultimately the pain may be severe. In the first hour or two there may be nothing objectively evident upon examination and even the pinpoint portal through the skin may be obscure.

If the fluid is inert (water), there may be no sequelae so long as circulation is not impaired and infection does not ensue. However, if the injection is chemically reactive, the patient must be hospitalized and observed hourly while receiving concomitant antibiotics and sometimes steroids and low-molecular-weight dextran. When the injection is known to be toxic to tissues even in the absence of any objective findings, the involved tissue planes should be decompressed by fasciotomy and the skin left open (Fig. 16-8). Swelling following these injections results from chemical cellulitis and vasculitis as well as increased tissue tension. Failure to adequately decompress the part early only increases the risk of gangrene or an ischemic contracture. This decompression attempts to preserve the venous return. It is virtually impossible to debride any liquid from the interstices of the tissues, and most chemical solvents will only aggravate the tissue injury. The extent of the extravasation of leaded paint will be evident upon roentgenograms. Other common sources for injection injuries of the hand are household aerosol containers and self-protective tear gas pens and Mace dispensers.[1]

GREASE GUN INJURY

These injection injuries have been recognized for several decades. The lubricant may enter the hand at pressures up to 15,000 pounds per square inch and initiate an intense foreign body reaction culminating in oleomas.[19,20] The treatment is immediate surgery to decompress the tissues and debride the foreign body from the tissue spaces (Fig. 16-9).

A thermal or cryogenic injury can also occur, depending upon the temperature of the injected material or its endothermic or exothermic reaction. Molten plastic injected under several thousand pounds of pressure and temperatures above 100° C produces severe thermal injury in addition to the mechanical effects of the injection itself.[2,4,7]

Drug abuse injuries have left a toll of septic and aseptic cellulitis and the resultant problems of abscess formation, congestion and cicatrix. In addition there have been severe vascular problems (Chap. 10) and neuropathies from the direct injection of nerves or their compression. Nerve entrapment results from the narcotized individual's lying upon his extremity or from direct pressure upon a subcutaneous nerve. Ischemic contracture (Volkmann's) occurs but can sometimes be forestalled by early decompression.

Electrical Burns

These injuries (Chap. 19) are truly complex, since coagulation of multiple tissues occurs and circulation is markedly embarrassed. As with severe injection injuries, the prime measures of treatment direct themselves to the preservation of circulation, prevention of infection and early debridement of obviously non-viable tissues. At times a hopeless case requires early amputation.

References

1. Adams, J.P., Fee, N. and Kenmore, P.I.: Tear gas injuries. J. Bone Joint Surg., 48A:436, 1966.
2. Baker, J.M.: Molten plastic injuries of hand. Plast. Reconstr. Surg., 15:233, 1955.
3. Bateman, J.E.: *Trauma to Nerves in Limbs.* W.B. Saunders, Philadelphia, 1962.
4. Brown, H.C., Williams, H.B. and Woolhouse, F.M.: Principles of salvage in mutilating hand injuries. J. Trauma, 8:319, 1968.
5. Burkhalter, W.E., Butler, B., Metz, W. and Omer, G.: Experiences with delayed primary closure of war wounds of the hand in Vietnam. J. Bone Joint Surg., 50A:945, 1968.
6. Chase, R.A.: Surgery of the hand. N. Engl. J. Med., 287:1174, 1227, 1972.
7. Desjacques, R. and Cognat, M.: Injection accidentelle a chaud de matiere plastique dans la main. Presse Med., 67:1878, 1959.
8. Kaufman, H.D.: The anatomy of experimentally produced high-pressure injection injuries of the hand. Br. J. Surg., 55:340, 1968.
9. Littler, J.W.: The physiology and dynamic function of the hand. Surg. Clin. North Am., 40:259, 1960.
10. London, R.S.: Simplicity of approach to treatment of the injured hand. J. Bone Joint Surg., 43B:454, 1961.
11. Mason, M.L. and Allen, H.S.: Indelible pencil injuries to the hands. Ann. Surg., 113:131, 1941.
12. Mason, M.D.: Fifty years progress in surgery of the hand. Int. Abst. Surg., 101:541, 1955.
13. Maxim, E.S., Webster, F.S. and Willander, D.A.: The cornpicker hand. J. Bone Joint Surg., 36A:21, 1954.
14. McCormack, R.M.: Crush, mangle and cornpicker injuries of the hand. In *Hand Surgery* (Flynn, J.E., Ed.). Williams and Wilkins, Baltimore, 1966.
15. McCormack, R.M.: Primary reconstruction in acute hand injuries. Surg. Clin. North Am., 40:337, 1960.
16. Posch, J. and Weller, C.N.: Mangle and severe wringer injuries of the hand in children. J. Bone Joint Surg., 36A:57, 1954.
17. Rank, B.K., Wakefield, A.R. and Hueston, J.T.: *Surgery of Repair as Applied to Hand Injuries.* Williams and Wilkins, Baltimore, 1960.
18. Robinson, D.W. and Masters, F.W.: Severe avulsion injuries of the extremities including the degloving type. Surg. Clin. North Am., 47:379, 1967.
19. Smith, M.G.H.: Grease gun injury. Br. Med. J., 2:918, 1964.
20. Stark, H.H., Wilson, J.N. and Boyes, J.H.: Grease gun injuries of the hand. J. Bone Joint Surg., 43A:45, 1961.

17 Amputations

Obviously an amputation may be as minor as the loss of skin and subcutaneous tissue from a fingertip or as major as the loss of the whole hand. The proper treatment varies with the complexity of the injury, the personal needs of the patient and the risk of future complications relative to the reparative procedure intended. No set rules can be established that will be applicable to all circumstances. At best, some basic concepts coupled with common sense will go further in providing proper treatment for the injured hand than the intimate knowledge of several very complicated and risky reconstructive procedures.

Partial Amputations of the Finger

Total and Subtotal Distal Phalangeal Amputations

Listed below is a myriad of procedures available for treating partial losses of the distal segment of the finger:

- Partial or total distal digital losses
  - Wound dressing only ("skillful neglect")
  - Primary wound closure
  - Split-thickness skin graft
  - Full-thickness skin graft
  - Replacement of avulsed tissue
  - Local flaps
- Volar advancement flap
  - Atasoy[1]
  - Snow[11]
- Lateral advancement flap
  - Kutler[7]
- Flaps from a distance
  - Cross-finger flap
  - Palmar flap
  - Cross-arm flap
  - Neurovascular island pedicle flap
  - Thoracic or abdominal pedicle flap

The simplest procedure is to do nothing—"skillful neglect." This type of management, often used in children, runs the risk of unsatisfactory scar contracture, dysesthesia and possible deformity (Fig. 17-1). It is not applicable except to the most minor of injuries or the most recalcitrant of individuals.

Many partial losses of tissue from the fingertip result from catching the finger in a closing door. Consequently the often battered and crushed remnant is brought along with high expectations for its successful replantation. The reattachment of such contused bits of flesh is uniformally unsuccessful

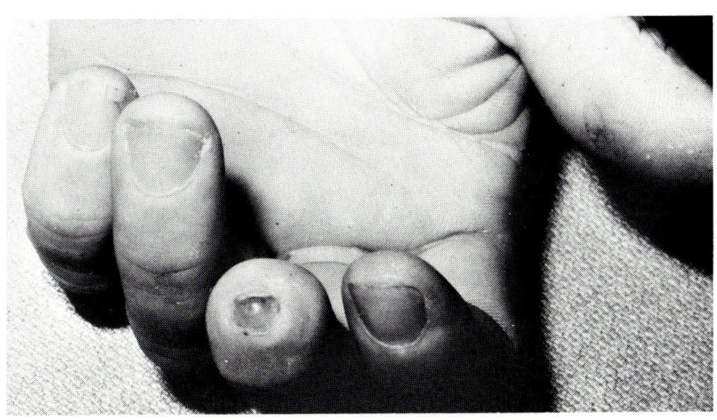

Figure 17-1. *"Beaking" or downward curving of the nail occurred following treatment of the avulsion injury of this man's long finger by simple dressings alone.*

and should not be attempted. However, some portion of the amputated skin may prove suitable for reattachment once the subcutaneous fat has been thoroughly removed. In general, a split-thickness skin graft taken from an inconspicuous area (hypothenar region or groin) will prove more predictable in its take as a free graft than a full-thickness graft recovered from the avulsed part.[9] Grafts to the volar surface which are taken from areas other than the palm or sole tend to hyperpigment, especially in dark-complexioned individuals (Fig. 17-2). Occasionally an unsightly scar will occur at the donor site on the flexor aspect of the forearm (Fig. 17-3).

The advantages of using split-thickness skin grafts are that they will take even when the bed is not optimal and will survive over small projections of bone, exposed tendon and subcutaneous fat.[6] The patient is not committed to a protracted course of treatment and in many instances may return to work within a few days. Should this initial repair prove inadequate, further reconstruction can be done electively on a healed wound (Fig. 17-4).

When the bone has been amputated sufficiently far proximally a simple closure may be all that is needed. This closure should be loose, and lateral "dog ears" need not be trimmed but allowed to shrink down as healing proceeds. The end of the bone should be quite smooth and any remnants of nail matrix should be excised or repositioned in their proper locations (Fig. 17-5). Usually the digital nerve ends are ligated with fine nylon (6-0) if they are readily evident in the wound. Full-thick-

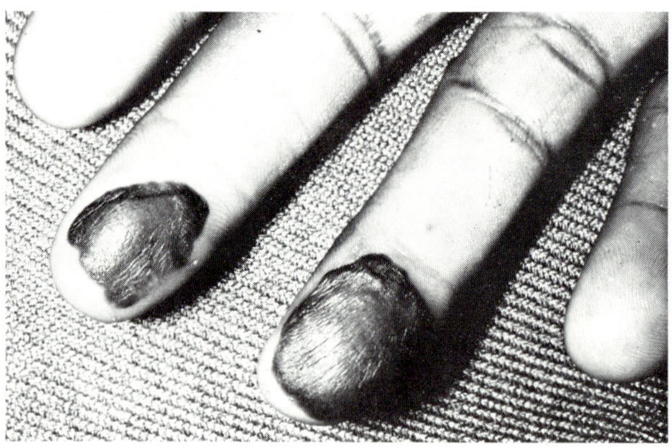

Figure 17-2. *Hyperpigmentation resulted in skin grafts from the groin placed on the fingertips of this young black girl.*

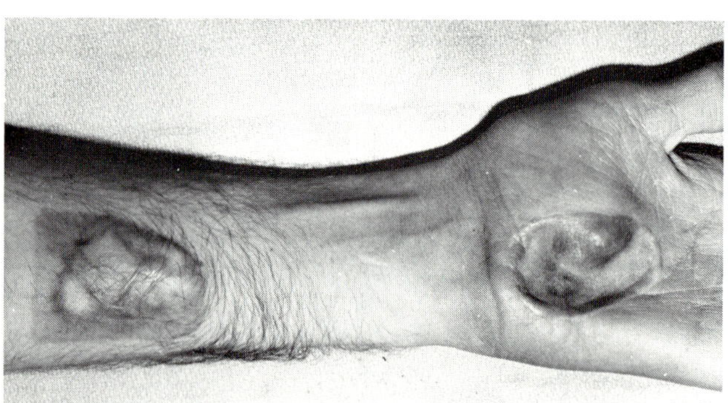

Figure 17-3. *A very deep graft taken from the volar aspect of the forearm for the palm resulted in a conspicuous and symptomatic scar.*

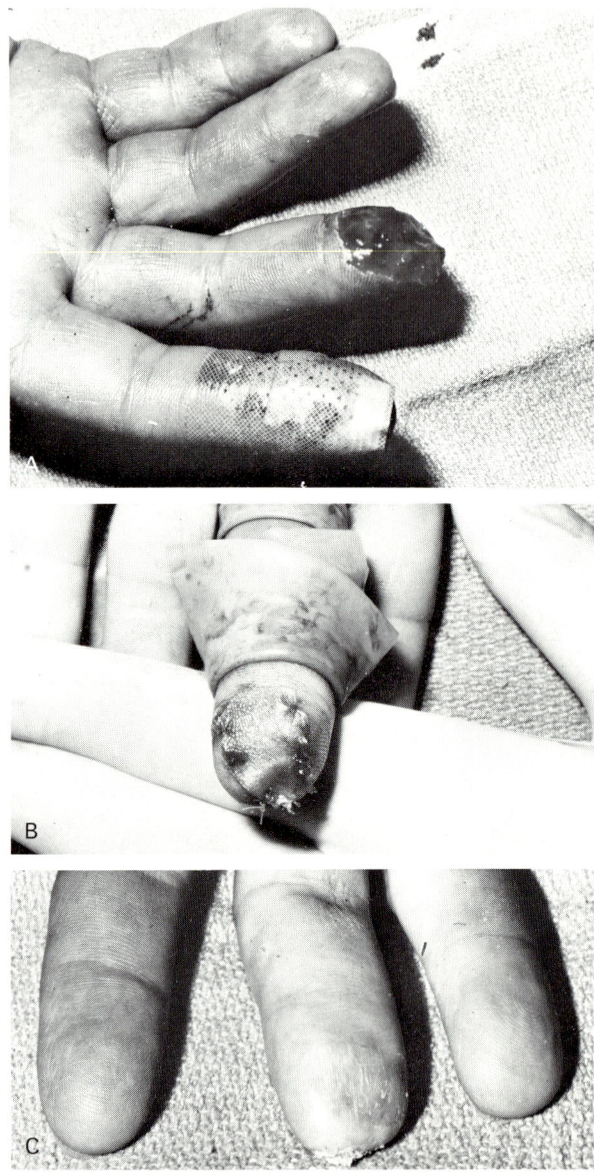

Figure 17-4. *A superficial avulsion of the long fingertip is repaired by a split-thickness skin graft from the hypothenar area. An excellent cosmetic and functional result is obtained.*

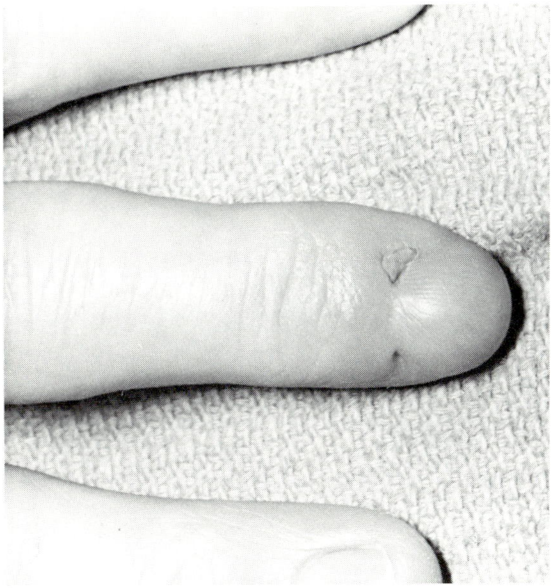

Figure 17-5. *The fingertip had been reconstructed with a palmar flap. The nail matrix had not been completely ablated, resulting in two painful nail horns. These were subsequently excised.*

ness skin grafts taken from the antecubital fossa (Wolfe's grafts) are not recommended since they do not share with split-thickness skin grafts the predictability of survival on the traumatized bed. The advantages gained in terms of future pliability, freedom from contracture, and greater durability by the use of a full-thickness skin graft and a thick partial-thickness graft are negligible.

The technique for procurement and placement of a split-thickness skin graft is as follows:

1. The patient is comfortably recumbent with the injured hand at his side on an arm board.
2. Anesthesia is induced by use of an intermetacarpal block just proximal to the metacarpal head (Chap. 26). The area which will serve as a donor site (hypothenar region, forearm, upper arm or groin) is infiltrated with lidocaine also.
3. The arm is elevated for 3 to 5 minutes and a padded blood pressure cuff is applied to the upper arm. It is inflated to 300 mm Hg and the tubing is clamped.
4. The wound is cleansed with a non-irritating saline solution or even tap water rather than a germicidal solution.
5. A rubber dam (Penrose drain) 2.5 cm wide is wrapped about the digit from distal to proximal and held with a hemostat. The distal part is cut away to reveal the injury. The upper arm tourniquet is deflated.
6. The wound is inspected using loupe magnification, the remaining clots are lifted away and the small open vessels are electrocoagulated with a disposable ophthalmologic cautery. Larger vessels are ligated with non-reactive absorbable suture or nylon. The irregular ends of bone are trimmed back and the nail bed and matrix are restored to their normal position. Rents in the nail bed and matrix are repaired usually with fine (5-0 or 6-0) absorbable non-reactive sutures, polyglactin or polyglycolic acid.
7. The skin is removed from the donor area using a #10 scalpel blade, razor blade or small freehand skin graft knife (Goulian) (Fig. 17-6). The donor site is covered with a single layer of lubricated gauze and several thicknesses of soaking wet plain gauze.
8. The graft is placed on the defect and may be secured in a variety of ways. If the bed is irregular and extensive a tied-down dressing (Stent) might be preferable (Chap. 6). The easiest and most frequently used method is to secure the graft with non-encircling $\frac{1}{8}''$ porous paper strips (Fig. 17-7). A form-fitted piece of lubricated gauze is then applied and multiple thicknesses of soaking wet gauze are molded over the fingertip. To this is added a piece of sponge plastic (Reston) or rubber, and the whole is secured with a tubular gauze wrapping. The entire hand is usually placed in a splint or cast for a few days until the initial dressing is changed. The need for casting varies with the preference of the surgeon and the responsiveness of the patient. The digital tourniquet is removed once the dressing is secure and the more proximal padded tourniquet has been completely removed.
9. The patient is instructed to keep the part elevated and to report immediately if throbbing pain develops. The initial dressing is changed from 2 to 5 days following the injury. Subsequent dressings and splinting are dictated by the individual circumstances.

Certain fingertip amputations are quite suited to reconstruction by the use of local flaps. Perhaps

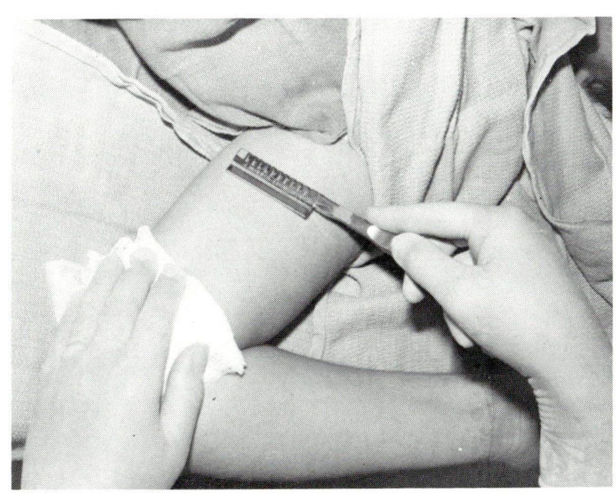

Figure 17-6. *A skin graft is procured from the medial upper arm with the Goulian knife.*

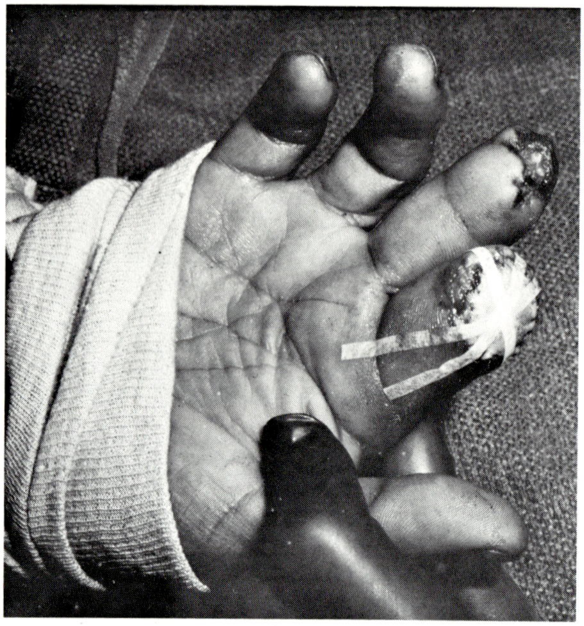

Figure 17-7. *Split-thickness grafts are easily secured by porous adhesive paper strips.*

the most popular of these is the classic Kutler[5,7] bilateral triangular advancement flap or its volar modification proposed by Atasoy[1] (Fig. 17-8). Caution must be exercised in developing these flaps to avoid compromising their circulation by undermining and making the closure too tight. Both methods tend to produce "beaking" of the residual nail from lack of underlying padding and support.

In some circumstances it may be advisable to advance a large segment of the volar surface of the finger.[11] Midaxial incisions are made bilaterally and the volar flap is raised as far proximally as necessary by detaching Cleland's and Grayson's cutaneous ligaments (Fig. 17-9). The next proximal joint is flexed slightly to gain length and, if need be, the neurovascular bundles can be skeletonized and a proximal spacing graft inserted. The joint is maintained in flexion until after the sutures are removed. This procedure has the advantage of transferring distalward volar skin that has finer sensibility than almost any other type of reconstruction. The procedure does pose a risk of injury to the neurovascular pedicles and of joint stiffness if the proximal flexion is too severe and too lengthy.

In general the shortcomings of local advancement flaps of whatever design are: (1) inadequate support of the regenerating nail and subsequent downcurving (beaking), (2) their tendency to become fixed to underlying bone and unyielding because of the loss of subcutaneous padding and (3) the tendency of the surgeon to make the closure too tight, thus increasing the amount of rigid scar.

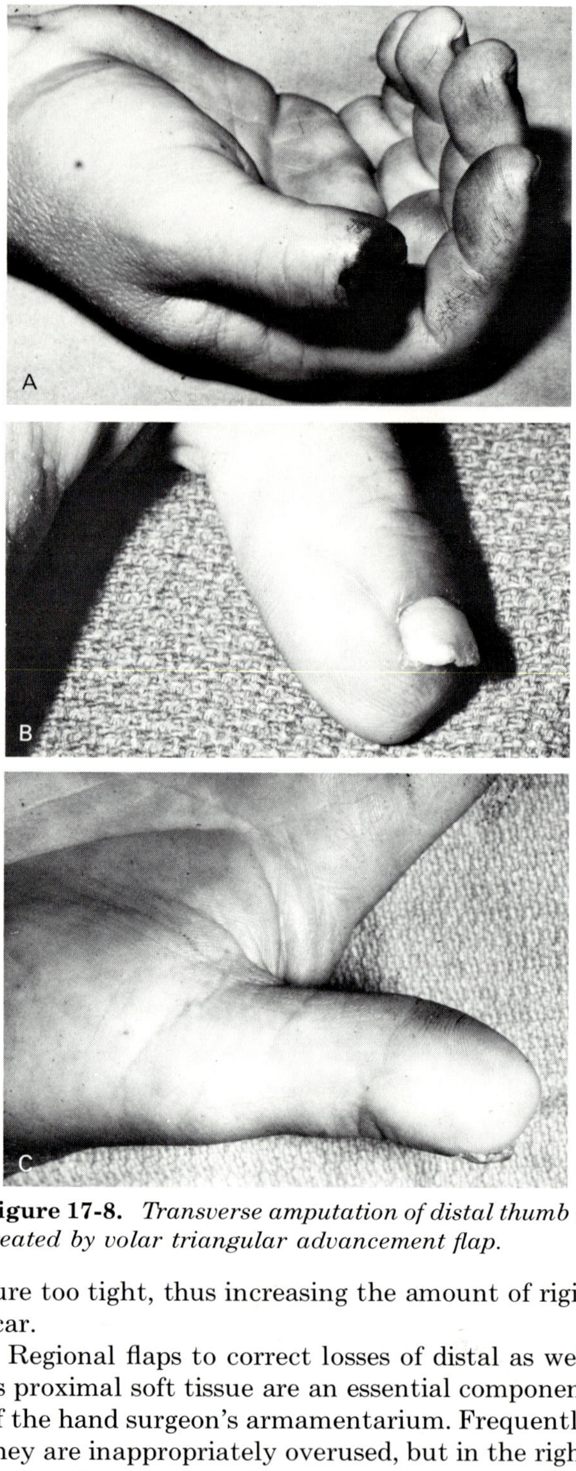

Figure 17-8. *Transverse amputation of distal thumb is treated by volar triangular advancement flap.*

Regional flaps to correct losses of distal as well as proximal soft tissue are an essential component of the hand surgeon's armamentarium. Frequently they are inappropriately overused, but in the right circumstances and with proper judgment they may be valuable adjuncts for primary treatment or secondary reconstruction. A good rule is not to use a flap when a split-thickness skin graft will suffice.

The palmar or thenar flap is one of the very useful but frequently abused regional flaps for fingertip reconstruction. Properly considered and executed, it provides well-padded volar-type skin

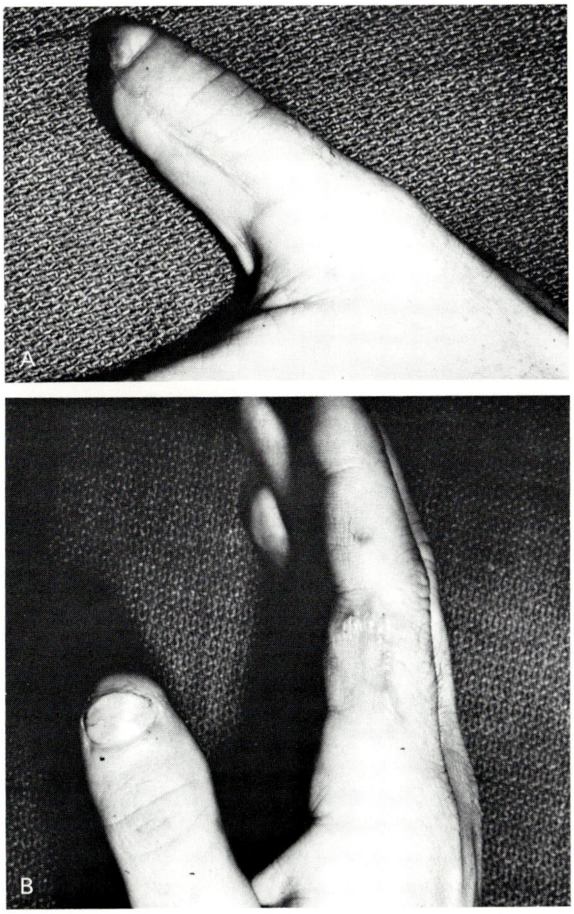

Figure 17-9. *Amputation of the distal thumb was reconstructed by advancing the volar surface of the thumb while flexing the interphalangeal joint. This did not produce as satisfactory a result as the cross-finger flap used for the identical injury on the other side.*

with substantial support to the regenerating nail. It may be used primarily or for later reconstruction. Little risk should occur to the patient with respect to digital stiffness and discomfort at the donor site. Generally patients over the age of 50 or those with joint injuries or arthritis should not undergo this type of procedure.

The procedure can be performed with general, infusion or regional block anesthesia.

1. A padded upper arm tourniquet is needed, and the arm should be exsanguinated by elevation prior to placement and inflation.
2. The digital tip in question is cleansed with an isotonic saline solution and debrided as previously described. The bony irregularities are removed and the nail elements resected or repositioned if they are distorted.
3. To determine the donor site for the flap, the digit is gently flexed toward the palm. The distal interphalangeal joint should be only slightly flexed and the proximal joint flexed to 80°. The flap is outlined on the palm or the thenar eminence, making it slightly larger than the corresponding defect. The flap is elevated with its base proximal in most instances. An excess of subcutaneous fat is removed with the flap, ensuring that adequate padding of the tip will be provided. The donor wound is either closed primarily or the injured fingertip is brought down into it.

   The flap is attached with half-buried mattress sutures and a piece of adherent plastic sponge (Reston) is placed over the dorsum of the finger. A wet dressing is placed in the palm about the fingertip and a cast is usually employed for 3 to 5 days. After that a restraining tape strip over the injured finger, which is padded at the proximal interphalangeal joint, suffices. The patient may then wash and cleanse his hand.
4. Division of the flap is done with local anesthesia at 9 to 12 days after application. Usually the final trimming and insetting is not done for 24 to 48 hours after the release. The donor site is closed primarily or allowed to heal secondarily. It is *not* grafted.

A cross-finger flap may be preferable to a palmer flap but involves an uninjured finger, exposing it to the risk of infection, stiffness and scarring. These flaps are designed in many forms to fit the circumstances of the injury. Basically a flap of skin is unfurled from the dorsal aspect of the adjacent finger and hinged along the adjacent axial border of the finger. The injured finger is then positioned to extend the flap over the defect (Fig. 17-10). A skin graft is required for resurfacing the donor defect. A helpful trick in placing the skin graft is to sew it reverse side up to the adjacent border of the injury and then run a fine nylon suture around its remaining periphery to attach it to the donor site of the flap. The flap is usually secured to its recipient area with half-buried mattress sutures. Fourteen to 20 days of immobilization are needed before the flap can be divided. If early division is elected, the procedure should be done in stages. Usually the distal and proximal thirds of the flap are severed and 24 to 72 hours later the division is completed. A day or two should intervene before the tailoring and insetting of the flap to allow edema to subside.

Only under unusual conditions should a primary neurovascular island pedicle be considered for the loss of the distal segment. Usually this opportunity transpires when multiple digits have been injured and a single pedicle with distal tissue remains on a digit that is otherwise totally destroyed (Fig. 17-11). Whenever a neurovascular island pedicle is

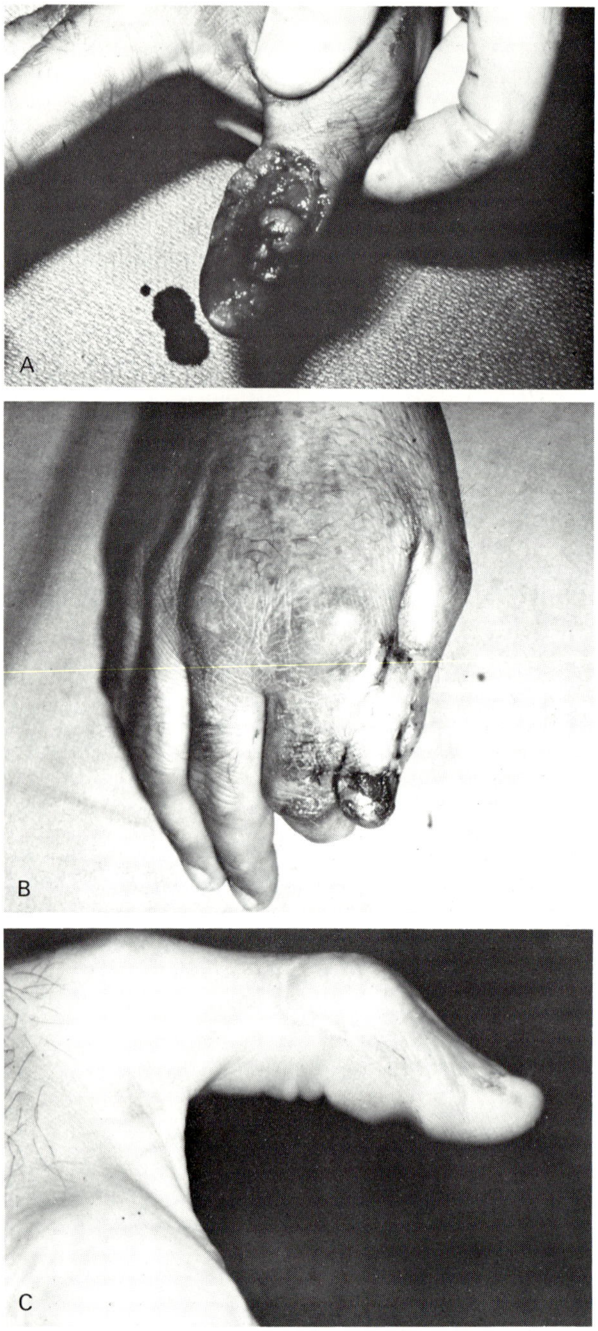

Figure 17-10. *This man suffered an injury to the dorsum of the proximal interphalangeal joint of the thumb with division of the extensor tendon and avulsion of a portion of the nail bed. It was repaired with an immediate cross-finger flap.*

transferred it must be done meticulously with great care to avoid kinking or occluding the arterial or venous circulation (Chap. 15) and must be routed so that later swelling will not engorge the flap.

To cover larger defects, especially partial degloving injuries of the fingers or multiple digital injuries, cross-arm, axillary, infraclavicular, and thoracic flaps may be employed. These are individually planned and tailored to fit the specific injury being treated (Chap. 9).

Digital length is of greatest importance in the thumb and index finger. Loss of hand function is often greater with traumatic shortening of the thumb than with any of the fingers. Once the index finger has been amputated through or proximal to

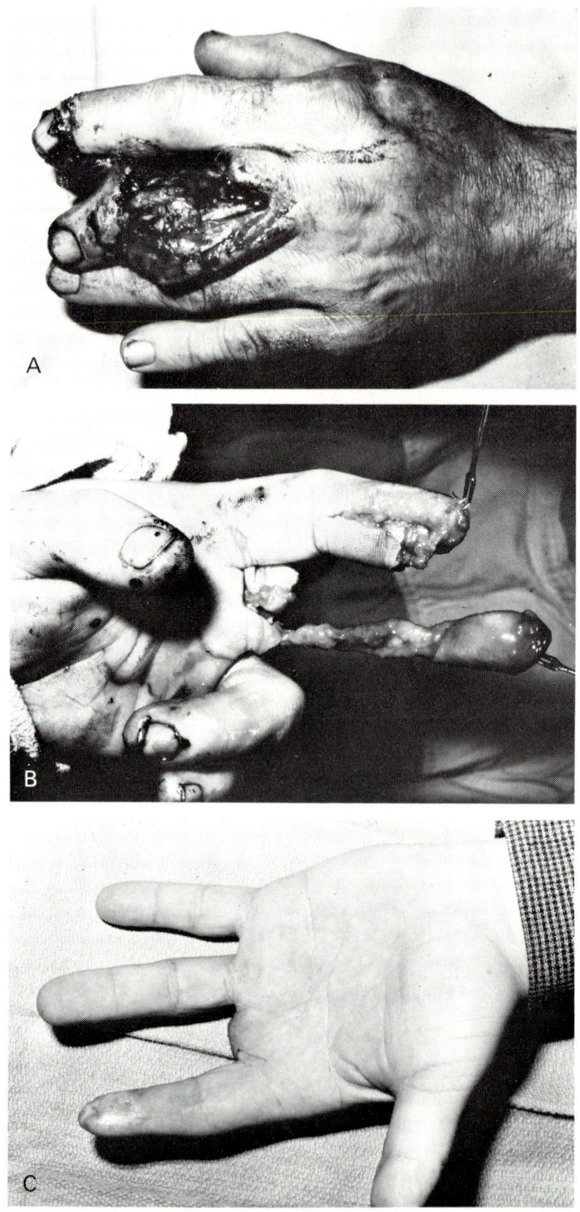

Figure 17-11. *This 30-year-old male sustained a crush injury to the index and long fingers with total comminution of the phalanges of the long finger. The tip of the long finger was transferred on a neurovascular pedicle to replace the mangled and avulsed index fingertip.*

the distal interphalangeal joint, most individuals transfer the manipulations formerly assigned to the thumb and index finger to the thumb and long finger. The residual index finger becomes an awkward barrier to dexterity. Under these circumstances, a ray amputation of the index finger may be indicated. Similarly, when the index finger has been irreversibly traumatized at the proximal phalangeal level or near the metacarpophalangeal joint, a primary removal of that ray may be the best procedure.

The preferred incision for ray amputation is a racket-shaped incision at the metacarpophalangeal joint level (Fig. 17-12). The limb of the incision extends proximally in the thumb web to expose the first dorsal interosseous muscle. The muscle is detached through its tendon distally and the periosteum of the metacarpal is opened. The bone is divided obliquely as near to its proximal expansion as possible. The extensor tendons are divided and removed distally. The flexor tendons are pulled out and divided as far proximal as possible as the wrist is flexed. The distal tendon of the first dorsal interosseous is then inserted into the base of the proximal phalanx of the long finger to strengthen its abduction. The structures of the radial and ulnar neurovascular bundles are ligated individually with fine nylon and the digital nerves tucked into the intrinsic muscles. Usually a small Penrose drain is passed through the proximal incision into the depth of the wound. After closure of the skin wound a layer of lubricated gauze is applied to the incision, and a soaking wet gauze dressing with sponge padding is placed over it. The entire hand and wrist are splinted for 10 to 14 days in a boxing-glove cast. The drain is removed on the fifth day and the cast reapplied. When the skin sutures are removed the fingers are allowed to flex but no digital abduction is permitted for another week.

Ray amputation of the little finger is performed in a similar manner except the abductor digiti minimi is transferred into the adjacent proximal phalanx of the ring finger (Fig. 17-13).

Loss of the long or ring fingers at or near the metacarpophalangeal joint leads to the prospect of an incompetent palm, that is, small objects will have the tendency to fall out of the hand when held in the palm with the fingers flexed. The simplest procedure to correct this problem is subperiosteal resection of the metacarpal providing the patient's activities do not dictate maintenance of palmar breadth. To achieve a cosmetically improved and better functioning hand, the index finger may be transferred to the long finger site or

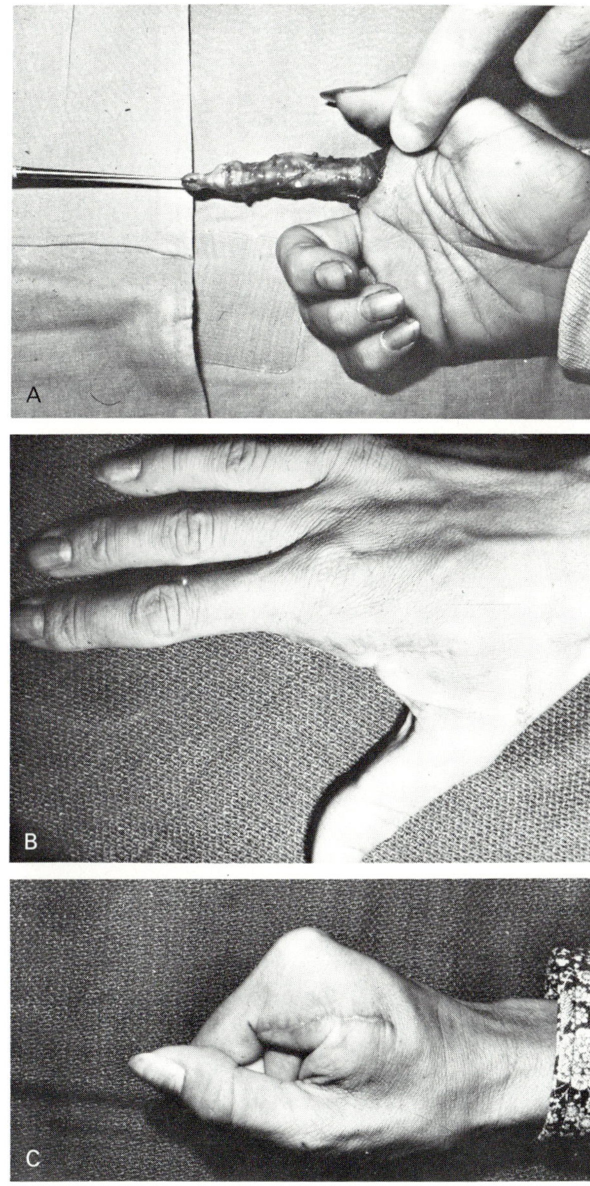

Figure 17-12. *This 30-year-old seamstress degloved her right index finger in a power lawnmower. Immediate ray amputation was done, transferring the first dorsal interosseous muscle into the base of the long metacarpal. Function and cosmesis are excellent.* (*Also see Fig. 16-6.*)

the little finger moved to the ring position[3,10] (Fig. 17-14). This means a considerable period of immobilization (6 weeks) until the metacarpal transfer heals, a factor which must be recognized when electing this additional step. On occasion with merely resection of either the long or ring ray plus their intrinsic musculature it is possible to close the resultant gap by repair of the intermetacarpal ligaments distally.

Most female patients and many males who are

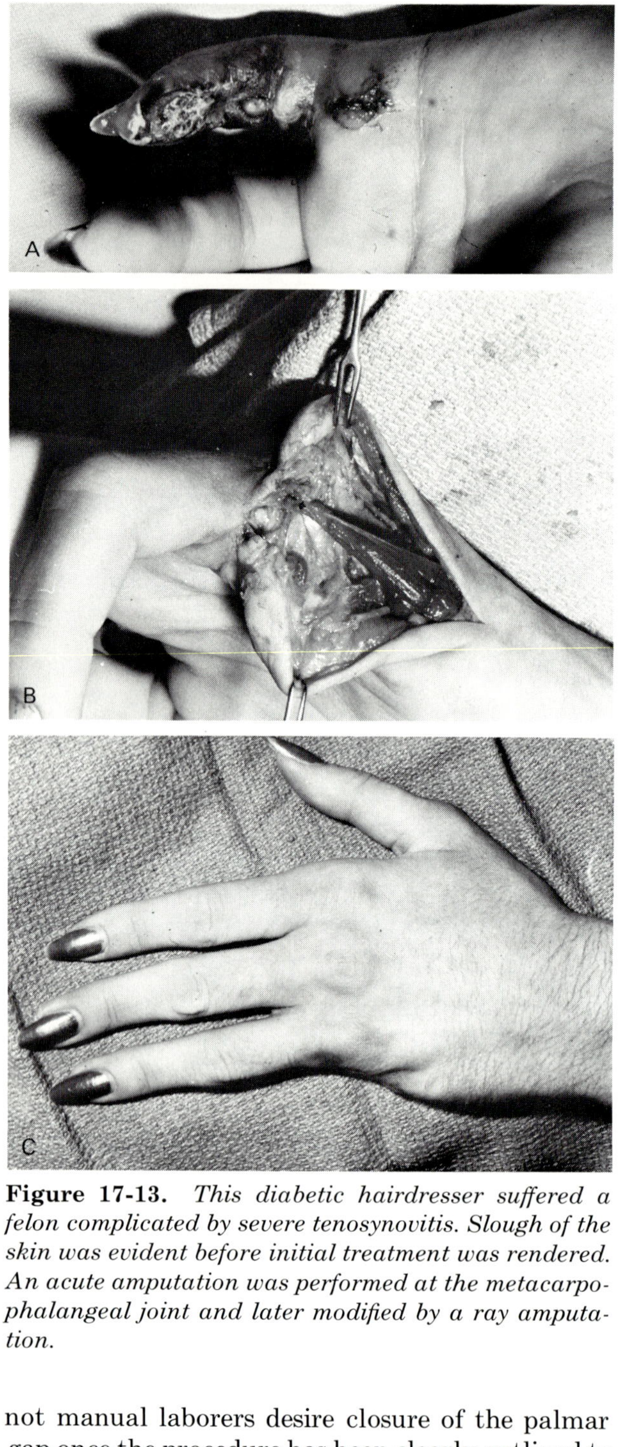

Figure 17-13. *This diabetic hairdresser suffered a felon complicated by severe tenosynovitis. Slough of the skin was evident before initial treatment was rendered. An acute amputation was performed at the metacarpophalangeal joint and later modified by a ray amputation.*

not manual laborers desire closure of the palmar gap once the procedure has been clearly outlined to them.

Certain technical points should be observed in the performance of this operation:[10]

1. A dorsal and volar wedge of skin should be removed at the site of the amputation.
2. The skin incision in the new web space must be interdigited to avoid a linear contracture.
3. The new metacarpal length must be sufficient to provide a contoured transverse arch.
4. The interosseous muscles on the resected metacarpal are removed without damaging those remaining.
5. The ligated digital nerves should be buried in the intermetacarpal space to avoid symptoms from any subsequent neuromas.
6. The intrinsic muscles are freed from the radial side of the index finger or the ulnar side of the little finger by elevating the periosteum sufficiently to permit the lateral movement of the transfer to its new location.
7. The donor metacarpals should be beveled to minimize any radial or ulnar projections of the margins of the palm.
8. A portion of the resected bone should then be fashioned into a intramedullary bone graft to stabilize the two metacarpal segments. Further longitudinal stability is achieved with a Kirschner wire which spares the metacarpophalangeal joint.
9. The flexor tendons of the amputated finger are pulled out and divided as short as possible, allowing them to retract into the forearm.
10. The position of the transferred ray is adjusted by flexing the fingers simultaneously and securing its head by a Kirschner wire directed across the transverse arch of the palm.
11. Fine suction drains are placed beneath the skin and into the metacarpal space after the intermetacarpal ligament is repaired.
12. The hand is immobilized in a bulky dressing within a plaster shell once the skin wounds are closed.
13. Usually the suction drains are removed on the second or third postoperative day.
14. The wrist and metacarpophalangeal joints are immobilized by a cast for 5 to 6 weeks, during which time the distal positions of the finger are free to move.
15. The Kirschner wires are removed at 5 to 6 weeks after the operation.

Complications that result from this procedure are: non-union, malrotation, stiffness and hematoma.

Non-union results from failing to use a intramedullary bone graft, making the osteotomy too far distally, and providing inadequate interosseous fixation. Malrotation may occur from inadequate fixation or improper alignment. Stiffness reflects trauma to the extensor tendons either during surgery or from the interosseous fixation.

Thumb Amputations

The thumb accounts for 40 to 50 per cent of hand function and the surgeon must guard its

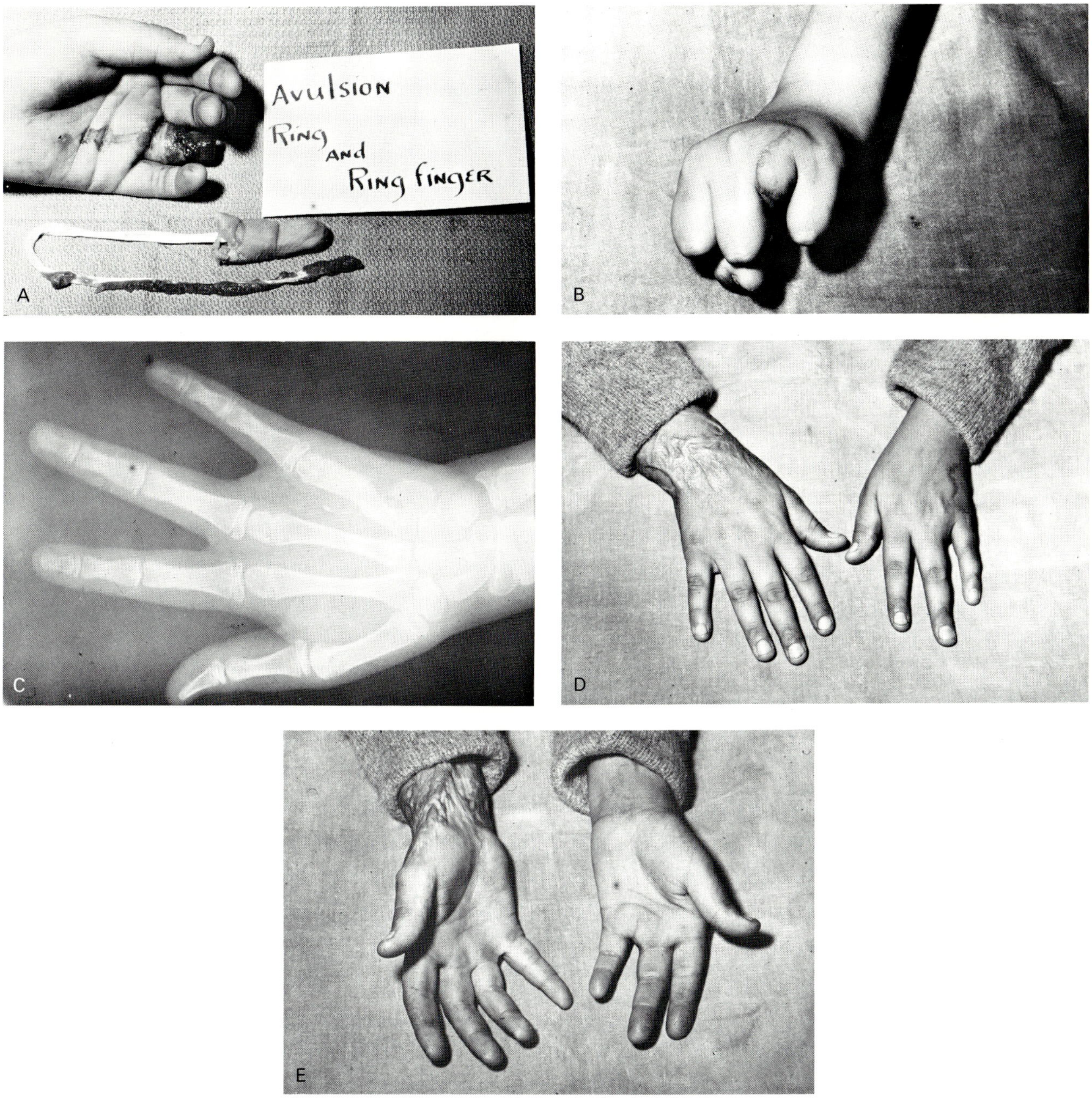

Figure 17-14. *This young boy sustained a subtotal avulsion of his ring finger. The initial amputation handicapped him as it resulted in an incompetent palm. Transfer of the little finger ray to the metacarpal of the ring finger was carried out as described in the text.*

length carefully (Fig. 17-15). However, length should not be maintained foolishly at the risk of infection or possible compromise of residual hand function.[4] Bales and his associates have suggested that the simplest procedures to repair the injured thumb, often using local flaps, are frequently the best.[2] Some patients make surprising functional recoveries despite substantial loss of thumb length. Certain individuals may compensate for amputations well into the proximal phalanx (Figs. 17-16–17-18).

The same local procedures are available for immediate thumb reconstruction as have been described previously with respect to other fingers:

Expansion of first web
- Soft tissue revision only
- Resection of residual index metacarpal if present

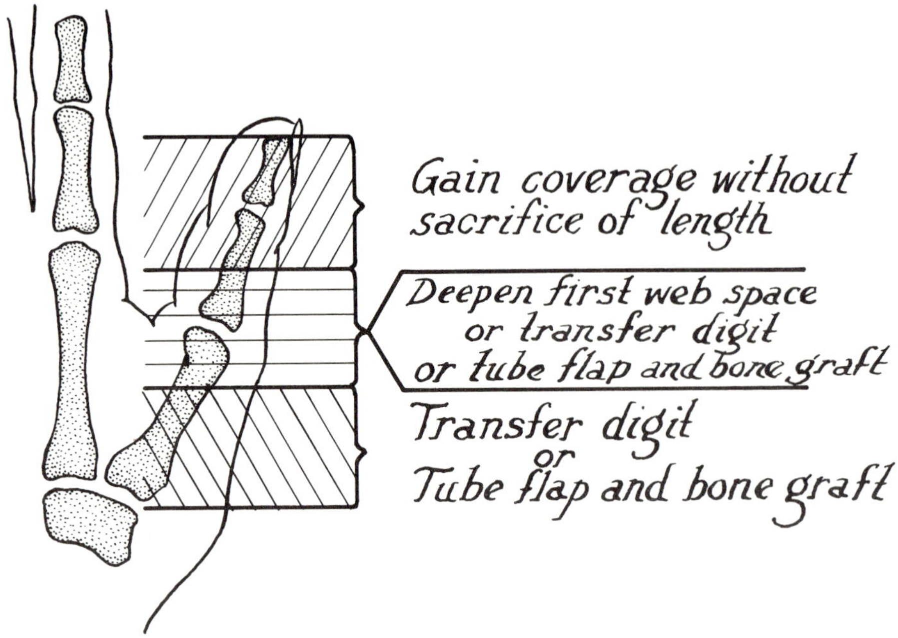

Figure 17-15. *Considerations for thumb reconstruction depend upon the level of amputation.* (*Redrawn from Chase, R.A.*[4])

Composite reconstruction
  Free bone graft, neurovascular island pedicle and infraclavicular flap
Pollicization
  Index digit transfer
  Ring or little finger transfer

An adequate first web space is needed for competent thumb function. Should the thumb be short, a secondary procedure to open that web by a Z-plasty, free graft, dorsal rotation flap and graft or a distant flap may be utilized. At times, the adductor must be freed from its insertion on the third metacarpal to allow sufficient web expansion (Chap. 21). If there have been multiple injuries and the index finger has been amputated, resection of its residual metacarpal enhances the functional breadth of the web.

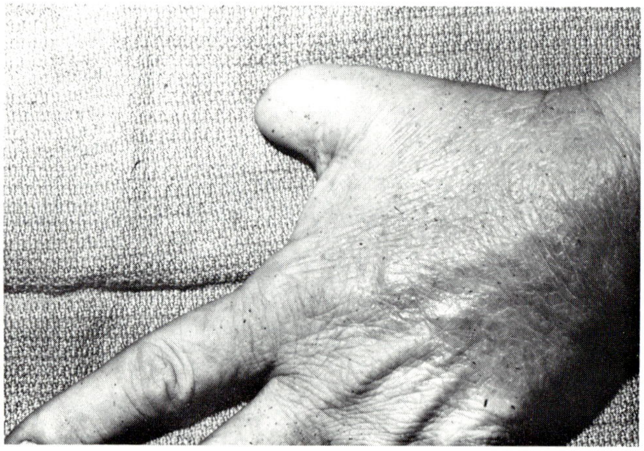

Figure 17-16. *This elderly carpenter refused any additional surgery except initial wound closure when he avulsed a portion of his minor thumb. Although the web space could be expanded he compensates very well for his loss.*

Stein and Morgan have proposed an intricate reconstructive procedure for thumb lengthening which employs a free bone graft, a neurovascular island pedicle and a tubed deltopectoral flap.[12] This is a secondary procedure which avoids pollicization and yet provides a somewhat sensitive post for lengthening the thumb.

An iliac bone graft is obtained and a standard neurovascular pedicle flap prepared from the ring finger (Chap. 15). The injured end of the thumb and its concomitant scar are resected. The bone graft is positioned and fixed internally with crossed Kirschner wires. The neurovascular pedicle is brought out to the volar surface of the bone graft, taking care to avoid twisting the vascular stalk. A medially based pedicle is then tubed in the opposite infraclavicular area. Prior to insertion of the bone graft and the thumb into this pedicle, the donor site on the side of the ring finger is repaired with a split-thickness skin graft taken from the hip near the site of the bone graft.

The thumb is then brought up to the tubed pedicle so that the bone graft lies within it. The neurovascular island forms the volar aspect of the thumb and the tubed pedicle the sides and dorsum.

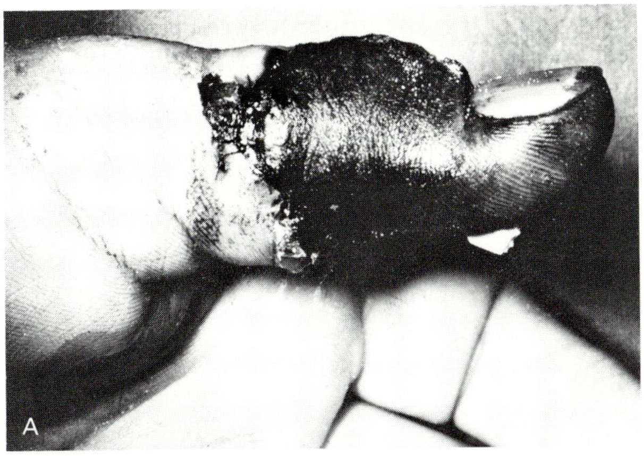

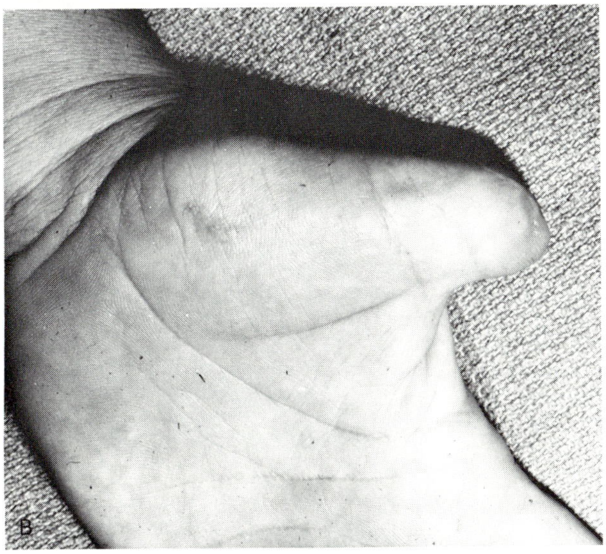

Figure 17-17. *Gangrene developed in the distal portion of this lady's thumb after she crushed it while moving a piano. Ultimately amputation was done through the proximal phalanx and has provided her with a serviceable thumb.*

The arm is immobilized at the side for a few days and then under careful supervision movement of each shoulder is begun. At $2\frac{1}{2}$ to 3 weeks the pedicle is divided and the tip revised and closed. The thumb is protected for 6 more weeks and at 8 to 12 weeks, once roentgenographic signs of healing are noted, the Kirschner wires are removed. The neurovascular pedicle enhances the circulation to the bone graft and adds sensibility to the working surface of the thumb post. Deepening of the web, if contemplated, should be done prior to reconstruction. Waiting until after the island pedicle has been transferred risks injury to the transferred neurovascular bundle.

If the thumb amputation spares the metacarpophalangeal joint, the choice of reconstruction may be: (1) lengthening by a tubed flap and bony post, as described, (2) use of the residual index finger if it is damaged and (3) transfer of the middle and distal phalanges of the ring finger. This last type of transfer spares the index finger but does not permit the transfer of a dorsal vein. The use of the index finger allows at least one and at times two dorsal veins to be preserved. Also the use of the index finger maintains independent distal phalangeal flexion, a feature which has to be provided the other digits by transfer of the individual profundus tendon into the flexor pollicis longus at the wrist. In all instances the extensor tendons must be shortened and the extensor indicis and extensor communis transferred into the extensor pollicis longus.[8]

The classic technique of index finger transfer employs five steps: (1) the selection of appropriate skin incisions, (2) the development of the neurovascular pedicle, (3) the dissection and mobilization of the finger, (4) the stabilization of the transferred finger and (5) the adjustment of balance.[8]

INCISION

The incisions surround the base of the index finger unless the need to expand scars within the web limits such placement. If there is severe scarring of the web area and at the base of the thumb, resurfacing of the web with a pedicle graft may be necessary as a preliminary step. The dorsal veins should be protected in the performance of the initial incisions.

The length of the thumb required is diagrammed on the index digit. The volar neurovascular bundles and dorsal musculature are exposed as the flaps at the digital base and web space are raised.

NEUROVASCULAR PEDICLE

The restraining septae of the palmar fascia are divided to free both neurovascular bundles. The proper volar digital artery to the radial side of the long finger is divided and ligated near its origin. The proper digital nerves can be lengthened by inspecting the common volar digital nerve with low-power magnification and carefully splitting its sheath longitudinally to separate the individual nerves. Any dorsal veins that can be preserved should be left so that congestion of the digit is minimized.

MOBILIZATION OF THE FINGER

The conexus intertendineus (junctura) between the extensor tendons should be divided. The two

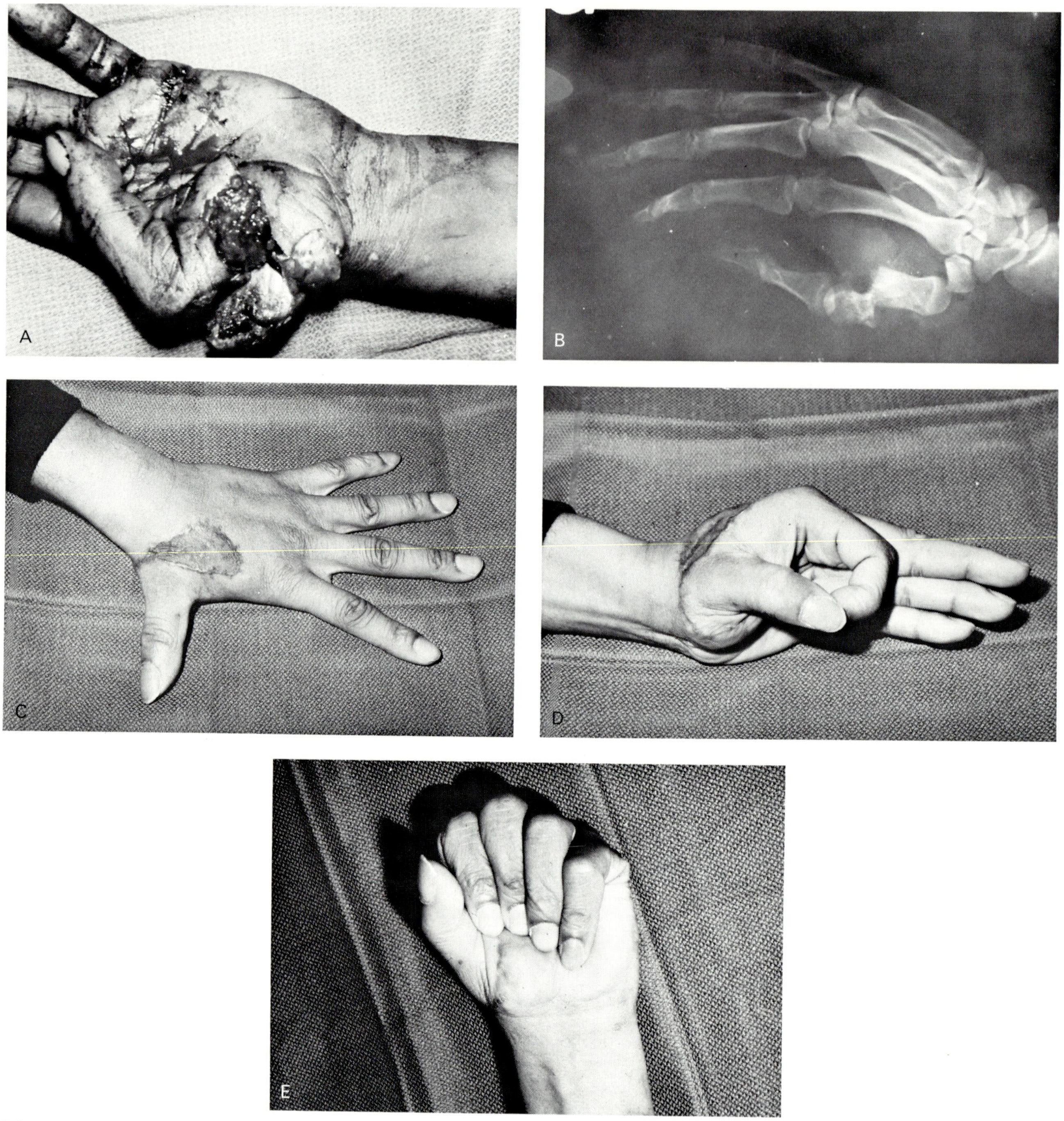

Figure 17-18. *A young man sustained a punch press injury to the basal joint of the thumb. The proximal portion of the metacarpal was totally free in the wound. It was removed and the extensor and flexor systems were shortened. A pseudoarthrosis was established between the residual metacarpal and the trapezium which provided pain-free motion.*

interossei (volar and dorsal) are divided through their musculotendinous junctions and the metacarpal is exposed. The intermetacarpal ligament is divided and the radial periosteum is incised. The metacarpal is divided near its base and the excess shaft resected subperiosteally. The residual fascia between the interossei of the second and third metacarpals is divided.

STABILIZATION

If there is residual first metacarpal fixation of the transfer, stabilization is best accomplished by a bone graft taken from the resected metacarpal shaft and contoured to fit into the opposing marrow cavities. The distal bony shaft is then placed on the bone graft and positioned in the proper degree of pronation. The length of the new thumb must be carefully estimated. The tendency is to make the reconstruction too long. Ideally the natural thumb comes nearly to the proximal interphalangeal joint of the index finger. Once the thumb is positioned, the bony juncture is secured with crossed Kirschner wires.

ADJUSTMENT OF BALANCE

The extensor indicis proprius is divided near its union with the extensor communis tendon and the proximal portion rerouted along the course of the extensor pollicis longus. It is then resutured into the extensor tendon at an appropriate tension permitting opposition to the little finger tip. The extensor digitorum communis is divided more proximally and transferred into the extensor pollicis longus.

The reconstructed thumb must be immobilized in the position of function for 8 to 10 weeks. At that point active motion is gradually instituted, with the patient encouraged to exercise the hand in warm soapy water with a sponge. Active motion and assisted active motion should be emphasized.

Transfer of the ring finger can be done in a similar fashion. Since it is not possible to transfer a dorsal vein along with the finger, attention should be given to the possibility of a dorsal microvascular anastomosis at the conclusion of the transfer. Usually this transfer encompasses a portion of the proximal phalanx and the two interphalangeal joints. To provide independent distal phalangeal flexion the profundus tendon is usually united with the proximal flexor pollicis longus and the superficialis tendon shortened to allow it to function more efficiently. The extensor communis tendon and the extensor pollicis longus are joined dorsally. Thus the prospect of diminished venous drainage and multiple procedures to flexor tendons make the other transfers less desirable than the index finger, which is favored by proximity and more suitable anatomy.

Multiple Amputations

At the time of the acute injury nothing must be discarded that will aid in later reconstruction. Length must be maintained, edema minimized and infection prevented. The best opportunity for useful reconstruction later stems from careful planning and conservative surgery at the time of the initial injury. Within the badly mangled hand parts of one digit may be found that can be used to cover or partially restore another (Fig. 17-19).

Once the hand has healed after multiple amputations, consideration can be given to constructing a thumb cleft or to adding a simple prosthesis so that the thumb or an active digit may be used in effective pinch (Fig. 17-20). The more simple the reconstruction or the prosthesis, the more likely the patient is to use it.

A satisfactory grasping mechanism depends upon the presence of a cleft between two opposing poles which are rotated opposite one another or can adduct parallel to each other[15] (Fig. 17-21). Such a cleft can be developed by resecting a shortened metacarpal and in addition performing a rotational osteotomy on the metacarpal of the little finger to place it more favorably for thumb or thumb post opposition.

Complete amputation through the carpus usually requires prosthetic replacement if the patient desires it. Residual movement at the radiocarpal joint is especially useful for prehension, utilizing an open-end socket with a palmar post.[13] Similarly, for amputations at the wrist a prosthesis can be fitted that allows useful pronation and supination.

Bilateral hand amputation provides a circumstance which might be benefited by the Krukenburg operation. Through this procedure the surgeon can maintain useful sensibility and provide vigorous prehension. The best results are obtained when 60 to 75 per cent of the forearm remains with a normal soft tissue cover. An active pincer action is created by opposing the radial ray with the ulnar ray. Good soft tissue with adequate sensibility is rotated into the cleft. Strength should not be compromised by making the limbs too long, but when they are too short insufficient distal separation will result.

Swanson has had one of the greatest experiences

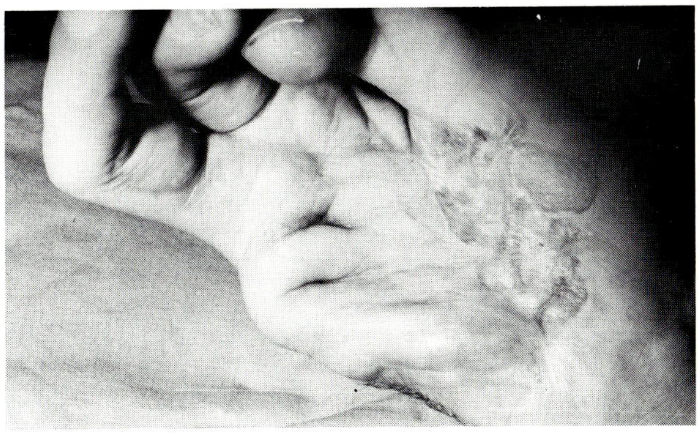

Figure 17-19. *This young man had a blast injury to his hand necessitating amputation of the ulnar two rays. The dorsal skin of those digits was used to replace skin avulsed from the palm.* (*See Fig. 16-2.*)

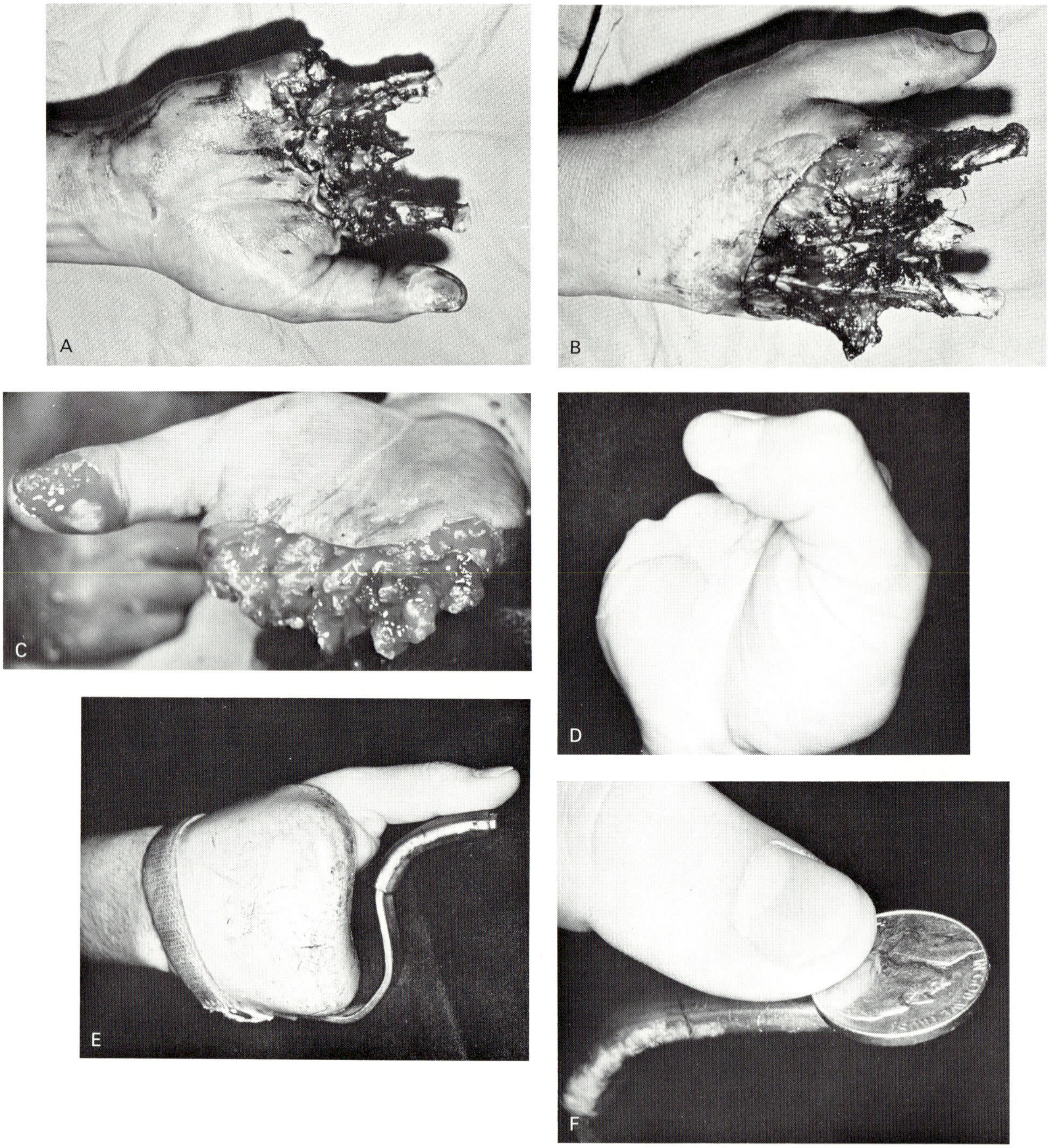

Figure 17-20. *A cornpicker injury produced an amputation of all four fingers plus extensive soft tissue loss over both the palm and dorsum* **(A,B).** *After good debridement and completion of amputations at the level of metacarpophalangeal joints* **(C)** *sufficient soft tissue remained over the bone to permit split-thickness skin graft coverage. The final result, achieved at the first repair, was a mitten hand with a normal thumb* **(D)** *which has been attached to a simple functional prosthesis* **(E,F).** (*Courtesy of Harold Bales, M.D.*)

with the Krukenburg procedure in the United States.[14] His technique is divided into several steps: (1) the dorsal and volar skin incisions, (2) separation of the flexor and pronator muscles, (3) division of the dorsal muscles and (4) wound closure (Fig. 17-22).

INCISIONS

The dorsal skin incision is made longitudinally toward the ulnar side, developing a triangular flap proximally to surface the apex of the web. The longitudinal volar incision lies toward the radial aspect of that surface.

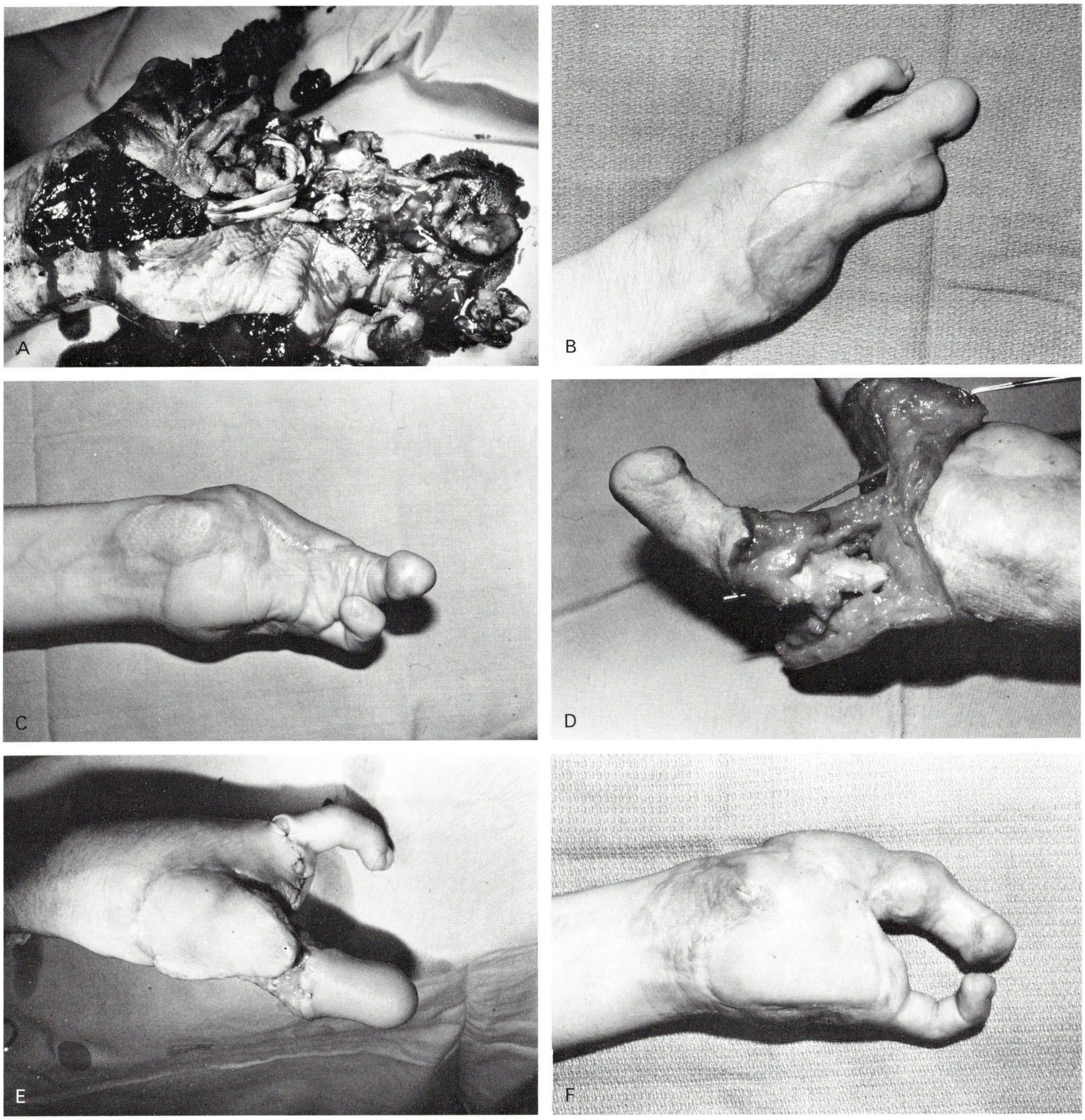

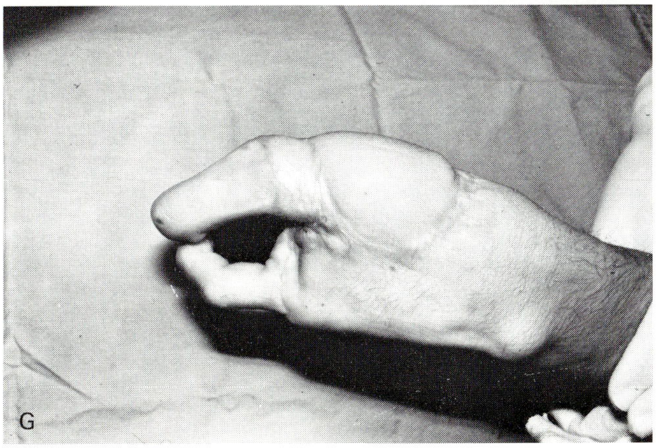

Figure 17-21A. *Initial crush injury from a punch press.* **B:** *Healed hand prior to resection of metacarpal III and placement of abdominal flap.* **C:** *Following resection of metacarpal III and placement of abdominal flap.* **D,E:** *Intraoperative views of "pollicization" of ring finger to residual stump of metacarpal II.* **F,G:** *Postoperative pinch achieved by repositioned digits.*

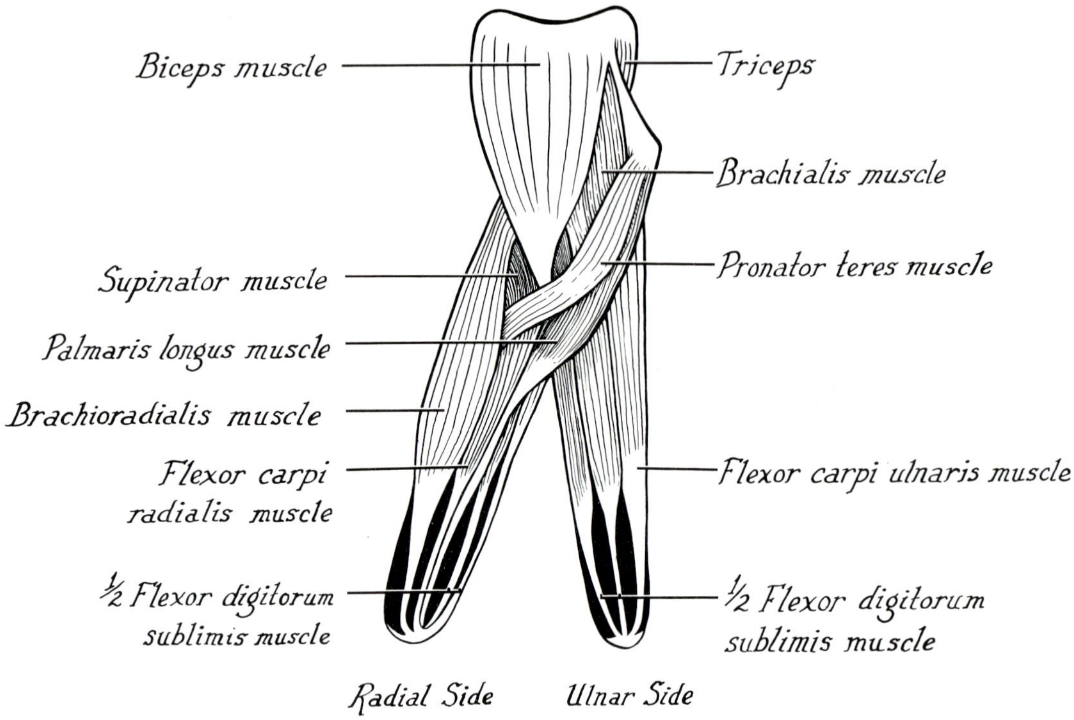

A

Flexor Surface

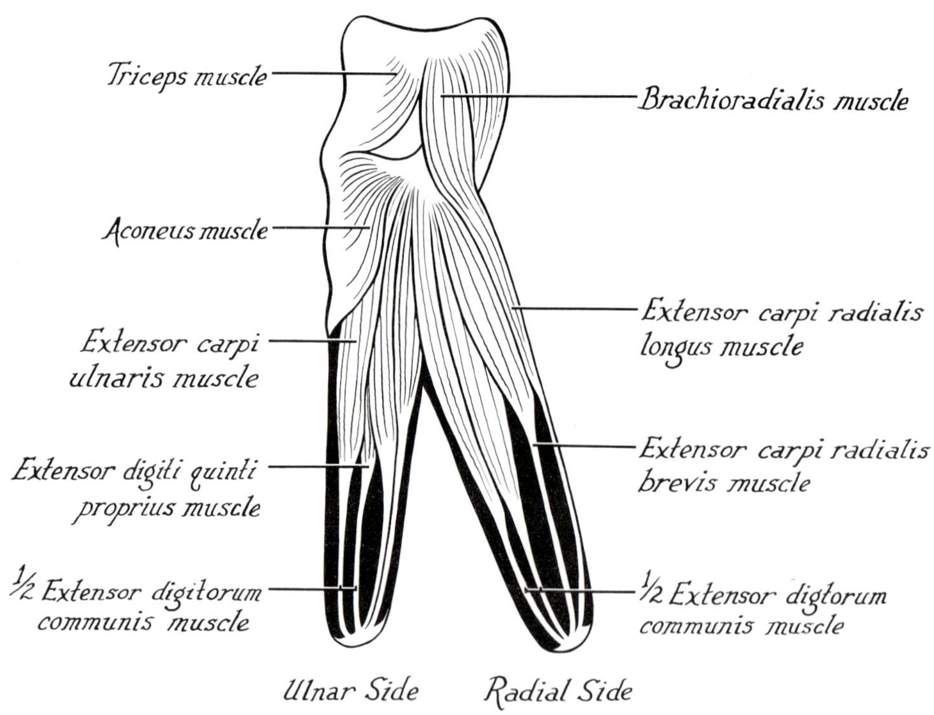

B

Dorsal Surface

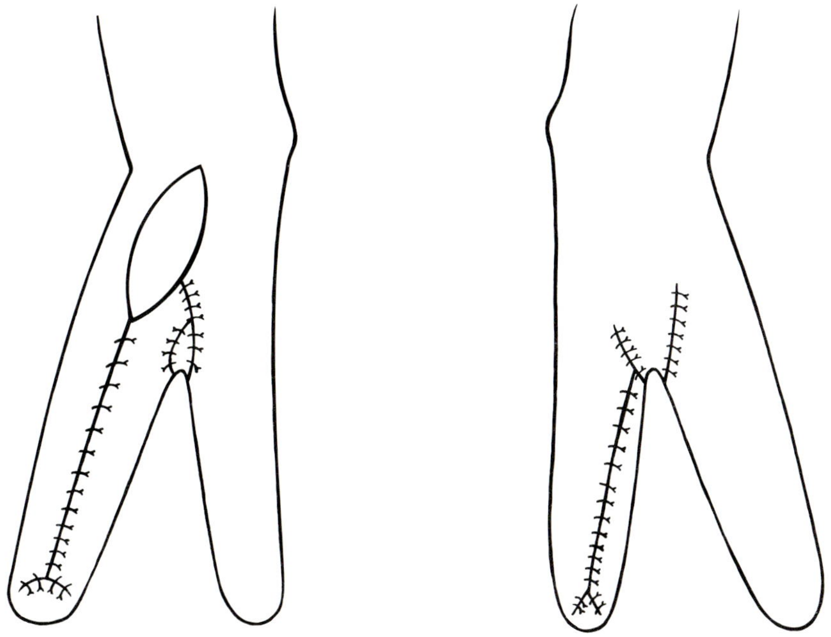

Figure 17-22. *Swanson technique for construction of a pincer forearm (Krukenberg procedure).*

VOLAR AND DORSAL MUSCLE SEPARATION

The muscles that are transferred to, or maintained on, the radial side of the forearm are: the radial wrist flexors and extensors, the flexor digitorum superficialis of the index and long fingers, the comparable portions of the extensor digitorum communis, the pronator teres, the palmaris longus if present, and the brachioradialis. The remaining muscles are inserted on the ulnar component of the forearm. At times, the pronator quadratus and flexor digitorum profundus are too bulky to permit easy closure of the wound and must be resected. In addition, the flexor pollicis longus, abductor pollicis longus, and extensor pollicis brevis may be resected to reduce bulk, but the important pronator teres must be preserved. After the muscle distribution has been performed the interosseous membrane should be freed along its ulnar border while protecting the interosseous neurovascular bundle. The limbs will now separate 5 to 12 cm. If the tips will not touch, osteotomies of the radius and ulnar are required.

WOUND CLOSURE

The skin closure is done after the tourniquet has been removed and is placed to avoid the opposing surfaces. Split-thickness skin grafts may be needed near the apical flap.

The dressing is applied with the limbs separated at least 6 cm. After 2 to 3 weeks active abduction and adduction can be started and use of the limb in guarded physiotherapy gradually increased.

References

1. Atasoy, E., Ioakimidis, E., Kasdan, M.D. Kutz, J.E. and Kleinert, H.E.: Reconstruction of the amputated finger tip with a triangular volar flap. A new surgical procedure. J. Bone Joint Surg., 52A:921, 1970.
2. Bales, C.R., DeMuth, R.J., Tooze, F.M. and Graham, W.P.: Thumb length preservation following soft tissue injuries. J. Trauma, 18:901, 1975.
3. Carroll, R.E.: Transposition of the index finger to replace the middle finger. Clin. Orthop., 15:27, 1959.
4. Chase, R.A.: Functional levels of amputation in the hand. Surg. Clin. North Am., 40:415, 1960.
5. Fisher, R.H.: The Kutler method of repair of finger tip amputations. J. Bone Joint Surg., 49A:317, 1967.
6. Frazier, T.G. and Graham, W.P.: Finger tip injuries. Pa. Med., 74:51, 1971.
7. Kutler, W.: A new method for finger tip amputations. J.A.M.A., 133:29, 1947.
8. Littler, J.W.: Neurovascular pedicle method of digital transposition for reconstruction of the thumb. Plast. Reconstr. Surg., 12:303, 1953.
9. Patton, H.S.: Split skin grafts from hypothenar area for fingertip avulsions. Plast. Reconstr. Surg., 43:426, 1969.

10. Peacock, E.E., Jr.: Metacarpal transfer following amputation of a central digit. Plast. Reconstr. Surg., 29:345, 1962.
11. Snow, J.W.: The use of a volar flap for repair of fingertip amputations. A preliminary report. Plast. Reconstr. Surg., 40:163, 1967.
12. Stein, F. and Morgan, L.R.: The use of the Bakamjian flap in reconstruction of the hand. J. Bone Joint Surg., 54A:909, 1972.
13. Swanson, A.B.: Levels of amputation of fingers and hands—consideration for treatment. Surg. Clin. North Am., 44:1115, 1964.
14. Swanson, A.B.: The Krukenburg procedure in the juvenile amputee. J. Bone Joint Surg., 46A:1540, 1964.
15. Weckesser, E.C.: Reconstruction of a grasping mechanism following loss of digits. Clin. Orthop., 15:69, 1959.

18 Contractures

Mobility of the hand is reduced in many conditions by the development of contractures. These may restrict motion in any plane and may be functionally disabling. Once a contracture is established, there may be secondary changes in otherwise normal tissues so that there is an aggravation of the disability and correction becomes progressively difficult. In Dupuytren's fasciitis, for instance, the prime abnormality is inherent in the fascia, but with time there may be irreversible foreshortening of volar skin and periarticular soft tissues. Correction then is a compound and complex task far in excess of simple fasciectomy. The same holds for contractures arising primarily in skin (burns), muscles (Volkmann's contracture), tendons fixed by adhesions and joints frozen by ligamentous shortening.

Appreciation of the magnitude of the impact of contractures should strengthen appreciation of the importance of their prevention and early correction. Basic principles in the management of disorders of the hand must be tailored to the avoidance and reduction of contracture. The best possible circulation must be maintained to prevent insidious or rapidly developing ischemic fibrosis. Surgical wounds must be planned properly and wounds of injury modified to minimize the risk of restricting scar. Immobilization must be instituted to allow tissues to heal and form adaptable scars. Mobilization of joints and muscles must follow at the earliest moment consistent with proper wound healing. The patient must be educated to appreciate the importance and the parameters of proper immobilization and mobilization. Where necessary he must be given adequate help to implement them.

Competence in the field of physiotherapy is indispensable for the education and aid needed by many patients. Active and passive work and appropriately prescribed dynamic splints, applied with perseverance, constitute the principal media for preventing and overcoming many problems. The motivation and the confidence of the patient are prime factors in success and sometimes require a great deal of time to develop. The apprehensive fearful patient is reluctant to use his injured hand and is far more prone to problems of scar and contracture than the responsible and willing patient. When the management of fixed contractures is surgical, it is important that the patient not only wants the surgery but is willing and able to take the time and accept the responsibility to fulfill his role in the convalescence.

The factors predisposing to scar formation and aggravation of a contracture must be recognized (age, associated metabolic disorders, predilections to stiffness by existing concomitant collagen disorders, paralysis, low pain thresholds, anxiety states, etc.).

The tissues commonly responsible for specific contractures are the skin, fascia, periarticular tissues, muscles and tendons, and bones and joints. Contractures caused by some specific disorders are dealt with in other chapters—burns, congenital deformities, bones and joints, Volkmann's contracture, and tendon adhesions. The surgical procedures of grafting, wound closure and pedicle coverage are described in Chapter 6.

Cutaneous Contractures

Contractures of the skin are most common on the flexor aspect and in the webs so that there is a limitation to digital and wrist extension and hand spreading. On the dorsum of the hand and digits, loss of skin substance or too tight a wound closure can result in an extensor and adduction contracture.

Contractures limited to the skin can be caused by inadequate "cloth" or a tight linear scar (Figs. 18-1, 18-2). The former requires the addition of skin (more "cloth"), whereas the latter necessitates resection of the tight bond and lengthening of its axis (Fig. 18-3). Additional skin can be provided by free graft, local flap or pedicle from a distance. The free graft is usually a thick split-thickness skin graft (0.02 in). It must be applied to the defect when its size is maximal; for the dorsum this is in flexion and for the volar aspect it is in extension. These positions must be held for at least a week until a take is completely assured. Internal fixation with Kirschner wires may be the only way to hold the desired position effectively. If the graft is greater than 6.25 cm^2 and there is the slightest doubt of adequate hemostasis upon release of the tourniquet, the application should be delayed at least 12 hours. Since most of these grafts contract about 50 per cent, the lateral extension of the graft should be adequate and whenever possible should reach the lateral midaxial line. Skin "darts" should be used freely to break up straight lines of scar. The uncertainty of take of full-thickness skin grafts limits their usage.

A skin deficit on the volar aspect of a digit often can be filled by a cross-finger pedicle flap (Chap. 6) (Fig. 18-4). Web space contractures between the fingers may be corrected by the excision of the scar and closure with a rotation flap from the side of the proximal phalanx of an adjacent digit. Defects

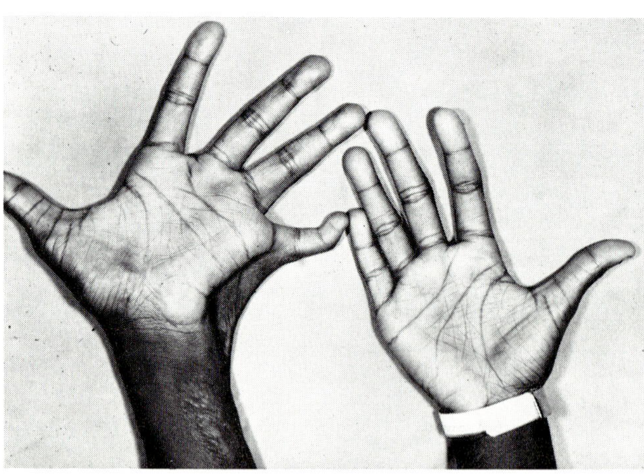

Figure 18-1. *Web contracture of ulnar border of wrist with growth disturbance produced by a burn scar in a young girl.*

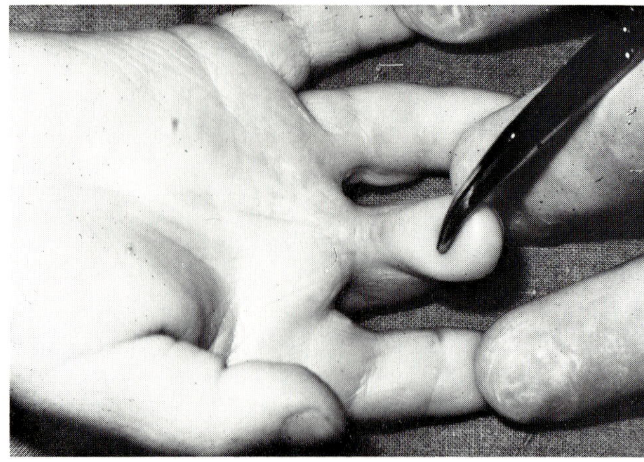

Figure 18-2. *Severe flexion contracture of volar aspect of a digit that occurred after a burn injury.*

created on the dorsum of the hand following the excision of scar cannot usually be covered by rotation flaps because of the lack of excess skin and the tautness of existing skin when the fist is closed. Therefore defects here usually require split-thickness skin grafts as described for the flexor aspect of the digits. Occasionally a distant pedicle flap is needed, particularly when padding is important. However, this invariably means that several procedures will be necessary before adequate tailoring and cosmesis are achieved. The most common source of a distant pedicle is the thoracicoabdominal area. Temporary disability is the longest and the cost of hospitalization the highest with this approach to the problem.

When the contracture stems from a tight longitudinal scar, correction is usually possible by excision of the scar and lengthening of the wound by Z-plasty technique. When there is a combination of lack of cloth and a tight longitudinal scar, consideration should be given to combining a rotation flap with free skin grafts. This is particularly useful in correcting web contractures of the fingers and thumb.

Once tissues have healed, an elastic glove can help immeasurably to retard the formation of hypertrophic scar and recurrent contracture.

Some generalized skin disorders cause contractures. The most notable of these is scleroderma which in the progressive type produces such tightening of the skin (hidebound) that a stiff claw deformity of the hand may result. This is due to a marked thickening of the connective tissue and may be accompanied by subcutaneous calcification, osteoporosis and destruction of distal phalanges. These advanced changes may be preceded by Raynaud's phenomenon. No effective treatment of the basic disorder exists.

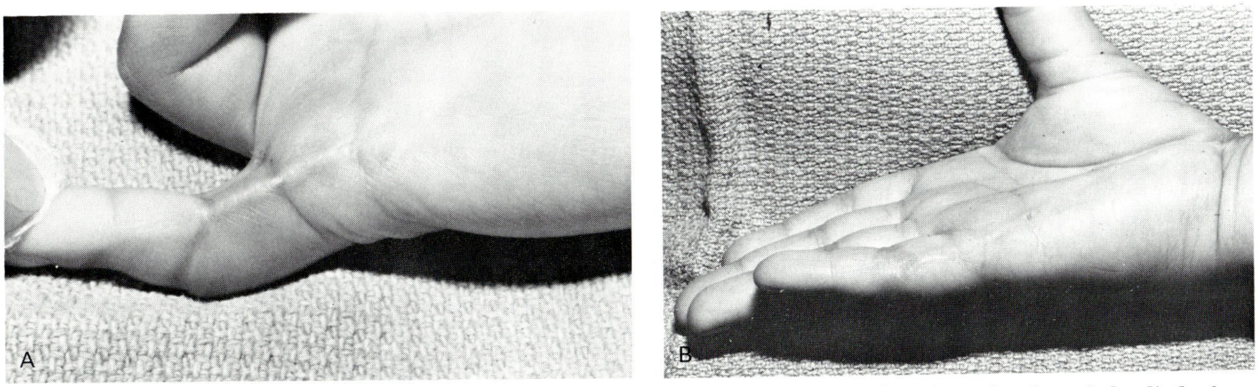

Figure 18-3. *Volar skin contracture occurring in a longitudinal wound on the ulnar border of the little finger. Release required a skin graft.*

Musculotendinous Contractures

The extrinsic and intrinsic musculotendinous structures are the prime cause of contractures in a variety of circumstances, especially after trauma. The contracture is caused by a reduction in length, elasticity or mobility of one or more units. The tendon is primarily responsible for a contracture when it is adherent and has lost its amplitude or when it is reconstituted and has lost substance. The muscle is primarily responsible when it has become fibrotic and lost elasticity or when the fascia around the muscle has thickened and shortened.

Any direct injury or inflammatory process in the bed or substance of either tendon or muscle can invoke these changes. Ischemia initiated by venous congestion or by arterial compromise can also lead to adherence and foreshortening of these motor units (Volkmann's, Chaps. 10 and 16) (Fig. 18-5).

The restrictions imposed on motion by contractures from these musculotendinous units can be considered as "plus states." Accordingly, there are flexor and extensor plus states and intrinsic and extrinsic plus states, depending on the anatomical area involved. The level of involvement is determined clinically by the joints affected. If more than one joint is crossed distal to the point of abnormality any one joint can be positioned to gain length (laxity) and allow movement in the opposite direction of the other joints. However, all joints cannot be moved simultaneously through a normal range in the same direction. Plus states produce the same effect as tenodesis or static tendon transfer.

The treatment of plus states is dependent upon whether there is merely an adherence or a foreshortening of the motor unit. Adherence is treated by tenolysis and, if possible, immediate mobilization. Foreshortening is treated by division, by lengthening or by transfer to substitute for the unit causing the deformity. Frequently a major problem rests with the type of bed and cover of the motor unit. When inadequate, these must be replaced by pedicle tissue. At times the answer lies in "simplification of function" by arthrodesis, tenodesis and reduction of the number of joints in the cantilever system.

Extensor Plus States[4]

When the forearm musculature is involved, it is generally necessary to divide and liberate the tendon of the affected motor unit. Dynamic control is preserved by transferring a new motor into the tendon.

If the problem lies distal to the muscle, then the treatment involves lysis of adhesions, division or lengthening of the tendon or replacement of the tendon by a transfer or a tendon graft. Binding of the tendons within their sheaths by the retinacular system of the wrist requires removal of the retinaculum or its elevation as a flap and transfer deep to the tendons (Fig. 18–6).

Tenolysis of the extensor hood over the phalanges has a poor prognosis because the limited excursion and weakness of extensor power favor the reformation of adhesions. If such a tenolysis is undertaken, immediate and supervised mobilization is paramount. The judicious instillation of triamcinolone at the time of operation may be efficacious.

Shrinkage of the middle extensor hood in the absence of adhesions prevents simultaneous flexion of all three joints of the finger. This can be effectively overcome by tenotomy and sagittal band retinaculotomy. Its performance under local anesthesia establishes immediately the adequacy of the procedure. The skin incision is made lateral to the

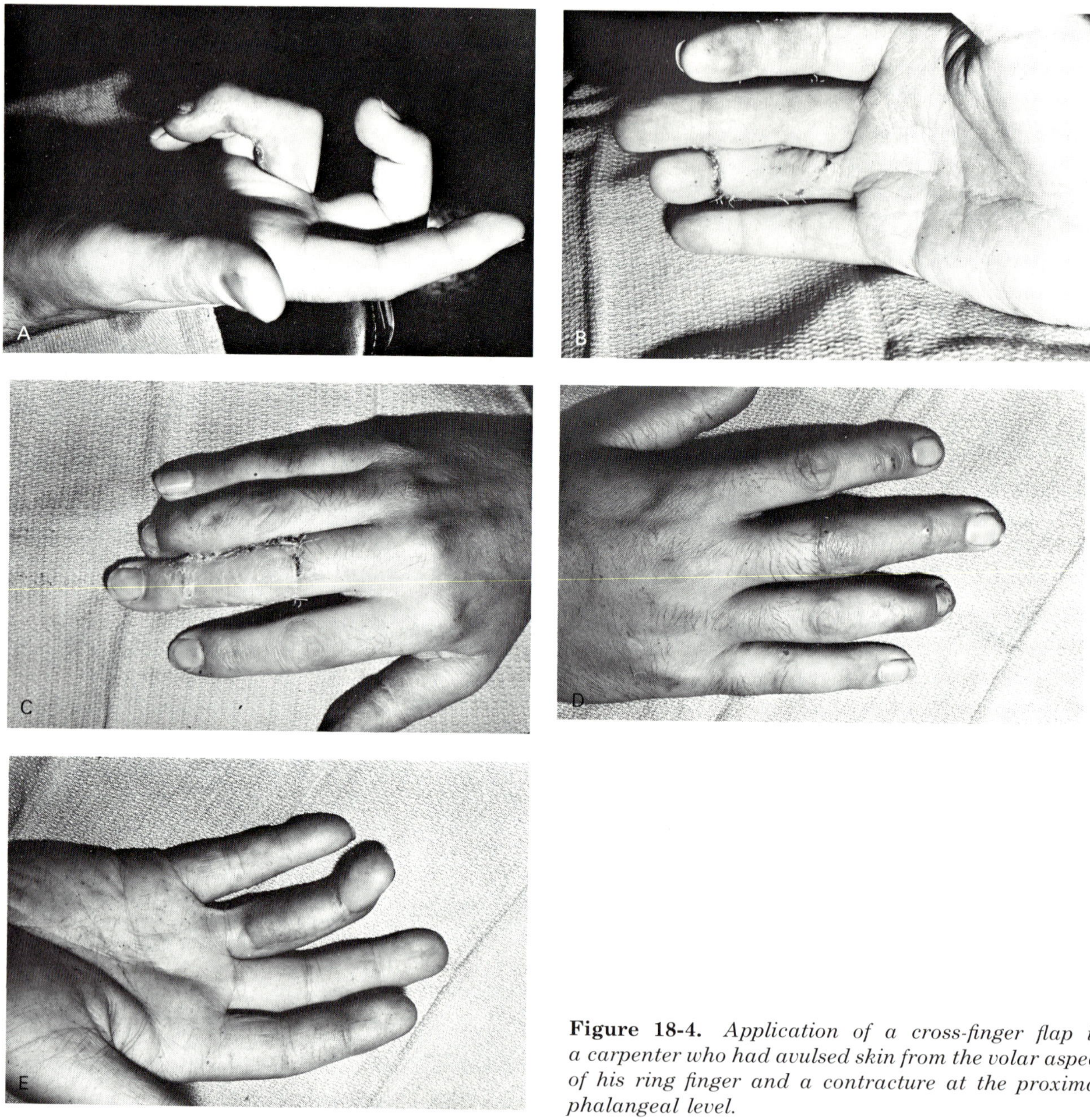

Figure 18-4. *Application of a cross-finger flap in a carpenter who had avulsed skin from the volar aspect of his ring finger and a contracture at the proximal phalangeal level.*

apex of the metacarpal head. The middle extensor tendon is notched in a staggered fashion at 2 or 3 levels. The notching extends past the midline of the tendon so that no single middle extensor tendon fiber remains in continuity over the length of the proximal phalanx. If inadequate range of motion follows the initial tenotomies, then the ulnar sagittal band is notched. At times the radial sagittal band must also be notched (Figs. 18-7, 14-17).

Flexor Plus States

The prime difference in flexor plus disorders from extensor plus states lies in the retinacular sheath systems of the wrist and digits. Otherwise the principles and procedures for operative treatment are comparable.

The carpal canal cannot be bypassed as the extensor retinacular sheath system can. Lysis of one or two adherent tendons has a favorable prognosis but involvement of all nine flexor tendons in the canal markedly reduces the chances for successful tenolysis unless there is a reduction in the number (total mass) of tendons. Such reduction usually means resection of the superficialis tendons. The concomitant existence of a painful neuroma of the median nerve limits the patient's capacity to mobilize the hand after tenolysis. The flexor pollicis

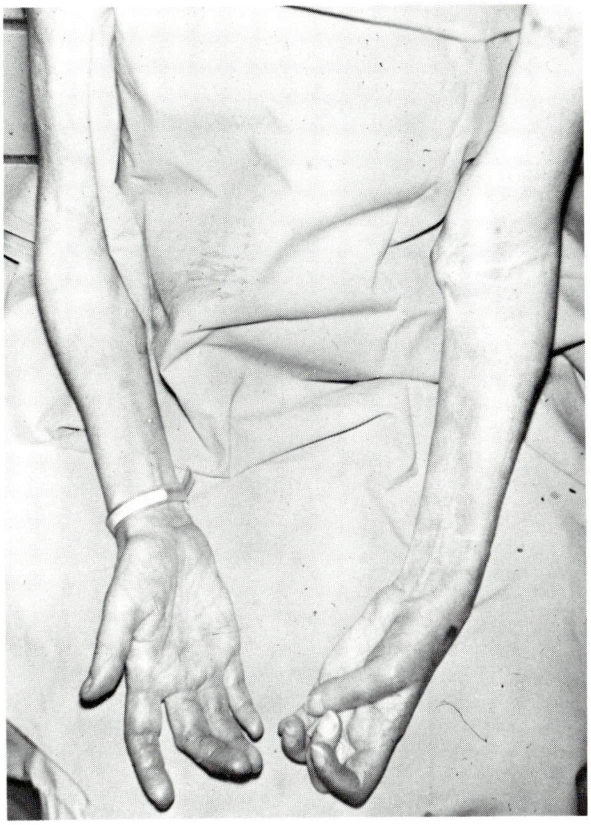

Figure 18-5. *Moderately severe Volkmann's contracture of left hand and forearm following a supracondylar elbow fracture in an elderly inmate of a state mental institution. This is an "intrinsic minus" hand.*

longus is the flexor tendon most amenable to lengthening. It is usually lengthened at the musculotendinous junction outside the carpal canal by a long oblique or long Z incision. This tendon is the only one which can be successfully transferred out of the carpal canal; it can be rerouted through the substance of the thenar musculature.

Adherence of flexor tendons within the digital sheaths is one of the most common factors causing flexor plus. The choices of surgical treatment are usually: (1) flexor tenolysis with preservation of the pulleys, (2) tenolysis and resection of one or more pulleys and one of the two tendons (e.g the superficialis) and (3) tendon resection and a staged tendon grafting preceded by the placement of a silicone rod for pseudosheath formation.

A common contracture is caused by adherence of the superficialis to a fracture callus of the proximal phalanx. The differentiation of flexion contracture of the proximal interphalangeal joint caused by this phenomenon from an intrinsic joint contracture is impossible preoperatively in the presence of a normal roentgenogram. Section of the superficialis tendon proximal to the short vinculum usually results in complete motion of the digit. The amplitude and power of the flexors are advantages in treating flexor plus states.

In some instances, the contracture of the flexor sheath in the digit is the sole or contributing factor to the limitation of digital extension. In such cases, the involved portion of the sheath must be divided or resected.

Intrinsic Plus States

The consequences of fibrosis of the intrinsic muscles usually involve the function of the interossei and adductor of the thumb. Shrinkage of the interossei makes it impossible to extend the metacarpophalangeal joints and to flex the interphalangeal joints simultaneously. Hence the condition is diagnosed by passively extending the metacarpophalangeal joint and demonstrating resistance to interphalangeal joint flexion. Likewise, flexion of the interphalangeal joints prevents extension of the metacarpophalangeal joint (Fig. 18-8). This problem is commonly generated by posttraumatic congestion, hemorrhea, and ischemia within the fascial compartments of the interossei. Proper appreciation of this fact makes it possible to prevent these changes by early emergency fasciotomy of these compartments.

Treatment consists of sectioning the lateral extensor tendons (intrinsic bands) or removing a triangle from the lateral wings of the extensor hood (Littler release) (Fig. 18-9). Bilateral midaxial incisions or a dorsal longitudinal incision are used for exposure. Active motion is begun immediately.

The generalized intrinsic plus state of the hand in Figure 18-10 should be contrasted with the intrinsic minus hand of the patient with unopposed extrinsic muscle action in Figure 18-5.

ADDUCTOR CONTRACTURE

Fibrosis of the adductor of the thumb and thickening of its fascia may cause an adduction contracture of the thumb web. At times the fascia alone causes the contracture while the muscle remains elastic. Therefore, the benefits of fasciotomy are established at operation before proceeding to myotomy.

Myotomy is usually done at the origin of the adductor on the middle metacarpal, taking care to preserve its innervation. To prevent recurrence of the contracture postoperatively, dynamic splinting or fixation of the thumb metacarpal in abduction

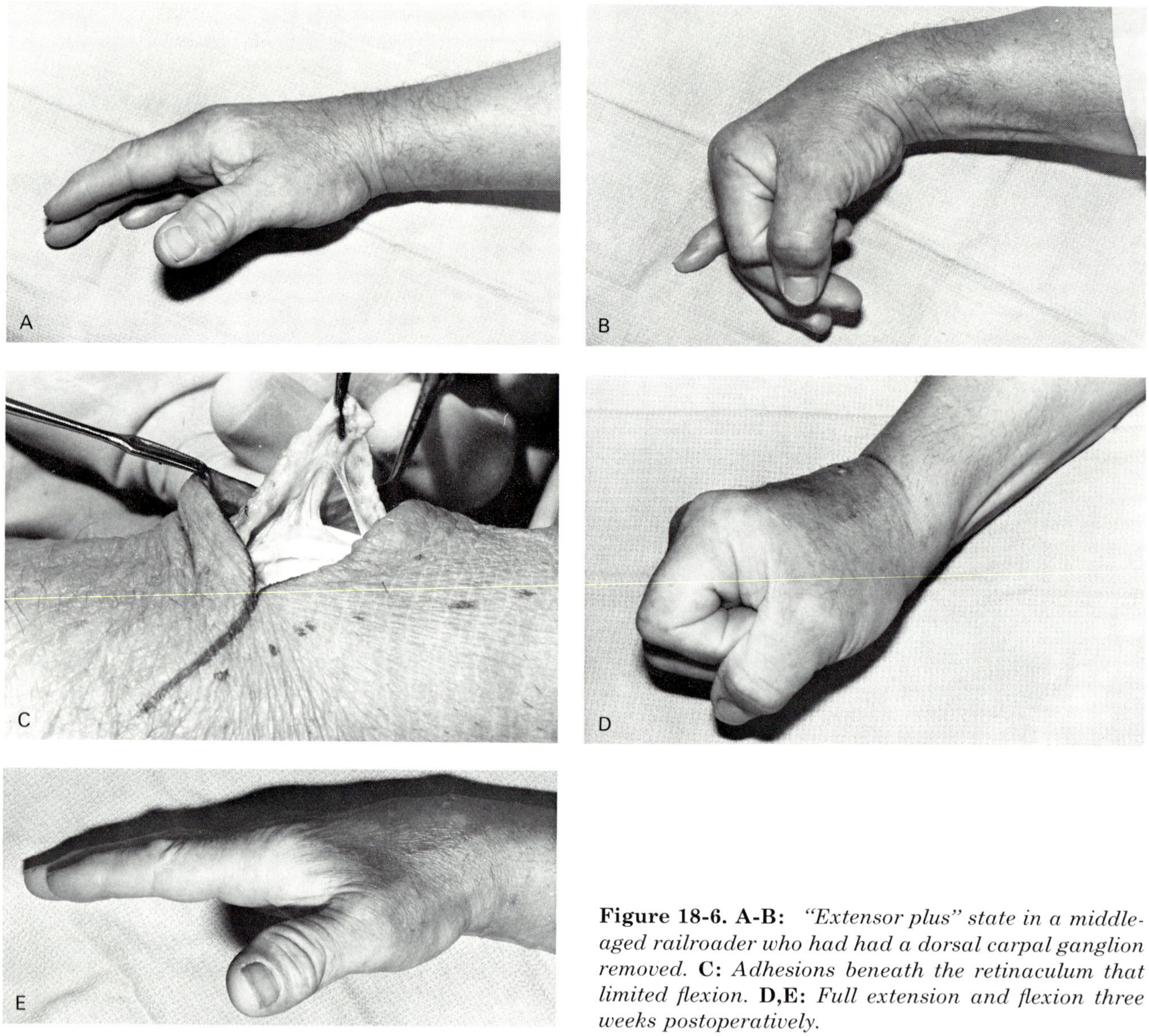

Figure 18-6. A-B: *"Extensor plus" state in a middle-aged railroader who had had a dorsal carpal ganglion removed.* **C:** *Adhesions beneath the retinaculum that limited flexion.* **D,E:** *Full extension and flexion three weeks postoperatively.*

with Kirschner wires is usually necessary for 3 to 6 weeks. The surgical approach to the fascia is through the dorsum of the thumb web. If the skin is also tight, the incision is curved completely toward the index metacarpal so as to raise a flap based radially on the thumb metacarpal. A split-thickness skin graft is then needed to close the gap when the thumb is positioned in full abduction. Adductor myotomy at the middle metacarpal is done through a midpalmar incision parallel to the thenar crease (Fig. 15-23).

BLOCKING OF INTRINSIC EXCURSION BY THE INTERMETACARPAL LIGAMENT[10]

In this condition there is scarring between the interosseous and lumbrical tendons just distal to the intermetacarpal ligament. As a consequence the excursion proximally during simultaneous metacarpophalangeal flexion and interphalangeal extension is blocked and the effort to overcome this is painful (Fig. 18-11).

This fibrosis is usually the result of any trauma at the level of the metacarpophalangeal joint. A tear of the collateral ligament is a common cause of the problem.

The condition must be suspected in any patient with a history of trauma about the metacarpophalangeal joint who complains of intractable pain while making a fist. The diagnosis is confirmed by the production of pain with simultaneous forceful flexion of the metacarpophalangeal joint and extension of the interphalangeal joints. The Bunnell test for intrinsic plus will be positive if the

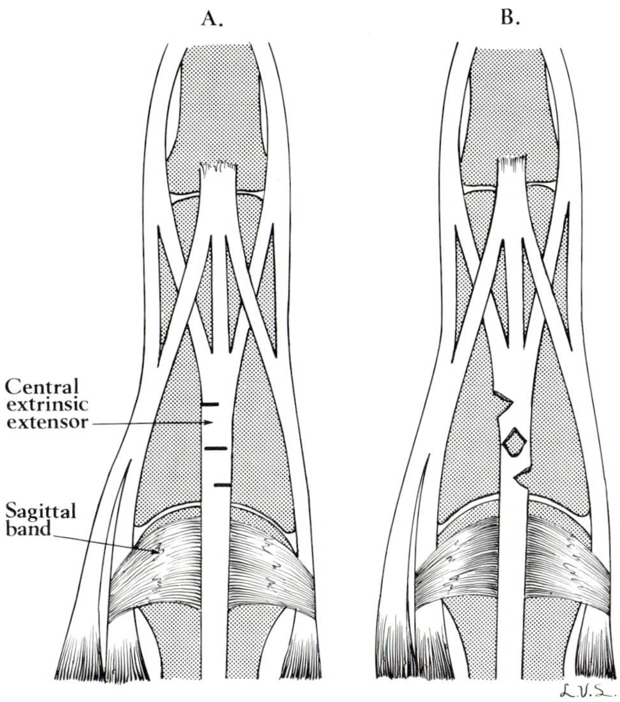

Figure 18-7. *Release of the extensor plus at the level of the middle extensor tendon (central extrinsic extensor) by staggered tenotomies. Retinaculotomy of the sagittal bands is optional. (Reproduced from Kilgore, E.S., et al.[7] by permission of the publisher.)*

intrinsics are adherent to the intermetacarpal ligament. If the precipitating factor was a ligamentous injury, pain will also be produced by placing the ligament on stretch (spreading the fingers when the metacarpophalangeal joints are flexed). Sometimes patients complain of swelling and aching at night.

The problem is treated by resecting the distal half of the intermetacarpal ligament and freeing the interosseous and lumbrical tendons distally (Fig. 18-11). The surgical approach is through a dorsal longitudinal incision over the web. Postoperatively the hand is mobilized immediately to prevent adherence of the intrinsic tendons.

Any lysis procedure designed to liberate joint movement and tendon excursion must be followed by immediate postoperative active movement. The placement of 20 to 40 mg of triamcinolone in the wound during surgery may be helpful. Pending healing of the skin wound, exercise should be supervised closely (even daily) by the surgeon, with adequate elevation and attention to splinting of the wrist and digits during the intervals between such exercise.

Joint Contractures (Chap. 21)

The pathological changes of bone and periarticular soft tissues about a joint are frequently the sole cause of a contracture in extension or flexion. As a rule, the roentgenograms will define bony but not soft tissue etiology. There is often a combination of bone and soft tissue factors.

The bony factors are usually post-traumatic deformities such as dislocation and displaced fracture, deformities of non-traumatic arthritis and

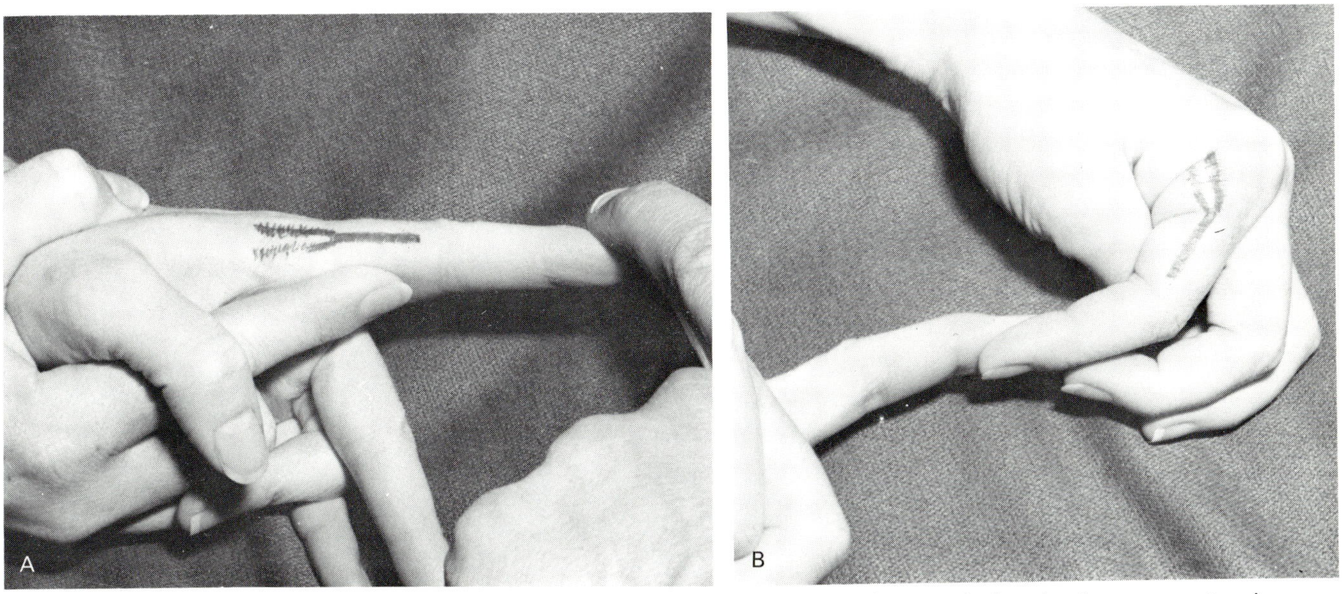

Figure 18-8. *A positive intrinsic plus test. The contracted intrinsic mechanism precludes simultaneous extension of the metacarpophalangeal joint and distal joint flexion. Likewise, when the distal two joints are flexed the metacarpophalangeal joint cannot be extended.*

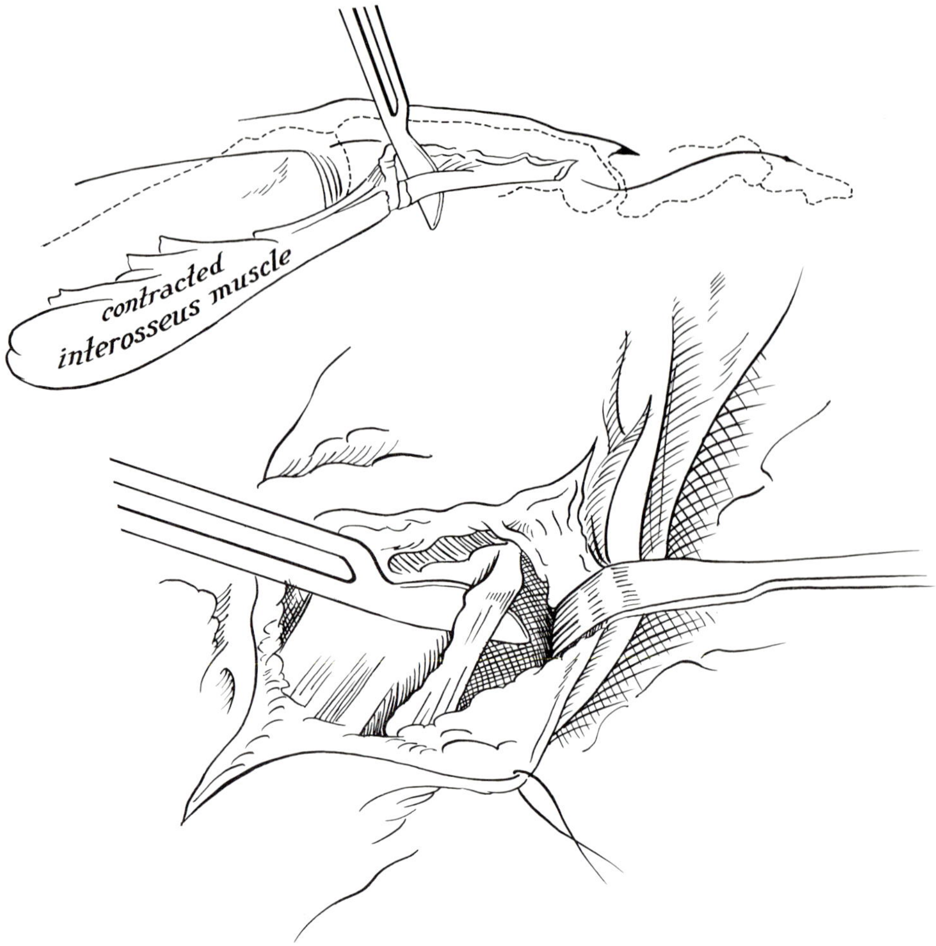

Figure 18-9. *Diagrammatic release of contracted interosseous muscle by lateral band resection.* (*Redrawn from Littler, J.W.*[8])

congenital anomalies. Acute traumatic deformities are often curable by appropriate reduction and immobilization followed by mobilization (Chaps. 11, 12). Fixed post-traumatic and non-traumatic contractures generally require appropriate surgical correction by some form of resection arthroplasty or functional arthrodesis. Sometimes this involves nothing more than the resection of a prominent lip of bone while at other times it involves implant arthroplasty.

The periarticular soft tissue changes causing contractures involve the joint capsule, volar plate, and collateral ligaments. Any one or all may be involved in a specific case. A contracture in exten-

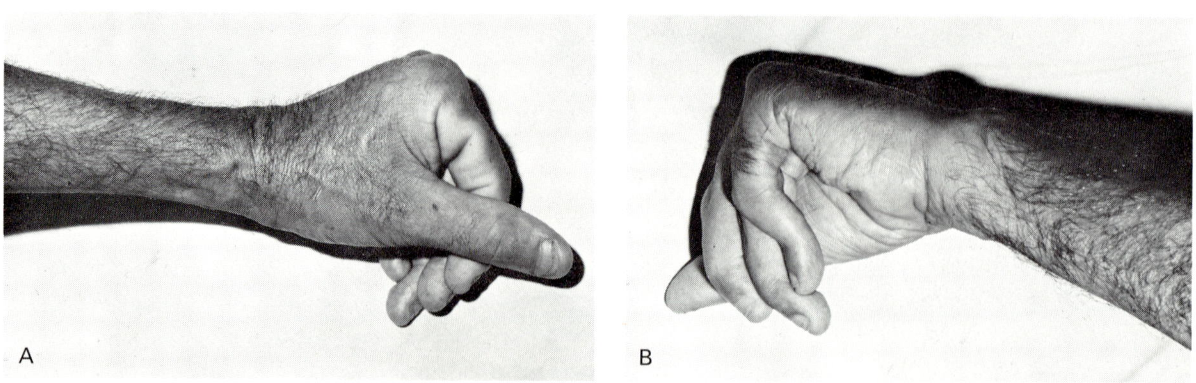

Figure 18-10. *"Intrinsic plus" hand.*

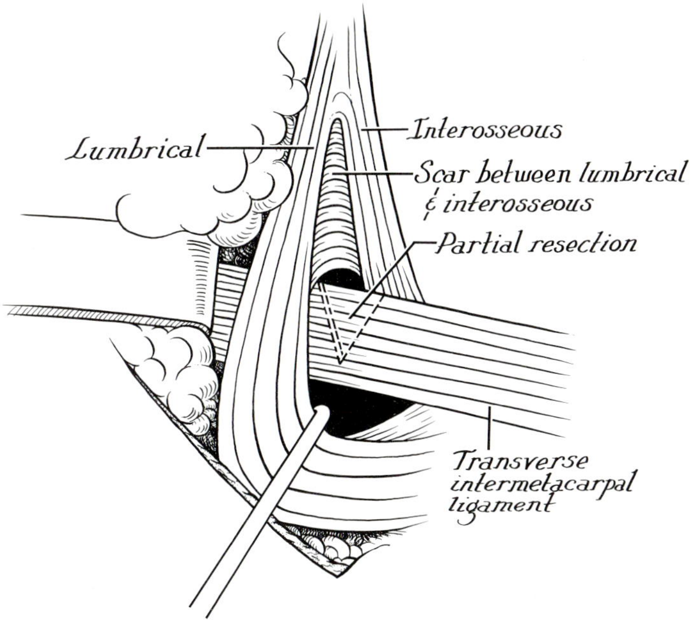

Figure 18-11. *Scarring between interosseous and lumbrical tendons which produced pain on clenching of the fist. Release of the distal scar and subtotal resection of the intermetacarpal ligament will usually relieve the problem.* (*Redrawn from Watson, H.K. et al.*[10])

sion usually means that the dorsal capsule and dorsal half of the collateral ligaments have to be assessed for tightness and surgically released. The volar plate may also be at fault when it is displaced into the joint, acting as a block under the wheel, or when it is adherent and thickened by scar so it has no excursion. A contracture in flexion usually means that the volar half of the collateral ligaments has to be assessed for tightness and released, and the volar plate has to be freed of adherent scar (e.g. contracture of the checkrein ligaments on the lateral aspects of its leading edge). In some cases, it is best to excise a triangle of the collateral ligaments with a #11 scalpel rather than to merely incise them. Instead of merely lysing the volar plate, it can be held with a strong single plastic surgical hook and resected with a curved #12 scalpel (Fig. 18-12).

All procedures consisting of joint lysis require immediate and progressive postoperative mobilization under close supervision of the surgeon so that active mobility will be maintained at the same time that the skin wound is healing. Adequate wrist and digital splinting and elevation are necessary between exercise periods. A small amount of local steroid (20 to 40 mg of triamcinolone) in the wound at surgery is sometimes helpful when tightness and scarring are marked.

Specific Diseases Associated with Contracture

Certain diseases invariably are associated with contractures. Many of these may be intractable to any form of treatment and may be aggravated by injudicious surgery.

A number of primary congenital conditions produce joint deformities in extension or flexion—arthrogryposis, symphalangism, etc. Others produce soft tissue contracture—camptodactyly and clinodactyly (Chap. 23).

Aging is a factor in the production of soft tissue and joint changes leading to contractures in extension or flexion. For the most part this is brought about by changes in the fascia manifested by the tightness and firmness of the soft tissues and osteoarthritis. Associated alterations of periarticular soft tissue, cartilage and neighboring bone can lead to marked stiffness (Chap. 25).

Any serious infection of part or all of the hand can lead to induration and scarring of the structures directly involved as well as neighboring tissues that are secondarily involved by fixed edema. All conditions that precipitate or are associated with any degree of ischemia or congestion will also produce fibrosis and contracture. The classic example of this is Volkmann's contracture (Chap. 10) (Fig. 18-5).

Specific collagen disorders also lead to contractures. The most pronounced of these is found in sclerodermatous hands wherein all tissues are involved, and particularly the skin which may be drawn tight as a drum (Figs. 7-28, 10-8).

Spastic contractures (Chap. 15) are seen in congenital, post-traumatic, postinfectious and degenerative encephalopathies. They may be amenable to functional improvement when limited in degree, but not when severe.

DUPUYTREN'S CONTRACTURE

Dupuytren's palmar and digital flexion contracture is a common functional, cosmetic and at times hygienic problem. On occasion tenderness impairs the patient's grasp but more often he complains of the awkwardness, frustration and embarrassment resulting from the inability to satisfactorily extend his fingers. He cannot shake hands, enter his pocket, put on a glove, wash his face, play golf and perform many other functions. The intertriginous maceration can be socially offensive.

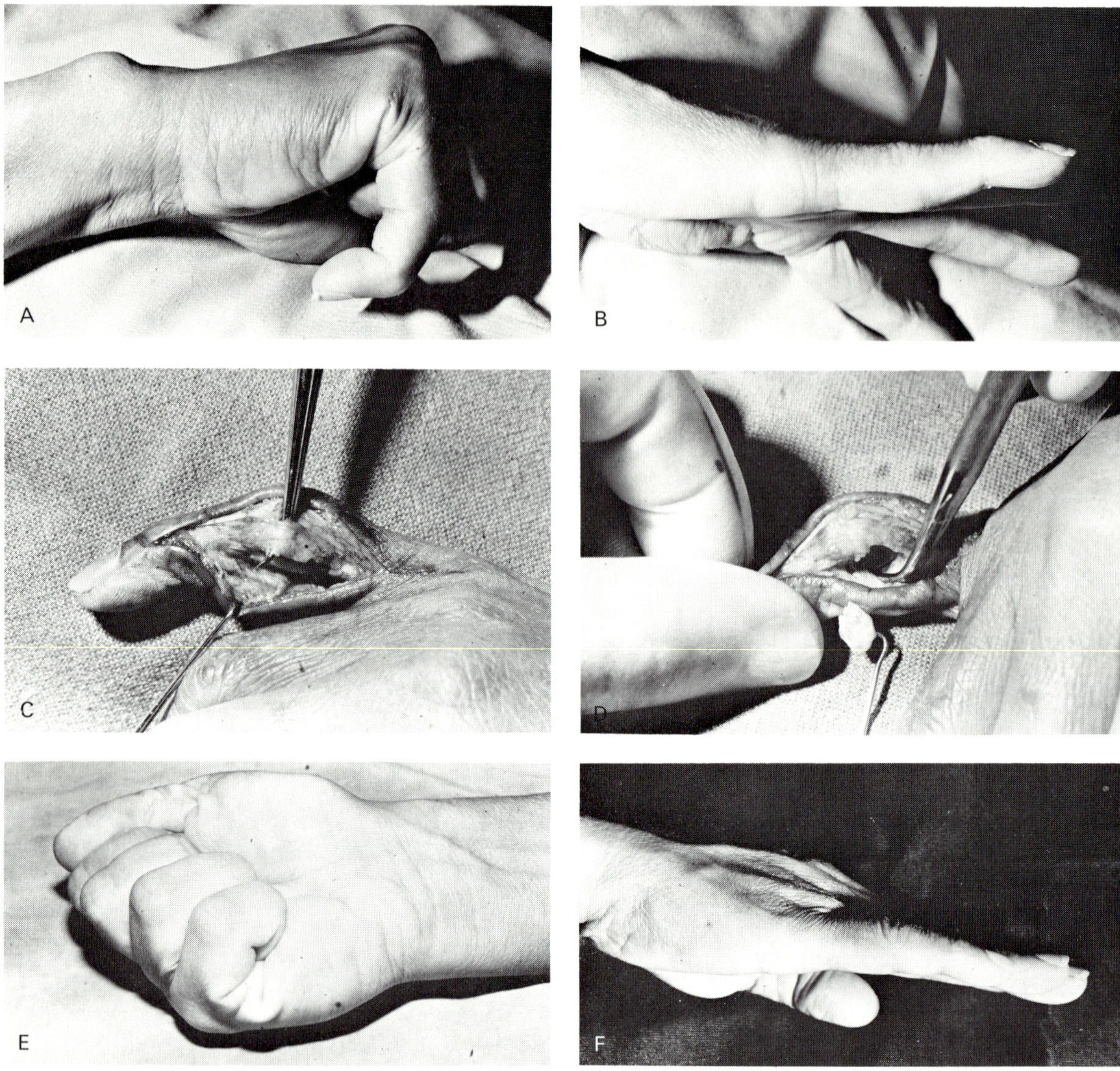

Figure 18-12. *Severe hyperextension injury to the proximal interphalangeal joint of the little finger. A tear of the volar plate resulted which blocked flexion. Resection of the volar plate* **(D)** *was done with considerable improvement in function.*

Etiology

In 1831 Guillaume Dupuytren, Baron of France, described the disease, and in 1832 published his famed article describing the contracture along with an operation for its correction.

The etiology is unknown. The indisputable factors often associated with this problem are age, sex, race and heredity. Allied but not consistent factors are chronic debilitating systemic disorders, e.g. diabetes, tuberculosis, epilepsy, cirrhosis. The role of trauma is disputed. Work by Davis[2] implicates the influence of the autonomic nervous system (sympathetics) by inducing ischemia through arteriolar spasm. This factor may contribute to the development of Dupuytren's disease in the above chronic disorders or following trauma. New research suggests that a specific cell, the myofibroblast, might be the cause. Induction of the contracture may result from the dermis rather than the fascia primarily.[3]

This fasciitis is primarily a disease of Caucasian males in the sixth to eighth decade of life. Approximately one-fourth of patients will have a positive family history. When it occurs in the youthful patient (e.g. in the third and fourth decades or rarely in the second decade) it is apt to be a more extensive process with repeated occurrences even after an adequate and proper fasciectomy. It is often unilateral and in the non-dominant hand, occurring as readily in sedentary workers as in manual laborers. Dupuytren's contracture is rarely if ever seen in pure Orientals or blacks.

Anatomy

The contracture may be bizarre and fail to coincide with anatomically distinct fascial elements, lending credence to the concept of dermal induction. Primarily it involves longitudinal bands of the palmar fascia (pretendinous bands) and vertical extensions of the palmar fascia to the skin superficially and the bone deep (vertical bands and septae). It also involves oblique and horizontal fascia of the webs (natatory ligament) but generally spares transverse midpalmar fibers, transverse palmar ligament between and deep to the pretendinous bands and proximal to the distal palmar flexion crease. In the fingers it involves primarily volar fascia deep to the fat pad of the proximal phalanges and lateral extensions to but not including Grayson's and Cleland's ligaments. It also involves vertical extensions to skin and bone (Figs. 18-13 and 18-14).

Flexion contracture of the thumb does not occur because of absence of a pretendinous band, but either adduction or abduction may be produced by involvement of the natatory ligament or the fascia on the radial margin of the thenar eminence (Fig. 18-15).

Established flexion contractures initiated by Dupuytren's fasciitis may be maintained only by this process. However, all too often secondary changes in the skin, periarticular structures (collateral ligaments), flexor tendon sheath, the extensor hood, Landsmeer's ligaments and even intrinsic and extrinsic muscles become contributing factors in the contracture and require surgical correction

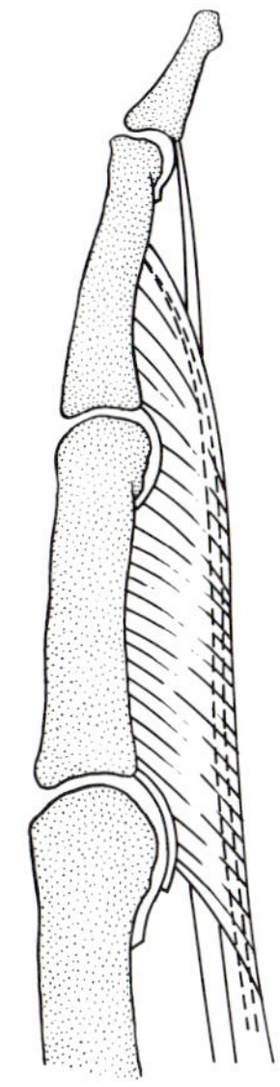

Figure 18-14. *Schematic representation of digital fascial sheets, contractures of which produce digital flexion deformities.*

for complete release. The skin involvement is variable, from no involvement to pinpoint infolding of the skin or infiltration of the skin and loss of all subcutaneous fat over a broad area. In the latter case the skin may be markedly shrunken with total loss of elasticity, requiring skin replacement at the time of fasciectomy.

The neurovascular bundle is never compromised by this fibrosis but may be easily injured by the unwary surgeon. At the base of the finger and at the proximal interphalangeal flexion crease the fibrous cord may spiral around the bundle as it passes distally. The color of the neurovascular bundle may be identical to that of the fascia, but in contrast to the fascia, which can be tensed by traction, the structures of the bundle remain soft and pliable.

Knuckle pads, plantar fasciitis and penile faciitis

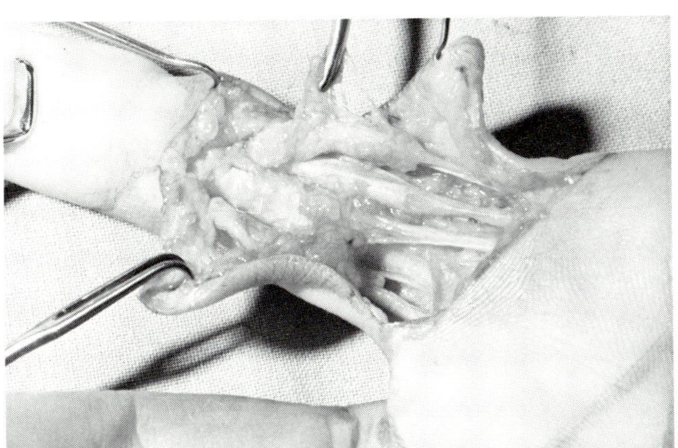

Figure 18-13. *Lateral extension of Dupuytren's fasciitis into the ulnar aspect of the little finger.*

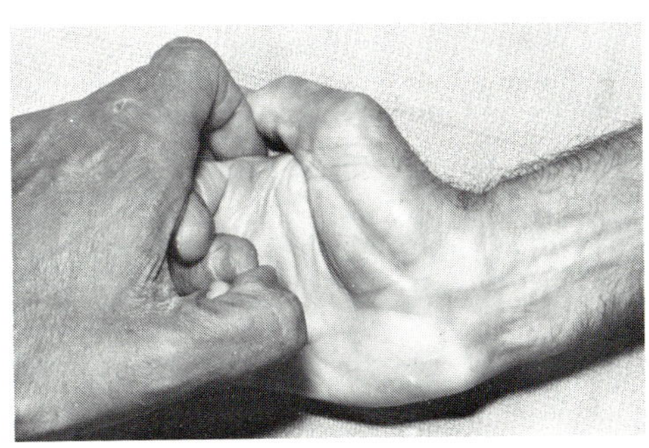

Figure 18-15. *Marked involvement of the thenar muscle area by Dupuytren's disease in a musician who was severely handicapped by his bilateral palmar and digital faciitis.*

(Peyronie's disease) are seen as related entities in association with or independent of palmar fasciitis. The knuckle pads usually are seen over the dorsum of the proximal interphalangeal joints but may also occur over the metacarpophalangeal joints (Fig. 22-9). Usually this is a subtle thickening of the dorsal fascia but occasionally it is a marked cosmetic problem.

Treatment

As in all surgery of the hand, the treatment of Dupuytren's disease must be adapted to the needs and tolerances of the patient. Every Dupuytren's contracture does not require surgery. The surgeon's role may be to assure the patient that he does not have cancer and that any treatment is entirely elective and should be on his demand. He should be made aware of the idiosyncrasies of the disease cited above and should be persuaded to consider surgery when a contracture is progressing rapidly and before the palmar involvement is surgically overwhelming. He should be appraised of the average duration of temporary disability following surgery, which runs 2 to 7 days for a fasciotomy and 4 to 6 weeks for a fasciectomy.

NON-OPERATIVE TREATMENT

The non-operative treatment of Dupuytren's fasciitis is the injection of the acutely inflamed palmar nodule with triamcinolone and an anesthetic (lidocaine). This is difficult and requires that the patient be supine. The surgeon uses a 26-gauge hypodermic needle on a tuberculin syringe and injects slowly. About 0.25 cc (5 mg) can be injected into these nodules. This can be repeated at 7- to 10-day intervals until relief occurs, or until three injections have been given. The benefits gained by local injections may be completely subjective. Injections must be into the nodule and not into the palmar fat for atrophy can result from the infiltration of normal tissue.

Hueston[6] has described the release of the contracture by forced rupture of the longitudinal element 15 minutes after injecting with trypsin, hyaluronidase and lidocaine. He has reserved this treatment for patients who are not suitable surgical candidates. Other non-operative measures (e.g. systemic vitamin E or radiation) have not proven effective.

SURGICAL TREATMENT

The two forms of operative treatment are fasciotomy and fasciectomy.

Fasciotomy can be done through a longitudinal or transverse incision. The former results in a closed wound, the latter in an open wound which may or may not require a split-thickness skin graft. Gonzalez[4] has advocated the latter for most cases and reports full return of function by 21 days in 83 per cent of the patients who had digital contractures.

For the patient whose disease is limited to a discrete pretendinous band without overlying skin involvement, single or multiple subcutaneous fasciotomies may be useful. A short longitudinal incision adjacent to the band is opened by careful dissection and under direct vision the tensed band is completely divided. Extension of the digit tends to close the wound. The morbidity of this procedure should be negligible and within a few days the patient should regain full use of the hand. This is the procedure of choice for the poor-risk patient or one for whom the duration of convalescence must be brief.

Fasciectomy is the generally preferred surgical treatment. This does not imply the total extirpation of the palmar fascia, which is impossible without ruining the hand. If the fasciitis is confined to a solitary nodule the excision is limited to that area only. However, more extensive disease with flexion contractures necessitates the resection of all of the fascia involved without injury to the neurovascular or musculotendinous structures.

In hopeless cases of severe digital contracture, amputation must be considered. This situation most commonly occurs with the little finger.

Technical Considerations in Surgery for Dupuytren's Contracture. The basic principles governing surgery of the hand must be meticulously followed in the performance of fasciectomy. The use of loupe magnification and a proximally placed arterial tourniquet is essential. All vessels must be identified so that the major ones can be spared and the minute ones electrocoagulated with a needle-point cautery.

The selection of the incisions is dictated by the extent of the disease. These should be designed and marked before inflating the tourniquet. Removal of a solitary palmar nodule is easiest through a short transverse incision. Access to a longitudinal band and vertical septae in the palm is facilitated by a long zigzag incision which may be extended into the digit (Fig. 6-10). A long transverse midpalmar incision supplemented distally by short longitudinal or zigzag counterincisions is used to remove multiple pretendinous bands. Wakefield[9] and others prefer a midline incision which can be interrupted by Z-plasties at the flexion creases. Knuckle pads, if excised, are removed through a short transverse elliptical incision, sparing the deep veins.

Extensive undermining and the construction of long thin flaps risk skin necrosis. At all times the fascia dissected must be kept under tension. This is done by placing the digits in extension and by holding the fascia with a suitable hook or clamp. Fat must be reflected and carefully preserved as each segment of diseased fascia is traced out. Excessive thinning or perforation of the skin can be avoided by close observation of both sides of the flap. The dissection should be done by meticulous spreading and cutting with the small blunt-tipped scissors. At times en bloc dissection is best, at other times segmental dissection. Beware of tenting and cutting nerves and vessels. "Soft tissue" must be retracted and not cut. Strand by strand, only the fascia which can be flicked with a scissors tip when taut is divided. In the web and near the proximal interphalangeal joint the fascia may spiral around the neurovascular bundle.

There is often a fine line between advisable and excessive surgery, the latter aggravating the patient's initial disability. If upon completion of the fasciectomy the proximal interphalangeal joint cannot be extended or the distal interphalangeal joint flexed, the following procedures can be undertaken providing there is some laxity to the dorsal skin and the surgery up to this point has not jeopardized the digital circulation. Through the same incision or short midaxial counterincisions the volar half of the collateral ligaments of the proximal joint may be incised and the volar plate freed. Following this the joint can be carefully manipulated into extension and on rare occasions held there with a Kirschner wire for 2 to 3 weeks. For liberation of the extended distal interphalangeal joint and correction of the buttonhole deformity, Littler has incised (even resected) Landsmeer's ligament or preserved this ligament and furled the lateral bands together dorsally after dividing them over the middle phalanx. An alternative procedure is to free a slip of lateral band and weave it across the dorsum of the proximal interphalangeal joint[8] (Fig. 14-15**C**).

In rare instances the final restraint to the liberation of the contracture is a foreshortened musculotendinous unit of the superficialis or profundus muscles, making the proximal interphalangeal joint recoil excessively into flexion. For this flexor tenotomy must be considered, with or without lengthening. At times arthrodesis is the best solution to correct the contracted joint.

Amputation is reserved for the hopeless contracture that defies surgical correction and for problems of severe intertrigo in patients under custodial care. Most commonly a ray amputation of the little finger is performed. On occasion the filleted little finger is used as a skin flap for resurfacing the palm.

Although most wounds lend themselves to closure with running or interrupted nylon sutures in the skin only, it is necessary to leave others open or to skin graft.[1] When primary split-thickness skin grafting is done some form of tied-over dressing (Stent) must be used. Delaying the grafting and avoiding the use of sutures minimize the chance of bleeding beneath the graft.

An open wound or a small drain is occasionally elected in the case of the patient with a livid palm or with marked hypertension where hematoma can readily occur in spite of good hemostatic technique.

The integrity of the fingertip circulation should be checked by release of the tourniquet after partial application of the dressing and before the fingers are completely covered and sterility lost.

The dressing should conform to that described in Chapter 4. Wetness and gentle even compression without venous impairment are of paramount importance in removing blood from the wound and reducing postoperative swelling and induration. The dressing should be changed in 3 to 4 hours after surgery if considerable oozing has been expected. Otherwise the dressing is usually changed in 3 to 4 days, at which time the extent of desired digital movement can be directed by the condition of the wound. Some form of wrist splint is usually necessary for a week or two. Digital swelling must be controlled at all costs.

Drains can usually be removed at 3 to 4 days and thereafter replaced with a zinc oxide dressing. A tied-down dressing (Stent) should remain for 5 to 7 days.

Mobilization is selectively initiated at 3 to 4 days but not delayed longer than a week. Squeezing a sponge in soapy water may start even before the removal of sutures at 10 to 14 days. The removal of nylon sutures may be delayed for 2 to 3 weeks.

When cicatrix threatens the result postoperatively, injections of triamcinolone at weekly intervals are sometimes beneficial. Occasionally a reverse knuckle bender dynamic splint should be prescribed.

The immediate complications of surgery involve the skin, neurovascular structures and the bones and joints. Nerves and vessels are injured by cutting or stretching. The former is prevented by meticulous technique and the latter by avoiding the simultaneous manipulation of the metacarpophalangeal and proximal interphalangeal joints in extension. The atrophic skin may be torn by undue stretching. Joint capsules may be torn and phalanges fractured by unwarranted force. When the severance of a nerve is recognized, a neurorrhaphy should be done primarily. The effects of vascular spasm are counteracted by relieving tension, reopening the wound and instilling lidocaine perivascularly.

Late complications consist of skin sloughs and joint stiffness. The former are treated by debridement and appropriate grafting. The latter may be an intractable problem even if the patient is highly motivated.

Recurrence of the fasciitis may occur at exactly the same site. More often, however, this type of fasciitis is mistaken for postoperative scar. True recurrences are most common in young patients with Dupuytren's disease. De novo fasciitis of unoperative fascia occurs subsequent to surgery at all ages. The indications for reoperation correspond to those for primary surgery. Replacement of the involved dermis by skin grafting diminishes the chance of recurrence.

References

1. Carroll, R.E. and Conolly, W.B.: Open wound technique for Dupuytren's contracture. J. Bone Joint Surg., 52A:1068, 1970.
2. Davis, J.E.: On surgery of Dupuytren's contracture. Plast. Reconstr. Surg., 36:277, 1965.
3. Gabbiani, G. and Majno, G.: Dupuytren's contracture fibroblast contraction. An ultrastructural study. Am. J. Pathol., 66:131, 1972.
4. Gonzalez, R.L.: A simplified surgical approach in the treatment of Dupuytren's contracture. In *Symposium on the Hand* (Cramer, L.M. and Chase, R.A., Eds.). C.V. Mosby, St. Louis, 1971.
5. Harris, C. and Riordan, D.C.: Intrinsic contracture of the hand and its surgical treatment. J. Bone Joint Surg., 36A:10, 1954.
6. Heuston, J.T.: Enzymatic fasciotomy. Hand, 3:38, 1971.
7. Kilgore, E.S., Graham, W.P., Newmeyer, W.L. and Brown, L.G.: The extensor plus finger. Hand, 7:159, 1975.
8. Littler, J.W.: Principles of reconstructive surgery of the hand. In *Reconstructive Plastic Surgery* (Converse, J.W., Ed.). W.B. Saunders, Philadelphia, 1964.
9. Wakefield, A.R.: Dupuytren's contracture. Surg. Clin. North Am., 40:483, 1960.
10. Watson, H.K., Ritland, G.D. and Chung, E.K.: Post traumatic interosseous-lumbrical adhesions. A cause of pain and disability in the hand. J. Bone Joint Surg., 56A:79, 1974.

19 Burns and Cold Injury

By the nature of its use for prehension and protection the hand commonly falls prey to the different types of burns: thermal, frictional, electrical, chemical and radiation. Depending upon the type and depth of the burn swelling, cicatrix, necrosis and even malignancy follow, endangering function. "Prophylactic" treatment is often urgent to preserve existing function, and if delayed (in some instances, even a few hours) will set the stage for irreversible stiffness and deformity. While the "life-threatening" burn of the patient is being managed the "economic life-threatening" burns of his hands must be simultaneously treated with equal zeal. The focus should be not merely on the hand but on all joints of the upper extremity.

The factors influencing the recovery from a burn are: (1) extent, depth and location of the burn, (2) etiology of the burn, (3) age and general health of the patient, (4) associated injuries, (5) degree of edema and local sepsis, (6) quality of care and cooperation of the patient and (7) preexisting hand disorders.

The knowledge of the mechanism of injury is essential in determining the type of burn and assessing its depth and the extent of the injury. The depth of skin involvement is determined by: erythema (first degree), blistering (second degree), absent sensation (third degree) and charring (fourth degree) (Figs. 19-1, 19-2). Diagrams in the patient's record are valuable graphic notations of the character of the burn and the progress of its treatment.

Burns threaten function initially by the development of swelling (transudation of protein-rich fluid), infection, pain and tissue loss, and subsequently by cicatrization and stiffness. The goals in treatment are the prevention of anatomical deformity and stiffness and the restoration of optimal function.

Thermal Burns

Most burns of the hand result from heat or friction. The extent and depth of the heat burn are determined by the expansiveness of the heating agent, its heat-holding capacity, the duration of contact with it and the thickness and resistance of exposed skin. In most cases the depth of a burn is proportional to the extent of surface involved, particularly in the case of liquid or flame burns.

Palmar skin which is keratinized and thick is less prone to the deep second- and third-degree burns common to the dorsum of the hand. The location of the burn predisposes to disability by contracture (in the palm and webs), tendon disruption (dorsum of the proximal interphalangeal joint) and loss of subcutaneous padding (fingertips).

Flame burns usually involve the dorsum of the hand, which is employed in shielding the face, whereas immersion in hot liquids injures both surfaces. These are either second- or third-degree burns. Hot tar spilled on the hand is alarming and looks terrible but it cools so rapidly that it rarely produces third-degree burns. It is readily removed with ether. The hand burned by hot grease is much less alarming in appearance. However, because of its heat-retaining capacity deep second- or third-degree white waxy burns result. Water spillage may be only first degree in depth.

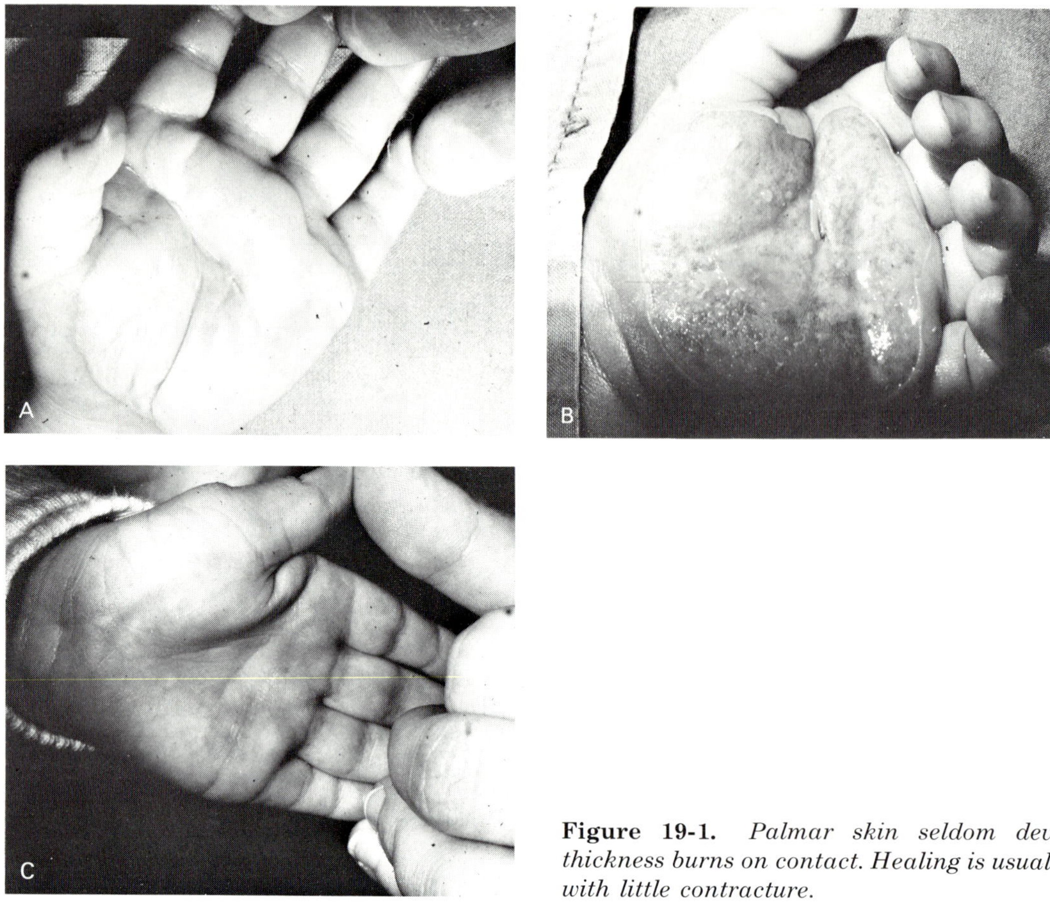

Figure 19-1. *Palmar skin seldom develops full-thickness burns on contact. Healing is usually excellent with little contracture.*

Protective withdrawal following contact with hot surfaces or sparks reduces the likelihood of severe burns. This protective withdrawal is not possible in the development of friction burns which are usually very deep (often third degree).

The age of a patient with burns of the hand can be a factor in contributing to loss of function and anatomical deformities. Infants, poorly motivated adults and many elderly patients tend to hold the wrist flexed and the fingers and thumb flexed into the palm. This "position of injury" is the position of rest and pain, which when established results in serious limitation of function. Infants and young children are usually unable to cooperate in a program of active motion; therefore more dressings and splints are needed but still may not prevent deformities. Elderly patients are often too weak to move their hands actively and their deformities may occur insidiously.

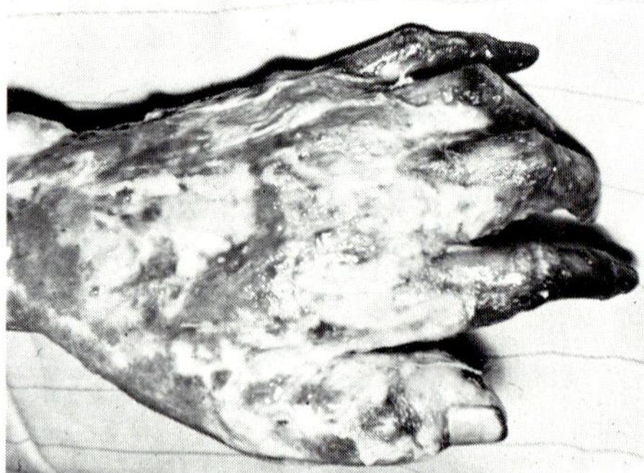

Figure 19-2. *Fourth-degree burns involve the tendons and bones of the digits.*

Associated burns or other injuries of the upper extremity or elsewhere usually impair the patient's or physician's ability to implement the ideal management of the burned hand (Fig. 19-3). The presence of these other injuries should not be allowed to unduly delay the institution of urgent measures in treating the burned hand. Preexisting disorders of the hand at times are detrimental in the recovery of the burned hand. Anemia, diabetes, hepatic and renal disorders can greatly complicate the management of burns if these problems are not amenable to prompt correction.

The surgeon and his staff must be experienced and, equally important, aggressive in ensuring that progress is maintained in salvaging function. Results are predicated upon quality of care and responsiveness of patient.

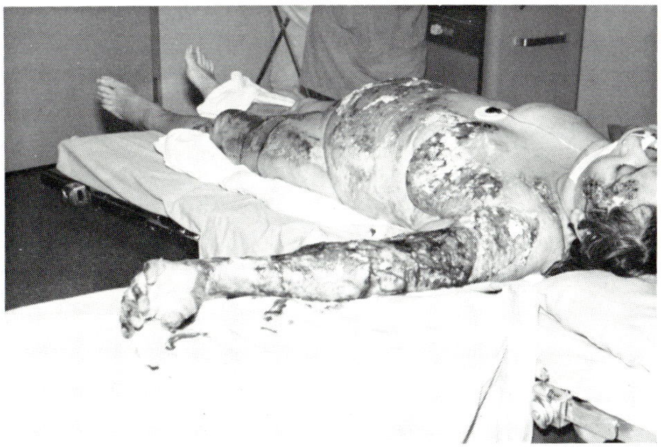

Figure 19-3. *This patient had residual left hemiparesis from previous stroke. The left upper extremity was amputated since it comprised the bulk of the third-degree burns.*

Treatment

The management of thermal injury is usually urgent to restore mobility (hopefully within 1 to 3 weeks). The factors requiring immediate attention are: (1) control of pain, (2) control of swelling, (3) debridement and (4) prevention of infection.

In the emergency treatment of the burn, the hand should be immersed in iced water. Proprietary preparations, butter and similar topical agents should not be applied. The part should be elevated and wrapped with a clean cold compress and the patient transported for expert definitive management.

FIRST-DEGREE BURN

If treatment is necessary at all mild analgesics and continuous cold compresses should suffice.

SUPERFICIAL SECOND-DEGREE BURN

Unless blisters are already bulky or broken they need not be debrided and can be allowed to dry. A dressing should be applied, consisting of fine mesh Xeroform gauze followed by loosely meshed non-constrictive plain gauze. However, when the blister has been debrided and the burn is more than 2.5 cm in diameter, biological dressings are preferred for the control of pain. These include allograft, xenograft (pig skin) and amniotic membrane[3] (Fig. 19-4). When these are not available, the appropriate substitutes for biological dressings are twice-daily applications of: (1) the painless antibacterial creams (silver sulfadiazine), (2) emollients (zinc oxide ointment or an ointment made up of: silver nitrate—1 part, balsam of Peru—5 parts, hydrous lanolin—30 parts, and amber petrolatum—30 parts), and (3) detergents (povidone-iodine).

When epithelialization has occurred and oozing ceases, skin comfort and softness may be maintained by twice-daily applications of a very thin coating of 0.025 per cent flurandrenolide cream after bathing. Lanolin may also be used provided the skin is well hydrated by immersion in water prior to the application.

Hanging of the hand and the assumption of the "position of injury" must be avoided. This may require splinting at night with tailored isoprene or padded plaster[9] (Fig. 19-5). Above all, the digits and wrist (as well as the shoulder and elbow) must be made to pass through a full range of motion hourly during the day. Early active motion can be extremely effective in preventing loss of function and the development of anatomical deformities in the burned hand. The ideal time to start active motion is immediately after the thermal injury and preferably before the development of maximal edema. It is far easier to maintain motion in a burned hand as edema develops than it is to restart motion in a hand that is swollen, stiff and painful from "fixed edema."

The benefits of early active motion are obvious. Motion maintains muscle strength, reduces edema that results in fibrosis, scarring and loss of function, prevents the shortening of collateral ligaments and other capsular structures and prevents the adherence of tendons to each other and to surrounding structures. This is important when tendons are surrounded by the protein-rich fluid of a burn wound.

The patient should be told what is desired with active motion and why it is important. The "why" should emphasize that active motion can reduce loss of function and anatomical deformities. With the wrist held in 25° to 30° of extension, flexion and extension of the digits and rotation of the thumb should be demonstrated. These motions should be repeated as completely as possible by the patient. At least once each day the hand should be washed and loose crust and eschar removed. This is easily accomplished in a body whirlpool where the patient can keep his hands in front of him while washing.

During periods of inactivity the burned hand should not be allowed to assume undesirable positions. The most common and least desirable attitude for the burned hand is that with wrist flexion. This can be prevented by a simple volar splint that immobilizes the wrist in approximately 20° exten-

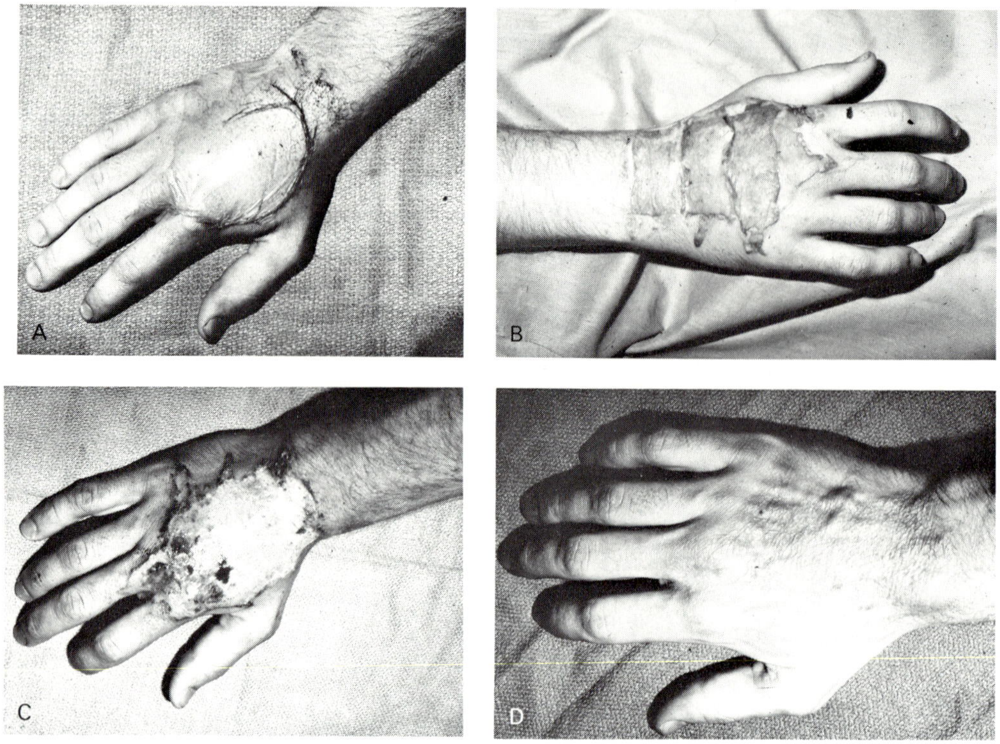

Figure 19-4. *This young man sustained a deep dermal burn from contact with hot grease* **(A).** *The wound was treated with allografts* **(B). C** *shows the appearance of the wound 8 days after injury at the time of removal of the second allograft. Excellent healing occurred and fully normal function was present at 3 months* **(D).**

sion. With this position, the pull of extensor tendons will be eased and the metacarpophalangeal joints will tend to assume a flexed position because of the effects of gravity plus the pull of the long flexor and the intrinsic muscles. It is also easier to achieve active extension of the interphalangeal joints and rotation of the thumb with the wrist slightly extended. If the patient tends to maintain the interphalangeal joints flexed and the thumb adducted after the wrist is splinted in extension, an addition to the splint is indicated to maintain the

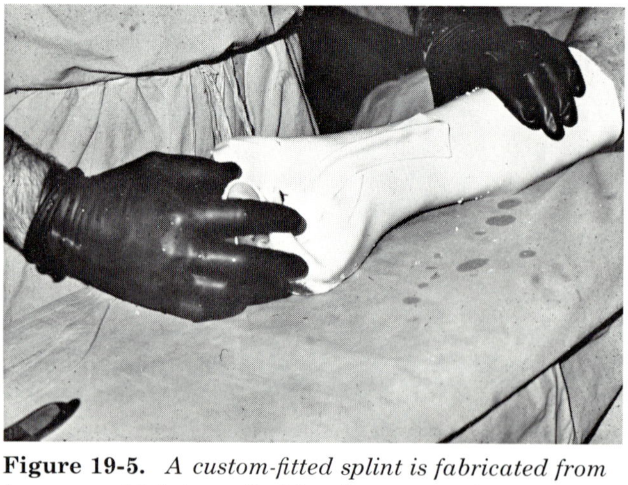

Figure 19-5. *A custom-fitted splint is fabricated from isoprene which is malleable when warmed.*

metacarpophalangeal joints flexed with the interphalangeal joints extended and the thumb abducted as widely as possible.

DEEP SECOND- AND THIRD-DEGREE BURNS

A deep second-degree burn is often indistinguishable in its clinical course from a third-degree burn. The restoration function is well served by treating some second-degree burns as full-thickness burns (Fig. 19-6). Deep partial-thickness burns of the flexor aspect of the forearm and medial upper arm frequently progress to full-thickness skin losses.

The greatest deterrent to function in these burns is congestion. Protein-rich fluid extravasates and pools in the loose spaces of the hand, primarily the dorsum. The metacarpophalangeal joints are drawn into hyperextension and the thumb is adducted. Disguised, underneath all the swelling, is a clawhand. Unattended, this readily becomes a fixed clawing with disastrous impairment of prehension. Much can be done to prevent this clawing by appropriate splinting, elevation and active motion. The proper splint is molded from isoprene to hold the wrist in 25 to 30° of extension, the thumb abducted and the metacarpophalangeal joints of the fingers well flexed.

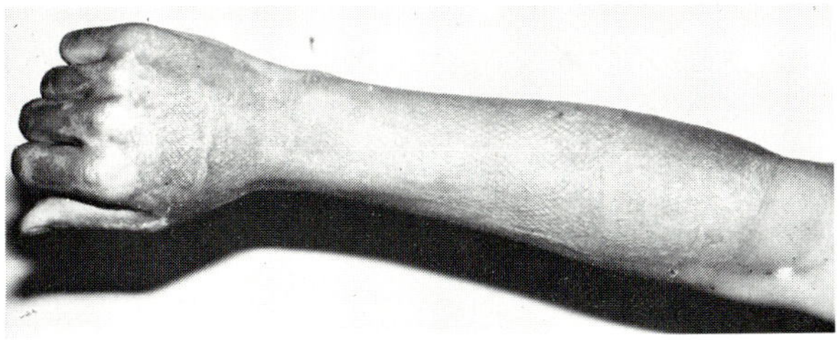

Figure 19-6. *This deep partial-thickness burn of the forearm was treated by tangential excision and overgrafting with meshed split-thickness skin grafts.*

Throbbing pain and the development of numbness herald excessive congestion marked by brawny induration. Then escharotomy becomes an emergency and often is done at the bedside (Fig. 19-7). The releasing incisions must not injure veins, nerves or tendons and should be made whenever possible in a way (zigzag) to avoid future contracting scars.

The claw deformity will be released if the metacarpophalangeal joints of the fingers are allowed to flex by a transverse incision immediately proximal to them and a zigzag incision in the thumb web. Maintenance of adequate flexion of the metacarpophalangeal joints and abduction of the thumb may require the placement of four Kirschner wires longitudinally across the metacarpophalangeal joints and one between the thumb and index metacarpals. When the extensor hood mechanism is compromised and the proximal interphalangeal joint seems likely to lose its mobility and enter into a claw deformity, this joint may be fixed in slight flexion by the use of a small Kirschner wire. Such internal splints remain until grafting is completed and mobilization is begun. Alternative splinting preferred by some surgeons is the use of a "hay rake."[4]

Additional releasing incisions are often necessary on the sides of the digits and the forearm and arm. However, these must not be so close together (particularly when they are deep) that they compromise the circulation to otherwise viable skin. Above all, the releasing incisions must extend through the fascia of any compartments (either flexor or extensor) in which the tissues are under excess tension.

Every effort is made to avoid infection. Patients who have not had tetanus prophylaxis within a year should be given tetanus toxoid, and if they have never been immunized human hyperimmune serum should be given.

Although grafting is the ultimate protection against infection, pending closure of the wound topical and systemic antibacterial agents are needed in most instances. The choice of topical antibacterial agents depends upon the preference and experience of the surgeon and the availability of biological dressings.

Systemic antibiotics are usually considered necessary in the initial management of patients with thermal injuries. Also, they are indicated prior to and immediately after grafting to prevent streptococcal infections from destroying the grafts. Since many granulating wounds also contain staphylococci which may be penicillin resistant, it is necessary to use an antibiotic that is effective against both gram-positive organisms. Both methicillin and clindamycin are satisfactory. Systemic antibiotics should be started 12 to 24 hours prior to grafting and continued for at least 2 to 3 days. If the wounds are not completely covered at this time the antibiotics may be continued longer.

The surgeon must be aggressive in his excision of the eschar and set his timetable to achieve enough grafting to permit vigorous daily motion within 10 days of the burn. Delays of 3 to 4 weeks in waiting out the viability of deep second-degree burns entail a certain risk of infection and intractable stiffness

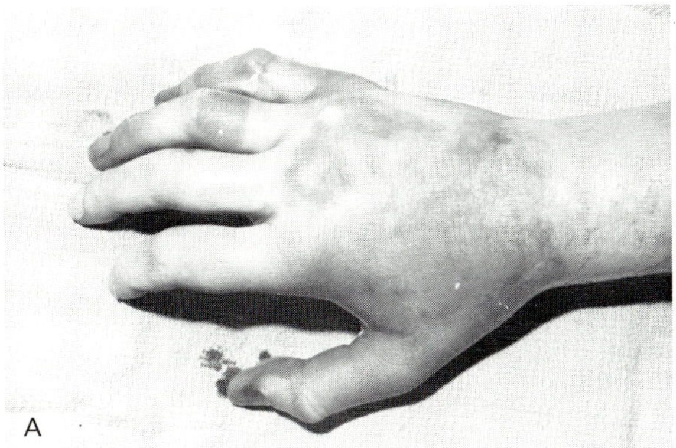

A

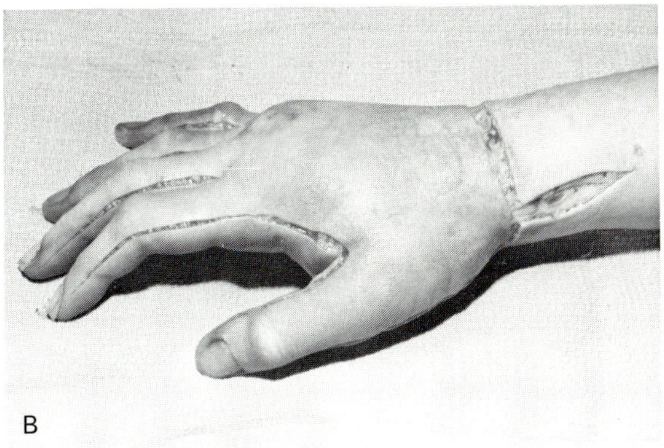

B

Figure 19-7. *This full-thickness burn occurred following prolonged immersion in hot water* **(A).** *Despite escharotomies* **(B)** *and removal of the dorsal skin when the patient was first seen 36 hours after her burn, necrosis of the fingers still occurred.*

from scarring. Furthermore, the quality of the regenerated epithelium is often unsatisfactory. The surgeon must not be reluctant to excise second-degree burns.

It is impossible to be dogmatic in the technique and requirements of debridement. The surgeon must be experienced and adaptive to the needs of the wound. In the main, however, the debridement will be most effective if done under tourniquet control at a level just beneath the dermis, using magnification for pinpoint control of hemostasis with electrocautery. Thrombosed veins should be excised. Multiple darts should be made along the wound margins. The wound is covered with fine-meshed gauze and a moistened dressing with the hand in the position of function. Enzymatic debridement with ointment from bacillus sutilains is still unproven and may increase the risk of sepsis.

Primary grafting is seldom done because of the high incidence of failure caused by oozing under the graft. The graft is taken coincident with the debridement and stored in Ringer's lactate solution in a sterile container in the operating room refrigerator. It is then applied 12 to 48 hours later under optimal conditions, at which time hemostasis and the best chance for graft survival exist. The thinner the graft (0.10 to 0.15 in) the greater is the assurance of a take. The thicker the graft (0.15 to 0.25 in) the better is the cosmetic and functional result.

Grafts may be postage stamps or in mesh or sheet form (Fig. 19-6). The surgeon's choice is governed by his assessment of the problem and the availability of skin for grafting and by the condition of the bed of the burn wound. Inasmuch as tied-down dressings (Stent) are not needed at the time of delayed grafting, suturing may not be needed and is contraindicated if it produces bleeding under the graft.

Immobilization is essential for at least 48 hours after grafting. If a dressing is applied during this time it should be continuously moistened to enhance drainage away from the wound. Open treatment requires constant attention to the removal of subgraft serous accumulations, using the surgeon's method of choice. One preference is to puncture the graft with a small hypodermic needle or #11 scalpel blade rather than to roll out the serum from beneath the graft with a cotton applicator.

Ideally, after 48 hours the graft is sufficiently adherent to initiate exercise and hydrotherapy. Again on an hourly basis, the patient exercises his hand maximally. At least twice a day his hand is immersed in warm water for no more than 30 minutes. This makes the hand more comfortable and permits the easy removal of any crusts. Active assisted passive range of motion can be encouraged during this hydrotherapy, and is especially necessary when metacarpophalangeal joint flexion is less than 20° and thumb abduction is less than 45°.

Concomitant functional splinting with custom-molded isoprene is needed for periods of rest. The splint should ensure wrist extension of 20 to 30°, thumb abduction of 40° and metacarpophalangeal joint flexion of at least 40°. In the course of overcoming a claw deformity, the splint must also fully extend the proximal interphalangeal joints.

Continuous, controlled, dynamic pressure wrapping should be initiated as soon as the graft is secure, in order to modify (decrease chondroitin sulfate A) the developing scar and avert hypertrophy with the development of secondary contracture.[10,11] The simplest material for this is a removable elastic bandage. For the hand or finger alone, a surgeon's rubber glove is ideal. Tailor-made gloves can be fabricated for the whole arm (Jobst Institute, Inc., 653 Main St., Toledo, Ohio 43694). There should be a proper distal-to-proximal pressure gradient of 35 to 55 mm Hg. Compression can be applied over or under a padded isoprene functional hand splint.

Extensive burns of the hand that are patchy with scattered islands of good surviving skin (especially volar) among lakes of eschar are sometimes more effectively debrided by multiple daily dressing changes at the time of immersion in a whirlpool for exercising. The gauze dressing draws away the eschar as it separates and the viable skin is preserved. This technique is acceptable in preference to extensive surgical debridement providing a satisfactory range of motion is maintained, and syndactyly is not developing in ungrafted raw areas of adjacent fingers.

FOURTH-DEGREE BURNS

The sooner that charred portions of the hand are surgically debrided the better. As a rule such burns are incurred during a state of coma, which often means that there are extensive body and even inhalation injuries. At some times, the patient is comatose by virtue of alcohol, drug overdose or some other disease (cerebrovascular accident). In these circumstances the burn is confined to the part of the extremity which was continuously in contact with the agent of heat (a hot radiator).

These burns invariably involve tendons and bones of multiple digits and sizable portions of the body of the hand. It may be very difficult to salvage enough skeletal length to reconstruct any prehensile function (Fig. 19-2). The risk of clostridial infections is higher in these individuals than in patients with burns of lesser depth who are in better health.

Functional Disability

All tissues and structures of the hand can be directly or indirectly altered by thermal burns. The greatest impairment arises from stiffness, caused by scarring and the contracture of skin, shrinkage of synovial, capsular and ligamentous tissues. The adherence and disintegration of the extensor mechanism, the fibrosis of intrinsic musculature, chronditis, arthrodesis of joints and web syndactyly further complicate the end-result.

Characteristic deformities develop which may be interrelated or totally independent of one another. The *claw deformity* is common, with hyperextension of the metacarpophalangeal joints and flexion of the interphalangeal joints. Hyperextension of the metacarpophalangeal joints follows overdistension of the dorsal skin secondary to subcutaneous edema. The interphalangeal joint flexion occurs from the tension of the long flexors. The acute claw deformity can usually be relieved by rapid operative or non-operative control of the edema. When the edema becomes "fixed" there is secondary fibrosis of all soft tissues, especially skin, fascia and periarticular structures.

The correction of "fixed" clawing involves: (1) replacing the dorsal skin and (2) extensor tenolysis. In some instances a tenotomy is required, necessitating a secondary tendon reconstruction and (3) metacarpophalangeal joint capsulotomy starting on the ulnar side to avoid ulnar drift, but often requiring division of radial collateral ligament. This is usually done by splitting the central slip. Metacarpophalangeal joint surgery is seldom needed in children (Fig. 19-8).

Internal fixation with a longitudinal Kirschner wire is advised whenever capsulotomy is done concomitantly with resurfacing or in a patient whose intrinsic musculature is weak or in whom motivation is inadequate. The wires are generally removed in 3 to 4 weeks. When Kirschner wires have not been used immediate mobilization is necessary.

The *buttonhole deformity* follows destruction of the extensor mechanism over the proximal interphalangeal joint. The hood may be totally destroyed or merely attenuated. The choice of reconstructive procedure (Chap. 14) depends upon the condition of the proximal interphalangeal joint and the overlying skin. This skin must be full thickness and pliable. The articular cartilage must be healthy and the joint must be mobile.

An *adduction contracture* of the thumb is instigated by dorsal edema in the same manner as metacarpophalangeal joint hyperextension is produced. Contracture of the dorsal skin and fascia of the muscles in the web may "fix" this deformity. The release in the acute phase is by non-operative or operative measures previously described in this chapter. Release of the fixed phase requires resurfacing of dorsal skin. A flap of dorsal skin based on the thumb metacarpal is raised and allowed to slide radially as the web is opened. The residual defect is grafted. The fascia in the thumb web is divided and sometimes the adductor pollicis must be released from its origin on the third metacarpal through a separate volar incision (Fig. 19-9). Its innervation must be preserved. The spread of the web is dynamically maintained with a spreader bar. Two 19-gauge hypodermic needles are passed transversely through the necks of the thumb and index metacarpals and the hubs are left as sockets facing one another to receive and hold the ends of a Kirschner wire cut to the appropriate length and having the desired spring. This fixation is maintained for 3 to 6 weeks.

Rigidity of the interphalangeal joints in extension is caused either by lack of skin or by pericapsular contractures. Often the proximal interphalangeal joint is in full extension and a secondary mallet deformity has developed at the distal interphalangeal joint. Subsequent to this a swan-neck deformity occurs with further extension of the proximal interphalangeal joint. In most instances the stiffness of the proximal interphalangeal joint is relieved once satisfactory skin coverage is attained; however, if the quality of the skin is good arthrolysis may be all that is required. Stiffness of the interphalangeal joint of the thumb or the distal interphalangeal of the fingers in extension may warrant arthrodesis in 15 to 20° of flexion (Chap. 13).

Severe *flexion and web contractures* result from contracture of the skin. Release is generally by transverse division of the involved scar so that the limits of the wound meet the axis of joint rotation. Great care is exercised to avoid injury to neurovascular structures by cutting or stretching. A suitable graft is placed after spreading the incision so that the wound generally forms the configuration of a diamond. Tied-down dressings (Stent) for

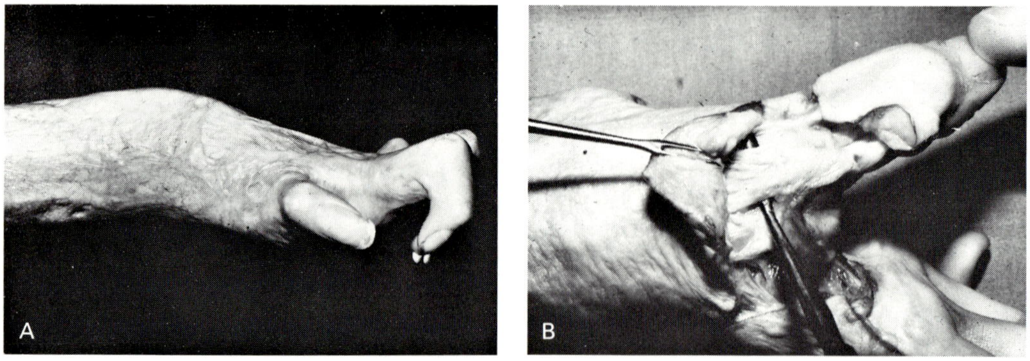

Figure 19-8. *The severe clawhand was produced by deep dermal burns that were allowed to heal* **(A).** *The thickened subcutaneous dorsal scar resembles a tendon* **(B).**

full-thickness and split-thickness grafts are indispensable. The surgeon's judgment will dictate the cover to use. If he elects pedicle coverage, it will generally be developed by a local rotational flap. However, a distant flap may be preferred in some instances for the thumb web and palm. In preparing a bed in the palm, it may be preferable to excise than to incise the scar. When free skin grafts are used on palmar surfaces for the release of these contractures, full-thickness skin taken from the non-hair-bearing area of the groin is preferable to split-thickness skin. In pigmented individuals the hyperpigmentation of a graft may be avoided if it is obtained from the ulnar aspect of the palm or the instep. Skeletal fixation is employed frequently to hold the interphalangeal joints and thumb web in the desired position for 3 to 4 weeks.

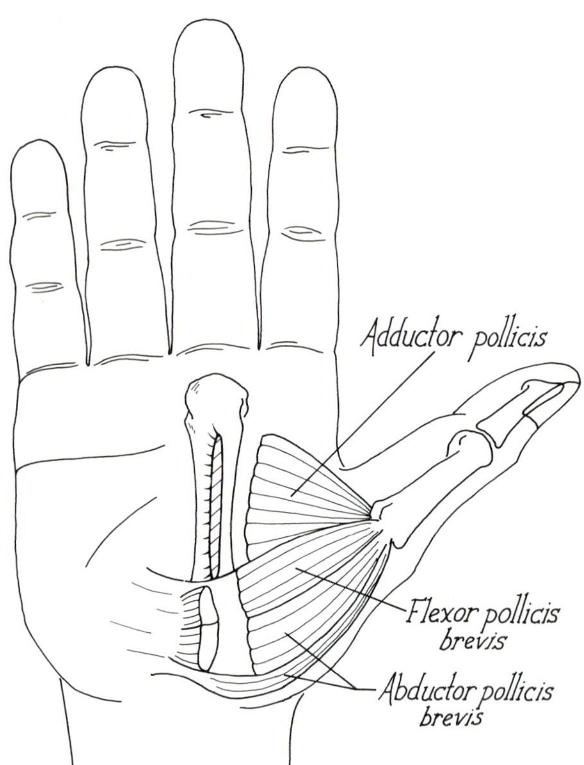

Figure 19-9. *The adductor pollicis was released at its origin for first web contractures. Occasionally the other thenar muscles must be released also.*

Other problems causing cosmetic or functional disability relating to the skin are pigmentary changes, limited endurance to wear and tear when too thin and poorly padded, hypersensitivity, grotesque hypertrophic scarring and nail deformities. These conditions may justify selective resurfacing. There is no technique to restore cosmetically normal nails.

Carcinoma occasionally develops in healed burn scars. The susceptibility of the injured tissues is increased by repeated trauma. The latent period for the appearance of the carcinoma may be brief (acute burn scar carcinoma) or more usually many years after the original injury. These squamous cell carcinomas are commonly associated with distant metastases in the absence of regional lymph node involvement.[15]

Amputation is indicated when the digit or hand is an impediment to the patient's functional, social and economical well-being and beyond hope for salvage.

Frictional Injury

Frictional injury is incurred by motion, generally at high speed, of the skin compressed upon an unlubricated hard surface. In sliding down a rope or hill, in skidding and falling from a motorcycle or in being dragged by a horse or car, the skin moves on the hard surface. This injury produces a straightforward loss of tissue by mechanical abrasion and avulsion without the occult dimension of thermal injury. When, however, the skin is trapped by the high-speed roller of a press, there may be little or no loss of substance but a waxy-white third-degree burn from the heat of friction with somewhat indistinct limits of injury (Fig. 19-10).

When abrasion and avulsion, not heat, are the factors of trauma, the need for debridement may be less and the wound may at first require little more than thin split-thickness grafting for closure. Where, however, heat is the prime factor in the injury, the treatment should follow the precepts of burn management already discussed—usually prompt debridement and grafting. In either case there may be marked destruction of deeper tissues, challenging secondary reconstruction or making it impossible (Fig. 16-7).

Electrical Burn

The electrical burn is produced by electricity causing coagulation of tissues. The hand is the most frequently injured part of the body. The mechanics of the burn are twofold: (1) by arc heat (e.g. a crossed circuit) and (2) by conduction within the tissues. The voltage may be high or low (less than 1000 volts) in the first instance, but is usually high in the second. The arc burn deposits carbon which blackens the skin. This invariably accentuates the anxiety initiated by the frightening exposure to the noisy unexpected flash. More often than not there is no burn at all, or if present it is less than third degree and does not affect subcutaneous tissues. Standard thermal burn treatment should be instituted with prompt reassurance to the patient.

With the conduction of electricity through the tissues there must be a point of entry and of exit. Here arcing at temperatures reaching several thousand degrees produces the greatest tissue coagulation. Centrally there is charring and peripherally a white waxy ring is surrounded by a reddish halo. The electrical current is primarily conducted along blood vessels which have the least resistance. Changes occur in the vessel walls, predisposing to thrombosis and at times delayed hemorrhage extending considerable distances from the points of entrance and exit of the current. This accounts for secondary ischemic changes which are often hidden and are responsible for the "iceberg" magnitude of the tissue affected. Often the extent of ischemia is immediate and easily recognized in debridement by the experienced surgeon. At other times it is delayed (Fig. 19-11). This has led to the erroneous philosophy of late rather than early debridement. It is far better to do an early debridement anywhere from 1 to 5 days after injury, with a second look for additional non-viable tissue 24 to 48 hours later before covering the wound. This removes devitalized tissues and reduces dead space and the likelihood of infection. It also hastens the opportunity for reconstruction and minimizes hospitalization and disability.

As stated by Peterson[12] the duration of contact with the current and its voltage are the prime factors causing tissue damage. He gives the factors in tissue destruction and vascular damage as follows:

Voltage
Current (amperage)
Resistances at entry point
Resistances at exit point
Duration
Pathway
Type of current
Patient's susceptibility

Regarding debridement, Peterson's description is classic: "In the excision of electrical burns of the hand, the bloodless field provided by a pneumatic

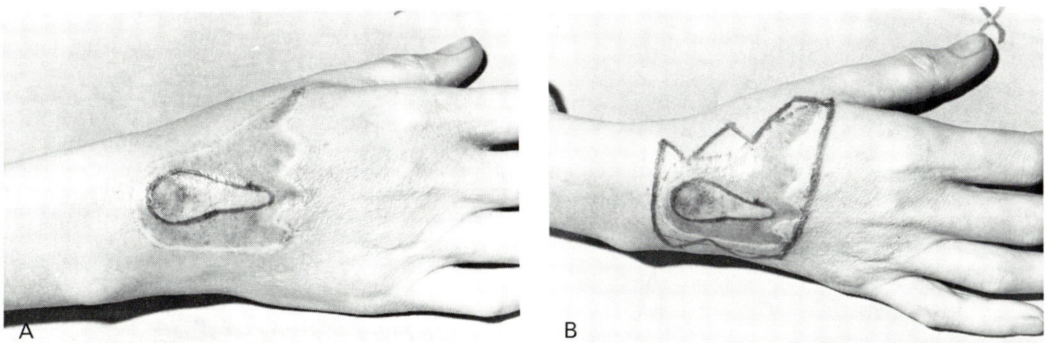

Figure 19-10. *This lady caught her hand between rollers at work. She developed a friction burn of the dorsum of her hand which was excised and grafted immediately. The outline shows the area of full-thickness injury. The area excised and grafted is shown in* **B.**

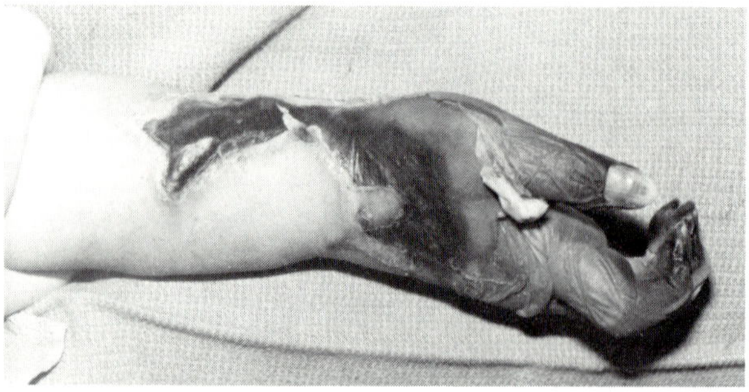

Figure 19-11. *This lady lost the entire hand from a severe electrical injury.*

tourniquet has distinct advantages in determining the extent of deep necrosis. Damaged tendon, muscle, nerve and joint capsule are readily identified. In the severest injuries, these structures may be charred or obliterated. Coagulated muscle has the light brown color of milk chocolate. Necrosed tendons, areolar tissue and fascia lose their glistening appearance and appear dry. Fat is an opaque pinkish-gray compared with its normal yellow. Nerves may be swollen, soft friable, and gray tan in color, or thin and tapered."[12]

The wrist, elbow, and shoulder joints are often closed by the tetanic contractions of musculature, facilitating the arcing of current between their surfaces. This results in additional skin burns. Fasciotomy may be needed before any other treatment with these injuries.

Ugland[13] states that "permanent damage to peripheral nerves by strong electrical currents does not extend beyond the areas of the local tissue damage." His experimental studies show that dysfunction of peripheral nerves induced by strong electrical current is reversible in the areas not coagulated by thermal injury. Thus it is imperative that secondary ischemic fibrosis of salvageable nerves be prevented by appropriate early decompression. Arteriography is helpful in confirming the magnitude of circulatory impairment suspected clinically in some of these cases.

The maximum salvage of function is aided by early wound closure. Except in the debridement of punctate arc burns, simple wound approximation is rarely accomplished. In most instances closure by grafts is necessary. The surgeon must choose between the merits of simple free grafting and pedicle grafting, which may enhance the local circulation.

Chemical Burns

These injuries result from the effects of topical exposure. They are of two types: (1) One may have a purely chemical coagulation necrosis of the skin. If the reaction is exothermic a thermal injury is added. (2) Some chemicals such as picric acid penetrate the skin without any obvious lesion, but affect the subcutaneous tissues by causing vasculitis and neuritis.[1]

In the first group, coagulation of the skin with symptomatology is immediate. In the second, onset is usually insidious and progressive. The immediate treatment in both types is to stop the exposure and to wash the area copiously with water. This should be continued over a long period in some instances such as lye (NaOH) burns, which may require 24 hours of irrigation. In some cases specific antidotes are available and can be injected locally to neutralize the effect of the chemical (10 per cent calcium gluconate for hydrofluoric acid burns)[8] (Fig. 19-12).

Burns caused by alkalis (calcium hydroxide, sodium hydroxide, potassium hydroxide and calcium oxide—lime) result from saponification and the exothermic conversion of protein to alkaline albuminates. These changes increase the permeability of the skin, favoring deeper penetration of residual lye and the extension of the injury. In the case of inorganic acid burns, the injurious effects result primarily from the free ions (hydrogen and the accompanying anion) which can be more easily lavaged. Certain anions may at times be specifically neutralized. This is especially true of fluoride in hydrofluoric acid burns seen commonly with glass etching and brick reclaiming. This anion is the most electronegative element as well as one of the smallest; consequently it diffuses rapidly. It can be neutralized (sometimes several times) by subcutaneous injection of a small amount of 10 per cent calcium gluconate at the site of injury.

After the initial period of lavage, second- and third-degree burns caused by chemicals are managed in the same fashion as burns from other sources.

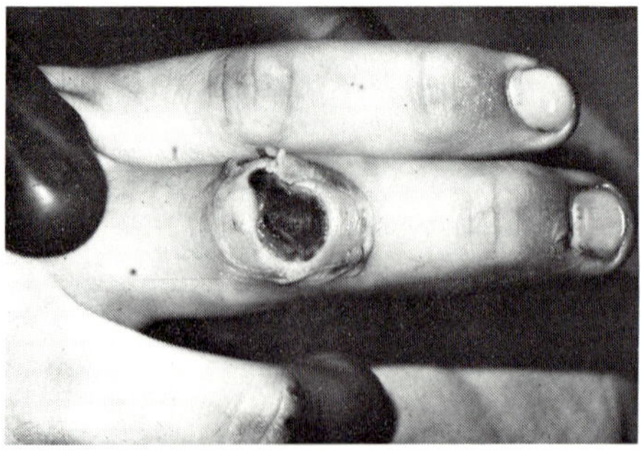

Figure 19-12. *Untreated hydrofluoric acid burn of dorsum of proximal interphalangeal joint is shown.*

Solutions known to cause neuritis and vasculitis industrially by carelessness or by leakage into protective work gloves are picric acid, formalin and chromic acid. Elemental yellow phosphorus, unlike red phosphorus, is volatile and soluble and causes burns. This element is neutralized by irrigation with 1 per cent copper sulfate solution and the burn is treated in routine fashion.

Radiation Burns

With the realization of the hazards of radiation and its long-term malignancy-producing potential there has been less exposure of the hands. Characteristically radiation burns have not been recognized until 10 to 20 years after they occurred, when skin changes became manifest. These were seen as occupational burns on the index and long fingers of dentists and their technicians and on the dorsum of the hands of surgeons and radiologists doing fluoroscopy. Patients have developed these problems in response to the treatment of dermatological disorders (eczema and warts). Fair-skinned people exposed to actinic rays of the sun have a tendency to form premalignant and malignant changes on the dorsum of the hand and fingers (Chaps. 7, 22).

The characteristic changes consist of atrophy and telangiectasia of the skin and subcutaneous tissues, ridging of nails, mottled pigmentation and hyperkeratosis, which may be mistaken for aging. Ultimately the premalignant keratoses transform into Bowen's disease, squamous cell carcinoma, basal cell carcinoma and, rarely, sarcomas and melanomas.

Acute radiation dermatitis is seen much less commonly and usually is the result of unrecognized and unexpected exposure to radiation (Fig. 19-13). It varies from mild to massive (Table 19-1). The inflammatory reaction is usually manifest within hours and may completely disappear after several weeks or, in massive burns, may progress to extensive tissue necrosis of the hand. Depending upon the magnitude of the reaction, the patient will have varying degrees of pain and stiffness. In the mild and moderate cases these symptoms usually do not appear until the end of the latent period between the initial and second phase of erythema.

The treatment of chronic radiation dermatitis depends upon the etiology and the degree of skin changes. If the cutaneous changes are superficial and are due to solar radiation, 5-fluorouracil (5FU) is used. A solution of 2 to 5 per cent 5FU in propylene glycol is applied b.i.d. for 10 to 14 days. This results in an erythematous desquamation that heals in 7 to 10 days, often with complete disappearance of the actinic process. However, a carcinomatous ulceration is treated by excision with an adequate margin and appropriate closure (Chap. 22).

The acute radiation injury is accompanied by great psychological distress and anxiety in the patient and often in his medical attendants. The surgeon must be realistically empathetic in his supporting role. One of the principal immediate problems is the control of pain. This may require morphine or dihydromorphinone.

Table 19-1. *Radiation Exposure (modified from Hansen and Edgerton[7])*

ACUTE	APPEARANCE	REMISSION	REAPPEARANCE	SIGNS AND SYMPTOMS	ULTIMATE STATE
Mild	Hours	Yes	7–21 days	Minimal. Slight swelling and stiffness	Pigmentary changes
Moderate	Hours	Yes	Less than 7–21 days	Blistering and superficial ulceration	Telangiectasis Atrophy Keratosis
Severe	Hours	?	May be continuous from onset	Blistering, severe pain and slough of tissue	Intractable ulceration and stiffness
Massive	Immediate severe inflammatory reaction progressing to necrosis of all tissues in depth				Requires amputations
CHRONIC	May be no immediate local evidence of radiation effect			Many years after exposure, presenile atrophy telangiectasia and hyperkeratosis	Ulceration, stiffness, and loss of cutaneous durability

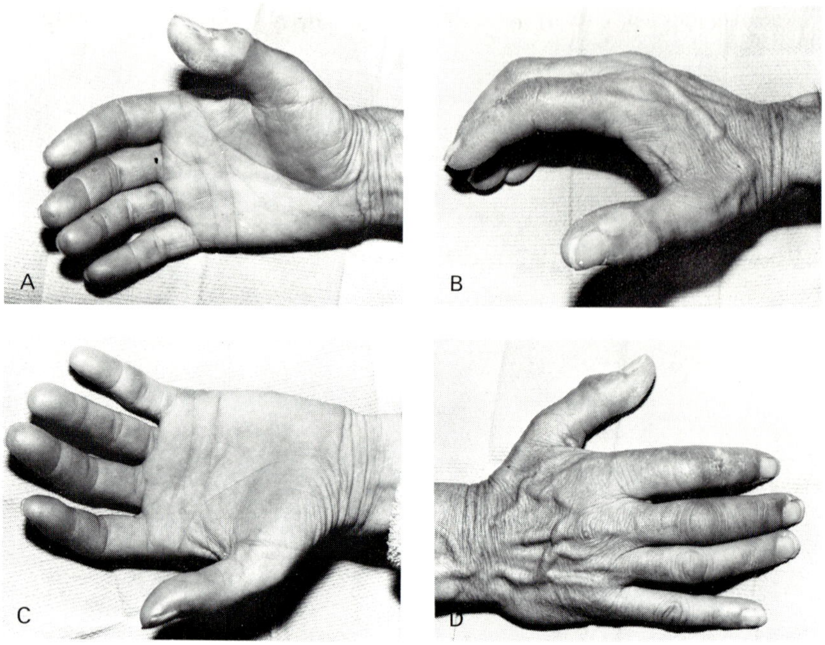

Figure 19-13. *This man's hand was directly exposed to 14,000 to 16,000 R while he was working with a malfunctioning leak detector. After a period of desquamation he developed stiffness and repeated minor skin ulcerations.*

The choice of facilities for treating this burn is governed by the severity of radiation exposure and the stability and responsiveness of the patient. Anything greater than a mild acute injury may require hospitalization to properly manage pain, edema and skin care. Elevation, functional splinting, active motion as tolerated are instituted immediately. Small blebs may be allowed to dry but large blisters should be debrided and covered with zinc oxide or silver sulfadiazine and a soft, loose dressing. Broad-spectrum systemic antibiotics and tetanus prophylaxis should be given to avoid suprainfection.

Beyond these general measures, the plight of the surgeon and the patient is expectancy. If the edema and blistering progress to ulceration of the skin, then the depth of the burn exends to a point where amputation of part or all of the hand must be considered just as in the case of the massive acute radiation injury. When the superficial weeping ceases and the inflammation stabilizes the edema will recede. The surgeon must await the development of the typical late radiation changes of the skin before determining the need for new skin coverage. The technique for skin replacement follows the principles outlined for thermal burns.

Occasionally an accidental injection of radioactive material occurs. Such an event presents trapped material, usually liquid, in the extracellular space. The magnitude of the potential burn is a function of the dosage, the half-life of the material and the capacity of the body to excrete it. These factors make it worthwhile to consider: (1) the application of an arterial tourniquet and immediate transfer to the hospital for care, (2) obtaining a sample if necessary from the tissues, for assay by a radiobiologist (barring this, photographic film may be used as an emergency measure), and (3) weighing the merits of incising and flushing the involved tissue versus intra-arterial perfusion.

Cold Injury

Frostbite is a vasoconstrictive state which may progress to microvascular thrombosis and irreversible ischemia with gangrene.[14] Inflammatory changes develop during this process along with edema and bleb formation. Frostbite results from exposure to cold and its severity is directly related to the degree of cold and the duration of exposure. Systemic cooling, diminished peripheral perfusion and oxygenation aggravate the magnitude and severity of frostbite.

The susceptibility of a patient to frostbite is influenced by: (1) exposure to cold, (2) preservation of existing body heat, (3) capacity to produce internal heat, (4) ability to perfuse and oxygenate his tissues. Therefore prophylaxis is of the utmost importance in preventing this injury with potentially disastrous consequences to the hand. Prophylactic measures include:

1. Protection of the hands by avoiding exposure, chilling winds and contact with freezing metal. Cotton or silk gloves should be used whenever metal must be handled.
2. Adequate total body insulation, including all parts of the head and neck, is necessary, as is the avoidance of excess physical activity which forces an increased loss of heat through the skin (sweating) and through hard breathing. The latter seriously depletes the body's heat reserves and reflexly induces peripheral vasospasm, aggravating the problem. Both of these actions can contribute to dehydration with subsequent hemoconcentration and impairment of blood flow. Attention to the needs for rest and freedom from anxiety must be observed. Alcohol, a peripheral vasodilator, is a deterrent rather than an advantage since it increases heat loss and later accentuates rebound vasospasm. Clothing should be loose fitting and mittens should be of soft flexible leather, e.g. deerskin not horsehide, with inner mittens of wool. Fingernails should be trimmed and frequent hand washing avoided.
3. Both a good state of health and a high caloric intake (primarily fats and carbohydrates in an appealing form) must be maintained.
4. In addition to the foregoing measures, adequate perfusion can be maintained by an external source of heat such as blowing on the hands or burying them in the axilla and by adequate attention to good hydration. With threatened frostbite smoking should be avoided.

Clinically there are two forms of frostbite, superficial and deep. The former involves only the skin and its adjacent subcutaneous tissue. It is often heralded by the acute cessation of local discomfort due to cold. A welcome warm feeling may follow. This should be recognized promptly and immediate measures taken to warm the part and subsequently to keep it warm and dry.

Slightly deeper frostbite is followed by skin changes consisting of blistering within 48 hours and some generalized edema. There may be some discomfort for several weeks from the effects of swelling, e.g. throbbing and dysesthesia. In the wake of this may be extreme hypersensitivity to exposure to cold.

Deep frostbite must be treated by hospitalization. All tissues including bone may be involved.[6] The entire hand swells and delayed massive blistering ensues. There is considerable pain from the onset which gets worse in the form of hypersensitivity as the swelling and blisters recede. Patients who have cryofibrinogenemia are susceptible to frostbite.[2] Cryofibrinogen precipitates more readily in the presence of heparin, contraindicating the use of this anticoagulant for treating frostbite in these patients.

The injured part should be at rest and any constrictive garment or jewelry removed. If there have been injuries such as fractures these should be splinted and dressed but not reduced or operated upon until the patient is evaluated in the hospital. Active rewarming may begin with the administration of hot liquids and wrapping the patient in prewarmed blankets. Smoking and alcohol should be avoided.

Once the patient is hospitalized, rapid rewarming is done by immersion in warm water (40 to 44° C) for 20 minutes; longer immersion serves no purpose. As rewarming proceeds the patient will develop enough dysesthesia to warrant analgesics. If a tub is not available, blanket or body rewarming may be substituted but may require longer.

Exercise and "thawing" in cold water or rubbing in snow should be avoided, as should exposure to excessive heat. The skin should be protected and infection avoided by meticulous sterile technique, systemic antibiotics, and prophylaxis against tetanus. Large blisters should be debrided and the wound covered with either lubricated meshed gauze or biological dressings. No elective debridement should be done until the tissues are well demarcated and have begun to separate.

Golding et al.[5] have found that sympathectomy at 24 to 48 hours after thawing produced a more distal level of demarcation, faster resolution of edema, less pain and a future improved awareness of cold in the sympathectomized limb.

As soon as possible after rewarming there should be guarded progressive active motion. However

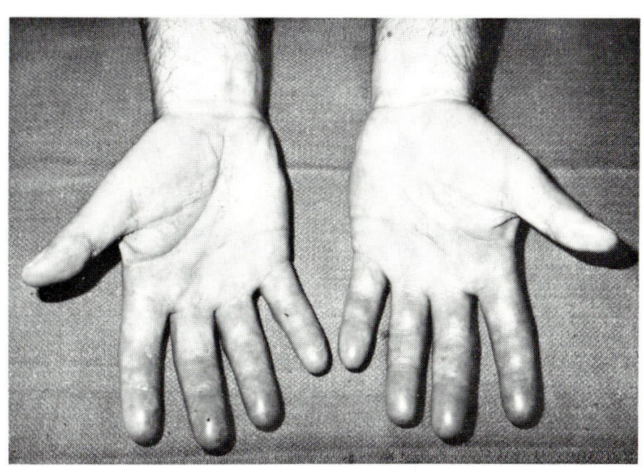

Figure 19-14. *Atrophy of the skin and subcutaneous tissue followed deep frostbite.*

there must be no passive manipulation or massaging of the injured tissues. Proper treatment of even serious cases may result in good preservation of tissue and function with surprisingly minimal disability (Fig. 19-14). Sequelae consisting of paresthesia and vasospasticity remain in some cases. In children there may be cold-induced focal phalangeal necrosis with destructive changes of the digital joints (especially distal interphalangeal joints) consisting of collapse or angulation.[6]

References

1. Calabretta, A.M. and Graham, W.P.: Chemical burns. Pa. Med., 77:62, 1974.
2. Colocho, G. and Graham, W.P.: Cryofibrinogenemia in patients with cold injury. Rev. Lat. Am. Chir. Plast., 17:27, 1973.
3. Colocho, G., Graham, W.P., III, Greene, A.E., Matheson, D.W. and Lynch, D.: Human amniotic membrane as a physiologic wound dressing. Arch. Surg., 109:370, 1974.
4. Evans, E.B., Larson, D.O., Alleston, S. and Willis, B.: Prevention and correction of deformity after severe burns. Surg. Clin. North Am., 50:1361, 1970.
5. Golding, M.R., deJong, P., Sawyer, P.N., Hennigar, G.R. and Wesolowski, S.A.: Protection from early and late sequelae to frost bite by regional sympathectomy. Mechanism of "cold sensitivity" following frost bite. Surgery, 53:303, 1963.
6. Hakstian, R.W.: Cold induced symmetrical focal phalangeal necrosis in childhood. Presented at A.S.S.H. 26th Annual Meeting. San Francisco, March 1971.
7. Hansen, F.C. and Edgerton, M.T.: Radiation burns. In *Hand Surgery* (Flynn, J.E., Ed.). Williams and Wilkins, Baltimore, 1967.
8. Iverson, R. and Laub, D.R.: Hydrofluoric acid burn therapy. Surg. Forum, 21:517, 1970.
9. Johnson, C.J. and Graham, W.P. III: Use of thermoplastic splints in the treatment of burned hands. Plast. Reconstr. Surg., 44:399, 1969.
10. Larson, D.L., Aliston, S., Evans, E.B., Dobrkovsky, M. and Linaris, H.A.: Techniques for decreasing scar formation and contractures in the burn patient. J. Trauma, 11:807, 1971.
11. Larson, D.L.: The prevention and correction of burn scar contracture and hypertrophy. Shriners Burns Institute, Galveston, 1973.
12. Peterson, R.A.: Electrical burns of the hand. J. Bone Joint Surg., 48A:407, 1966.
13. Ugland, O.M.: Electrical burns. A clinical and experimental study with special reference to peripheral nerve injury. Scand. J. Plast. Reconstr. Surg., Suppl. 2, 1967.
14. Washburn, B.: What is it—how to prevent it—emergency treatment. N. Engl. J. Med., 266:974, 1962.
15. Wein, A.J., Graham, W.P. III and Royster, H.P.: Malignant change in chronic wounds. Ind. Med., 41:12, 1972.

20 Infections

General Principles

Infection of the hand is infrequently seen in the private practice of hand surgery and is a rare complication of well-done surgical procedures. Infections are commonly the product of neglect by indigent patients. Once established, they can lead to severe disability unless urgent attention is given to fundamental practices that enhance circulation. Limited host resistance, virulence of an organism and the presence of dead space are the most prejudicial factors favoring the establishment of an infection. Elevation, immobilization and the release of tension are the most crucial factors in treatment.

Almost any organism can produce infection in the hand. Fifty per cent of these infections are caused by Staphylococcus aureus and 15 per cent by beta-hemolytic streptococci. The other most common organisms are Aerobacter aerogenes (10 per cent), enterococcus (10 per cent) and Escherichia coli (5 per cent). The incidences of infecting organisms are as follows:

Staphylococcus aureus	50 per cent
Beta-hemolytic streptococcus	15 per cent
Aerobacter aerogenes	10 per cent
Enterococcus	10 per cent
Escherichia coli	5 per cent
Multiple organisms	70 per cent

Approximately 25 per cent of cases fail to yield a specific organism on culture. In view of this, in all intractable infections a broad selection of culturing techniques and an adequate time period for growth should be employed.

Less common infections and their causative organisms are:

1. Bacterial: These include the gram-positive clostridia and anthrax bacillus, the gram-negative Proteus, Pseudomonas, gonococcus, Pasteurella and brucella, and mycobacteria causing tuberculosis and leprosy. Of this group, the leprosy infection is the most common.
2. Chlamydiae: These obligate intracellular parasites are probably of gram-negative origin and give rise to cat-scratch fever.
3. Viral: These include herpes simplex and herpes zoster and the virus causing miter's nodule.
4. Fungal: These produce the superficial and deep mycoses.
5. Protozoal: Leishmoniasis is the most common protozoal infection manifested in the hand.
6. Metazoal: A host of these worms cause such diseases as trichinosis, filariasis, loiasis, onchocerciasis, cutaneous larva migrans, dracontiasis and gnathostomiasis.
7. Miscellaneous: Erysipeloid is caused by Erysipelothrix rhusiopathiae or insidiosa; glanders is produced by Pseudomonas mallei.

The hands may become infected from the organisms residing on the patient's skin or coming from the nose, mouth, perineum or a hematogenous source. Soil and animal environment and vector contact are other sources. Urban machinery is rarely a source of bacterial contamination. The mode of entry varies from no recognizable injury to obvious skin penetrations. On rare occasions the hand may be seeded by bacteremia secondary to a focus of infection in the respiratory, gastrointestinal or genitourinary systems.

Incidences of the various hand infections are listed below:

Cellulitis and lymphangitis	28 per cent
Paronychia and eponychia	25 per cent
Furuncle, carbuncle	18 per cent
Wound infection (non-operative)	12 per cent
Felon	8 per cent
Tenosynovitis	3 per cent
Pyoderma	1 per cent
Osteomyelitis	1 per cent
Miscellaneous (non-pyogenic)	4 per cent

As can be seen, cellulitis and lymphangitis as a group are the most common infections of the upper extremity; together with paronychia and eponychia they comprise over 50 per cent of infections of the hand. However, from these, other tissues or tissue may become infected. Most infections become established through a vicious cycle consisting of contamination of a dead space, tissue reaction, tissue tension, circulatory impairment, and eventual necrosis with abscess formation.

Cellulitis is the inflammatory response to pathogenic invasion and is manifested by pain (often throbbing) and tenderness, redness, heat and swelling. This may be localized or widespread. Tissue tension is of paramount surgical concern. With sufficient tension and tissue necrosis an abscess forms. Its development is usually the result of microvascular thromboses which may be enhanced by the local effects of toxins and anoxia. The prime purpose of drainage is to improve the venous return by decompressing the tension from the abscess. As a consequence, the improved circulation will hasten the resolution of the infection.

The hand is unique in its predisposition to the establishment and spread of infections. It is composed of many spaces which rapidly become congested, causing extension of the infection throughout the space. With increasing tension the infection passes into adjacent spaces. Such spread may be directly, as is seen with extension from the distal pulp space to the bony phalanx or from bone into a joint. In other instances the spread may be through fascial planes, along tendon sheaths, or through lymphatics. It may also be hematogenous.

The tissues with the least resistance to infection are those with the most limited blood supply, notably nail folds, tendon sheaths, joints and bones. Circumstances favoring the establishment of infection are: (1) venous and lymphatic congestion following trauma and tight surgical closures, dressings or casts, (2) dead space created by hematoma, seroma or devitalized tissue, (3) retained foreign body, especially one that promotes a chemical inflammatory response, and (4) arterial insufficiency.

A good history is indispensable when evaluating a patient who has a potential or established infection. In addition to determining the source and type of contamination, the history must reveal any pertinent factors of general health.

The usual symptoms and signs of infection are pain, heat and redness. Throbbing pain is an urgent symptom, and in the hand with normal sensibility the only symptom of consequence in the usual infection. The rapid appearance of inflammation within hours usually signifies a streptococcal infection. This is in contrast to a staphylococcal infection, which usually takes 3 to 6 days to develop. Streptococcal infections more often have a systemic effect than do staphylococcal infections. The recognition of infection in a denervated part of the hand requires closer observation.

Heat and redness signify the existence of infection in a wound. Swelling and tenderness may indicate infection of the deeper tissues. Voluntary guarding against movement is a companion to involvement of a tendon sheath or joint. When fever and leukocytosis exist, the process is usually extensive throughout the hand and forearm. Fluctuation is a late sign.

Hemorrhagic vesicles may occur with rapidly progressing streptococcal infection. Suppurative vesicles which appear insidiously accompany staphylococcal involvement of the skin. Multiple tiny clear vesicles which are painful herald the appearance of a herpes infection.

The usual investigations that are diagnostically helpful consist of: (1) cultures, (2) gram stain, (3) biopsies, (4) roentgenograms, (5) serologic tests and (6) skin tests.

The differential diagnosis of infection invokes a consideration of many other conditions associated with inflammation. There may be non-infectious myositis crepitans, non-infectious tenosynovitis, arthritis and acute calcification. Gout, dermatitis and systemic or local allergic reactions may also be confused with infection. The latter is most often seen in butchers' and fish-handlers' wounds, in which there is reaction to implanted foreign protein. Certain tumors (osteoid osteoma) and injected chemicals may cause general or local inflammatory reactions.

The total functions of the infected hand must be kept in mind while treating the infection. The amputation of a badly infected digit may preserve function in the rest of the hand by preventing generalized infection and stiffness.

The need for hospitalization is dictated by the severity of the infection and the availability of adequate facilities and supervision for proper management. In general, infections of tendon sheaths or other deep spaces or infections associated with marked edema are best treated in the hospital.

Most infections are generated out of neglect and are, therefore, preventable. Tissue defense should be maintained by ensuring good blood flow and adequate blood volume. Constriction by clothing, jewelry, dressings, casts, skin and fascia must be avoided. The extremity must be comfortably immobilized and elevated above the heart.

In the care of an open injury and in elective operations, aseptic technique and antisepsis should be observed. Dead space is reduced with the aid of irrigation (even with tap water) by floating away clots and other debris. Normal skin may be painted with 1 per cent iodine or povidone-iodine which should then be washed away with alcohol. Both these solutions should be kept out of the wound. Hydrogen peroxide (3 per cent) is the best agent for softening and removing dried blood. Chemically irritating foreign bodies and bulky ones that cause tension should be removed as early as possible.

Dead space should be controlled and drainage ensured whenever there is a risk of infection by the placement of a drain if the wound is deep and the contamination is widespread. The drainage can be maintained by coating the skin surface with zinc oxide or a continuous moist dressing to prevent crusting and sealing of the wound.

Prophylactic local and/or systemic antibiotics should be used on all penetrating contaminations and all open injuries which impair normal circulation or predispose to swelling or dead space. Continuous catheter antibiotic drip into such wounds should be maintained for 2 to 3 days (bacitracin 50,000 u/500 cc at 5 cc/hr with 1 gm of lidocaine).

Patients who have never had tetanus immunization should receive human tetanus antiserum (250 units) if contamination of the wound has been from the soil, animals, mouth or feces. The need for booster immunization depends upon the nature of the contamination and the time of the patient's last immunization. It should probably not be given more frequently than at yearly intervals.

The initial choice of antibiotics (Table 20-1) should be empirical and their administration started at the suspicion of infection, unless the infective process is already well localized (paronychia or furuncle) or is about to drain spontaneously. The antibiotic may be subsequently changed according to the dictates of the culture. Non-operative treatment is followed when the part is still soft and the venous return is satisfactory. Throbbing pain, if present, is usually minimal and will be controlled by elevation and splinting.

Non-operative treatment consists of rest, elevation, splinting and antibiotics. There must be no joint and muscle activity. At times the undisciplined patient requires confinement to bed to ensure this inactivity. The hand must be consistently elevated above the heart for the control of swelling. In bed, this may be achieved by keeping the patient supine while his forearm and hand are propped against pillows. Suspension by a noose must be avoided. A loosely padded circumferential cast which immobilizes the wrist is mandatory in most instances of infection, even those confined to the digit. If need be, this may be extended over the hand in a boxing-glove fashion. In patients who are difficult to discipline (e.g. infants and alcoholics) a long-arm cast with the elbow at a right angle must be used so that the extremity can then be safely tied up for elevation. All immobilization must be done in the position of function.

Surgery is performed for purposes of diagnosis and treatment. It is diagnostically necessary when the existence of infection is likely but not proven by any discharge. It is therapeutic in providing decompression and sequestration.

The patient should be recumbent during the incision and drainage to avoid syncope. An upper-arm tourniquet should be applied before any incision is initiated, inflated to 100 mm Hg above the systolic pressure after maximal elevation of the extremity. Exsanguination of the arm, by wrapping, should not be done for fear of spreading the infection. The anesthetic should be tailored to the circumstance and adequate for painless surgery. A proximal nerve block or general anesthetic is necessary. Ethyl chloride spray gives inadequate freedom from pain and should not be used.

Incisions should be made for two reasons: (1) relief of tissue tension and (2) diagnosis and drainage of an abscess. At times the two purposes are served by a common incision; at other times, a longer incision or subsidiary incisions are needed to ensure the release of venous congestion. For drainage of an abscess, the location of the incision is *always* directly over the point of maximal tenderness and/or maximal fluctuation (thinning of the overlying tissues). Wounds should be parallel to nerves, arteries or veins which must be saved. To avoid secondary contractures, zigzag wounds across flexion creases or in web spaces are desirable. Once the skin is incised, deeper dissection should be con-

Table 20-1. *Choice (empirical) of Antibiotics in Hand Infections*

SUSPECTED ORGANISM	ANTIBIOTIC	
	1ST CHOICE	2ND CHOICE
Staphylococcus	Cloxacillin Methicillin Clindamycin Cephalothin (i.m. or i.v.) Cephalexin (p.o.)	Erythromycin Penicillin
Beta-hemolytic streptococcus	Penicillin	Erythromycin Ampicillin
Gram-negative organisms	Gentamicin Carbenicillin	Neomycin
Mixed flora	Cephalothin Penicillin Streptomycin	Tetracycline

ducted gently with a blunt instrument to avoid iatrogenic trauma to vital structures. After drainage is established, irrigation, using a fine plastic catheter and a solution of antibiotics, may be beneficial. The catheter may be secured by a suture and the irrigation continued postoperatively for 2 to 3 days. Debridement of necrotic tissue should be adequate without compromise of viable tissue with important function (e.g. nerves and vessels) or the exposure of uninvolved tendon sheaths and joints.

No infected wound should be approximated with any tension at all, or closed without adequate drainage. An open wound that can develop healthy granulation tissue and be grafted secondarily will serve the cause of hand function far more than a septic wound that is closed. A drain consisting of a gauze wick or fashioned from a surgical glove or plastic tube should fit loosely in the wound and be left for a minimum of 2 to 3 days. At times more than one drain is needed, especially where catheter irrigation with antibiotics is used and through-and-through flow is desired.

The abatement of redness and tenderness signals the resolution of sepsis, and the softening of tissues the resolution of the inflammatory response. Failure in this regard makes residual infection and even residual abscess formation suspect. The antibiotic treatment must then be continued and better drainage provided.

Prompt recognition and treatment should clear most infected hands of sepsis in 6 to 8 days. If recognized and treated expeditiously, half of infected hands will not need surgical drainage. However, it is better to incise early without finding pus than to permit tension to develop in the tissues and the spread of infection. Delay can lead to involvement of tendon sheaths and bone as well as to necrosis and ulceration. Inadequate after-care with compression of the median and ulnar nerves occurs when swelling is excessive. Muscles also may become fibrotic, leading to the Volkmann's type of contractures.

Specific Infections

Vascular Infections

LYMPHANGITIS AND LYMPHADENITIS

Although infection may involve the deep lymphatics, only superficial lymphangitis can be recognized clinically. The distinguishing feature is a red streak on the dorsum of the hand and the volar surface of the forearm. Since deep lymphangitis is rarely recognized early, it often progresses to marked brawny edema with systemic symptoms.

The onset of superficial lymphangitis is rapid (within hours) and is invariably streptococcal in origin. Lymphadenitis develops secondarily when the infection is neglected. Involvement of the deep lymphatic system follows other deep infection and, unlike superficial lymphangitis, is usually associated with throbbing pain and tenderness from the tension of the tissues. The treatment of both superficial and deep involvement of the lymphatics is absolute rest, immobilization in the position of function, and elevation. Hospitalization may be mandatory. Antibiotics are empirically administered to treat streptococci until specific cultures and drug sensitivities are available (Table 20-1).

Brawny edema is a serious problem and requires urgent consideration of extensive fasciotomies to improve the circulation. Intractable lymphadenitis may require either drainage of a local abscess or biopsy.

When there is chronic edema the disability is often prolonged and sometimes permanent. Elastic sleeve and glove compression or the use of an alternating pressure gradient may be helpful in relieving this swelling.

PHLEBITIS

Septic phlebitis can occur in association with an extensive infection of the forearm and hand, but most commonly follows intravenous injections. When localized to the site of an intravenous catheter, and in the absence of systemic symptoms and signs (fever or embolization), septic and non-septic phlebitis are indistinguishable. The stigmata are induration, tenderness, and sometimes redness overlying a superficial vein or deep tenderness on compression of the forearm and arm.

Most phlebitis can be prevented by meticulous aseptic technique and the early removal of any indwelling venous catheters. Treatment requires elevation, immobilization and antibiotics. If septic emboli occur, the vein must be ligated proximally and resected distally. This problem is frequent in drug addicts and severely burned patients.

Cutaneous and Subcutaneous Infections

CELLULITIS

Cellulitis develops at a variable rate, depending upon the organism. The contamination may occur through an insignificant portal of entry, but usually occurs through an easily recognized wound.

Cellulitis which develops slowly usually is the product of neglect with failure to immobilize an injured part and to control congestion, leading to fixed edema. Therefore, the response to treatment may be slow. Fasciotomy must be undertaken when the induration is brawny, progresses with treatment or is associated with nerve palsy.

Cellulitis which progresses rapidly over a period of hours suggests the development of a necrotizing fasciitis (hemolytic streptococcal gangrene). This is a critical situation requiring immediate decompression and debridement with massive doses of intravenous antibiotics (Fig. 20-1). Ulceration caused by microaerophilic streptococci (Meleney's ulcer[7]) and progressive synergistic bacterial gangrene are other streptococcal infections which require intensive treatment. The latter is a dual infection of non-hemolytic streptococci and Staphylococcus aureus. These rare infections are prevalent in patients whose defense mechanisms are diminished secondary to antineoplastic chemotherapy or diabetes mellitus.

FURUNCLE AND CARBUNCLE

These occur in the hair-bearing skin of the hand and arm and with neglect may develop into a widespread cellulitis. Recurrent furunculosis is frequently an indication of lowered resistance due to chronic illness or physical and emotional fatigue. These infections are caused by Staphylococcus aureus. Recognized early, they may be aborted with rest, immobilization and elevation, and systemic (not topical) antibiotics. Once the abscess is well localized and pointing, antibiotics are generally unnecessary.

Drainage may be spontaneous or surgical. It is facilitated by compresses of water or zinc oxide ointment until expulsion of the necrotic core. Adequate drainage can be produced through a linear or zigzag incision. Stellate incisions with undermining should not be used because they lead to excessive scarring.

PYODERMA AND COLLAR-BUTTON ABSCESS

Pyoderma is an intradermal abscess. When the blister is suppurative the organism is usually the

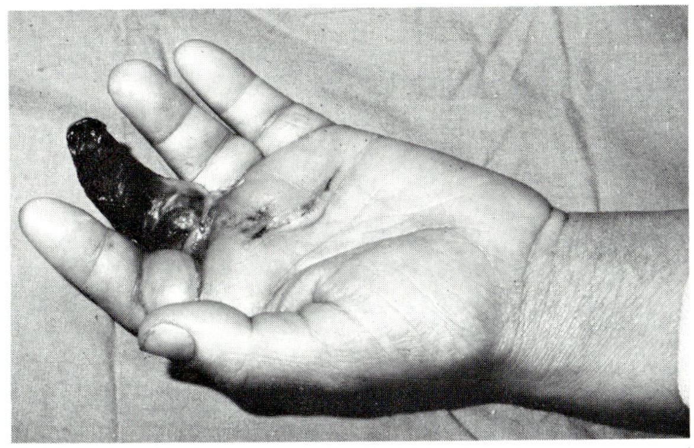

Figure 20-1. *Streptococcal gangrene and necrosis of the middle finger of a lady whose husband treated her distal digital insect bite by cauterization with a silver nitrate stick. She developed streptococcal septicemia and a midpalmar abscess.*

staphylococcus, and when the contents are watery the infecting agent is the streptococcus. Staphylococcal pyoderma can usually be treated by excising the blister and applying moistened compresses of water or zinc oxide to the wound. The streptococcal pyoderma should be treated similarly with the addition of systemic penicillin (Fig. 20-2).

A pyoderma may connect with a deep abscess by a sinus to form a dumbbell-shaped space—a collar-button abscess which may be subdermal or deeper. Such an abscess frequently occurs under a callus of the distal palm. This is suspected when the zone of inflammation is large compared to the size of the infected vesicle.

Treatment must ensure adequate drainage of the deep component of the abscess once the pyoderma is unroofed. The extent of the deep component may be assessed by probing and selective pressure to express pus through the communicating sinus. If the sinus is inadequate for drainage it must be enlarged and a drain inserted when the cavity is deep.

PYOGENIC GRANULOMA

This tumor, a variety of hemangioma, usually develops under a chronically moist dressing, and may be 2 to 20 mm, or more, in diameter.[6] Sometimes it forms about a suture knot or other foreign body which must be removed. Pain may be prominent, especially when it arises about the nail (Fig. 20-3). Small lesions (3 to 4 mm) will resolve rapidly upon exposure to the air. Lesions with a sizable base (greater than 6 mm) should be removed flush with the skin. The base of larger pyogenic granulomas should be grafted with a thin split-thickness graft to prevent recurrence. If, in spite of these measures, the lesion persists or recurs unusual infections (fungus) or tumors (melanoma, keratoacanthoma, squamous cell carcinoma) must be suspected, and appropriate cultures and biopsies must be performed.

ABRASIONS, BURNS AND GRANULATING WOUNDS (CHAP. 19)

When these wounds are chronic and suppurative they should be rendered suitable for split-thickness skin grafting as soon as possible by appropriate surgical debridement and the use of topical antibacterial agents (silver sulfadiazine). The common flora are staphylococci, streptococci and Pseudomonas.

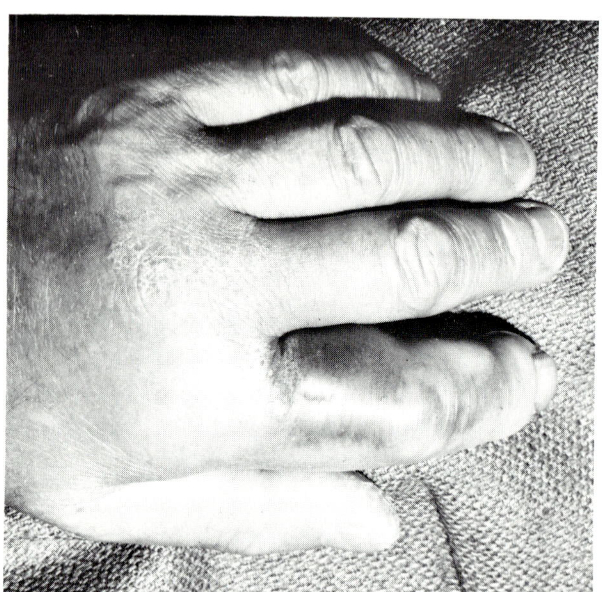

Figure 20-2. *Streptococcal pyoderma illustrating hemorrhagic bullae of index finger in a diabetic who neglected a minor scrape.*

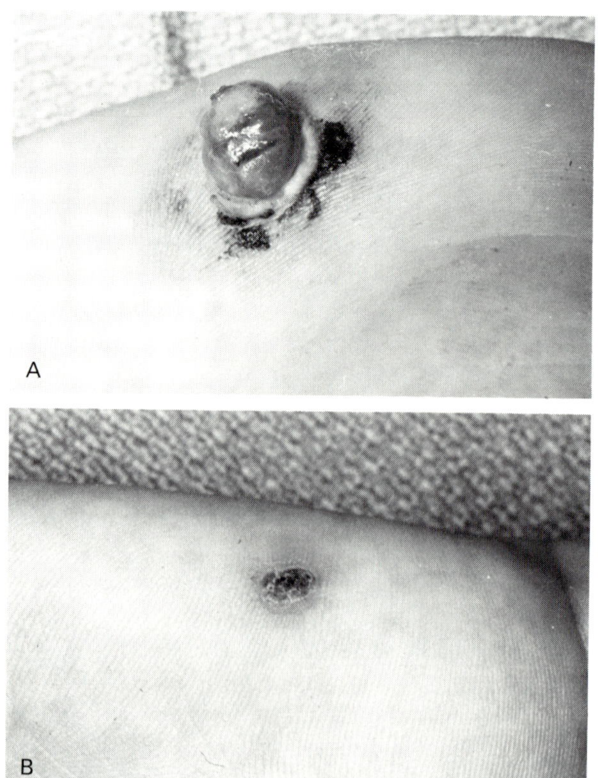

Figure 20-3. *Pyogenic granuloma of the palm following a minor puncture wound that was chronically macerated by a Band-Aid and petrolatum.*

OTHER INFECTIONS AND INFESTATIONS

See Chapter 7 for discussion.

Infections About the Nail

The soft tissues about the fingernail are often traumatized, and the rigidity of the nail pressing upon inflamed tissue aggravates the inflammatory process. Chronic inflammation and repeated infections often reflect long-standing fatigue and emotional strain which must be recognized.

ACUTE INFECTIONS

The usual pathogens of periungual infections are staphylococci and in certain chronic cases fungi. *Paronychia* (whitlow) is an inflammatory involvement of the fold on the radial or ulnar side of the nail, and eponychia, involvement of the basal fold. The *run-around* infection involves both areas. A *subungual* abscess floats the fingernail off its bed whereas a *subeponychial* abscess, usually the result of a splinter or puncture wound, is confined to the space between the nail bed and the bony phalanx. Occasionally a *paraeponychial* abscess is seen in the soft tissues proximal to the nail fold. These infections may be associated with a diffuse cellulitis which can extend into the volar fat pad, mimicking a felon. The rapidly developing tissue tension of these infections causes pain and frequently leads to abscess formation.

An attempt should be made to abort the early infection by appropriate elevation, immobilization and antibiotics. An abscess that is draining should be kept continuously moist with water or zinc oxide until all pain and tenderness have subsided.

Incision and drainage of a paronychia or eponychia must be painless. This is ensured by the use of a needlepoint knife (#11 scalpel) to incise the point of maximum tenderness in the skin fold; anesthesia is not necessary as long as the incision does not cause bleeding. The blade is held flat against the nail and enters the abscess through the non-viable and insensitive epidermis. The incision is adequate when pus is expressed and pain is relieved (Fig. 20-4).

An intermetacarpal nerve block is needed to explore an abscess which has not already pointed. Local or topical anesthesia will not suffice. The "trapdoor" incision is disfiguring and unnecessary for adequate drainage of an eponychia or paronychia. A small stab wound directly into a paraeponychial abscess avoids scar contracture of the nail fold itself. A subungual abscess is drained by removing only the base of the fingernail without incising the skin. The distal nail plate is not disturbed. A tiny loose pack of fine meshed gauze is inserted to separate the matrix from the eponychial fold for several days. The subeponychial abscess is approached through the tip of the finger by incising between the nail matrix and the bone. The distal portion of the fingernail directly over the abscess is notched or removed transversely. A minute foreign body should be searched for in these infections.

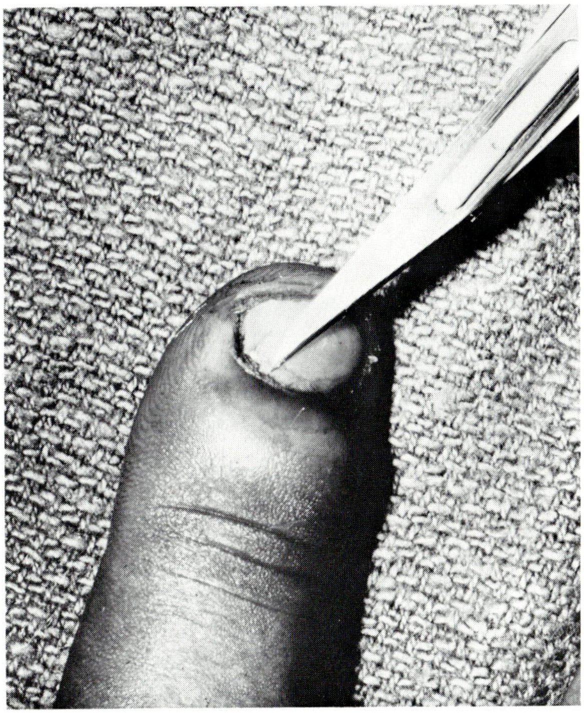

Figure 20-4. *Drainage of a paronychia with a #11 scalpel held flat against the nail. This should be painless and should not produce bleeding.*

CHRONIC INFECTIONS

There are two categories of this problem: (1) that occurring in the patient under chronic nervous strain and (2) that occurring as an occupational affliction. Successful treatment of the former problem requires adequate attention to the underlying emotional state and the relief of the sources of psychological strain. As a rule these patients do not develop the corrugated nails seen in patients whose infections are occupationally related. Their tissue problem is more a superficial inflammatory reaction of the nail fold. Local treatment consists of the topical application 2 to 3 times a day of Neosporin ointment, povidone-iodine ointment (Betadine), or drying with tincture of benzoin.

Occupational paronychial and eponychial infections are often seen in dishwashers. The nail fold may thicken and harden with scar tissue. Pain is not prominent unless an abscess forms. The telltale mark of this occupational problem is the corrugation of the nail. The chronic whitlow with scarring and induration of the nail fold is perpetuated by fungal and low-grade bacterial infections. The most common pathogens are Candida albicans and Staphylococcus aureus.

This industrial problem cannot be arrested unless the finger is kept dry. The patient must avoid dishwater and detergents, as well as maceration from perspiration inside plastic and rubber gloves. If such gloves are used, a cotton liner should be worn. Prolonged topical and systemic antibacterial and antifungal therapy may be beneficial. The antifungal agents used are griseofulvin systemically and nystatin or tolnaftate topically (Chap. 7). The complete removal of the deformed nail, followed by protracted avoidance of moisture, has resulted in regrowth of a normal nail over several months.

On rare occasions the resection of the dense scar of the eponychial fold is indicated. An eponychial skin flap is raised to the insertion of the extensor tendon and the scar is removed. Magnification is necessary to avoid injury to the matrix with resulting deformity of the nail. An alternative to temporary disability in the dishwasher whose problem is intractable is the resection of the entire nail and its matrix, with closure of the wound by a split-thickness skin graft.

Any intractable inflammation about the nail which has been rendered ideal treatment raises the suspicion of a neoplastic process such as a melanoma (Hutchinson's melanotic whitlow). An adequate biopsy is then necessary.

Space Infections

The multiple spaces (Chap. 2) of the hand which are created by the fascia and at times lined with synovium are targets for infection because: (1) their circulation is limited, and (2) their circulation is easily occluded by congestion. Infection often results from minor puncture wounds. The pathogenic organism is usually Staphylococcus aureus or streptococcus.

Treatment depends upon the stage of the infection. An incipient infection without significant signs and symptoms should be treated with elevation, immobilization and antibiotics. If there is an open wound a dressing moistened with water or zinc oxide is added. The same treatment may obtain if there is slight to moderate congestion, providing the part is observed hourly for the arrest of the process and its resolution. Strong analgesics should not be given since the appearance and progression of throbbing pain determine the need for surgical decompression. When the infected space is already moderately tense, incision should be undertaken before fluctuation becomes manifest. Once a space has been incised, continuous irrigation with antibiotics should be considered (*Septic Tenosynovitis,* below).

As soon as there is evidence of control of the infection (subsiding of drainage and inflammation), active motion must be initiated to prevent stiffness.

The proper management for specific space infections is as follows:

PULP SPACE (FAT PAD, ANTERIOR CLOSED SPACE, FELON) (FIG. 20-5)

Incision and drainage should always be at the point of maximum tenderness. Whether in the proximal, middle or distal pad, most of these abscesses point to the center of the pad. The preferred incision is a longitudinal midline incision directly over the abscess, sparing the flexion creases.[5] This preserves the digital nerves and avoids iatrogenic injury to the all-important circulation. Contrary to popular belief, the healed midline scar is not painful. Drainage of the infected distal pad by other incisions (fish-mouth, hockey-stick, through-and-through, lateral or transverse) has been disabling. Such incisions have invoked iatrogenic necrosis from ischemia, anesthesia of the tip of the digit and painful scarring (Fig. 20-6). Division of the vertical fascial fibers of the pulp, often

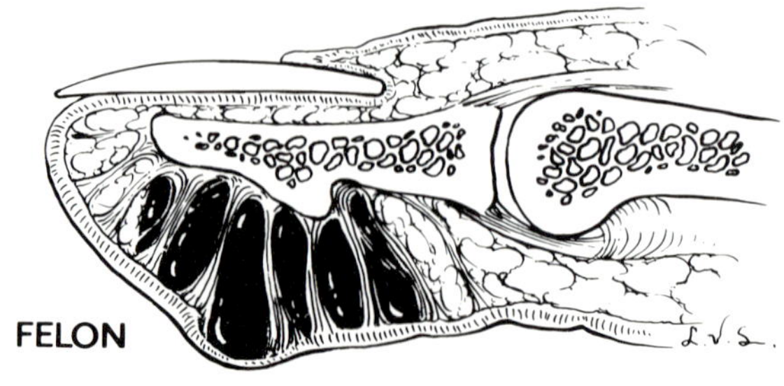

Figure 20-5. *Felon.* (*From Kilgore, E.S. et al.*[5])

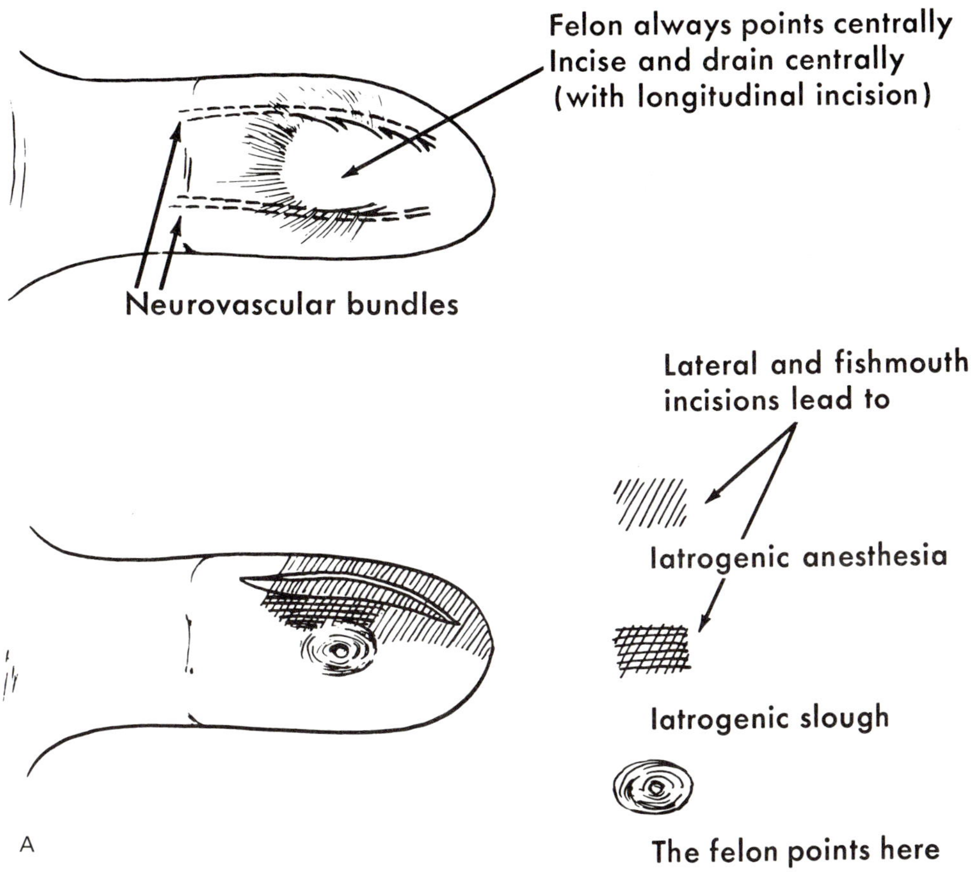

Figure 20-6A. *The correct incision for a felon to avoid iatrogenic injury is longitudinally in the midpulp over the point of maximum tenderness. (From Cramer, L.M. and Chase, R.A. (Eds.):* Symposium on the Hand. *C.V. Mosby, St. Louis, 1971.)*

recommended, can produce irreversible instability of the distal fat pad and is usually unnecessary (Fig. 20-7). Neglected pulp space infections may secondarily involve bone, the flexor tendon sheath, and the adjacent distal joint. Herpes simplex infections (Chap. 7) of the distal phalangeal area

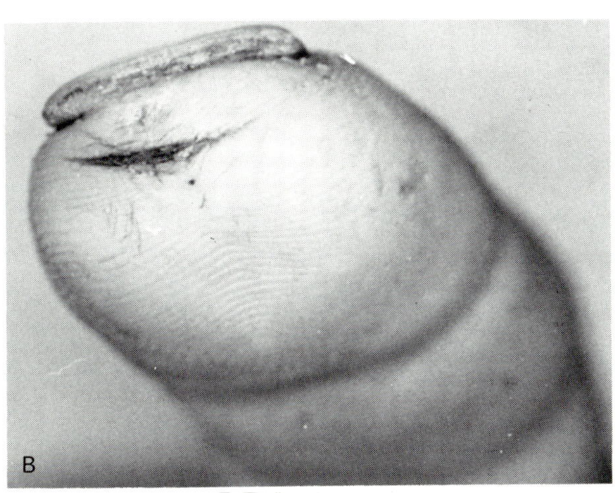

Figure 20-6B. *A disabling painful scar resulting from a modified fish-mouth incision 3 years previously.*

may be confused with a felon. Although the pain is intense, the tissues are soft, no abscess is present, and drainage will only aggravate the problem.

WEB SPACE

Infection of the web is usually caused by a puncture wound or the extension of infection from a callus of the distal palm, the lumbrical canal or the thenar space. These infections point dorsally and should be drained dorsally by a longitudinal incision between the fingers and a sagittal zigzag incision over the thumb web. If neglected, web space infections may lead to rigidity of the metacarpophalangeal joints in extension, or to adduction contracture of the thumb.

MIDPALMAR SPACE

This space may be infected by direct puncture or by the extension of infection from adjacent spaces (flexor sheaths of the index, long and ring fingers,

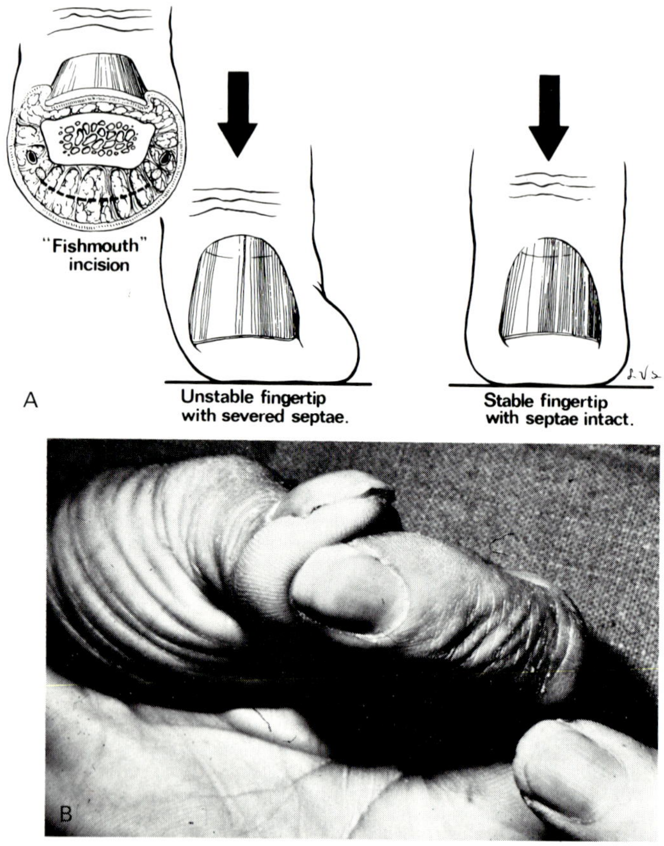

Figure 20-7A. *Disabling instability of the distal pad can result from division of all the septae.* **B.** *The loss of stability of the fat pad of the thumb after division of septae has made pickup of small objects difficult.* (*From Kilgore, E.S. et al.*[5])

the lumbrical canals, and the radial and ulnar bursae) (Fig. 20-8). The unyielding palmar fascia causes great tension to develop in this space, forcing the maximal edema to appear on the dorsum of the hand. However, the point of maximal tenderness is in the midpalm, where the incision should be placed transversely (Fig. 6-1). Gentle blunt dissection must be used to open this space to avoid injury to the many vital structures it contains. A drain or irrigating catheter may then be placed in the depths of the abscess.

THENAR SPACE

Infection in this space results from direct penetration or extension from the flexor sheath of the index finger. It usually points dorsally in the thumb web and appears as a web space abscess. When it points over the thenar musculature, it must be drained there, avoiding injury to the recurrent motor branch of the median nerve (Fig. 20-9).

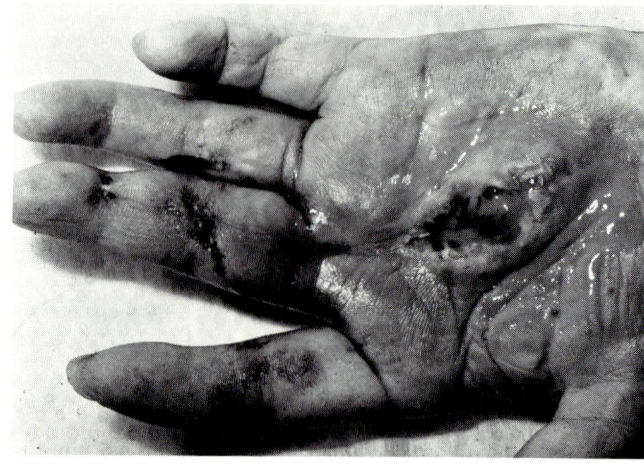

Figure 20-8. *Rupture of a neglected tenosynovitis into the midpalmar space resulted in a totally stiff and functionless hand.*

HYPOTHENAR SPACE

These infections also result from penetrating injuries. They should be drained wherever they point, using careful blunt dissection after the skin wound has been made.

SPACE OF PARONA

Infection within this space usually results by extension from the radial or ulnar bursa. Drainage should be along the ulnar side of the distal forearm deep to the flexor tendons and the ulnar artery and nerve. The incision should lie parallel to and between the flexor carpi ulnaris and the ulnar styloid. Beneath the skin, blunt dissection should be performed to avoid injury to the dorsal branch of the ulnar nerve and to the main ulnar nerve and artery. A drain or continuous irrigation is needed for this area.

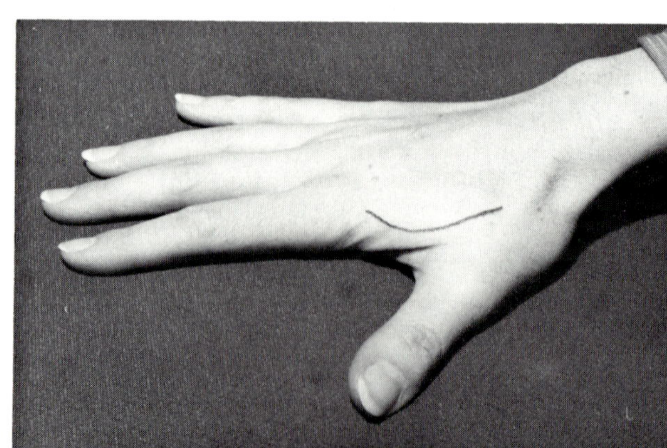

Figure 20-9. *A dorsal first web incision draining a thenar space infection.*

DORSAL SUBAPONEUROTIC SPACE AND SUBCUTANEOUS SPACES

Beneath the loose skin on the dorsum of the hand are the superficial subcutaneous and deep subaponeurotic spaces, which readily fill with edema fluid or pus. They are separated by the aponeurosis of the long extensor tendons to the fingers but freely communicate with one another. Both dorsal spaces may become infected by extension from spaces in the palm via the web spaces.

Infection of these spaces is usually accompanied by tenderness. The absence of tenderness helps to differentiate dorsal edema from infections.

These infections may point anywhere on the dorsum of the hand. Drainage should be established through one or more incisions. With extensive infection multiple separate incisions are needed. These usually consist of a longitudinal incision on the ulnar border, a zigzag incision over the thumb web and a transverse incision over the heads of the metacarpals. Once the skin is divided, careful blunt dissection is used to spare the veins, nerves and tendons. Drains and catheters for irrigation are inserted. The distal transverse incision reduces the chance for a claw deformity as long as the metacarpophalangeal joints are immobilized in flexion.

Infections may extend into the extensor tendon bursae and the distal forearm. Under such circumstances a counterincision is necessary at the proximal limit of the inflammatory process to institute through-and-through irrigation. At times the whole dorsum of the hand and forearm must be opened.

SEPTIC TENOSYNOVITIS

The flexor and extensor tendon bursae, which are poorly vascularized, are easily infected by puncture wounds and minor lacerations, especially at the joint creases where protective padding is limited. Since there is no obstruction to the spread of infection with continued active motion, a bursa usually becomes totally involved from its distal to its proximal limits. Unless promptly attended at the inception of infection, serious disability results through the development of secondary adhesions and stiffness and even tendon necrosis.

Staphylococcus aureus and streptococcus are the most common infecting organisms; however, unusual pathogens must be kept in mind—gonorrhea, syphilis, tuberculosis, Pasteurella, etc. The diagnosis is usually made by the pain produced in stretching the inflamed bursa. This can be done actively or passively. The examiner must not confuse the diagnosis by producing pain through pressure or tension on other inflamed tissues.

The best clinical test for flexor tenosynovitis is the instantaneous production of pain when the finger is extended by lifting on the nail alone (Fig. 20-10). This will avoid diagnostic confusion with infections limited to tissues other than the bursa. An empty bursa resulting from retraction of a divided tendon yields a less dramatic response to this test.

With rest, elevation and antibiotics, it is safe to observe the early case for several hours. When these non-operative measures fail, or the process is already advanced, decompression is mandatory.

The bursa is opened distally through a short sagittal wound in the midline of the middle phalangeal fat pad. A similar counterincision is made in the distal third of the palm. A plastic irrigating catheter is inserted 1.0 to 1.5 cm into the bursa through the distal wound and secured with a suture.[2] A drainage catheter is inserted a similar distance through the counterincision. A culture is obtained and the sheath is thoroughly irrigated (Fig. 20-11) with an antibiotic solution, as previously described. The antibiotic drip is continued for 2 to 3 days, with the patient flat in bed and the extremity continuously elevated.

Phlegmonous tenosynovitis usually requires opening the bursa throughout its length through a midaxial or volar zigzag incision. The necrotic tendon is excised. The subsequent reconstruction by a

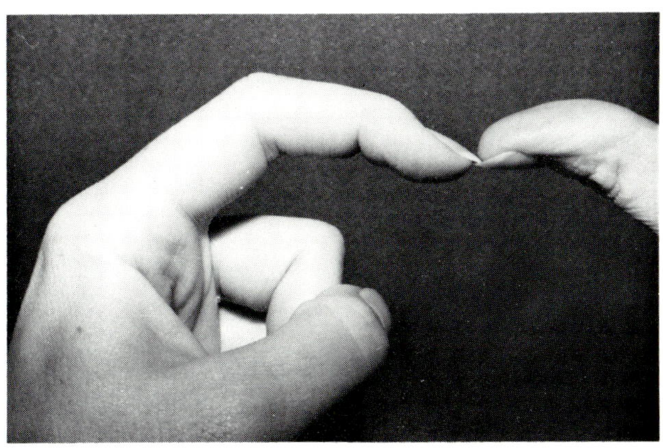

Figure 20-10. *The critical test of flexor tenosynovitis is passive stretching of the synovium. To do this the examiner must extend the digit by lifting the patient's fingernail without pressing skin or fat.*

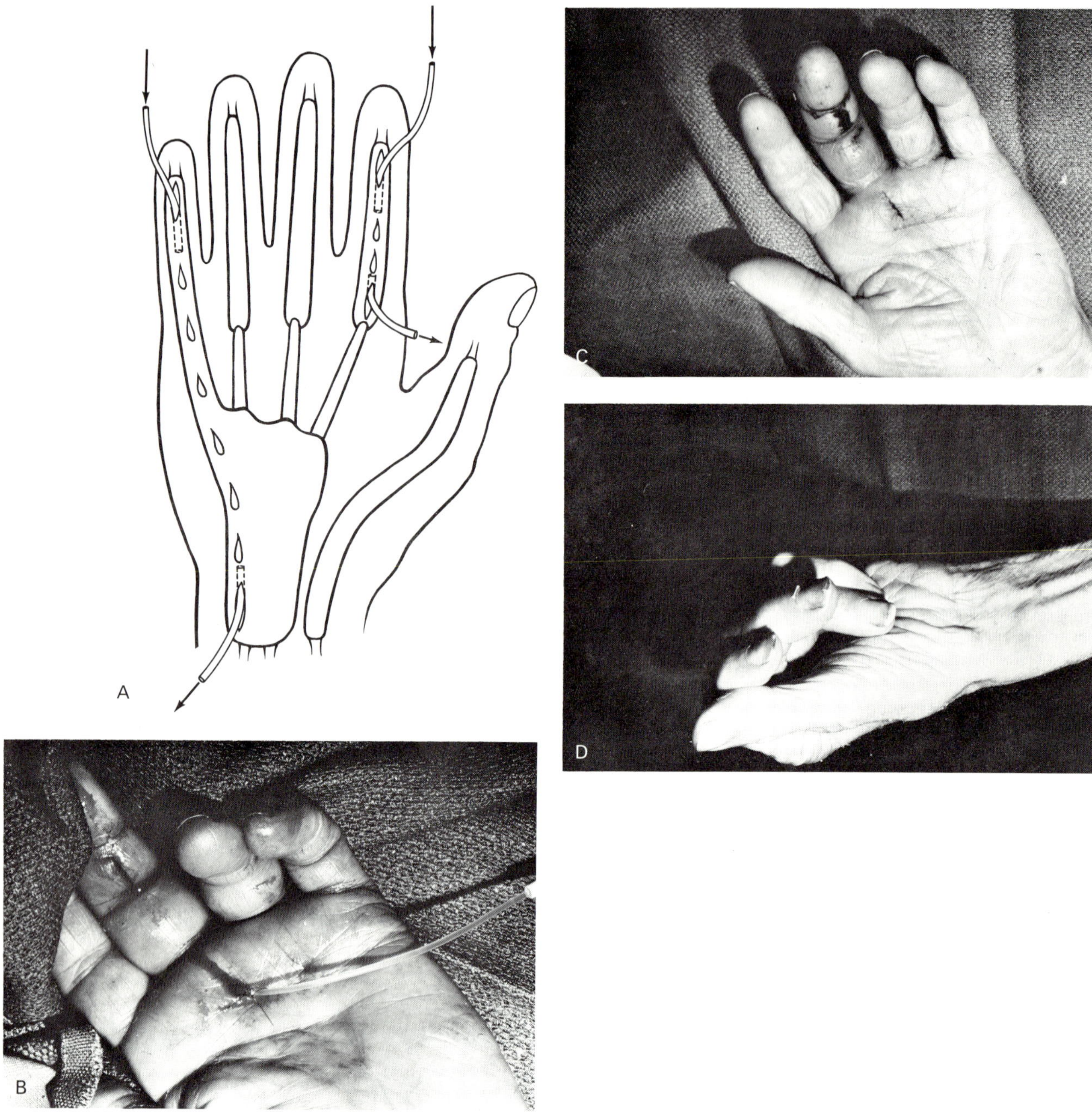

Figure 20-11A. *The through-and-through irrigation of the infected tendon sheath using fine plastic catheters is accomplished via proximal and distal midline incisions. These do not cross the joint creases. Usually the irrigant is introduced distally.* **B.** *Flexor tenosynovitis in an elderly woman receiving chemotherapy for lymphoma. The irrigating catheter was introduced through the proximal incision. The catheter should be placed through the distal wound to facilitate drainage when the hand is elevated.* **C.** *Eight days after drainage and three days after cessation of irrigation.* **D.** *Active flexion eight days after drainage. Full extension was possible a few days later.*

tendon graft is usually preceded by the insertion of a silicone tendon prosthesis. All reconstruction must await the complete resolution of induration and the return of satisfactory joint mobility. Hopeless cases which jeopardize existing hand function usually require early amputation.

Bites (Animal or Human Tooth Wound Infections)

A wound inflicted by a tooth inoculates the hand with a variety of organisms, the prime pathogen of which is an anerobic streptococcus. Tissues with limited blood supply have low resistance and, therefore, contamination of the synovial surfaces of a joint or tendons must be managed as a serious problem from the onset. Wounds into the knuckles from fist fights enter the joint and are self-sealing. The relative anaerobic state of the synovial tissue favors the growth of the pathogen. Continued joint activity and dependency of the hand aggravate the rapidly developing congestion and infection. Stiffness and destruction of the joint are usually the consequence of neglect. Because of the reluctance of patients to acknowledge a fight, any wound over a knuckle about which a vague history is given should raise suspicions of its having occurred from a human tooth. Roentgenographic examination should be done for all of these injuries initially and in follow-up.

Accidental puncture wounds from tacks and pins, contaminated with saliva, may produce similar infections among upholsterers and seamstresses. Animal and human bites into tendon bursae also favor these infections, whereas bites in well-vascularized tissues are unlikely to do so.

Fresh wounds about joints and tendon sheaths should be immediately managed as though severely infected with appropriate immobilization, elevation, local and systemic antibiotics and tetanus prophylaxis. Divided structures should not be repaired and the wound should not be closed. Deep wounds into soft tissues should be drained. All of these wounds should be dressed with gauze moistened with water or zinc oxide. Hospitalization is mandatory for the irresponsible patient in order to maintain elevation and immobilization properly.

Established infections from bites are treated by decompression of brawny edema and better drainage of any abscess. Such cases usually need continuous irrigation with antibiotic solutions.

Animal bites may invoke infection due to Pasteurella multocida.[3] This gram-negative rod, sensitive to all common antibiotics, initiates a cellulitis which progresses rapidly to cause pain and even abscess formation within 24 hours. The response to proper treatment is usually rapid and complete.

Septic Arthritis

Septic arthritis has to be differentiated from non-infectious desmitis and arthritis such as gout or rheumatoid arthritis. This differentiation is usually made by appropriate roentgenograms, laboratory tests and responses to treatment.

Infection usually follows an open injury but may be hematogenous. If neglected or misdiagnosed, destructive changes, osteomyelitis, tenosynovitis and stiffness may result. History is of paramount importance and should reveal the existence of an open injury or infection elsewhere in the body. A confirmation of the diagnosis follows a positive culture. Suspicion of the diagnosis exists from serial roentgenograms which show loss of articular cartilage (thinning of a joint) and evidence of osteomyelitis. All fresh open injuries into joints should be treated with elevation, immobilization, and intra-articular and systemic antibiotics. Established infection should be treated empirically with the antibiotic chosen according to the history and the gram stain; this should be changed if indicated by the results of the culture.

The duration of antibiotic administration depends upon the disappearance of the acute inflammatory reaction and the failure of recrudescence after one week of active motion. Tuberculosis and fungal infections, which may have minimal acute signs, invariably require months of treatment and serial evaluations clinically and radiographically. Uncommon infections, such as gonorrhea or syphilis and inflammation due to tumors, must be suspected in recalcitrant cases.

Following resolution of an infection a symptomatic joint may warrant arthrodesis or arthroplasty.

Osteomyelitis

Osteomyelitis can occur in any bone. It commonly occurs in open injuries and infections of the distal phalanx, in bones adjacent to infected joints or bursae, at amputation stumps and about compound fractures. On rare occasions it is hematogenous. The usual infecting organism is the staphylococcus.

The infection is suspected by the presence of swelling, persistent bone pain (percussion tenderness), and lytic changes or sequestration on roentgenography. Osteomyelitis with a probable sequestrum must be suspected in the absence of any other explanation for persistent drainage and recurrent abscess formation. Demonstration of a sequestrum may require tomography or image-intensified roentgenograms. Not until a sequestrectomy has been performed can a resolution of the infection and an early end to the need for antibiotics be expected.

A sequestrectomy must be complete and include all granulation tissue and poorly vascularized bone. When the sequestrum lies at the tip of a digit a fish-mouth incision is the best approach. When it is in the body of a phalanx a dorsal-lateral incision is generally favored. Elsewhere the surgical approach should be chosen for its simplicity and the accessibility of the bone without endangering function. Upon removal of diseased bone the cavity should be packed with tightly woven gauze (umbilical tape). The packing may be replaced, but is not totally removed until the space it occupies is filled with healthy granulation. Packing is generally not necessary after sequestrectomy of the fingertip through a fish-mouth incision.

After sequestrectomy, and in the absence of a sequestrum, antibiotics and immobilization are relied upon to control the infection. Immobilization is continued until the bony pain has subsided and there is no longer evidence of continued osteolysis. Antibiotics may be discontinued if there has been no recrudesence after one month of mobilization. Digital amputation is considered whenever the treatment of infection in one digit jeopardizes the function of the whole hand through stiffness. Whenever osteomyelitis is intractable, unusual pathogens as well as tumors must be excluded.

Miscellaneous Bacterial Infections

LEPROSY

Hansen's acid-fast bacillus has not been cultured in vitro with certainty, yet it is one of the oldest and most insidious infectious diseases. It still afflicts millions, primarily in tropical and subtropical countries. Of the two types of leprosy, lepromatous and tuberculoid, both may involve peripheral nerves.[1] This involvement corresponds to the most superficial location of nerves, the median nerve just proximal to the carpal tunnel and the ulnar nerve at the olecranon. This susceptibility is caused by a lowered temperature of the nerve in these exposed areas.

The lepromatous type occurs in patients who have a low resistance and is characterized by an enormous superficial bacterial infestation. Neuritis occurs with diffuse even thickening of the nerve which, if painful, may be relieved by internal neurolysis. Tuberculoid leprosy occurs in people with strong resistance. Organisms are difficult to demonstrate, but reactions to their presence may be sufficiently intense to produce neural necrosis. The hand disability caused by leprosy is the result of anesthesia and intrinsic muscle paralysis. Ulceration of the digits results from the ischemia of pressure necrosis.

Two types of drugs are used in treating leprosy. Diaminodiphenyl sulfone (DDS) is specific against M. leprae, in doses of 400 mg a week, varying from 20 to 100 mg daily. Anti-inflammatory drugs such as corticosteroids and antimalarials (stibophen) and thalidomide are also used. Apparently thalidomide is effective in diminishing the development of deformities caused by leprosy[1] (Fig. 20-12).

The role of the hand surgeon is directed toward educating the patient to protect his insensible hands and through reconstructive measures to improve motor function.

TUBERCULOSIS

M. tuberculosis can infect all the tissues of the hand. Most cases are the result of hematogenous spread but direct inoculation does occur. A primary focus other than the hand must be sought but may not be present.

Tuberculosis should be suspected and ruled out in any case of an indolent inflammatory process. Whenever possible cultures of fluid or tissue biopsies should be obtained. These may take many weeks and even months to become positive. Typical as well as atypical mycobacterial infections should be suspected.

The skin lesions may be initially papular and secondarily ulcerated. Roentgenograms of the involved bones of the hand demonstrate periosteal thickening which is less than that seen with syphilis. Total joint destruction and ankylosis may occur

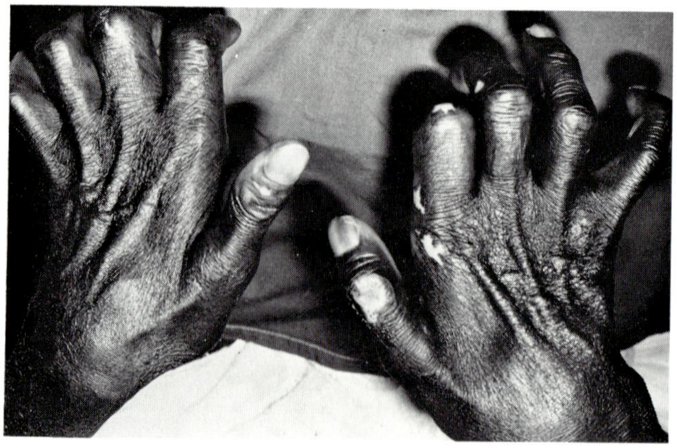

Figure 20-12. *Leprosy. Elderly black patient with marked intrinsic muscle atrophy and several subcutaneous nodules.* (*Courtesy of S.H. Miller, M.D.*)

primarily, or as an extension from adjacent bones or tuberculous tenosynovitis. The tenosynovitis is characteristically boggy and non-tender, and the synovial membrane is markedly adherent to the tendon which may be degenerated and even ruptured. This adherence is the prime stigma of this disease at surgery, helping to differentiate it from rheumatoid and non-specific villonodular tenosynovitis, in which the synovium peels more freely from the tendons. Free-floating "rice bodies" composed of coagulated fibrin are commonly found. Any tendon bursa may have isolated involvement by tuberculosis, but commonly it is diffuse about the carpal canal or the extensor retinaculum.

The treatment of boggy tenosynovitis is resection of all diseased synovial tissue and decompression of tendon sheaths. In treating tuberculosis of the skin, bone, joint or tendon sheaths, the appropriate chemotherapy is given for a period of 6 to 12 months. This consists of the following drugs in varying combinations: streptomycin, isoniazid and para-aminosalicylic acid. The involved part of the hand should be splinted for comfort and until the wound heals. Prolonged splinting may result in unnecessary stiffness.

CLOSTRIDIAL INFECTIONS

Clostridial infections are infrequent in healthy wounds with good circulation. Wound contamination from sewage, soil and animals is most apt to cause these infections. When suspected, immediate prophylactic measures must be instituted. These consist of proper drainage, debridement and the administration of the appropriate antiserum, local and systemic antibiotics.

Once infection is established, the surgeon must radically debride the wound and must ensure that the patient's vital signs are constantly monitored. If signs of toxicity develop, further debridement, including amputation, must be considered. Gas within the tissues may be detected by crepitation or by roentgenograms. Massive doses of intravenous penicillin (30 million units/day) as well as additional antiserum must be given. Activated zinc peroxide in a paste provides additional oxygen to the wound. If tetany develops respiratory support and muscle relaxants must be given. Human antitoxin (250 to 500 units i.m.) is administered with a booster dose of tetanus toxoid, 0.5 cc, in another location. Polyvalent antitoxin may be given for patients with gas gangrene but is ineffective if adequate local wound treatment has not been done.

ANTHRAX

The gram-positive spore-forming aerobic bacillus causing anthrax is a cutaneous and fecal contaminant of sheep, cattle and horses. It enters the skin through minor trauma and within 12 to 36 hours forms a papule. This progresses to a vesicle, pustule and finally a necrotic ulcer. The whole limb may become involved and septicemia can occur. Penicillin and other antibiotics are effective treatment and should be started promptly to forestall dissemination of the infection. Immunization is available for domestic animals and humans.

GONORRHEA

Gonococcal arthritis, tenosynovitis and rare dermatitis (keratosis blennorrhagica) are the result of hematological spread, usually from the genitourinary system.

The involvement of the hand usually develops in the second or third week after the primary genitourinary infection. It has a predilection for the joints and tendon sheaths that are most exposed to stress or that have been traumatized. The diagnosis requires the identification of the organism by smear or culture. This infection can be confused with gout or rheumatoid synovitis, particularly if the patient hides his venereal problem.

The treatment consists of drainage and irrigation of the involved tendon sheath and administration of systemic antibiotics. Penicillin in daily doses of up to 15 to 30 million units intravenously should be continued until complete resolution of the inflammatory process has occurred. Other antibiotics may be used if penicillin-resistant strains are encountered. These may include ampicillin, tetracycline or erythromycin.

BRUCELLOSIS

Small gram-negative aerobic rods gain entrance into the hand through minor skin trauma in workers handling infected animals (primarily cattle, hogs, goats). Spread is through the lymphatics. The infected limb may become swollen and develop lymphadenopathy. The usual presenting complaint is systemic involvement after the incubation period of 5 to 20 days. The diagnosis rests on the history, the recovery of the organism and rising agglutination titer greater than 1:100. The preferred antibiotics are either, or both, streptomycin or tetracycline.

TULAREMIA

The small gram-negative aerobic bacillus causing tularemia infects the hand by entrance through skin via minor injuries in patients who handle infected rodents. It may be transmitted also by insect bites or acquired by ingestion.

An ulcerating papule forms at the site of entry and regional suppurative lymphadenitis (bubo) may follow. The diagnosis rests upon history, smears, cultures, skin tests and agglutination titers. The treatment consists of antibiotics (streptomycin, tetracycline or chloramphenicol).

ERYSIPELOID

See Chapter 7 for discussion.

GLANDERS

These infections are produced by Pseudomonas mallei, a gram-negative aerobic rod which traverses the broken or unbroken skin of the hand, causing ulceration. This is followed by lymphangitis and adenitis. These infections, acquired from horses and mules, are often fatal. The diagnosis depends upon the history, smear and culture, and the rising agglutinin titers. The mallein skin test may also be positive. Sulfonamides are used for therapy.

CAT-SCRATCH FEVER

Chlamydiae, obligate intracellular parasites, are etiologic agents of cat-scratch fever. It is likely that they are derived from gram-negative bacteria. Cat-scratch fever is a benign self-limiting disease introduced with a scratch which develops into a papule, vesicle, pustule or crusted ulcer. Symptoms and lymphadenopathy may not appear until three weeks after the initial injury and usually subside within two weeks. The diagnosis is usually confirmed by the history and clinical course. Aspiration of the suppurative lymph nodes yields sterile pus. No specific therapy is available. On occasion the aspiration of fluid from within enlarged nodes lessens the symptoms.

Viral Infections

HERPES SIMPLEX AND ZOSTER

See Chapter 7 for discussion.

WARTS

See Chapter 7 for discussion

MILKER'S NODULE

Farmers and individuals who work in slaughterhouses, or who, in other ways, come in contact with infected cow's udders, contract this viral infection. It is caused by the vaccinia virus and produces lesions on the hands and forearms. These begin as slightly pruritic papules which develop into small (5 to 8 mm) bluish-red nodules. The central portion of the lesion becomes umbilicated and often ulcerates. Lymphangitis and lymphadenitis can occur. Usually this self-limiting disease clears within 6 to 12 months.

Fungal Infections

Fungal infections in man may be categorized into superficial (Chap. 7) and deep mycoses (Fig. 20-13) (Table 20-2). The superficial ones involve the skin and its appendages, usually about the nail. They are clinically less significant than the deep mycoses which may involve all tissues. Both types may be indolent and intractable.

Nearly any fungus may infect the hand once

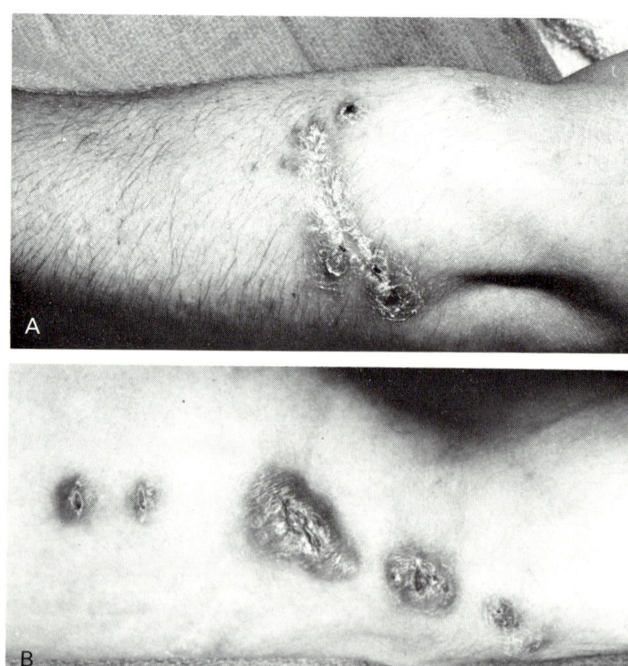

Figure 20-13. *The classic ulcers associated with sporotrichosis occurring on this farmer's forearm and arm after a minor skin injury.*

Table 20-2. *Deep Mycoses*

INJECTION	TREATMENT	PROGNOSIS
Actinomycosis	Penicillin Surgery (incision and drainage)	Good if limited to the skin
Blastomycosis	Amphotericin B 2-Hydroxystilbamidine	Good if limited to the skin
Coccidioidomycosis	Surgery (excision) Amphotericin B	Good
Sporotrichosis (Fig. 20-13)	Oral potassium iodide	Good
Maduromycosis	? Sulfones Surgery (even amputation)	Poor
Chromoblastomycosis	Surgical excision and/or amphotericin B	Favorable
Nocardiosis	Sulfisoxazole Cycloserine Surgery (drainage)	Poor

inoculated by trauma. Systemic and multiple organ involvement may or may not occur. The diagnosis depends on the identification of the organism by microscopy and culture. Deep mycoses are often associated with ulcerations and sinuses.

Protozoan Infections

Leishmaniasis, endemic to Asia and Latin America, enters the hand from the bite of a sand fly infected with L. tropica or brasiliensis. The primary lesion, "Oriental sore," may be dry or suppurative and ulcerated because of secondary infection. The diagnosis depends on the history and microscopic identification of the organism. This may be obtained from clean scrapings at the edge of the ulcer or by an appropriate culture.

Spontaneous healing may occur or the lesion may require surgical drainage or excision. Ethylstibamine is given, 0.2 gm initially i.v., followed by 0.3 gm i.v. daily for up to 16 doses. If this is unsuccessful amphotericin B may be indicated.

References

1. Brand, P.W.: Rehabilitation of the hand in leprosy. In: *Symposium on the Hand* (Cramer, L. and Chase, R., Eds.). C.V. Mosby, St. Louis, 1971.
2. Carter, S.J. and Mersheimer, W.: Infections of the hand. Orthop. Clin. North Am., 1:455, 1970.
3. Hawkins, L.G.: Local Pasteurella multocida infections. J. Bone Joint Surg., 51A:801, 1969.
4. Kilgore, E.S. and Graham, W.P.: Surgery of the hand. In: *Current Surgical Diagnosis and Treatment* (Dunphy, J.E. and Way, L.W., Eds.). Lange Medical Publications, Los Altos, 1973.
5. Kilgore, E.S., Brown, L.G., Newmeyer, W.L., Graham, W.P. and Davis, T.S.: Treatment of felons. Am. J. Surg., 130:194, 1975.
6. Lever, W.F.: *Histopathology of the Skin,* 5th Ed. J.B. Lippincott, Philadelphia, 1975.
7. Meleney, F.L.: *Treatise on Surgical Infections.* Oxford Publications, New York, 1948.

21 Stiffness

Stiffness is the loss of mobility, and is caused by a great variety of pathologic states; all categories of hand disorders are involved. It is seen as a consequence of degenerative states in hypertrophic osteoarthropathy after the sixth and seventh decades. It results from non-infectious inflammatory diseases including the collagen disorders. Stiffness follows trauma, infections and metabolic problems (e.g. gout), and it may be caused by tumors or can occur congenitally. Most commonly it follows edema and disuse. The causes of stiffness are therefore summarized as:

- Edema, inactivity and scar
- Specific disease states
  - Trauma
  - Degenerative arthritis
  - Infections
  - Collagen disorders
  - Metabolic disorders
  - Tumors
  - Congenital disorders
- Arthrodeses and tenodeses

Stiffness is the most common cause of disability after injury to the hand. When it is painless and the hand is in the position of function, disability may be minimal. However, the stiffness may be intractable and by itself the prime cause of pain on attempted movement. Its spontaneous resolution usually requires the motivation of the patient and the presence of muscle power. Every effort should be made to prevent it because, once established, stiffness may be time consuming and difficult to treat. The patient very often has the prime responsibility in this regard.

The physician and patient must realize the futility of trying to salvage motion in a hopelessly stiff or potentially stiff digit if so doing will seriously threaten the existing mobility of adjacent digits. This risk is highest when the long and ring fingers remain stiff in extension.

Edema, Inactivity and Scar

Edema produces stiffness on three bases: mechanical, chemical and neurogenic. These factors may act independently or in combination. The surgeon can treat most effectively the mechanical aspect.

Mechanically, edema develops by the curtailment of venous and lymphatic flow without simultaneous curtailment of arterial flow. Dependency of the extremity is the most common cause, and constriction of the part the second most common.

The biology of wound healing and the tissue reactions to foreign proteins and other substances incite edema through chemical means and osmotic influences. Neurogenic edema, often triggered by pain, is influenced by the sympathetic nervous system acting on specific end-organs. Edema is most apt to beget stiffness when it arises rapidly, a proclivity of any of the inciting factors.

Edema varies in its protein content, which is proportional to the rapidity of development. The higher the protein content, the greater is the tendency for the edema to become fixed and difficult to remove. Finally this leads to fibrotic thickening of tissues.

There are four factors in the mechanics of stiffness caused by edema: (1) an excess volume of water contained in the tissues which will not yield to attempted motion, (2) rigidity that is related to the "gelling" of the extravasated protein, (3) the shortening of ligaments secondary to their distension with fluid and (4) terminal fibrosis and fixed shortening, most notably of ligaments, fascia and skin. The edema enters the distensible spaces, particularly beneath the loose dorsal skin. Clawing of the hand results through hyperextension of the metacarpophalangeal joints. The thumb is adducted.

Inactivity alone may lead to stiffness by promoting stagnation of protein-rich fluid. The cellular response within the edematous and healing tissues leads to the fibrosis and scar which produce intractable stiffness.

The generation of stiffness from specific disease states is related to the edema, inactivity and scar which they generate or to the tissue alterations that occur.

Other Causes

Joints can be rendered immobile by the architectural disruptions that occur from trauma and other causes of arthritis. Adhesions and fibrosis of muscles from whatever cause can do the same. Shrinkage and loss of skin elasticity from any cause induce stiffness. Stiffness is also produced by design when the surgeon performs a functional arthrodesis or tenodesis.

Iatrogenic stiffness occurs and is usually a result of errors in omission and commission:

- Closure of the wound that should have been left open
- Closure of the wound too tightly
- Failure to perform a needed fasciotomy
- Failure to control dead space
- Inadequate immobilization
- Excessive immobilization
- Splinting joints in extreme flexion or extension
- Failure to educate the patient
- Failure to give antibiotics
- Failure to relieve throbbing pain mechanically

Stiffness Resulting From Musculotendinous Problems

This type of stiffness is most often due to a loss of elasticity or excursion of the muscle or tendon. It results from fibrosis, adhesions, atrophy and shrinkage. As a consequence, the effective length of the muscle-tendon unit is shortened. A static tightness is produced diagnostically by moving the joint which it crosses (e.g. extension tightens flexor muscle-tendon units and vice versa). This phenomenon is referred to as the "plus state" (intrinsic plus and extrinsic flexor and extensor plus).

Intrinsic Plus

Intrinsic plus is a common problem caused by excessive tightness of the intrinsic muscle and its tendon (lateral extensor tendon) entering the digit. This unit is tightened by extension of the proximal joint of the digit and is relaxed by flexion of this joint. It is also tightened by flexion of one or more interphalangeal joints. The common causes of intrinsic plus are fibrosis of the muscles from trauma, rheumatoid myositis and disuse.

Intrinsic plus is present when the interphalangeal joints cannot be flexed when the metacarpophalangeal joint is fully extended or when the metacarpophalangeal joint cannot be extended when the interphalangeal joints are fully flexed. To understand this, it must be appreciated that the intrinsic muscles flex the metacarpophalangeal joints and extend the interphalangeal joints. This action is determined by the relationship of the lateral extensor tendon to the axis of joint movement, namely, volar to the axis of the metacarpophalangeal joint and dorsal to the axis of the interphalangeal joint. Flexion of the metacarpophalangeal joint relaxes the intrinsics and allows the interphalangeal joints to flex, just as extension of the interphalangeal joints provides the relaxation needed for metacarpophalangeal joint extension (Fig. 21-1).

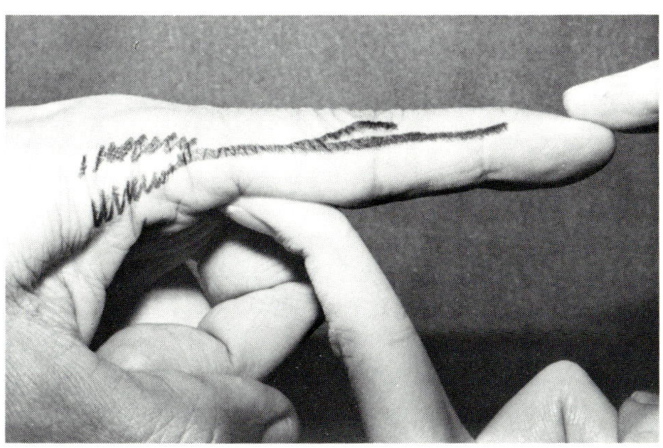

Figure 21-1. *Intrinsic plus is present when the metacarpophalangeal joint cannot be flexed while the interphalangeal joints are extended, and vice versa.*

Lumbrical Plus

This state occurs when the flexor profundus tendon is so long that the lumbrical fails to move sufficiently distal to relax its tension on the extensor hood. The consequence of this disturbed relationship (which also occurs if the lumbrical is shortened) is paradoxical extension of the interphalangeal joints with forceful attempts at profundus flexion. Passively the digit flexes with ease (Fig. 21-2).

Extrinsic Plus

Extrinsic plus occurs at the level of the forearm, wrist, hand or digits. The nature of the stiffness it causes is governed by the number of joints distal to the site of fibrosis. Insufficient length of the muscle-tendon unit prohibits simultaneous flexion or extension of all the joints. Therefore the relaxation needed for movement of one or more joints in the same direction requires positioning of the other joints in the opposite direction.

Anything that will produce fibrosis will cause an extrinsic plus deformity (usually trauma, infection or ischemia). The injury may be open or closed, operative or non-operative. Ischemic fibrosis (e.g. Volkmann's) may be generalized or confined to a limited muscle or tendon area (Chap. 18). Fibrosis limiting function after infection most commonly arises within the tendon sheaths. The diagnosis of this problem rests on defining the level of involvement and differentiating this fibrosis from intrinsic joint stiffness (Fig. 21-3).

The extrinsic plus state does not affect joints proximal to the level of involvement. Its differentiation from intrinsic joint stiffness may be impossible without surgery if the tendon is adherent immediately proximal to a joint. This difficulty is most often seen when either the extensors or flexors are adherent to the proximal phalanx and re-

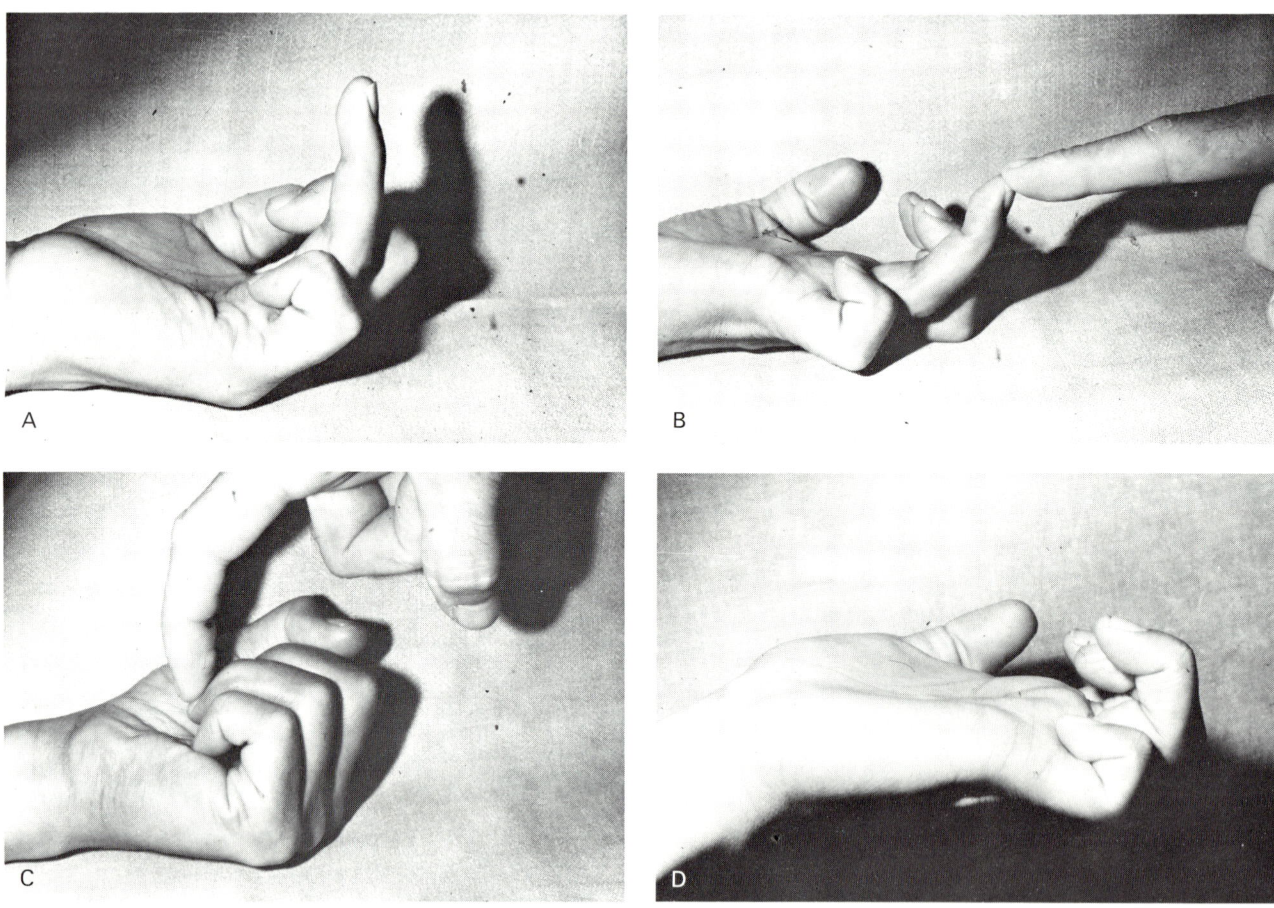

Figure 21-2. *With lumbrical plus, active flexion of the lengthened profundus tendon results in paradoxical extension of the interphalangeal joints* **(A).** *With continued profundus contraction the fingers cannot be passively flexed.* **(B).** *If the profundus tendon is relaxed the finger can be passively flexed* **(C).** *Division of the lumbrical solves the problem* **(D).**

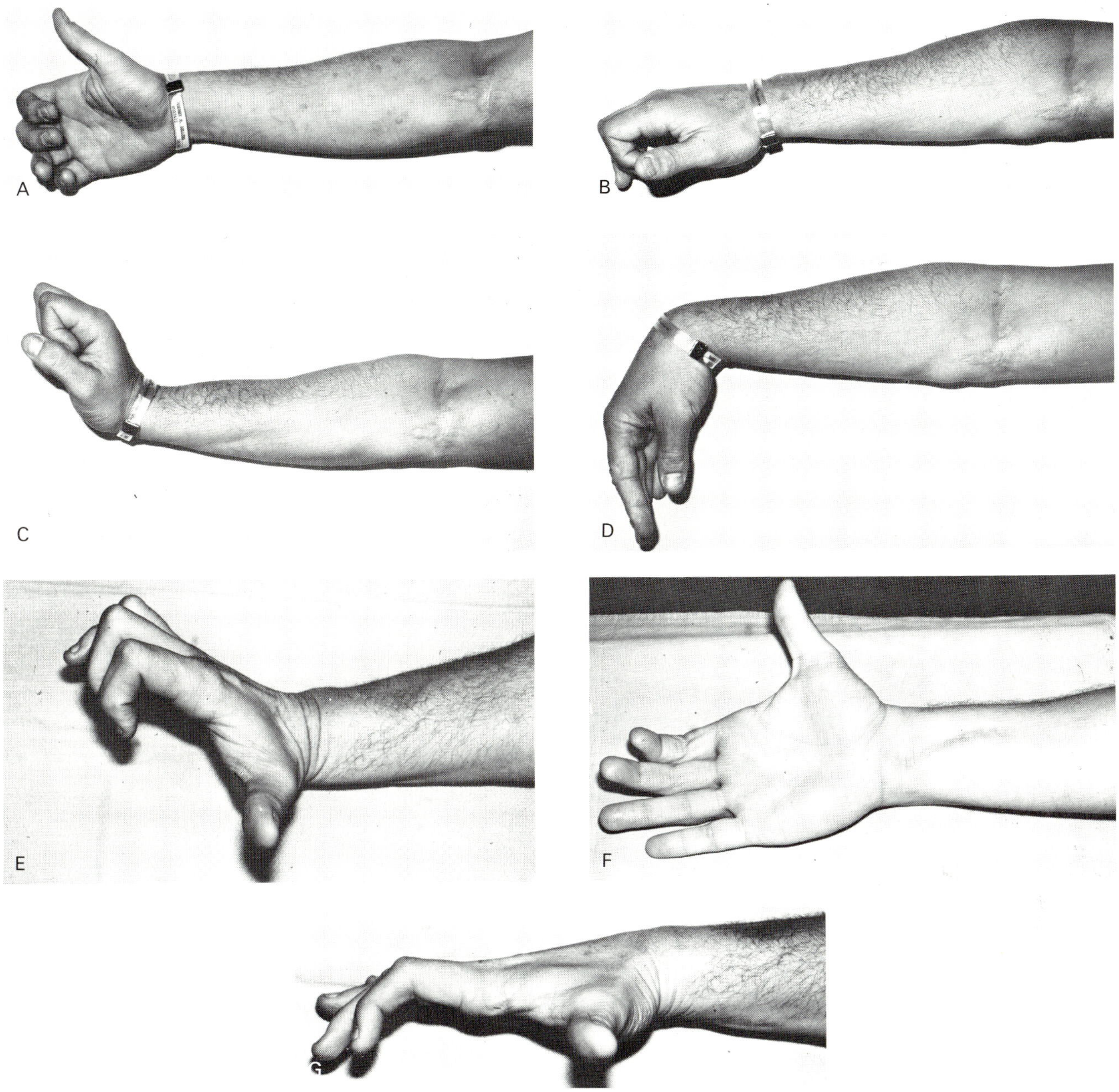

Figure 21-3. *At age 3 this 25-year-old male sustained a wringer injury to his right arm. Digital extension was limited with the wrist extended* **(A,B,C),** *and full extension could be attained only with the wrist fully flexed* **(D).** *Profundus and superficialis tendon lengthening was done, with improved extension* **(E,F,G).**

strict motion of the proximal interphalangeal joint (e.g. following fractures).

For several weeks or months after any tenorrhaphy, infection within any tendon sheath, or fracture adjacent to any tendon, extrinsic plus is a problem to be overcome by active and passive joint motion. When the problem is fixed, surgical measures are required. These include: tenolysis, complete tenotomy, tendon lengthening, tendon grafts (Chap. 14), tendon transfers (Chap. 15), resection of fibrotic tissue (Chap. 18) with or without the addition of new soft tissue cover (Chap. 6).

In its simplest form, tenolysis or tenotomy may offer immediate and dramatic movement of all affected joints. Supervised active motion must be initiated 2 to 3 days following the operation and regulated splinting continued until the wound is healed. As with the postoperative management of intrinsic joint stiffness, local triamcinolone injections and lidocaine anesthesia may be helpful.

Disability rating can be assigned if all reasonable measures of treatment have been rendered and there is no improvement in 2 to 3 months of effort by the patient.

Stiffness of the Wrist and Forearm

Trauma is the most common cause of stiffness of the forearm and wrist. Fractures about the wrist predispose to stiffness by distortion of the architecture and by the accompanying edema and hemorrhea, aggravated by pain. Once the stiffness becomes fixed, it may be intractable to any form of treatment including arthrolysis. Hence, placing the potentially stiff forearm and wrist in the functional position (Chap. 2) is of paramount importance at the time of immobilization. The most frequent gain of motion through surgery comes with resection of the distal 2.5 cm of the ulna (Darrach procedure) (Fig. 23-6). This removes the blockade of forearm rotation at the level of the distal radioulnar joint which is a common sequel to the shortening that occurs with fractures of the wrist and radial head and with rheumatoid deformity. To maintain stability, a flap of flexor carpi ulnaris can be used to minimize further subluxation. Wrist arthroplasty has been helpful in some cases (Chap. 24). Forearm stiffness is usually intractable to section of the interosseous membrane or division and resection of a synostosis.

If wrist and forearm stiffness is anticipated bilaterally, the position set for this should accommodate the basic eating and hygienic needs of the patient.

Treatment of Stiffness

Anticipation and prevention should lie foremost in the minds of the patient and his physician. This requires constant attention to: elevation, avoidance of constricting factors, adequate motion of joints, diminution of anxiety and control of pain and infection.

The development of a shoulder-hand syndrome from disease in the chest, neck or shoulder can be avoided by having the patient move all the joints of his upper extremity through a full range of motion several times a day. Painful problems, e.g. arthritis within the extremity, must be subjectively controlled enough to allow similar exertion. The patient must be educated repeatedly regarding the specifics of prevention of stiffness when he is convalescing from injury to his hand, infection or surgery. The physician must keep in mind and weigh the merits of postoperative immobilization versus the risks of stiffness. It is far better to have a crooked wrist and a supple painless hand than a perfectly reduced Colles' fracture and a totally stiff hand.

The golden opportunity for the prevention of edema and stiffness often lies with the first person to treat an injury or an acute inflammatory process. Experience is important in anticipating the inception and progression of the cycle of pain, edema, and stiffness. If the initiation of this cycle is suspected, all constricting jewelry and clothing should be removed from the upper extremity and immobilization and elevation instituted. Prophylactic antibiotics should be given when indicated.

If there is a serious question regarding the capacity of the patient to follow instructions, or a potentially serious problem exists (e.g. bite injury of the hand), the patient should be hospitalized for 12 to 24 hours.

The urgency of treating established edema when it is first seen must be paramount to all concerned. The immediate measures are those just cited in preventive care. In addition, relaxing incisions and the possible use of anticoagulants and antisludging materials must be considered. Other conditions which lead to the tension of tissues should be recognized and treated (e.g. arterial hemorrhage, skeletal derangements and foreign bodies).

Active joint motion should be initiated as soon as possible. As emphasized by Erik Moberg, active shoulder motion is effective in improving the circulation of the whole extremity. Edema can be reduced in the hand by having the patient wear a compressive glove. A surgeon's glove applied intermittently during the day at times of exercise helps to reduce edema. A tailored, knitted elastic glove with a gradient of pressure greatest distally can be worn for protracted periods. This will also force fixed edema out of the hand and reduce the thickness of scar tissue.

When stiffness seems unavoidable (e.g. severe burns or compression injuries), it is important to position the extremity for function and immobilize it accordingly. This may require internal fixation. Longitudinal Kirschner wires may be used to hold the metacarpophalangeal joints in flexion and the thumb abducted.

Non-operative Treatment of Established Stiffness

First and foremost it is necessary to establish adequate motivation within the patient. Muscle power must be developed, and this can be done only by concerted determined effort on his part. All the modalities available to induce active and passive movement must be employed in an integrated daily program at home. Physiotherapy facilities should be used when those at home fail or are inadequate (Chap. 4).

When pain inhibits movement, analgesics should be used and intermittent nerve blocks considered. Triamcinolone may be a valuable adjunct when injected with lidocaine about a painfully stiff joint at weekly intervals for 3 to 4 weeks.

The patient must be supine. After local anesthesia, 10 to 40 mg of triamcinolone are injected beneath the collateral ligaments and into the joint with a 26-gauge needle (Fig. 21-4). Immediately afterward, while the anesthetic is still effective, the joint is passed through its maximal range of motion actively and passively. Cautious manipulation is desirable and must be done without sudden force. This is particularly applicable to gain proximal interphalangeal joint extension for which active power is weak.

Dynamic splints may be useful (Chap. 4). When applied with tension, they should be used for a limited time (5 to 10 minutes). Without tension, they may be in place for protracted periods of time. They must not cause numbness, lasting pain or chronic edema.

Operative Treatment of The Stiff Hand

The surgical approach to stiffness depends upon the cause. If the stiffness is a result of skin contracture, an excision or transection of scar followed by appropriate free skin grafting or pedicle coverage may be necessary (Chap. 6). In the case of fascial hypertrophy and subcutaneous scar, appropriate sectioning or excision must be undertaken (Chap. 18).

Intrinsic joint stiffness may limit motion by bony or periarticular soft tissue abnormalities. The former can be defined roentgenographically. When present, the usual procedures to be considered are: reduction and alignment with or without repair of the volar plate, removal of a fragment of bone or other bony blocks, implant arthroplasty or fusion (Chaps. 13 and 24). Magnification is essential for the precision needed in operating upon these small joints.

Periarticular soft tissue causes of digital joint stiffness may be: tight collateral ligaments, fibrosis of the joint capsule and volar plate or displacement of the volar plate or tendinous tissue into the joint.

The treatment of adherent or dislocated volar plate may require its excision through a midaxial incision for the proximal interphalangeal joint and either a volar zigzag or dorsal midline incision for the metacarpophalangeal joint (Fig. 21-5). In gaining access to the joint, the dissection must be adjacent to the bone. The neurovascular bundle and flexor tendon sheath must be carefully retracted. A #12 curved blade is often useful in excising the volar plate. A small amount of triamcinolone can be instilled in the joint. The wound is closed with interrupted sutures. A cast is applied for 2 to 3 days, after which carefully supervised motion is allowed once or twice a day. Splinting must be continued for 7 to 10 days. By the end of 2 to 3 weeks, local triamcinolone may be readministered by injection and at times the joint is carefully manipulated following a local anesthetic block.

In some instances the capsule is so fibrotic and adherent that it must be incised. At other times the collateral ligament must be partially, subtotally, or, in rare instances, completely divided. This is done differently for the metacarpophalangeal joint and the proximal interphalangeal joint (the distal joint seldom needs such treatment). The metacarpophalangeal joint is approached through a longitudinal dorsal incision. The extensor tendon is split to enter the joint and, bit by bit, the collateral ligament on the ulnar side is carefully sectioned until the joint can be flexed without springing back into extension (Fig. 21-6). Occasionally the radial collateral ligament must also be divided. Leaving the radial ligament intact prevents ulnar drift.

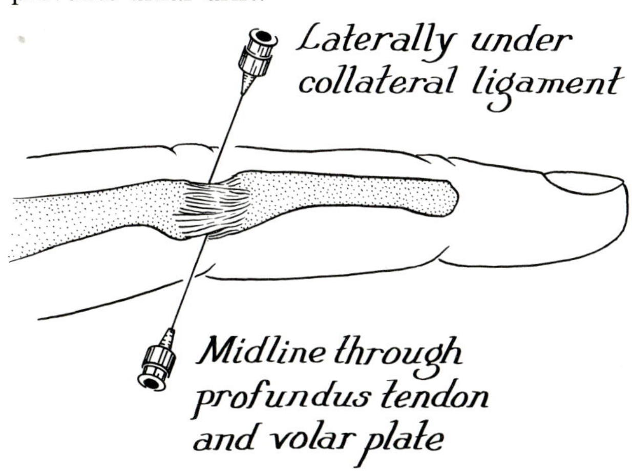

Figure 21-4. *The intra-articular injection of steroids for stiffness must be done gently with small volumes of solution after local anesthetic block. The injection is placed under the collateral ligaments perpendicular to their fibers or through the flexor sheath directly into the midpoint of the volar plate.*

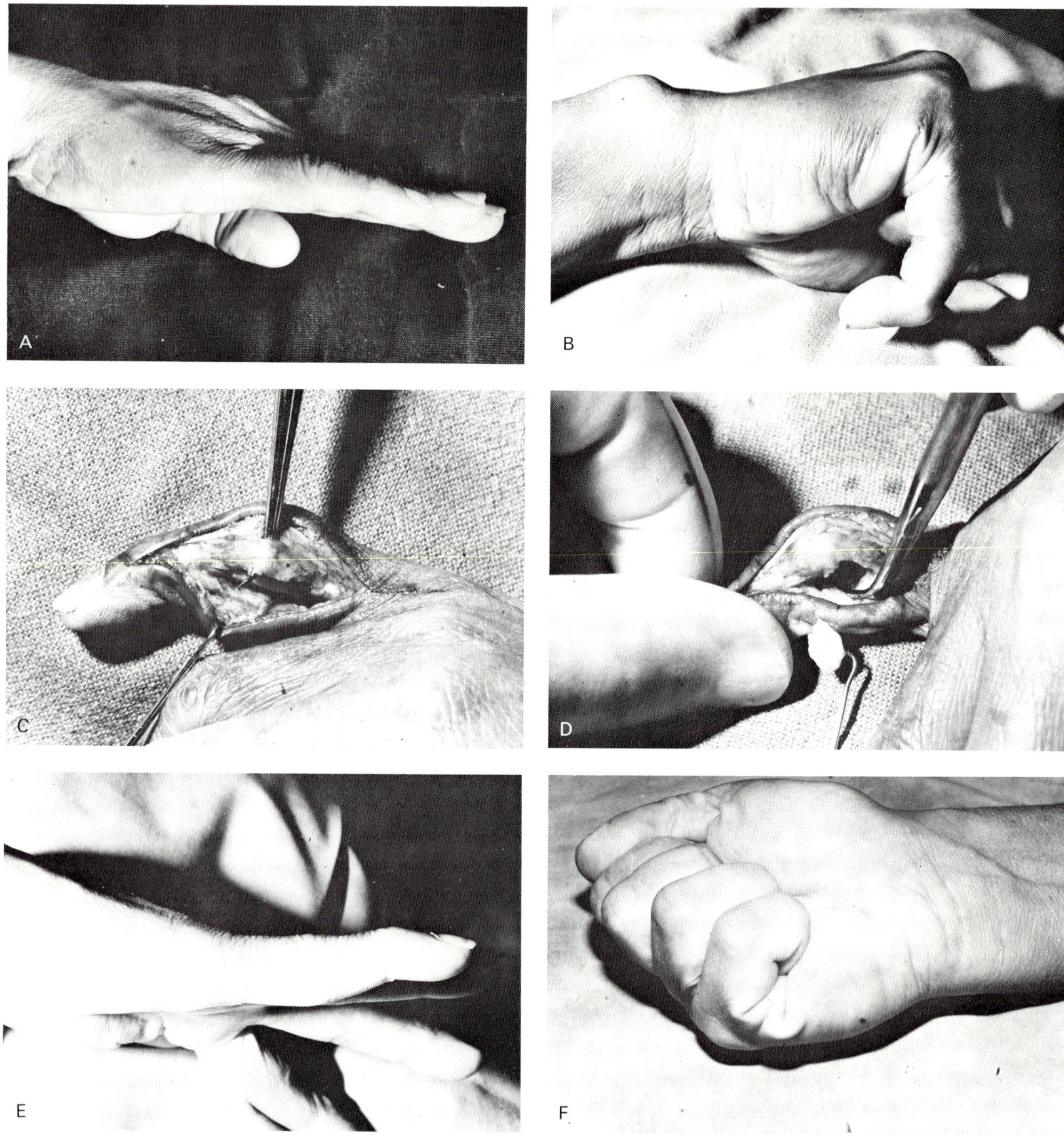

Figure 21-5. *This man had injured the proximal interphalangeal joint, following which the finger was splinted in extension* **(A)** *with loss of flexion at that joint* **(B).** *The stiffness of this joint was relieved by partial release of the radial collateral ligament* **(C)** *and removal of the volar plate* **(D).** *Complete extension was maintained* **(E)** *and full flexion was gained* **(F).**

The collateral ligaments of the proximal interphalangeal joint are for practical purposes divided into a volar and a dorsal half. When the joint is stiff in extension, the dorsal half is tight and needs to be sectioned. When the joint is stiff in flexion, the volar half is tight and needs to be divided (Fig. 21-7). In some instances it is best to excise a wedge of the offending ligament after exposing it through a midaxial incision. The extensor hood must be retracted and neither it nor the cartilage can be traumatized. In all instances the postoperative management is the same as that described for operations on the volar plate.

A flexion contracture of the proximal interphalangeal joint may be caused in part or wholly by a tight band of fascia (e.g. Grayson's, Cleland's or Landsmeer's ligaments) or by thickening of the flexor sheath. These thickened tissues must be divided and sometimes excised.

The adequacy of any of these procedures is repeatedly tested by manipulating the joint. Such manipulations must be done cautiously to avoid traction injury to the volar neurovascular structures. Keeping the more proximal joint flexed reduces the likelihood of this problem during the manipulation.

The joint should not spring back into the contracted position if the release is adequate. In a few instances the release of periarticular contractures is adequate and the recoil is caused by tightness in the musculotendinous unit. In this instance, it may be necessary to pin the joint with an oblique Kirschner wire in the desired position for 2 to 3 weeks. Consideration may also have to be given to a simultaneous extrinsic or intrinsic tendon lengthening or division (Chap. 14).

With prolonged stiffness there may be loss of skin elasticity which may hamper mobilization of the joint. In these circumstances the insufficiency of skin must be corrected with a pedicle flap prior to arthrolysis.

The prognosis is good when the patient is well motivated and has good muscle power and the mobilization is begun early, in 2 to 3 days after an

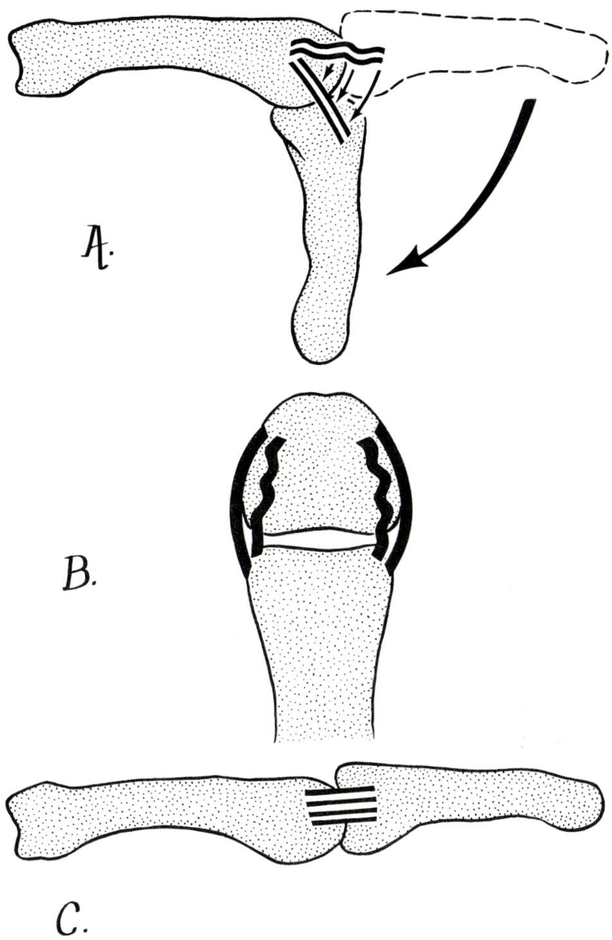

Figure 21-6. *Metacarpophalangeal joint. The collateral ligament is relaxed in extension, stretched in flexion* **(A).** *It must stretch to adapt to the flare of the condyle in flexion* **(B).** *Immobilization in extension allows the ligament to shorten* **(C).**

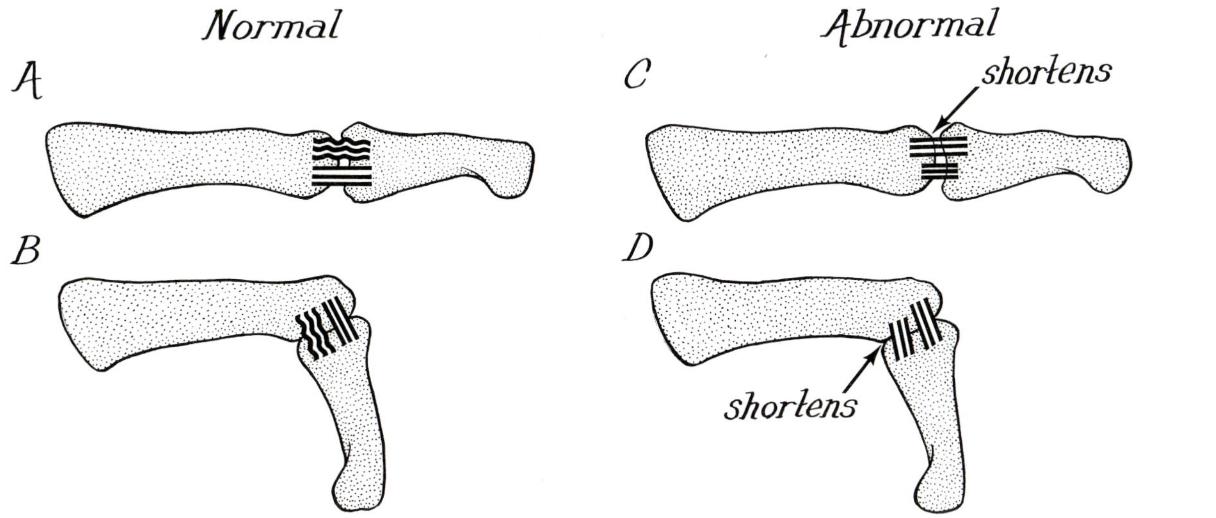

Figure 21-7. *Proximal interphalangeal joint. The dorsal half of collateral ligament is relaxed in extension and tight in flexion* **(A).** *The volar half is tight in extension and relaxed in flexion* **(B).** *Splinting in the extremes of positioning results in shortening of one or the other.*

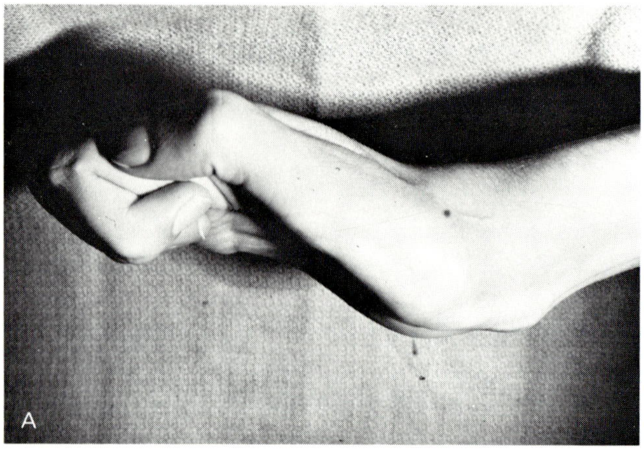

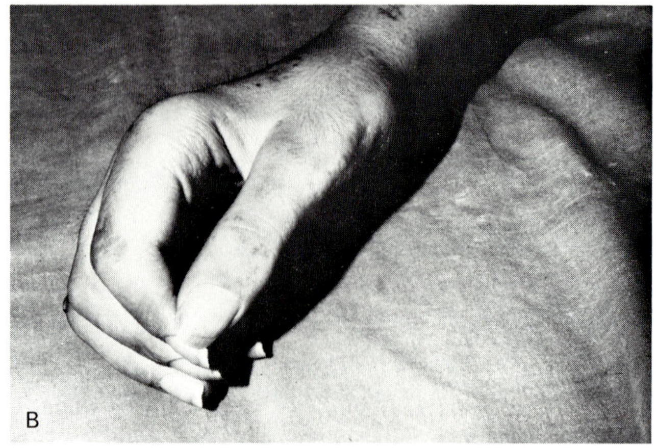

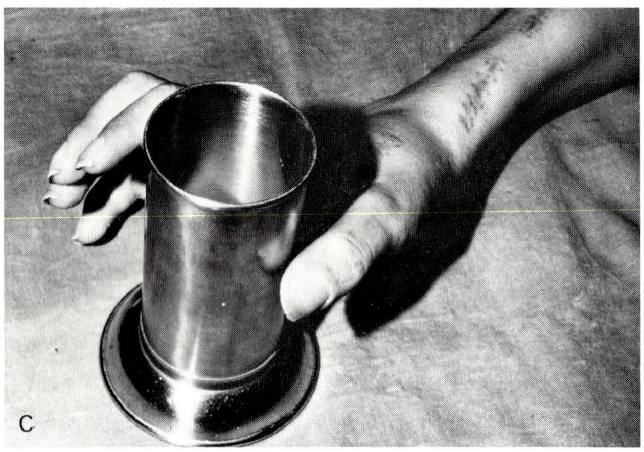

Figure 21-8. *This patient had a long-standing claw-hand* **(A)** *from complete median and ulnar nerve sections. A simplified helping hand was obtained by distal and proximal interphalangeal joint arthrodeses* **(B** *and* **C)** *along with tendon transfers.*

uneventful surgical procedure. The relative weakness of the digital extensors compared to the flexors makes it harder to overcome a flexion contracture at the proximal interphalangeal joint. The converse is true at the metacarpophalangeal joint.

In hopeless cases, when previous procedures have failed or muscle power, skin cover and patient motivation are lacking, arthrodesis in the position of function or selective amputation may be undertaken (Chaps. 13, 17) (Fig. 21-8).

22 Tumors

Tumors of the hand are commonplace. Very few are malignant, a fair number are benign neoplasms, but most are not neoplastic and are derived from the classic disease states: trauma, infection, inflammatory diseases, metabolic disorders, degenerative processes and congenital anomalies (Table 22-1).

Tumors of the hand occur at any age. Most malignancies originate from the skin and occur in the older age groups. The size of the lesion and the presence or absence of pain are not indicative of the likelihood of malignancy. Certain tumors are more likely to be found in the hand than in other parts of the body, e.g. glomus tumor and epidermoid inclusion cyst. However, this may reflect more their symptom potential in the hand than a preponderant incidence there.

Careful questioning and a systematic examination with evaluation of the circulation, innervation, musculoskeletal function, coupled with appropriately chosen roentgenograms (even angiography), will go far to provide an accurate diagnosis before operation. Transillumination in a darkroom and aspirations with an 18-gauge needle should be considered in the evaluation of a cystic lesion.

Treatment must always be tailored to the desires of the patient whom the surgeon should do his best to educate, without intimidation, to the prognostic realities of the tumor present. Under such circumstances, most patients choosing surgical treatment will do their best to adapt to its consequences.

The surgery of tumors requires precise technique to minimize the chance of recurrence and to avoid unnecessary loss of function from iatrogenic causes. The facilities and instruments must be ideal, and loupe magnification should always be available (Chap. 4). The incision is a critical factor to success. It should be long enough to give surgical access to adequately distinguish between what must be extirpated and what must be spared. The surgery will then be truly gentle. In the digit, this means placing the incision directly over the tumor (Chap. 6). Too many tumors have been incompletely removed and too many neurovascular bundles have been injured by the surgeon's insistence on the classic "midlateral" or "midaxial" approach to the digit.

The incidence of hand tumors varies somewhat by age and geographic distribution, with an order of frequency of:

Ganglion
Giant cell tumor
Epidermoid inclusion cyst
Fibroma
Hemangioma
Lipoma
Neurofibroma

Most statistics show a ganglion to be by far the most common tumor. The wart, nevus, giant cell tumor of the tendon sheath (xanthoma) and epidermoid inclusion cyst are almost equal to one another in incidence and collectively do not equal the incidence of the ganglion. Perhaps warts are truly the most common new growth in the hand; however, patients with warts are not often referred to the hand surgeon, so statistics from this specialty may provide a deceptively low incidence.

The discussion that follows will group tumors by

Table 22-1. *Non-neoplastic Disorders which Cause Tumors*

POST-TRAUMATIC
Hematoma, seroma, ganglion, epidermoid inclusion cyst, foreign body, neuroma in continuity or nerve stump neuroma, tendon stump, hypertrophic skin scar, bone stump or exostosis, knuckle bursa or aneurysm.
DEGENERATIVE STATES
Hypertrophic osteoarthropathy with Heberden's nodes, exostosis, ganglion and senile and seborrheic keratosis.
CHRONIC INFLAMMATORY STATES AND COLLAGEN DISORDERS
Rheumatoid disease causing synovitis as well as skin, subcutaneous and tendon nodules; non-specific villonodular tenosynovitis; Dupuytren's fasciitis; keratoacanthoma or Boeck's sarcoid.
INFECTIOUS CONDITIONS
Warts (verruca vulgaris), abscess or pyogenic granuloma, pseudoepitheliomatous hyperplasia.
METABOLIC DISORDERS
Gouty tophus and xanthoma.
CONGENITAL STATES
Hemangioma, ganglion, anomalous bone or muscle formation or arteriovenous fistula.

their anatomical location and origin with a further division into pseudotumors and benign and malignant tumors (Table 22-2). Certain lesions may be found in more than one anatomical area. If so, they will be discussed according to prime location or origin.

Pseudotumors

Skin and Fat

WARTS (CHAP. 7)

These lesions are virus induced and may resolve spontaneously or require treatment with salicylic acid plasters, liquid nitrogen or other topical agents as well as electrodesiccation. If warts are overtreated in breadth and depth by cryotherapy or electrodesiccation, iatrogenic nerve injury or excessive scarring may result (Fig. 22-1).

HYPERTROPHIC SCAR

This most often occurs in response to stretch stress following wounding and is most common after burns and lacerations. It may be almost keloidal in magnitude, but actual keloids are not seen in the hand. Patients may complain of pain if the scar is stretched or pressed. Scar hypertrophy following burns or injuries should be prevented by proper splinting and the use of elastic dressings (Chap. 19). Once thickened scars have developed and a progressive deformity is occurring or has been established, the surgical treatment requires a resection of the scar and resurfacing with a full-thickness skin graft or a pedicle flap (Chap. 6). A Z-plasty may be necessary. As an alternate to surgical revision, an attempt may be made to reduce the bulk of such scars by injecting triamcinolone into the scar (5 mg/cc). These injections are repeated 2 to 3 times at weekly intervals. Local pressure with a rubber glove or customized gauntlet should be used to further attempt to reduce the bulk; such a device may need to be worn for up to 6 months.

EPIDERMOID (INCLUSION) CYST

The pathogenesis of this common tumor of the volar surface of the digit or palm is an injury (e.g. puncture wound, laceration or surgical incision) which carries the germinative epithelial cells deep into the tissues where a nidus of skin growth is seeded and cannot desquamate (Fig. 22-2). Accordingly, as weeks, but more often months, pass, an "epithelial pearl" develops. It usually has a friable, glistening whitish capsule with cheesy contents. The cyst can easily be freed from its bed. The surgeon must strive for total removal without compromise of the wall to ensure against recurrence. Occasionally excision will be facilitated by leaving a small portion of the adherent, thin skin over the lesion to be used for traction during the dissection. Inclusion cysts are commonly found as painful (sometimes inflamed and/or purulent) small lumps on amputation stumps, especially when a remnant of nail has been left behind (Fig.

Table 22-2. *Tumors of the Hand*

	PSEUDOTUMORS	BENIGN TUMORS	MALIGNANT TUMORS
Skin	Warts (verruca vulgaris)	Nevus	Bowen's disease
	Hypertrophic scar	Keratosis	Basal cell carcinoma
	Rheumatoid nodule	Dermatofibroma	Squamous cell carcinoma
	Boeck's sarcoid	Keratoacanthoma	Melanoma
	Pyogenic granuloma		
	Pseudoepitheliomatous hyperplasia		
	Epithelial inclusion cyst		
	Keratinous cyst		
Fat	Hematoma and seroma	Lipoma	Liposarcoma
	Foreign body		
	Gouty tophus		
Fascia	Rheumatoid nodule	Fibroma	Fibrosarcoma
	Dupuytren's fasciitis	Giant cell tumor	Epithelioid sarcoma
	Knuckle pads	Xanthoma	
Joint	Ganglion	Giant cell synovioma	Synovial sarcoma
	Mucous cyst		
	Synovitis		
	Knuckle bursa		
Tendon	Tendon stump and callus		
	Rheumatoid nodule		
	Cyst		
Bone	Heberden's node	Enchondroma	Osteogenic sarcoma
	Exostosis	Osteoid osteoma	Chondrosarcoma
	Callus (fracture)	Osteochondroma	Ewing's tumor
	Bone cyst	Aneurysmal bone cyst	Metastatic tumors
		Giant cell tumor	
		Osteoblastoma	
Muscle	Hematoma	Leiomyoma	Rhabdomyosarcoma
	Hypertrophy		
	Duplication		
Vessels	Varix	Hemangioma	Hemangioendothelioma
		Involuting	Hemangiosarcoma
		Non-involuting	Lymphangiosarcoma
		Venous racemose aneurysm	Kaposi's sarcoma
		Lymphangioma	
		Glomus tumor	
Nerve	Neuroma	Neurofibroma	Malignant neurilemmoma
		Neurilemmoma	

22-3). In excising these, the underlying periosteum must be removed if the matrix of the nail extends to that depth. Such cysts may even form within the bone after a compound fracture or intramedullary drilling. If they expand sufficiently, pain and pathological fractures may result.

KERATINOUS CYST

This lesion is rare in the hand and is apt to be confused with an epidermoid inclusion cyst. The keratinous cyst occurs only in the hair-bearing skin and is therefore limited to the dorsum and is fixed to the skin. This contrasts with the inclusion cyst which is more prevalent on the volar aspect and frequently mobile and not attached to the skin. Keratinous cysts are treated by excision of the intact lesion.

PYOGENIC GRANULOMA

This overgrowth of granulation-like tissue rises above the surrounding skin (Fig. 22-4). It may be hypersensitive. The lesion is initiated by a

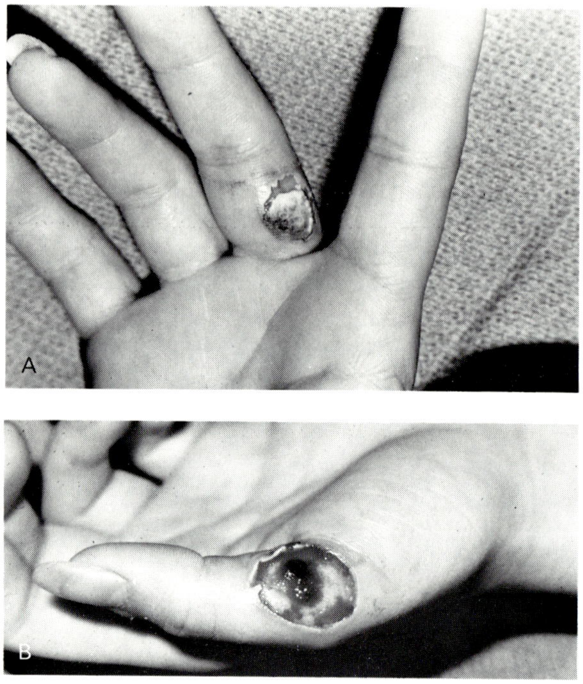

Figure 22-1. *Electrodesiccation of warts on this young girl's fingers led to injury to the volar digital nerves from the cautery as well as marked cutaneous scarring.*

wound of the skin which may be only a puncture wound. Its development is facilitated by inability of the granulation tissue to dry up, because the dressing is chronically saturated with serum from the granuloma. The treatment, if the lesion is less than 5 mm in diameter, is to allow it to desiccate by exposing it or by applying tincture of benzoin. The larger ones are best treated by scraping the

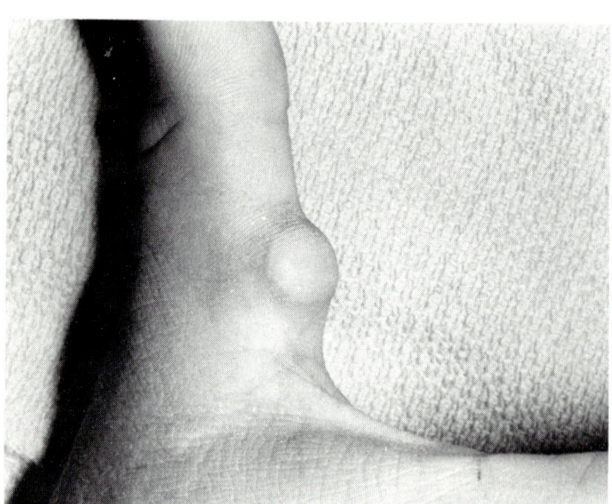

Figure 22-2. *This epidermoid inclusion cyst on the volar aspect of the thumb of a young carpenter had become secondarily infected.*

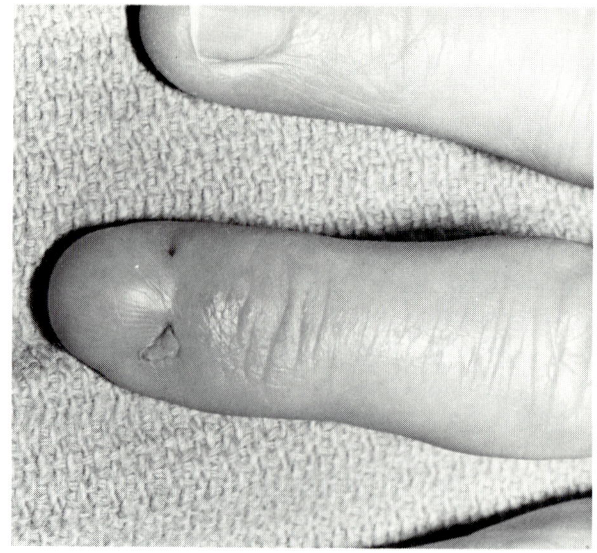

Figure 22-3. *Nail horns persisted on the tip of the index finger of this young woman who suffered a crushing injury to her fingertip one year earlier.*

granulation flush with the skin and grafting the base with a split-thickness skin graft.

RHEUMATOID NODULE

Twenty per cent of patients with rheumatoid arthritis have subcutaneous nodules (Fig. 22-5). Such lesions also involve the skin, fascia, bursae and tendons. They may be symptomatic when they block the motion of joints or tendons. Those in the skin are cosmetic rather than functional problems. They may be very large, particularly over the olecranon. They are adherent to their site of origin and care must be taken to avoid injuring neighboring structures of functional importance during their removal. The excision of large rheumatoid nodules may result in postoperative hematoma formation within the wound.

PSEUDOEPITHELIOMATOUS HYPERPLASIA

This overgrowth of epithelium occurs usually at the margin of a chronic ulcer. It is not premalignant but represents the ineffective effort of the epidermis to bridge the ulcer. Microscopically, the elongated epithelial pegs of well-differentiated cells extend into the dermis. The diagnosis is predicated upon the microscopic findings.

BOECK'S SARCOID

This condition of the reticuloendothelial system may involve the hand in two specific ways: (1) by

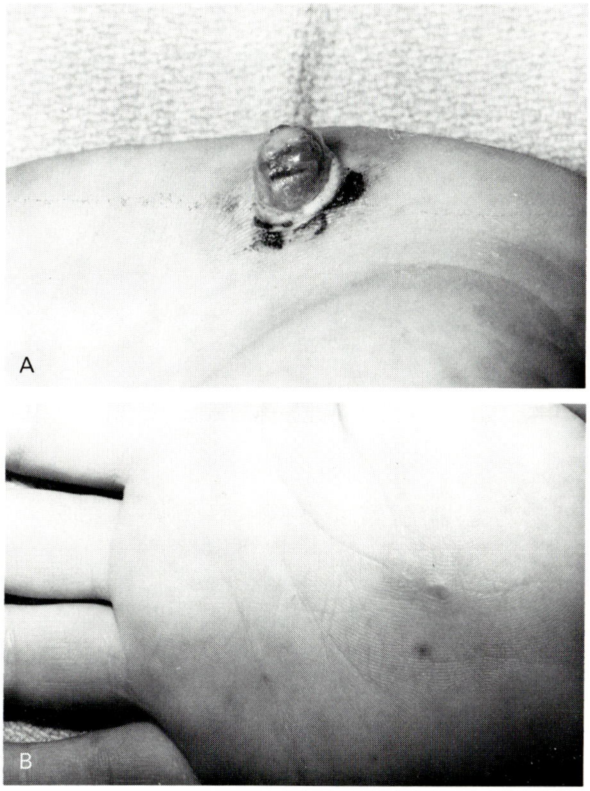

Figure 22-4. *This young boy experienced a pyogenic granuloma of his palm following minor injury, for which petrolatum was used as a dressing. The lesion responded to excision and the application of a small split-thickness skin graft.*

raised nodular lesions of the skin and (2) by fine cystic changes near the digital joints. A biopsy of the skin lesions shows non-caseating granulomas typical of this disorder.

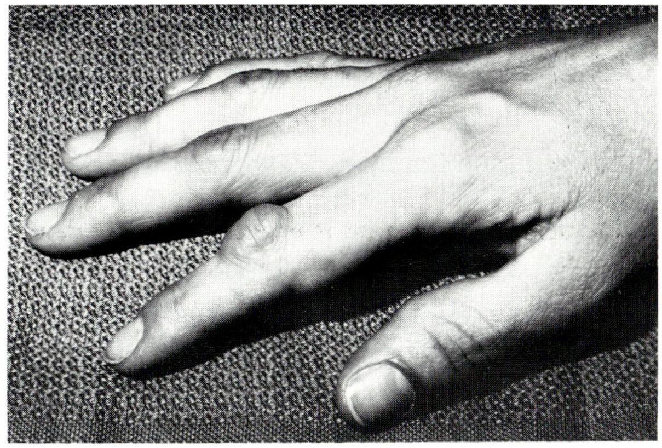

Figure 22-5. *These firm, intradermal rheumatoid nodules were the only manifestations of rheumatoid disease in this 30-year-old woman.*

HEMATOMA AND SEROMA

Trauma is the most common cause of localized swelling due to blood in the hand (Fig. 22-6). A seroma may follow within 2 to 3 weeks or more if a hematoma is not completely reabsorbed. The amount of bleeding is not necessarily related to the magnitude or severity of trauma. The friability of vessels, especially veins, and impaired coagulability of blood play an important role in the formation of these lesions. The dorsum of the hand, with its thin skin and concentration of veins, is the most frequent site of localized hematoma. Marked swelling may occur immediately after a contusion or laceration and truly frighten the patient. If the skin is thin and light, discoloration may be immediate. If the skin is thick and cushioned with fat, ecchymosis may not appear for several days. The volar surface of digits and palm are not spared hematomata, but here they usually follow greater violence (e.g. a fall on the outstretched hand or a crushing force to the digit). An arterial laceration, especially a partial one, will lead to a hematoma which may be obscured by the fascial space in which it occurs and the cushioning fat or muscle within the space (e.g. the thenar space).

The treatment of a hematoma is evacuation from an open wound if it can be gently expressed. However, it is injurious to try to remove blood in the tissues that is not a separate clot. The squeezing and scraping incident to such effort only traumatize the fat, muscles and nerves, and lead to more fibrosis. Caution should be exercised in converting a closed wound into an open wound to evacuate a clot unless the clot is expanding, the fascial space is brawny and there are symptoms and signs of beginning or progressive ischemia or palsy. Elevation, the removal of constricting dress-

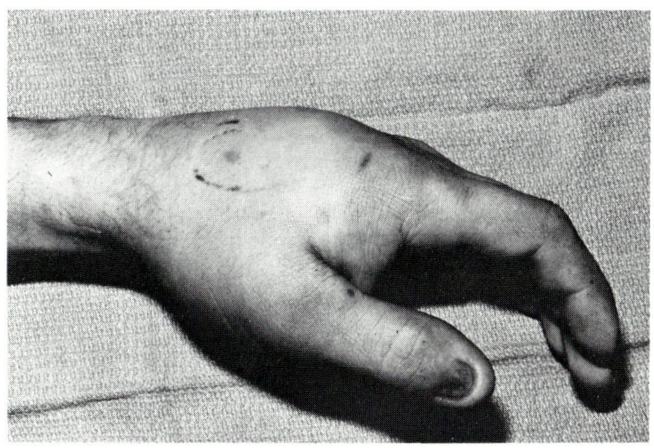

Figure 22-6. *The first web space of this young man's hand was contused by a rock drill, resulting in tearing of the first dorsal interosseous muscle and the occurrence of an extensive hematoma.*

ings, garments and jewelry, cooling of the hand and immobilization in the functional position are appropriate therapy within the first few hours of hemorrhage. Any coagulation defect (therapeutic anticoagulation) should be corrected until the bleeding has ceased and any need for surgical drainage has passed. Liquefaction of the hematoma and the formation of a seroma begin when fluctuation appears. Aspiration may then be undertaken with a large-bore needle and gentle compression applied thereafter with a sponge plastic or rubber under the bandage.

FOREIGN BODY

A foreign body of significant size can often be palpated (Fig. 22-7). Its existence is suspected by history. Small foreign bodies often stimulate a skin reaction of marked thickening (like a callus). The diagnosis and treatment are discussed in Chapter 9.

GOUTY TOPHUS (CHAP. 25)

These chalky deposits can be anywhere and sometimes very large (Fig. 22-8). However, as a rule function is not markedly curtailed. The blood uric acid is usually elevated above 9 mg/100 ml. The diagnosis is confirmed by laboratory tests and concomitant physical findings. At operation the tophus may be extensive enough to threaten the integrity of the extensor mechanism during the dissection.

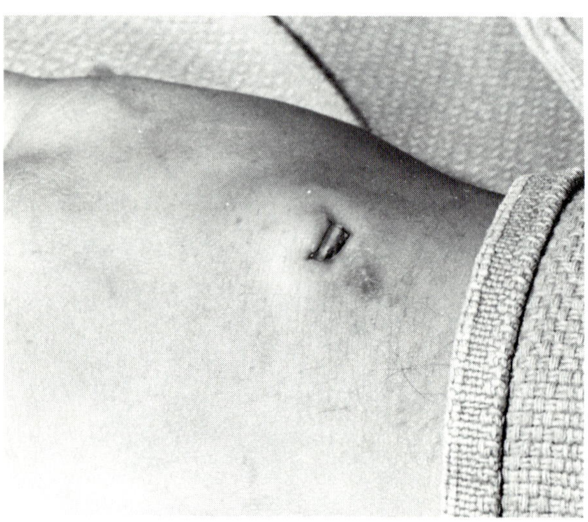

Figure 22-7. *This young girl had 3 months earlier thrust her hand through a plate glass window, sustaining a laceration on the dorsum. She experienced pain and discomfort in the area and felt a firm area beneath the skin. Ultimately the glass extruded spontaneously from the wound.*

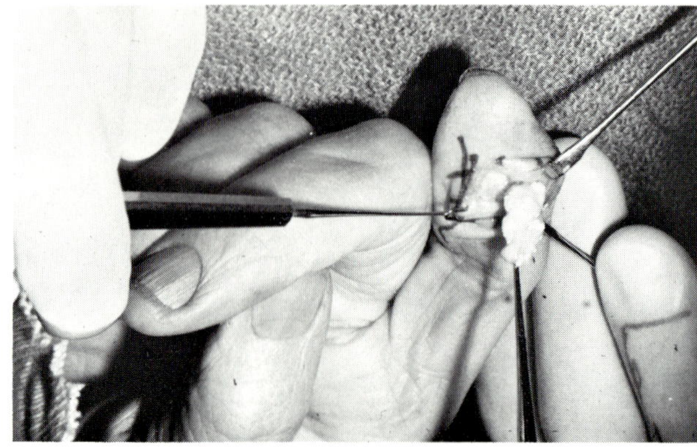

Figure 22-8. *This young woman had gouty tophi on the dorsal and volar aspects of her index fingertip. She desired a removal for cosmetic purposes. No other manifestations of gout were evident.*

Fascia

DUPUYTREN'S FASCIITIS (CHAP. 18)

This fascial hypertrophy of unknown etiology involves the palmar fascia. It is most commonly mistaken for a tumor when it consists of a nodule without any joint contracture. Such nodules occur most commonly in the midpalm over the ring and little finger rays and have been misconstrued as callus secondary to the pressure of gripping. They are generally quite firm and occasionally tender if the process is acute. The microscopic appearance is akin to that of a fibrosarcoma. Great discretion is necessary in the performance of any surgical treatment.

KNUCKLE PADS

These consist of a process similar to Dupuytren's fasciitis (Fig. 22-9). They are usually over the proximal interphalangeal joints, but may be present over any of the other digital joints. Great care must be taken to avoid injury to the extensor mechanism in removing these lesions, or severe secondary problems such as buttonhole deformity may result.

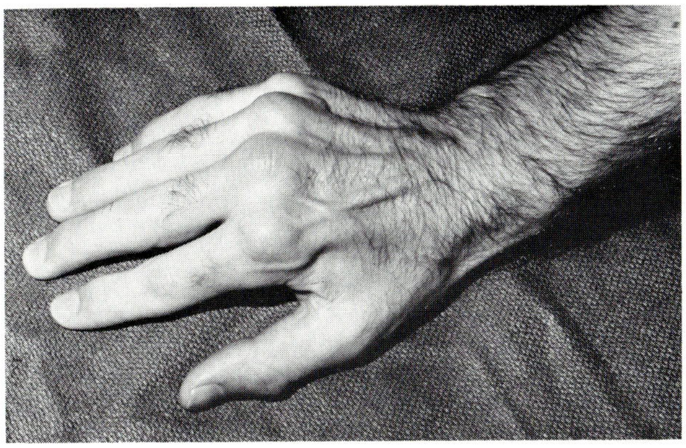

Figure 22-9. *This 30-year-old had had six previous operations for Dupuytren's contracture of both hands. He manifested knuckle pads on the dorsum of the metacarpophalangeal joints of all of his fingers.*

Joints

GANGLION

A ganglion is a synovial cyst arising from a joint or bursa of a tendon sheath (Fig. 22-10). It is the most common tumor of the hand, and develops as a consequence of herniation of the synovium from the joint or tendon bursa. The connecting stalk may be wide open or narrow. Its configuration may act as a check valve so that the fluid is locked in the cyst or the stalk may be completely sealed off. As a rule, the ganglion develops insidiously and the cyst wall gradually stretches along the path of least resistance ahead of the pressure gradient of the lubricating fluid it contains. When the cyst is completely sealed off, dehydration often concentrates the fluid, which may become solidified like jelly. The viscosity therefore varies greatly. In any case, aspiration usually requires a large-bore needle (18 gauge).

The lining is deceptive. As a rule the cyst is enveloped by multiple layers of an areolar type of tissue under tension and vessels or nerves may be stretched over the surface. The cyst wall itself, however, is usually delicate and easily torn. The stalk may be very long at times and traceable only by extremely precise dissection to its origin.

The most common ganglia occur about the wrist and arise on the dorsal or volar aspect usually more to the radial or ulnar aspect than in the midline. Those on the dorsum commonly arise from the radiocarpal joint and appear between the extensor carpi radialis and the digital extensors, which must be carefully protected during the dissection. Those on the flexor aspect commonly arise from the radioscaphoid joint and appear in close proximity to the radial artery, which they may envelop. There have been cases in which the ganglion has extended like a long worm a distance of 5 to 7.5 cm within the areolar sheath and parallel to the radial artery. A preoperative Allen's test is essential to ascertain collateral blood flow to the thumb. If this test shows poor collateral blood flow, the risk of thumb ischemia may contraindicate ganglionectomy. Ganglia on the radial side of the wrist, whether volar or dorsal, usually lie in close proximity to sensory branches of the radial nerve. The volar ones, in addition, are adjacent to the palmar cutaneous branch of the median nerve. These nerves tend to form intractable, painful neuromas and must therefore be diligently protected.

The dorsal ganglia arising from the extensor synovial bursae invariably appear distal to the extensor retinaculum. Here a ganglion must be distinguished from an extensor tenosynovitis. The ganglion is discrete, whereas the swelling of the tenosynovitis is over a broad area and often hourglass in configuration because of the constriction of the extensor retinaculum upon it. The ganglion of the tendon moves with excursion of the extensor tendon when the fist is opened and closed, whereas that arising from the joint does not. A dorsal boss over the index or long metacarpal or carpometacarpal joint is often mistaken for a ganglion and at times even has a small insignificant cystic area (really a bursa) over it. The ganglion can be transilluminated and aspirated for diagnostic purposes

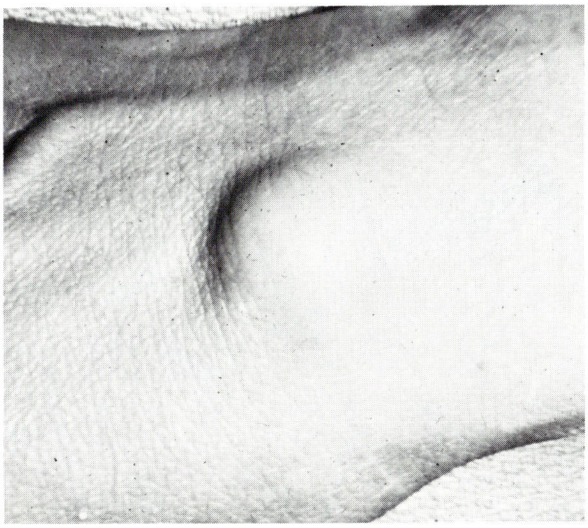

Figure 22-10. *Illustration shows a typical dorsal wrist ganglion.*

and a lateral roentgenogram will help define the bony boss.

The third most common ganglion is that of the flexor sheath of the fingers (Fig. 22-11). This manifests itself as "a pebble in a shoe"—a very hard, small mass. It is usually found at the distal margin of a proximal pulley and may be in the midline of the digit or off to the side. It can be aspirated when in the midline but not when it is displaced laterally, because of the risk of injury to the digital nerve and artery.

A ganglion develops by herniation of the synovial lining. Most cases are undoubtedly congenital; the fibrous portion of a joint capsule does not adequately contain the synovium under pressure of the synovial fluid. However, in some instances there may be a second factor of pumping action by the excursion of a joint or a tendon which causes a tight pinching of synovium and joint capsule or tendon sheath. This causes separation of the fibrous tissue of the capsule or sheath and allows the synovium to extrude and become trapped when the pinching is released.

At times, the awareness of a ganglion is directly related to some moment of particular stress or strain. The patient's attention is directed not to pain but to the lump. Undoubtedly, the synovial fluid pressure caused a sudden ballooning out of a preexisting ganglion. The osteoarthritic hypertrophic lipping about the distal joint is a factor in the genesis of a dorsal ganglion (mucous cyst) at that level.

Most patients have minimal or no symptoms from a ganglion. They may note some aching or a feeling of pressure when the position of the part places the maximum tension on the ganglion. The flexor sheath ganglion, however, may produce distinct pain with vigorous gripping or numbness or a Tinel's phenomenon when it is located so that pressure causes it to compress a digital nerve.

The diagnosis of a ganglion is made by obtaining the oily synovial fluid by aspiration or at operation. The diagnosis is suspected on the basis of the incidence of the tumor, its location, transillumination and, in many cases, a history of fluctuation in size as the ganglion fills and empties or ruptures.

A ganglion is treated to give reassurance to the patient that it is not malignant and does not portend arthritis or loss of function, to relieve pressure if it is symptomatic, and to reduce or remove the tumor for cosmetic reasons. Hence, all treatment is elective and surgery should be done only on the demand of the patient. The patient must choose between a bump on the dorsum of the wrist and a surgical scar which, at times, hypertrophies in spite of proper technique.

Most ganglia can be aspirated or perforated with a needle and compressed. Corticosteroids may then be instilled. This is a substitute for surgery often preferred by the patient. However, it is contraindicated where arteries and nerves are in jeopardy. Caution must be employed in keeping the injection within the ganglion so that cutaneous atrophy and depigmentation do not occur (Fig. 22-12). The recurrence rate is high because nothing has been done to remove the stalk or wall of the cyst.

Excision is not an office procedure. The incision must be carefully planned. It should be long enough to give the exposure needed without damage from the retracting of tissues. A transverse

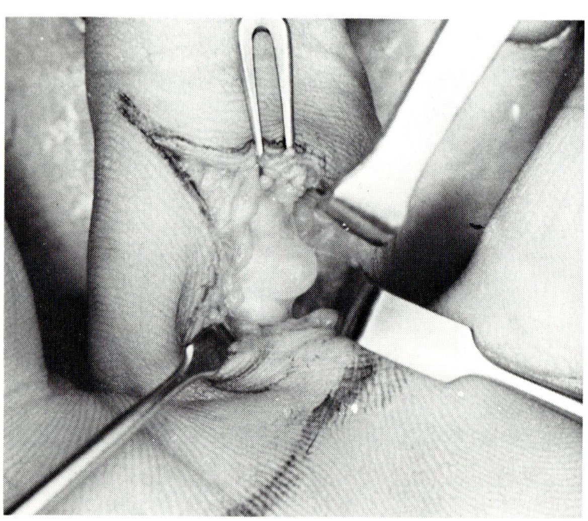

Figure 22-11. *This young man had a painful nodule near the metacarpophalangeal joint crease on the volar aspect of his hand. A small ganglion was found, arising from the tendon sheath in that area.*

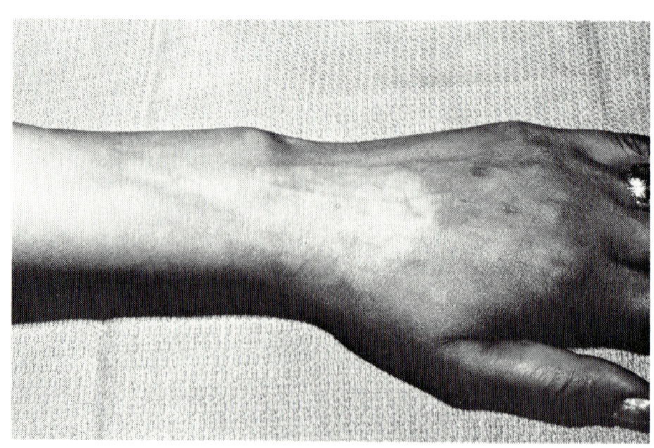

Figure 22-12. *This young black woman had a dorsal wrist ganglion injected with triamcinolone. Depigmentation of the skin followed. Eight months after the injection, the color had returned to normal.*

incision over the dorsum of the wrist gives the best cosmetic scar but runs the risk of some numbness distally and, if extreme care is not taken, of a symptomatic neuroma from injury to the dorsal sensory nerves.

Every effort should be made to keep the ganglion filled until it has been separated from surrounding tissue down to its stalk. This is usually a "peeling" process which must be done with tourniquet control and magnification. Once the origin of the cyst is defined, a rim of capsule of the joint or sheath of the tendon should be resected with the tented stalk. Any small satellite ganglia should be sought. The capsule and tendon sheath need not be closed or repaired. Methylene blue injected with a 30-gauge needle into the ganglion is helpful in tracing its stalk when difficulty is anticipated. The wound is closed with everting sutures of nylon and the part immobilized with a well-padded plaster splint which includes the wrist. Sutures are generally left in place for at least 2 to 3 weeks and immobilization is maintained for 7 to 10 days. The temporary disability for a working man following a wrist ganglionectomy is apt to be at least 3 to 4 weeks.

Recurrences are uncommon if the cyst is removed in toto; they are generally the result of technical problems. The ganglia that arise on the volar radial aspect of the wrist from a deep recess under the radial artery and abductor pollicis longus may have an inaccessible origin. Sometimes incompetence of the tourniquet allows blood to ooze into the field, obscuring vision and precluding adequate removal of the cyst.

Ganglia may occur anywhere about the digits but are more commonly seen on the dorsolateral aspects. They may be round and discrete or broad, flat or tubular, soft or hard and, rarely, tender. The most common of these is the mucous cyst. This is a dorsal ganglion of the distal interphalangeal joint which is associated invariably with some arthritic thickening or spur formation of the bone at the edge of the joint cartilage[8] (Fig. 22-13). The lesion is most common after middle age and at the radial or ulnar side of the mid-dorsum of the distal phalanx between the joint line and the eponychial fold. Mucous cysts transilluminate and may drain typical synovial fluid. The compression of the nail matrix by the cyst may be enough to cause a longitudinal furrow of the nail which may disappear if the cyst is removed (Fig. 22-14).

Recurrence is the most frustrating aspect of treatment. This can be minimized by adequate visualization under at least twofold magnification and by staining the ganglion and its extensions

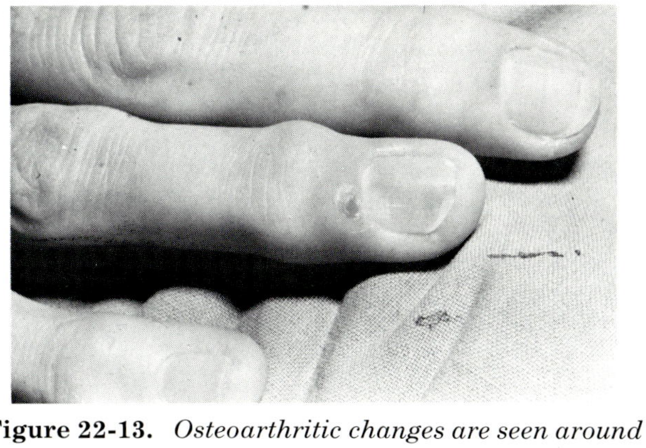

Figure 22-13. *Osteoarthritic changes are seen around the distal and phalangeal joint of this woman's finger. She has large Heberden's nodes and a mucous cyst.*

with methylene blue (Fig. 22-15). The technique for this is:

1. With the patient supine the extremity is elevated and an upper-arm tourniquet inflated.
2. An intermetacarpal block is performed just proximal to the head of the metacarpal (Chap. 26).
3. A 1″ wide rubber dam finger tourniquet (Penrose drain) is applied evenly to the base of the digit and held on the dorsum with a hemostat. The distal portion of the drain is cut away to expose the distal interphalangeal joint.
4. The upper-arm tourniquet is released and the skin incision is outlined with marking ink (Fig. 22-16). Usually this is an L-shaped incision which crosses the very crest of the eponychial fold and then proceeds along the dorsoradial or dorsoulnar sides of the distal and middle phalanges. If the skin is too adherent and excessively thin over the cyst, this area may be outlined for removal.
5. When the digit is anesthetized, a 30-gauge hypodermic needle is inserted through the midpoint of the distal flexion crease into the joint (a ½″ long needle must be inserted almost to its hub). A 2-cc Luer-Lok syringe containing a mixture of lidocaine, about 0.25 cc of hydrogen peroxide and 2 or 3 drops of methylene blue is attached to the

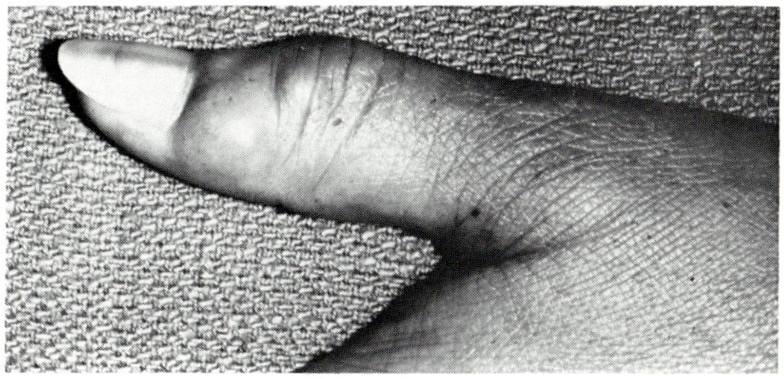

Figure 22-14. *The pressure of a mucous cyst at the distal interphalangeal joint level produces creasing of the nail.*

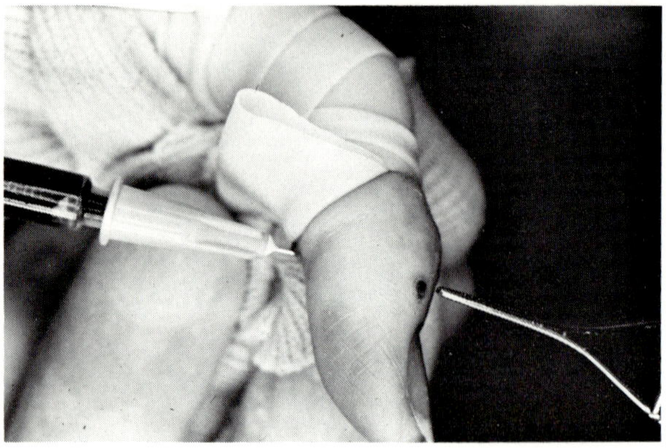

Figure 22-15. *Injection through the volar aspect of the distal interphalangeal joint with methylene blue and hydrogen peroxide produces a bluish discoloration of the dorsal digital ganglion.*

needle and injected into the joint. Force is not used for this and, as a rule, only 0.25 cc or less of the fluid can be injected. A bluish coloration of the cyst will usually ensue and the needle can be withdrawn.

6. The dissection then proceeds with the most meticulous care to avoid rupture of the cyst or injury to the blood supply of the skin flap. The cyst is freed from adherent tissues and dissected with its stalk to the parent synovial lining of the joint from which it extrudes.
7. A window of joint synovium is excised with the stalk and if, as is often the case, other unexpected synovial protrusions are exposed by the staining process, they too are excised (Fig. 22-17). This may necessitate elevating the extensor tendon with a blunt hook or probe to trace a dumbbell-shaped synovial protrusion beneath it to the other side of the tendon. Occasionally one or more tiny blue-stained cysts will be seen immediately under the tendon insertion on the distal phalanx. To avoid creating a mallet deformity by iatrogenic injury to the insertion, such cysts are best decompressed by needle puncture and not excised.
8. Careful resection of arthritic osteophytes (often demonstrated on one of several preoperative roentgenograms, e.g. A-P, lateral and oblique views), has been routinely recommended by some surgeons.[3]
9. Hemostasis is established with needlepoint electrocautery and tested by gentle compression of the digit.
10. The wound is closed with interrupted 5-0 and 6-0 nylon leaving the eponychium open for drainage. Occasionally a tiny skin graft is necessary. This can readily be removed from the adjacent dorsum or side of the finger with a razor blade or scalpel. It is secured by the dressing.
11. The single-layer dressing of fine mesh lubricated gauze next to the skin is covered with a layer of several thicknesses of flat, soaking-wet gauze on the dorsum only which is held in place by a sandwich of sponge plastic (Reston) followed by a padded splint for a week.

In excising these cysts, be mindful of the fact that the resection of the bone may initiate an arthritic flare which has been seen to progress to spontaneous joint fusion. Removal of the bony hump which has attenuated the extensor tendon may result in sufficient laxity to cause a mallet deformity.

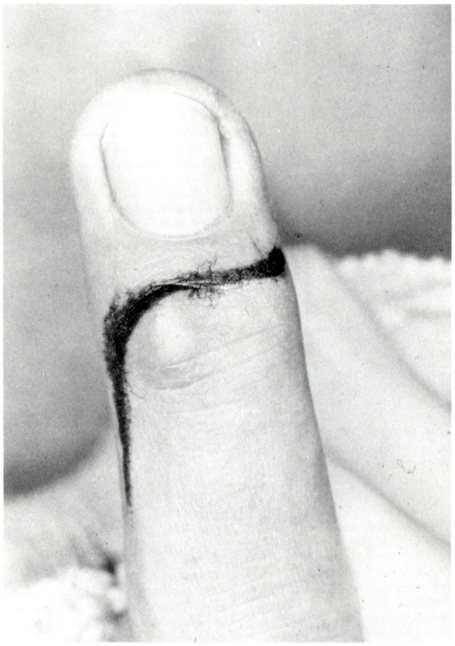

Figure 22-16. *An L-shaped incision is used for exposing the distal interphalangeal joint in removing a ganglion in this area.*

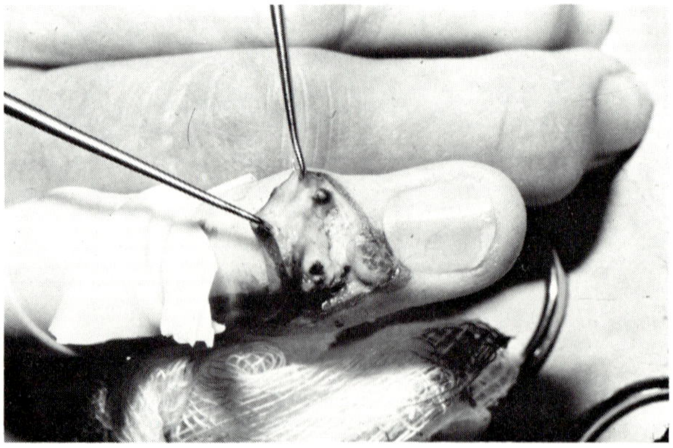

Figure 22-17. *The injection of the joint with methylene blue outlines daughter cysts that can be removed at the time of the excision of the symptomatic mucous cyst.*

SYNOVITIS

Synovitis manifests itself primarily as a pseudotumor about the dorsum of the wrist where the extensor tendon synovium is involved in a nonspecific, rheumatoid, or infectious (e.g. tuberculous) tenosynovitis. The tumefaction is usually that of the anatomical configuration of the extensor bursa. It may involve any one of the six extensor compartments, or all of them. There is often an hourglass appearance by virtue of the extensor retinaculum (non-specific synovitis—Chap. 8; infectious synovitis—Chap. 20; rheumatoid synovitis—Chap. 24) (Fig. 14-19).

KNUCKLE BURSA

This cystic swelling overlies the dorsum of the metacarpophalangeal or proximal interphalangeal joint and is invariably chronic, often with intermittent draining. The area is covered with skin thickened by underlying post-traumatic scar. Such cysts may occur following a laceration but sometimes result only from blunt trauma. They seldom become infected and may be resistant to spontaneous closure once drainage has begun. If chronic and troublesome to the patient, resection of the thick skin and closure without tension are usually successful. Sometimes an advancement or rotation flap is necessary. The extensor tendon constitutes the floor of this lesion and should not be disturbed. Injection with triamcinolone has not seemed to influence its resolution.

Tendon

TENDON STUMP AND CALLUS

Tendons present two common forms of pseudotumors. One is simply the tendon stump itself, which is most often palpable as a lump in the case of divided and retracted tendons on the dorsum of the hand or in the distal third of the forearm (both volar and dorsal aspects). Retracted stumps often are surrounded by a pouch of fluid which probably represents a liquefied hematoma. If the diagnosis is certain, no treatment other than reassurance is necessary.

Any injured tendon heals with callus formation. The added tendon bulk may be mistaken for tumor of other etiology. No specific treatment is necessary. In most instances, time will bring about a molding of the callus with reduction in its size.

RHEUMATOID NODULE

The substance of tendons is frequently involved in a rheumatoid degenerative process. This may or may not be in continuity with extensive synovial thickening from the same disease. Grossly the nodule lacks the typical color characteristics and strength of tendon. It may be white, grayish or light brown in color. The nodules are particularly symptomatic when they block excursion of a tendon through a tendon sheath. Occasionally the nodule is specifically confined to that part of the tendon which must pass under a tendon pulley and a triggering phenomenon ensues. Treatment is usually a combination of reducing the size of the nodule and sectioning of any restricting portion of the pulley.

TENDON CYST

On rare occasions a nodule is felt in a tendon, which on exploration turns out to be a cyst containing clear, serous fluid. The etiology is obscure, but trauma such as a needle injection is usually suspected and seems quite plausible. Treatment is only on demand by the patient and consists of exploration and decompression of the cyst without compromising the integrity of tendon continuity and strength. A #11 scalpel blade may be used to slit the tendon.

Bone

HEBERDEN'S NODES

These nodules occur about the distal interphalangeal joints in osteoarthritis and are most common in postmenopausal women. They are fusiform or knobby enlargements which are frequently painless (Fig. 22-18). At first there is no gross bony abnormality and the tumefaction is caused by mucoid degeneration of periarticular soft tissues. With time there is hypertrophic osseous lipping at the margins of the cartilage which can be identified radiologically. The process may be associated with mucous cysts and subsequent total destruction of the joint with secondary stiffness and angulations. There is no specific treatment to reduce the mass. In rare instances, for reasons of pain and cosmetic deformity, the distal joints have been fused and the bulky dorsal tissues reduced in size.

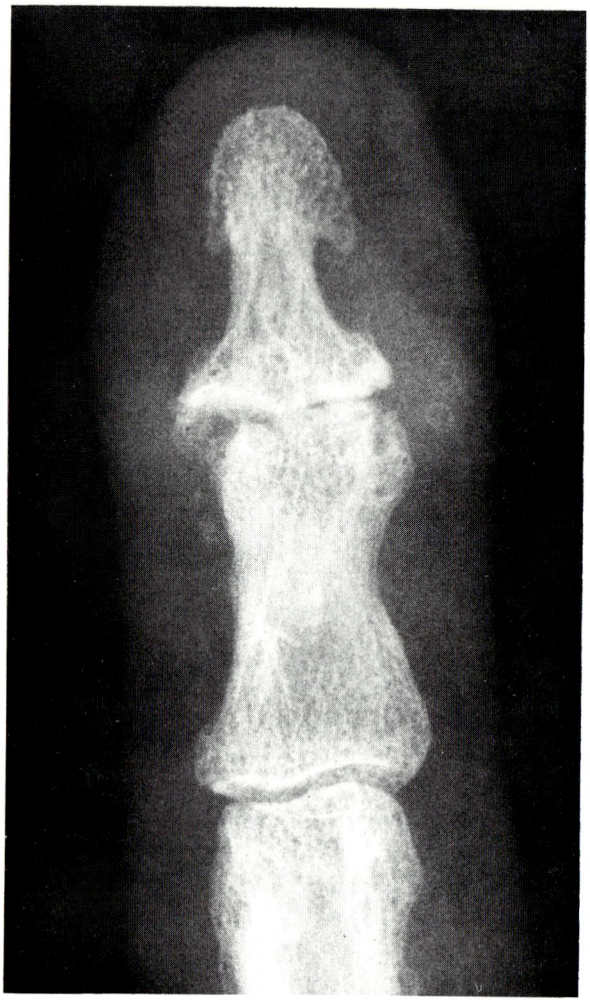

Figure 22-18. *This middle-aged woman had extensive osteoarthritic changes of her distal interphalangeal joints with large Heberden's nodes.*

EXOSTOSIS AND CALLUS

These are most commonly the result of callus formation or incompletely reduced fractures. They may be symptomatic if they serve as pressure points on the skin or a sensory nerve and may cause motor paralysis if they press on a motor nerve. Occasionally they are the sites of adherence or fraying of tendons. Treatment is justified for any of these reasons and consists of resection with an osteotome or rongeur.

MULTIPLE HEREDITARY EXOSTOSIS

This problem consists of an abnormality of the growth of the epiphyseal plate and the remodeling in that region. An increased dimension results in the metaphysis. The process frequently involves the forearm and as a consequence there is shortening of the distal end of the ulna and bowing of the radius (Madelung's deformity). There has been a high incidence of chondrosarcoma in these patients.

Treatment is unnecessary unless there is evidence of rapid change in size or a functional complication caused by encroachment of the exostosis on other tissues.

BONE CYST (SOLITARY)

This is an exceedingly rare lesion of the hand which tends to occur in the metacarpal and proximal phalanges. The cysts may replace the medullary cavity. There is a tendency to eccentricity of the cyst to one side or the other. These cysts are distinguished from the cysts of hyperparathyroidism which are generalized and not confined to the hand. They develop insidiously in youth, are unicameral and are frequently confused with enchondroma. They generally contain some yellow fluid without a clear-cut membrane around it. The treatment is dictated by size, deformity, and any symptoms (e.g. often a pathological fracture). It consists of curettage of the cavity and packing with a bone graft.

Muscle

Pseudotumors of muscle consist of post-traumatic hematomas, hypertrophy or congenital duplication. A hematoma is not usually a matter of diagnostic confusion inasmuch as there is usually a history of violence or puncture of the area. The most common circumstances which present a possibility of tumor are those of specific muscle hypertrophy in response to a patient's habits of effort or the existence of a congenital anomaly. The former can involve any muscle or group of muscles, e.g. hypertrophy of the flexor carpi ulnaris in the distal third of the forearm (Fig. 22-19). Congenital anomalies most commonly involve variations of the palmaris longus or the presence of any extensor brevis muscle on the dorsum of the hand.

Vessels

Pseudotumors of blood vessels are infrequent; however, occasionally a small, dark, firm mass is seen in a fat pad of the hand, e.g. the proximal phalanx, which is mobile and asymptomatic. At

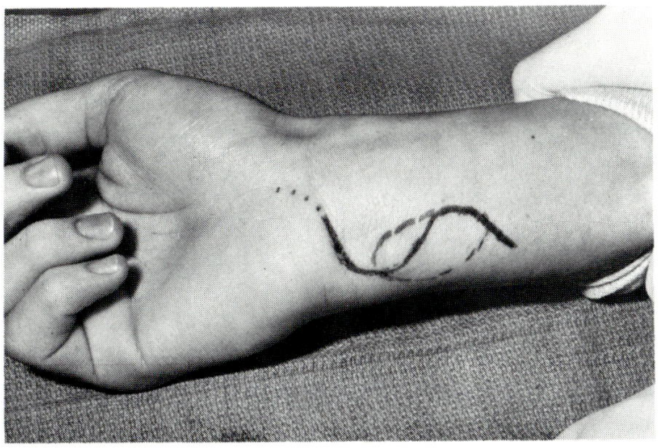

Figure 22-19. *A 24-year-old medical student, an avid weight lifter, had a large mass near the ulnar volar border of the wrist which, upon exploration, was found to be hypertrophied flexor carpi ulnaris muscle.*

operation it is a typical varix which may be partially or totally thrombosed and is easily removed and ligated from its parent veins. There is no recognized precipitating factor. Such lesions appear most commonly after the fourth decade (Fig. 22-20).

Aneurysms (Chap. 10) are usually easily diagnosed by physical findings of a pulsatile mass and a concomitant bruit (Fig. 22-21). They invariably follow an injury. Their location may be anywhere along the arterial system of the forearm, wrist and hand. Treatment is resection with or without an anastomosis or graft. The procedure is dictated by the status of collateral blood flow, which can be determined by the Allen's test or angiography.

Nerve

Pseudotumors of nerves are neuromas. These may be in continuity or on a nerve stump (Fig. 22-22). They may be asymptomatic or symptomatically crippling. They are caused by trauma, and their treatment depends on the symptoms they cause (Chap. 15).

Benign Tumors

Skin

NEVUS

A variety of discrete pigmentations are found on the hand and upper extremity, most of which are not strictly tumors and have no propensity to become malignant. The suspicion of malignancy in any of these lesions is raised only by an alteration in its size, color, elevation or ulceration of its surface (Fig. 22-23). If this occurs, a biopsy (preferably excisional) should be undertaken and an irrefutable diagnosis obtained histologically. Most excisions of pigmented lesions are done for cosmetic improvement (Chap. 7).

KERATOSES

Seborrheic Keratosis (*senile wart or basal cell papilloma*). This benign raised verrucoid lesion has a greasy feel and is asymptomatic (Fig. 22-24). It is plaque-like, light to dark brown in color, and varies greatly in size. It is entirely epidermal in origin and can be easily scraped from the surface of the skin with adequate local anesthesia. This lesion can become deeply pigmented and suggest a melanoma. Histologically it can sometimes be confused with basal cell carcinoma. It has no malignant potential.

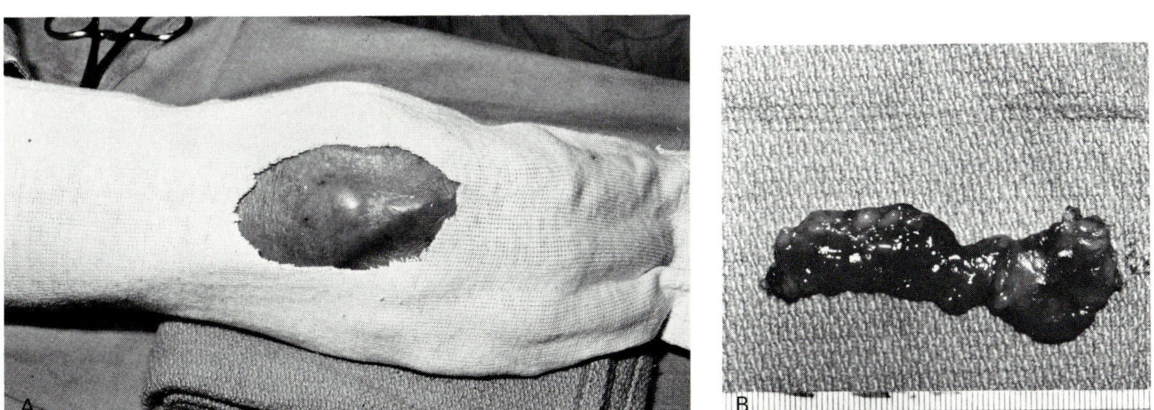

Figure 22-20. *This middle-aged woman had sustained minor trauma to the dorsum of her hand, resulting in the appearance of a hard nodule, which on resection was found to be a thrombosed varix.*

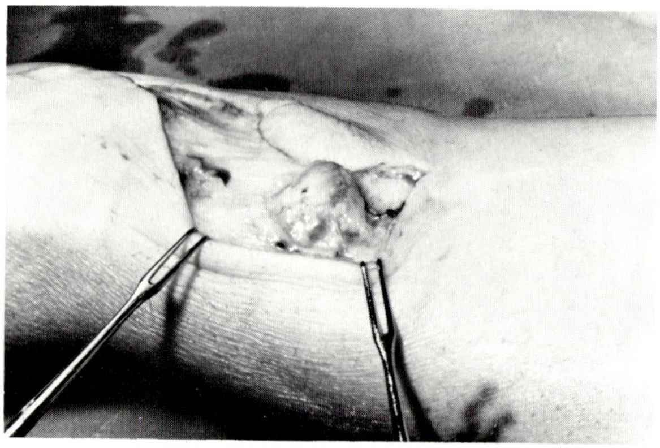

Figure 22-21. *This middle-aged white male had a minor injury to his wrist while skiing. Subsequently, he developed a slightly painful nodule in the area of the radial carpal joint which, upon exploration, was found to be an aneurysm of the radial artery.*

Senile Keratosis (*actinic keratosis*). This keratosis is a premalignant lesion of the fair skinned and occurs in areas of great exposure to the sun (dorsum of the hand). It is generally seen in the elderly and responds to topical treatment with 5-fluorouracil (Chap. 7).

SUBEPIDERMAL NODULAR FIBROSIS (DERMATOFIBROMA)

This benign tumor arises from the corium and represents a fibrous proliferation in response to minor trauma (e.g. an insect bite or hair follicle injury). It is usually pigmented (reddish or yellowish) and appears as a raised, firm nodule which is generally less than 1 cm in diameter (Fig. 22-25). The usual reason for removal is to establish the diagnosis and reassure the patient.

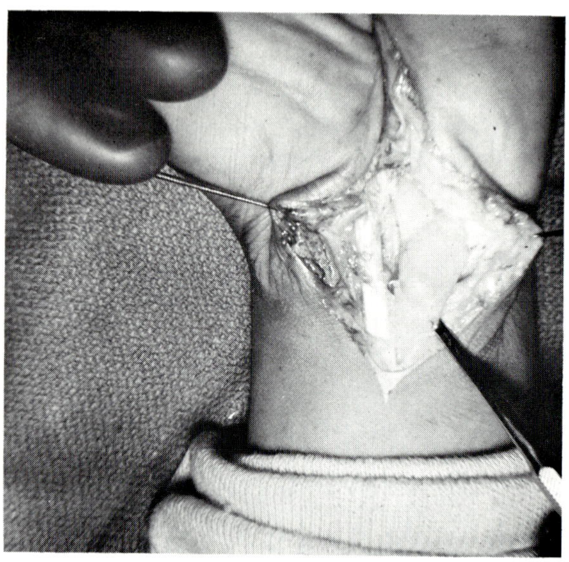

Figure 22-22. *Three years previously this male was wounded over the volar aspect of the wrist and a slightly tender firm mass appeared. Exploration of the wrist showed a neuroma in continuity with the median nerve.*

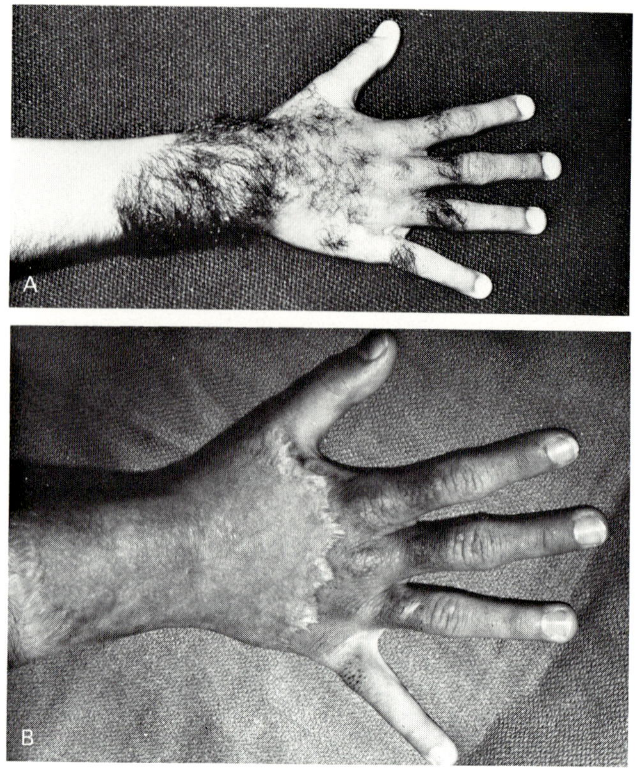

Figure 22-23. *This young girl was born with a pigmented hairy nevus of the dorsum of the hand which was excised in stages and replaced with thick split-thickness skin grafts from the buttock area.*

KERATOACANTHOMA

This benign lesion arises from the hair-bearing skin and grows with alarming rapidity (Fig. 22-26). It is an exophytic lesion which has a keratin plug overlying an area of acanthosis. Grossly it may cause fear of squamous cell carcinoma. Microscopically it shows no anaplasia even though mitotic figures are present.

The lesion generally reaches its maximum size (1 to 3 cm in diameter) in 4 to 6 weeks. After an additional 4 to 6 weeks, it begins to involute spontaneously. In 3 to 4 months from inception it disappears, leaving a slightly depressed and depigmented scar. Squamous cell carcinoma can be associated with this lesion so excision is the preferred treatment.

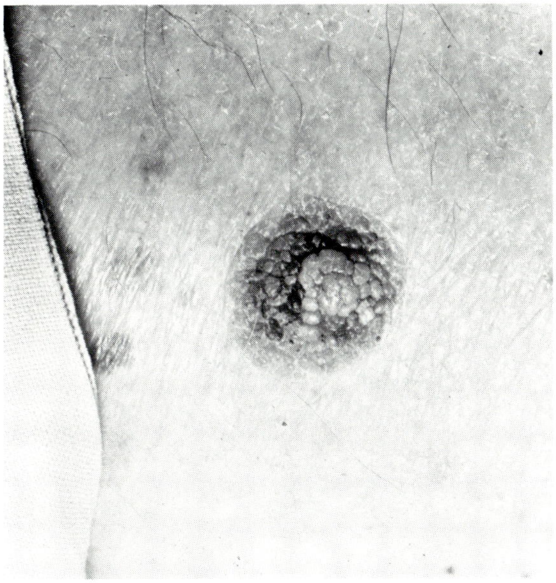

Figure 22-24. *This elderly white male had a waxy verrucoid lesion on the dorsum of the hand which he had removed for cosmetic purposes. The diagnosis was seborrheic keratosis.*

Fat

Lipoma is a benign tumor like any lipoma elsewhere and is found most commonly on the volar aspect of the hand (Fig. 22-27). The lesion is easily separated from the tissue around it unless it is intertwined around nerves and vessels. It is asymptomatic unless by its expansion it creates pressure on nerves. Excision should not be considered a simple problem until the lesion has been removed without any injury to surrounding nerves or vessels.

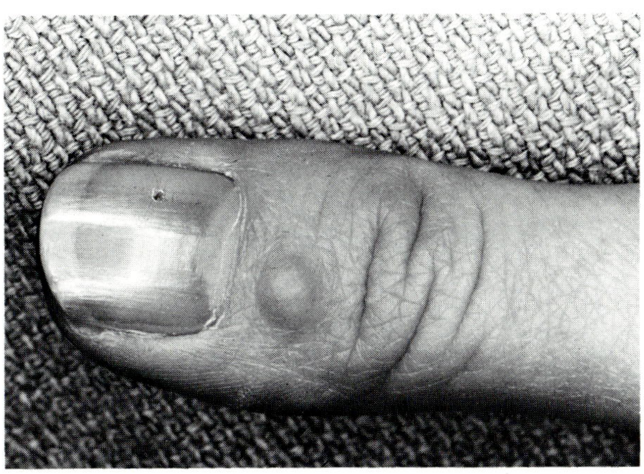

Figure 22-25. *This 30-year-old secretary had a firm nodule over the dorsal distal interphalangeal joint, with furrowing of the nail. Excision revealed a subepidermal nodular fibrosis.*

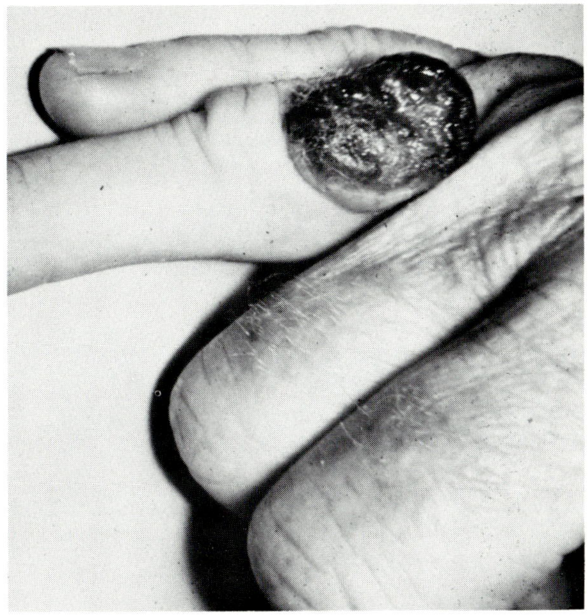

Figure 22-26. *This 50-year-old white female had sustained minor injury to the dorsum of her ring finger when she stuck herself with a rose thorn. The lesion enlarged rapidly over a 6-week period. Excision and skin grafting were carried out. The final diagnosis was keratoacanthoma.*

Fascia

FIBROMA

Rarely seen in the hand, these well-encapsulated, dense, fibrous tissue tumors occur on either the palmar or dorsal aspects of the fingers (Fig. 22-28). They must be differentiated clinically from ganglia, neurogenic tumors and epidermoid cysts. Bone or cartilage may be present within them. Complete surgical excision offers an excellent prognosis and recurrences should suggest the possibility of sarcomatous change.

GIANT CELL TUMOR

A giant cell tumor is a benign encapsulated tumor of unknown etiology resembling a xanthoma (Fig. 22-29). It arises from the white tissue of the hand, most commonly from the tendon sheath or collateral ligament but from the joint synovium as well (giant cell synovioma). It may also arise from fascia or bone. Whether or not trauma has any role in its etiology is debatable.

The clinical features of giant cell tumor are its firmness and its fixation to the deep fibrous structures from which it arises. The skin moves freely

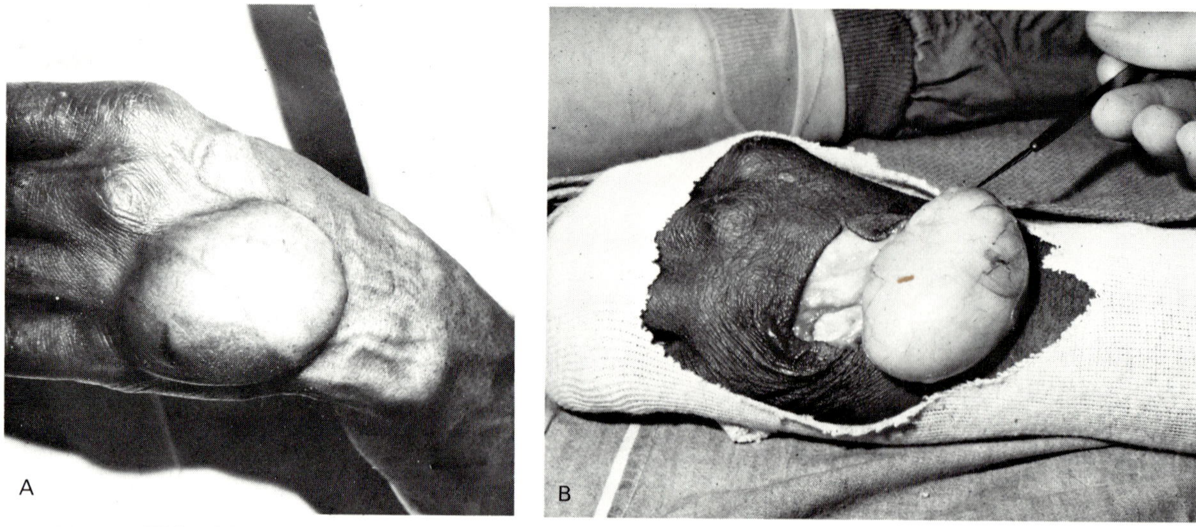

Figure 22-27. *This elderly female had a rubbery mass on the dorsum of her hand for many years. It was found to be a lipoma.*

over it. It is differentiated from a ganglion in that it does not transilluminate and does not yield fluid on aspiration.

The tumor occurs over a wide age span and, if not removed, may reach considerable size and extend widely into any part of the hand. It is most common on the volar and lateral aspects of digits. Its insidious growth allows it to extend between tissue planes and through narrow "windows" between anatomical structures. It may, for example, extend under the terminal tendon in a dumbbell fashion and enter the distal joint through a small space between the collateral ligament and the extensor tendon.

Giant cell tumors have a brown-yellow color and a fibrous consistency. The color facilitates its identification and the fibrous quality permits the surgeon to grasp it with a hook and apply considerable tension during dissection. The tumor is not invasive and a good plane is always obtainable between it and the surrounding tissues. The surface is multilobulated and frequently contains a nerve or artery which the tumor has displaced. The tumor is asymptomatic and usually does not impair function until it is of considerable size.

Unless it is completely removed it will recur. Therefore, meticulous dissection is essential. All of the brown-yellow tissue must be removed.

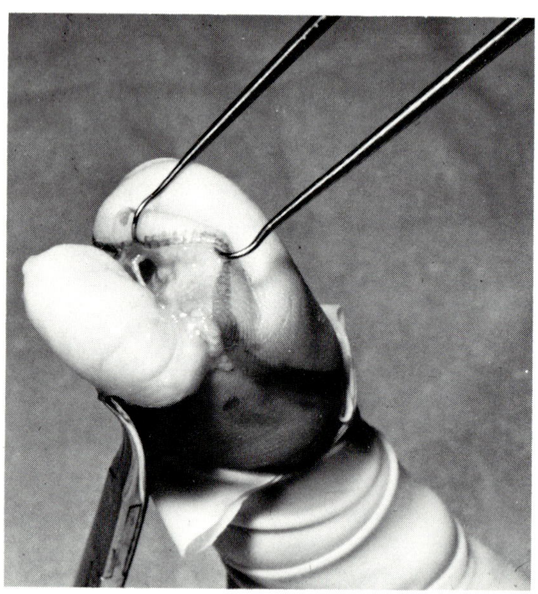

Figure 22-28. *This 26-year-old schoolteacher had a firm nodule within the distal fat pad of the thumb that was moderately tender on pressure. It proved to be a fibroma.*

XANTHOMAS

Previously, giant cell tumors and xanthomata were considered to be the same. Xanthomata are not strictly neoplasms and are associated with an increase in serum cholesterol. They tend to infiltrate widely, unlike giant cell tumors, which are encapsulated. Their removal is indicated only for cosmesis. Since the underlying metabolic disorder is not altered, recurrences are frequent.

JOINT GIANT CELL SYNOVIOMA

See *Giant Cell Tumor of Fascia* for discussion.

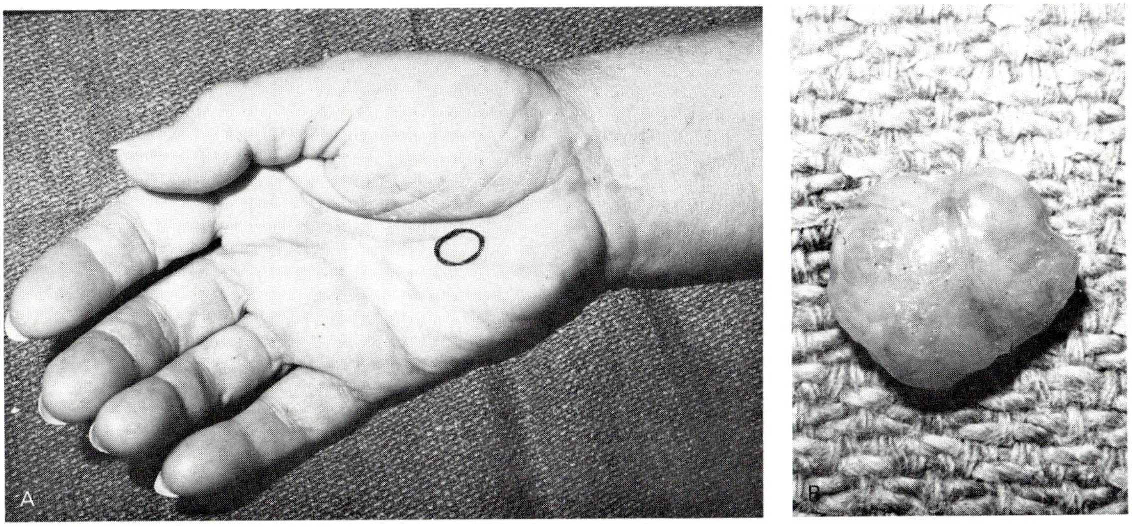

Figure 22-29. *This middle-aged white male had a slightly painful, hard mass in the hypothenar area of the palm for several years which gradually enlarged. Upon resection, it was found to be a giant cell tumor. No recurrence was noted.*

Bone

ENCHONDROMA

Ninety per cent of bone tumors of the hand are either solitary (Fig. 22-30) or multiple enchondromata (Ollier's disease). Most often their presence is recognized as the result of a pathological fracture; less commonly they are found serendipitously on roentgenograms taken for some other reason. The single lesions are usually found in the proximal phalanx with either the middle phalanx or the metacarpal as the next most frequent sites. Carpal bone involvement does not occur. The multiple enchondroma may be accompanied by multiple hemangiomas of the skin (Maffucci's syndrome).

The roentgenographic appearance of an enchondroma is characteristic. The lesion is usually eccentrically located with a margin of thinned sclerotic bone over it. Often tiny patches of calcified stippling are present within the central lytic area.

The surgical approach to the lesion should spare any dissection of the extensor or flexor tendons lest they adhere to the operative site in the bone. Hence, an incision on the lateral aspect of the metacarpal or phalanges is preferred in order that the tendon will be away from the osteotomy site. The window in the bone can be made with a drill or tiny osteotome. It should be just big enough to admit a small curette. The lesion has a cyst wall which is removed along with all the fibrocartilaginous debris. An incision in the forearm is then made over the olecranon and a small fragment of cortical bone is taken. This is cut into minute pieces with which the curetted bone space is packed. The wounds are then closed. A pathological fracture can be treated primarily in the same way providing it is not compound. The immobilization is in the position of function for at least 4 weeks. It may, however, take at least 4 to 6 months before the patient has enough active range of motion with strength to return to work.

OSTEOCHONDROMA (ECCHONDROMA)

These are the second most common tumors involving the bones of the hand (Fig. 22-30**A**). Their distribution is similar to enchondromata and they are usually detected by the patient as a prominence on a phalanx. The roentgenogram may demonstrate the common pedunculated projection or the rarer sessile protrusion. These outgrowths begin within the perichondrium and periosteum at the metaphyseal end of a bony shaft next to the epiphyseal plate. They are frequently noted in childhood, especially if the lesion produces pain with forceful use of the hand.

As these lesions occur in areas that may either limit function or cause pain, their excision may be indicated. Removal requires the resection of the surrounding periosteum and sufficient bone to minimize the chance of recurrence.

OSTEOID OSTEOMA

Osteoid osteoma is a painful benign tumor which usually occurs between the ages of 10 and 30 and

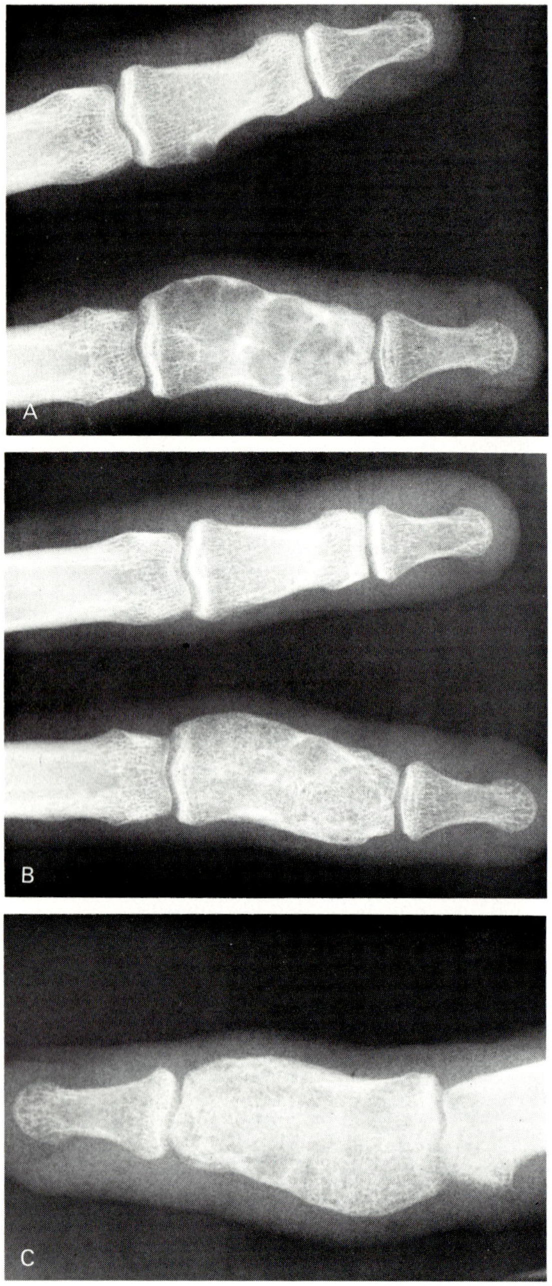

Figure 22-30. *This young white male suffered a pathologic fracture of the middle phalanx of the long finger during a basketball game. Roentgenograms revealed an enchondroma of that phalanx and an ecchondroma* **(A)** *of the adjacent middle phalanx. Following curettement of the fractured middle phalanx and packing with bone chips, remolding of the bone occurred* **(B,C)**.

involves primarily the proximal phalanx and metacarpal but may involve any bone of the hand.[1] The swelling, pain and increased heat suggest an infectious process. Relief of the pain, which is worse nocturnally, is usually achieved by aspirin. A roentgenogram reveals a lytic area surrounded by sclerotic bone. If this lytic area is in cortical bone, then there may be a pathognomonic central sclerotic spot (nidus) of osteoid and new bone surrounded by a clear halo which in turn is ringed by sclerotic bone. The treatment is excision or curettement of the lesion and packing with tiny chips of cortical bone, which brings prompt relief of the pain.

ANEURYSMAL BONE CYST AND GIANT CELL TUMOR OF BONE

Based on today's interpretation and classification, aneurysmal bone cyst is more common in the hand than the giant cell tumor of bone, with which it was confused for many years. Both lesions have the same history, findings and treatment. Often there is a history of minor trauma followed by rapid enlargement of the metacarpal or proximal phalanx. Roentgenograms reveal a greatly expanded, thinned cortex with a lacy network throughout the cyst.

The aneursymal bone cyst is exceedingly vascular and very soft, unlike the giant cell tumor which is firmer but equally as vascular. Biopsy of either tumor tends to produce bleeding and should be avoided. Both lesions tend to recur if the cavity is curetted insufficiently. The evacuated space is packed with bone chips after the lesion has been removed. A recurrence of the aneurysmal bone cyst may be treated by a low dose of roentgenographic therapy (800 to 1,000 rads). However, recurrence of the giant cell tumor necessitates a biopsy to rule out malignant transformation.

OSTEOBLASTOMA (OSSIFYING FIBROMA)

This benign lesion is rare and found usually in the first three decades of life (Fig. 22-31). Its clinical features are pain, swelling and slight tenderness with a well-circumscribed fusiform lytic lesion of bone.[9] The differential diagnosis is enchondroma, aneurysmal bone cyst or giant cell tumor.

The treatment is resection by curetting the cavity and packing it with tiny chips of bone. The tissue is friable and vascular and can be confused with aneurysmal bone cyst and giant cell tumor of bone.

Muscle

Leiomyoma is an exceedingly rare benign tumor which probably has no malignant counterpart in

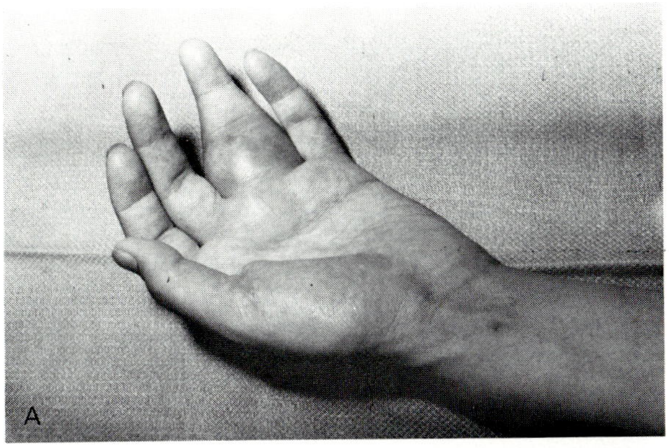

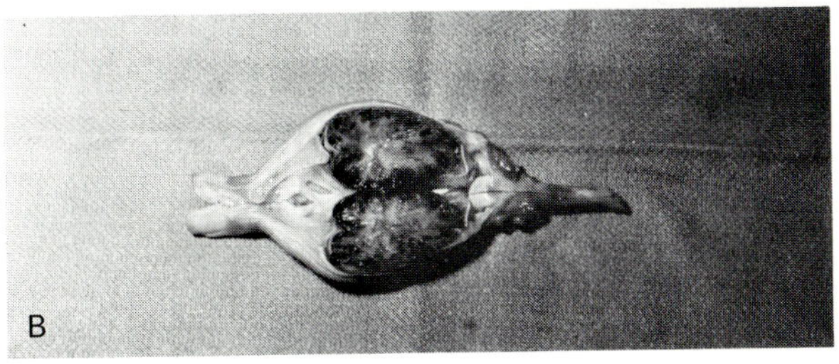

Figure 22-31. *This man developed a tender, swollen lesion of the finger with accompanying warmth. Roentgenograms were suggestive of an osteoblastoma and amputation of the finger verified this impression.*

the hand. It arises from smooth muscle of other than arterial origin. The few cases seen in the hand have been on the dorsum. The muscle cells are mature and the tumor responds to palpation or to cold by contracting into a hard knot that can be painful. The treatment is resection. The histopathology may resemble that of a venous angioma.

Vessels

HEMANGIOMA

Morris and Owsley[11] have classified hemangiomas into involuting and non-involuting types. The involuting hemangiomas are superficial or deep or a combination of the two. The non-involuting hemangiomas are port-wine stain, cavernous hemangioma, venous racemose aneurysm and arteriovenous fistula.

The involuting hemangiomata have been referred to as strawberry, nevus vasculosis, and capillary hemangioma (all superficial hemangiomata), strawberry nevus, capillary hemangioma, capillary and cavernous hemangioma (superficial and deep hemangiomata), and cavernous hemangioma (deep). To avoid confusion generated by the above overlapping terms, the classification of involuting and non-involuting hemangiomata is to be preferred.

The involuting hemangiomas are the most common and occur twice as frequently in girls as in boys. They appear at or shortly after birth, growing rapidly in the first 4 to 6 months. At this time involution starts and is usually complete by 6 to 7 years. The fair-skinned have a predisposition for the development of these lesions. The treatment is watchful waiting with encouragement and support of the parents. Surgical removal is rarely indicated since the residual scar following spontaneous resolution is less evident than that resulting from excision. Similarly dry ice, sclerosing solutions and radiation therapy are contraindicated for these hemangiomata.

The non-involuting hemangiomas are present at birth and untreated will persist indefinitely (Fig. 22-32). They do not have a period of rapid growth but tend to grow as the child does. Port-wine stains are never seen on the hands.

The cavernous hemangioma is a lesion that may be localized or extensive, scattered throughout the extremity. Malignant transformation is not a concern. Increased growth of this lesion can occur late in life. If the lesion is small and localized it may be surgically excised. The recurrence rate is high. For the larger lesions a compressive dressing (e.g. custom-fitted elastic gauntlet) may curtail enlargement and induce regression. This may have to be worn for several months. Prednisone, 5 mg t.i.d. for a month, may have a favorable effect with compression on diminishing the mass and symptoms of

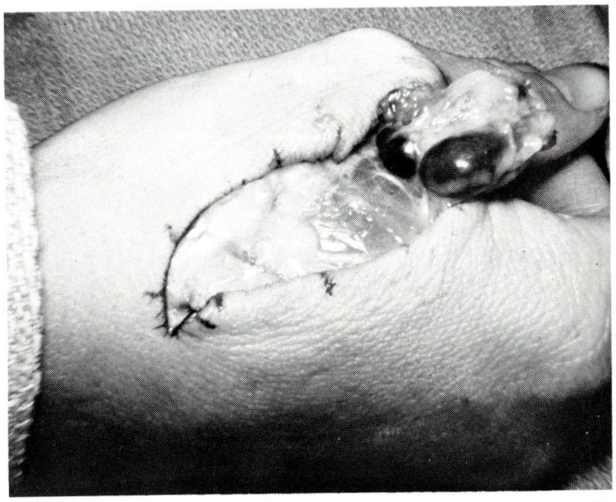

Figure 22-32. *This young woman had had a purplish discoloration of the first web space for many years. It gradually enlarged and became more uncomfortable to her. Resection revealed a cavernous hemangioma which did not recur.*

the hemangioma.[13] Surgical excision may be employed in instances of spontaneous ulceration and bleeding or excessive pain. This may be difficult if the field of dissection lies within the tumor. Preliminary angiogram is essential before extensive surgical undertaking. At times, amputation is necessary. Long-term therapy with steroids is not indicated for these lesions.

THE VENOUS RACEMOSE ANEURYSM

These uncommon lesions ramify throughout the involved extremity, often leading to overgrowth and deformity. When multiple arteriovenous communications exist, they are referred to as cirsoid aneurysms. At times amputation may be necessitated by the magnitude of the deformity and impending cardiac failure secondary to extensive shunting.

LYMPHANGIOMA

These lesions usually occur at birth or shortly thereafter and are manifest by the soft tissue swelling in the involved area. Simple lymphangioma is a localized lesion the treatment of which is excision. Cavernous lymphangiomata are either pure or mixed with hemangioma. Some of these are associated with congenital constrictive bands. The treatment is surgical. Prior to any attempt at resection of lymphangiomatous tissue that exists in the presence of a congenital band, the band should be eliminated by a Z-plasty. This relief of congestion may be the prime means of reducing the lymphedema. In some instances it is necessary to remove the skin with the tumor and subsequently graft the wound. The original skin may be used for this, following defatting.

An elastic gauntlet similar to that used for treating cavernous hemangiomas may be useful in the management of certain of these lesions.

GLOMUS TUMOR

A glomus tumor is a rare benign tumor arising from the normal arteriovenous anastomosis called the neuromyoarterial canal system of Sucquet-Hoyer (Fig. 22-33). The specific characteristic is the marked pain initiated by stimulation of the tumor with pressure at a precise trigger point. The tumor can occur in many areas, but is most symptomatic and incapacitating when it lies under the nail because of the absence of any surrounding padding.

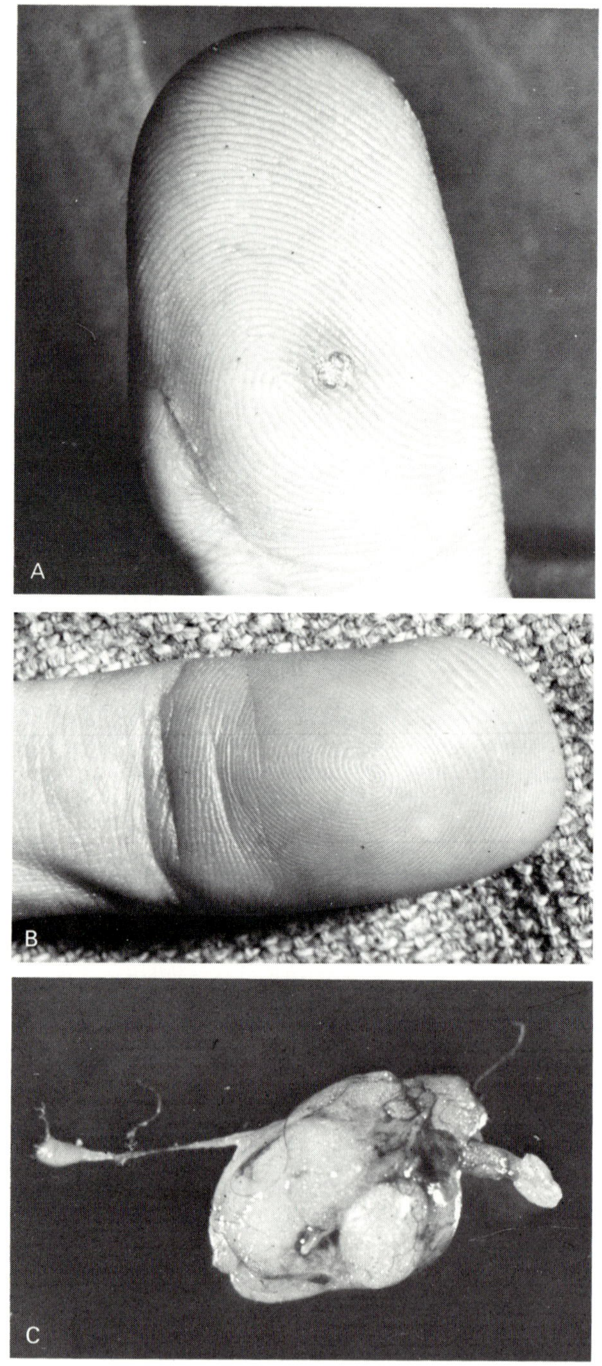

Figure 22-33A. *A young microbiologist had this painful lesion of the volar aspect of the thumb for several months. Excision revealed a glomus tumor.* **B,C.** *A young white male had a firm, tender nodule of the volar aspect of the thumb for approximately 1 year. It had gradually enlarged in size and increased in discomfort. Cross section of the resected speciman reveals the characteristic gross appearance of a glomus tumor.*

Here the pain may be excruciating. The distal phalanx may be scalloped because of pressure of the tumor.

At times this tumor is no more than 2 mm in

diameter. Its presence is suspected by the extent of pain at a trigger point anywhere on the hand when other causes of such pain are not likely (e.g. retained foreign body, neuroma, etc.).

The treatment is surgical. A bloodless field and magnification are imperative. When the tumor is subungual, the whole nail should be removed first and then a flap of nail bed elevated from the surface of the tumor, which is easily enucleated. The nail bed can then be sutured back in place and the sutures tied over a dressing for additional hemostasis if there is scalloping of the bone. A dressing and cast are applied for a week. Recurrences probably do not follow complete resection but possibly may occur if the resection is incomplete.

Nerves

NEUROFIBROMA

As an isloated tumor, a neurofibroma may be solitary or multiple. It involves a proliferation of the Schwann cells and is in continuity with peripheral nerves. When multiple, it may be part of the syndrome of von Recklinghausen's disease. The treatment is enucleation of the neurofibroma from normal funiculi if the tumor is in continuity with the major peripheral nerves, or total resection if it arises from a terminal trunk. The reason for treatment is generally dictated by the functional effect of the tumor or its cosmetic impact rather than by any symptomatology.

The functional impairment may be due to the bulk of the tumor compressing the nerve and causing neuropraxia or interfering with the normal capacity of the hand to grasp. There is a possibility of malignant degeneration in the tumors associated with von Recklinghausen's disease. The clue to this is the rapid increased growth of a mass. In this instance, a wide resection is necessary.

A variant of this group of tumors is neurolipofibromatosis. This involves a major nerve trunk, e.g. median or ulnar or both, over a considerable length of the nerve as well as some or all of its terminal branches. Tumefaction results in soft tissue enlargement throughout the course of the disease. Macrodactyly is seen[4] (Chap. 23). Pain is common and ranges from minimal dysesthesia to marked discomfort. In addition there may be paresis or palsy of motor or sensory function. The treatment is expectant and predicated on the need for decompression of the nerve within an anatomical tunnel. At times resection of the nerve and amputation of a macrodactylous digit or even the whole hand are necessary.

NEURILEMMOMA (SCHWANNOMA)

These small encapsulated benign tumors occur along the course of peripheral nerves (Fig. 22-34). They may be within the substance of a larger nerve rather than on the sheath. They occur with equal frequency in both sexes and at all ages. Usually symptoms result from the compression of the nerve and the tumor together against the phalanx, with dysesthesia or pain. Removal should be done with care, avoiding injury to the associated nerve.

Malignant Tumors

Skin

BOWEN'S DISEASE (CARCINOMA IN SITU)

See Chapter 7 for discussion.

BASAL CELL CARCINOMA (BASAL CELL EPITHELIOMA)

See Chapter 7 for discussion.

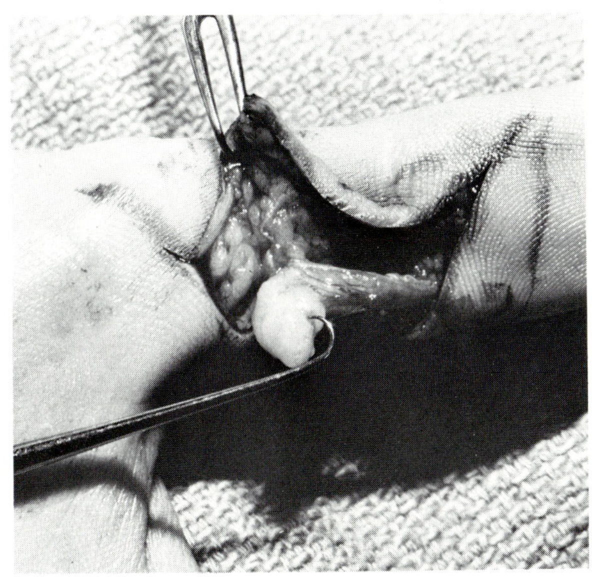

Figure 22-34. *This young female hospital attendant had multiple nodules within the distal and proximal phalangeal areas of the thumb. Upon removal, they were found to be associated with the distal nerves and were diagnosed microscopically as neurilemmoma.*

SQUAMOUS CELL CARCINOMA

This malignancy occurs most commonly on the dorsum of the hand where it results from chronic exposure to the actinic rays of the sun (Fig. 22-35). In the past, before the correlation was appreciated, exposure to roentgen rays by physicians, dentists and technicians and overexposure of patients in the treatment of warts and other skin disorders frequently led to this tumor. The carcinoma is of low-grade malignancy except when it arises in preexisting scars, burns, chronic ulcers, lupus erythematosus and poikiloderma.

The treatment in instances of carcinoma resulting from actinic exposure is local excision with an adequate cutaneous margin (1.0 cm). When the tumor is fixed to the underlying structures the resection has to include these and the depth will be governed by the histological and operative findings. Some form of reconstructive hand surgery is usually necessary under these circumstances (e.g. ray resection) (Fig. 22-36).

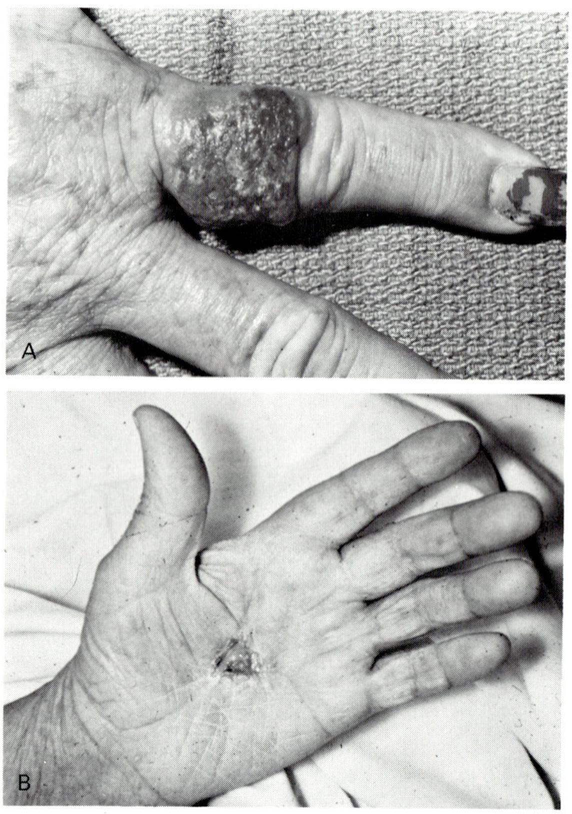

Figure 22-35A. *This 50-year-old white female had an ulcerated lesion on the dorsum of the index finger which was fixed to the bone and the underlying tendon. Biopsy revealed a squamous cell carcinoma.* **B.** *This elderly black female had an ulcerated lesion of the central palm for several years. Biopsy revealed a squamous cell carcinoma which was treated with radiation therapy. She eventually succumbed to rupture of the subclavian artery from massive necrosis of axillary and superclavicular nodal metastases.*

In the aggressive malignancies, surgery must be more radical locally. For squamous cell carcinoma regional lymph node dissection is indicated when nodes are palpable in the axilla and there is no evidence of distant metastasis. If the primary lesion is greater than 2.5 cm in diameter or fixed to the deeper tissues, a "prophylactic" lymph node dissection should be considered even in the absence of palpable nodes.

MELANOMA (CHAP. 7)

This uncommon lesion may occur anywhere on the hand but may appear about the fingernail and be mistaken for an infection (Hutchinson's melanotic whitlow) (Fig. 22-37). A history of trauma is often given but undoubtedly has no etiological bearing. Pain does not predominate but the fingernail may separate from its bed and crack. Disfigurement is often the only force compelling the patient to see a doctor, and by then the lesion may be exophytic and ulcerating.

There are three types of melanoma: lentigo maligna, superficial spreading and nodular. The first is a disease of the elderly, often reflected by changes in a mole of long-standing duration. Most commonly this is found on the face and only rarely may involve the dorsum of the hand or forearm. In the absence of deep invasion by this lesion, local excision (3 to 4 cm cutaneous margin) is generally curative.

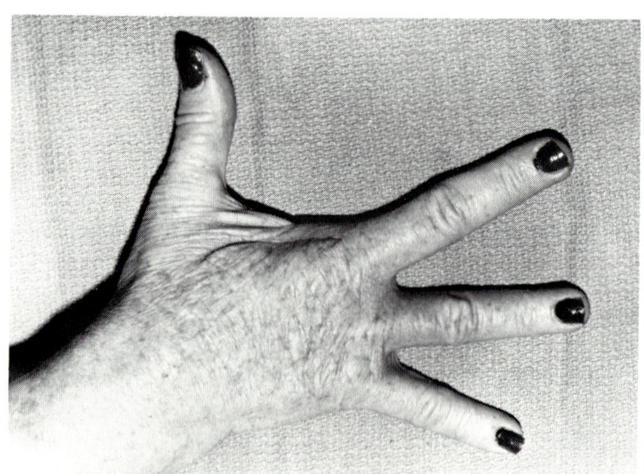

Figure 22-36. *The patient whose primary lesion was depicted in Figure 22-35A had a ray resection for removal of this fixed invasive tumor.*

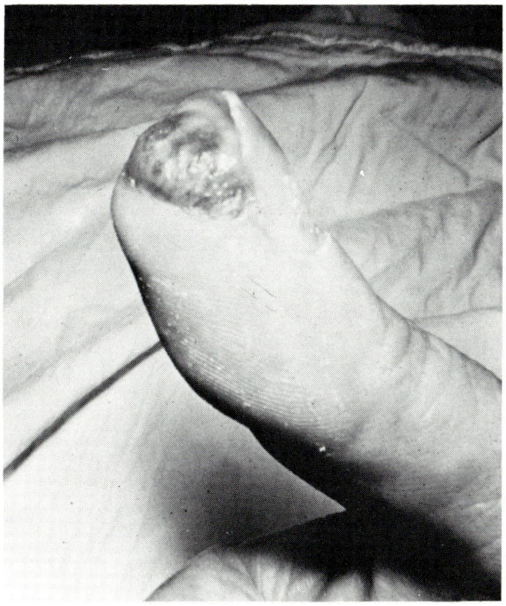

Figure 22-37. *This elderly white male had an ulcerated lesion beneath the nail of the thumb of his minor hand for several years. Biopsy revealed an amelanotic melanoma which required resection of the thumb.*

The superficial spreading melanoma also has a favorable prognosis if invasion does not occur. This lesion is limited to the superficial dermis but may develop areas of nodular melanoma within it. The wide local excision (cutaneous margin of 3 to 5 cm) of these lesions is often curative so long as there are no signs of deeper invasion of the dermis within the specimen.

Nodular melanoma is the most serious of the three. Clark has attempted to provide a prognostic and treatment-oriented classification for this type of melanoma.[2] The lesion is characterized by the level of its penetration through the dermis (Fig. 22-38). Not only can the patient's prognosis be anticipated by this histological assessment of the lesion, but a recommendation with regard to surgical treatment can be made (Table 22-3).[6,10,14] Regional node dissection (prophylactic) is advised for tumors exhibiting invasion of the dermis greater than 0.9 mm or Level III.

In all circumstances, local excision requires a wide excision (up to 5 cm from the margin of the tumor) and generally a ray amputation when the tumor arises in a digit (Fig. 22-39). For lesions on the arm and forearm, it is recommended that the deep fascia be left as a barrier when resecting the primary tumor. Regional node dissections are advised when nodal metastases are palpable and no evidence of systemic spread is found, or if the primary tumor is classified as invading to Level III or deeper.

Table 22-3. *Histologic Classification of Melanoma*

Level I	Tumor does not penetrate basement membrane
Level II	Tumor extends to the papillary dermis
Level III	Tumor extends to the interface between the papillary and reticular dermis.
Level IV	Tumor extends into the reticular dermis
Level V	Tumor extends into the subcutaneous fat

Fat

Liposarcomata are not common lesions. Often the diagnosis becomes evident only upon recurrence of a previously excised "lipoma." Surgical resection requires a bloc excision of the surrounding tissue and often risks injury to nerves and vessels. Usually the major nerves are spared unless the tumor is intimately wrapped around them. Amputation can be reserved for a later time should a second recurrence force that decision.

Fascia

FIBROSARCOMA

Fibrosarcoma is a rare tumor of the hand often manifesting itself as a superficial, slow-growing, hard fixed mass. It is capable of rapid growth from its inception and may grow to very large size, invading the skin and adjacent tissues.

Often there is a history of trauma preceding the appearance of the fibrosarcoma, but the exact etiology is not known. Hematogenous dissemination leads to the early appearance of pulmonary metastases. Lymphatic spread with regional lymph node involvement does occur. Congenital fibrosarcomas have been described. Radical excision or amputation is advised, as radiotherapy is of little value.

EPITHELIOID SARCOMA

This lesion had not been appreciated prior to 1970 when it was first described;[5] synovial sarcoma

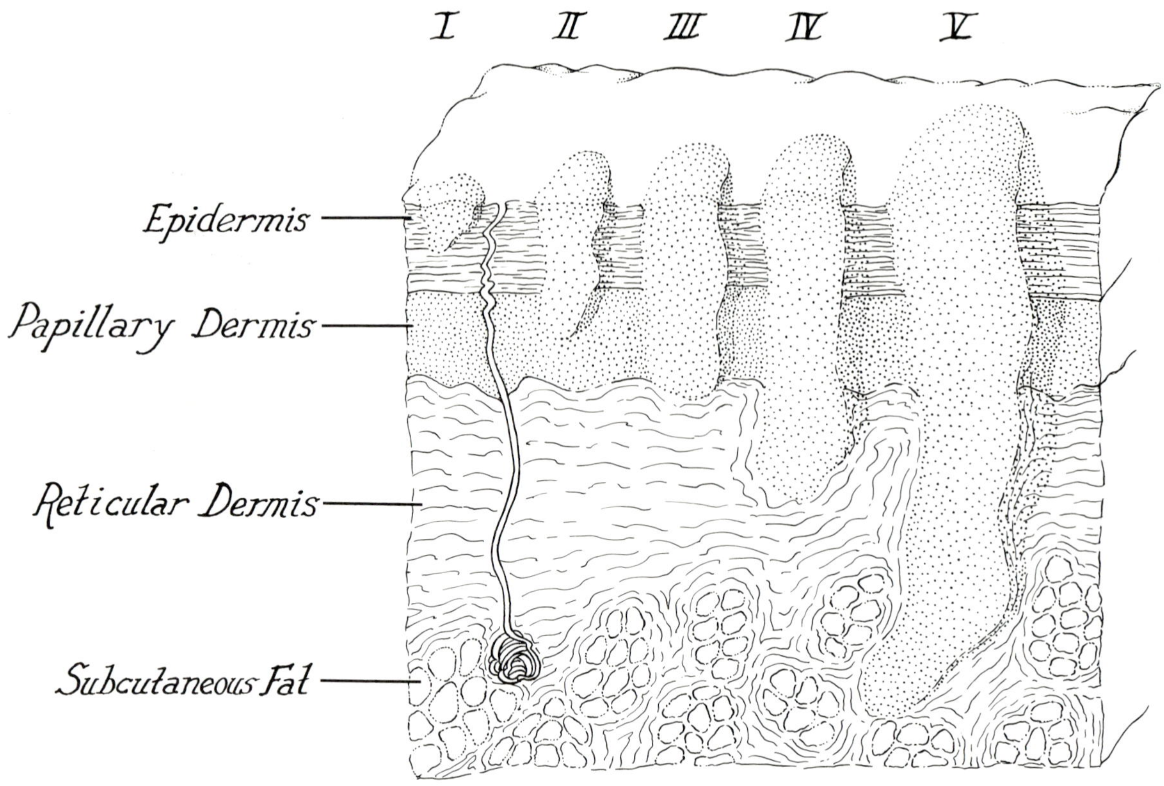

Figure 22-38. *Classification of the degree of invasion of melanoma through the dermis.* (*Redrawn from Franklin, J.D. et al.*[6])

was the most frequent diagnosis previously assigned. Most often the tumor arises as multiple hard nodules in the skin, but may originate deeper from the tendon sheath or fascia (Figs. 22-40, 22-41). Local recurrence and hematogenous spread are common. Metastases to the regional lymph nodes are also frequent.

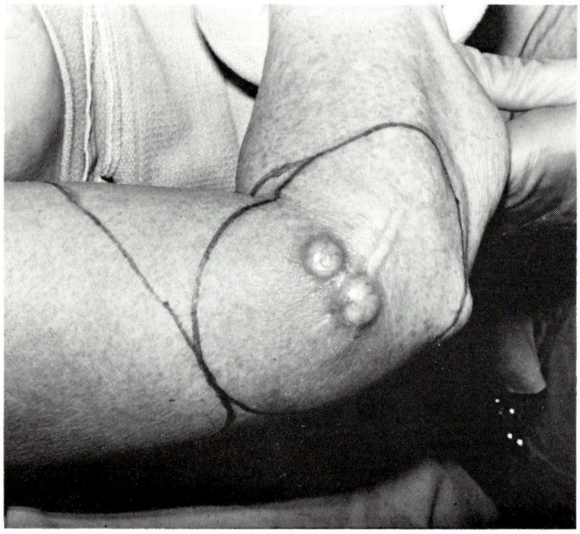

Figure 22-39. *Invasive melanoma of the elbow that had been previously inadequately treated was widely excised, with a concomitant axillary node dissection and skin graft.*

Depending upon the site of origin, wide resection or amputation may be indicated. Radiotherapy is effective in treating some local recurrences and regional metastases (Fig. 22-40**B**). Males between the ages of 20 and 30 show a higher incidence of this tumor than do females.

Joint

SYNOVIAL SARCOMA

These lesions are extremely rare in the hand and may pose great difficulty in proper diagnosis and treatment because of their slow growth, absence of symptoms and deceptively circumscribed appearance at operation. The synovial sarcoma, consisting primarily of anaplastic spindle cells, should be treated by amputation and regional node dissection. If the tumor is composed of pseudoepithelial elements and giant cells, amputation of the hand may not be necessary and a local radical excision may be adequate. A high incidence of recurrence accompanies the treatment of these lesions.

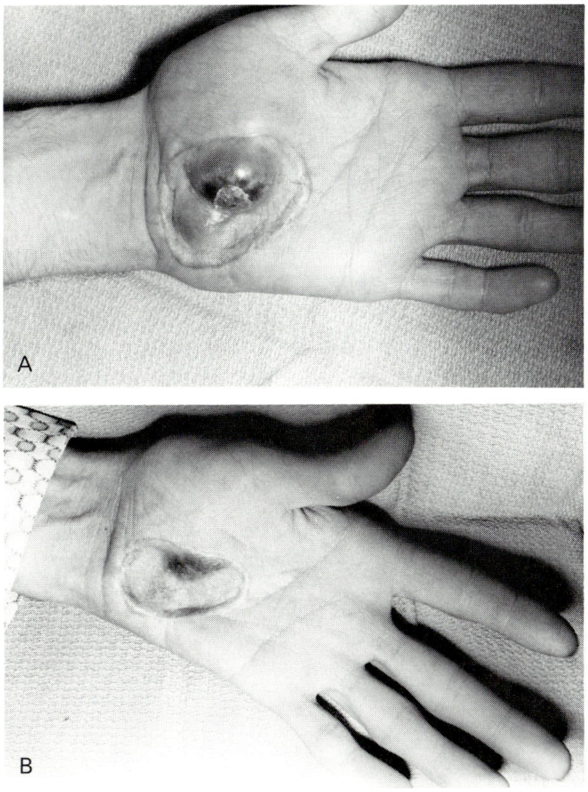

Figure 22-40. *This 26-year-old white male had had repeated resections of a lesion of the base of the palm over approximately five years. An epithelioid sarcoma was eventually diagnosed. He was treated locally with radiation therapy because of scalp metastases. Seven years after his initial operation, he succumbed to overwhelming metastases. No recurrence had developed in the radiated extremity.*

OSTEOGENIC SARCOMA

Fortunately this very malignant tumor rarely arises in the hand. It does, however, seem to have a better prognosis when it is found within the hand. The current treatment is extensive radiotherapy followed by amputation and prolonged chemotherapy.

On occasion osteogenic sarcoma will occur in the hands of individuals who have had extensive exposure to radiation in their work. It has also been reported to have metastasized to the hand.

CHONDROSARCOMA

This tumor usually arises from the periosteum or perichondrium of a chondroma, osteochondroma or enchondroma. It is rare in the hand and appears to arise more frequently from an enchondroma when multiple enchondromata exist.

The histological features of benign and malignant cartilaginous tumors are not sufficiently characteristic to make a clear-cut diagnosis without the help of the clinical findings. Therefore, it is important to note roentgenographic evidence of invasion and during surgery to observe any myxomatous softening as well as tissue invasion. These malignancies in the hand are of sufficiently low grade that a limited amputation of the involved section is usually adequate.

EWING'S TUMOR

This tumor rarely arises in the hand. It is a tumor of the medullary cavity which it involves completely. It is associated with fever, local heat and tenderness and a roentgenographic picture of erosion of bone. Sometimes the periosteum is stimulated to lay down striations of bone referred to as an "onion-skin appearance." Metastases to other bones are common.

The process is initially radiosensitive and the treatment is usually radiation therapy followed by amputation. The mortality is 95 per cent as distant metastases are often present at the time of the initial diagnosis.

METASTATIC TUMORS

The hand is a rare focus of metastasis from malignancies arising elsewhere in the body (Fig. 22-42). Virtually any tumor which spreads hematogenously can metastasize to the hand.[7] The most commonly reported are lung, breast and kidney tumors (Fig. 22-43). The phalanges and metacarpals are the usual sites, while the carpal bones and the radius and ulna are generally spared.

Although these tumors often manifest themselves in the hand when the patient has overwhelming carcinomatosis, they may occur sufficiently early in the course of the disease to require amputation or radiotherapy for relief of pain. A biopsy is necessary to establish the diagnosis.

Muscle

Rhabdomyosarcoma is a rare malignancy that seems to occur primarily in the first four decades of life (Fig. 22-44). It is highly malignant and all of the 12 patients reported by Potenza whose tumors arose in the hand died.[12] Amputation is recom-

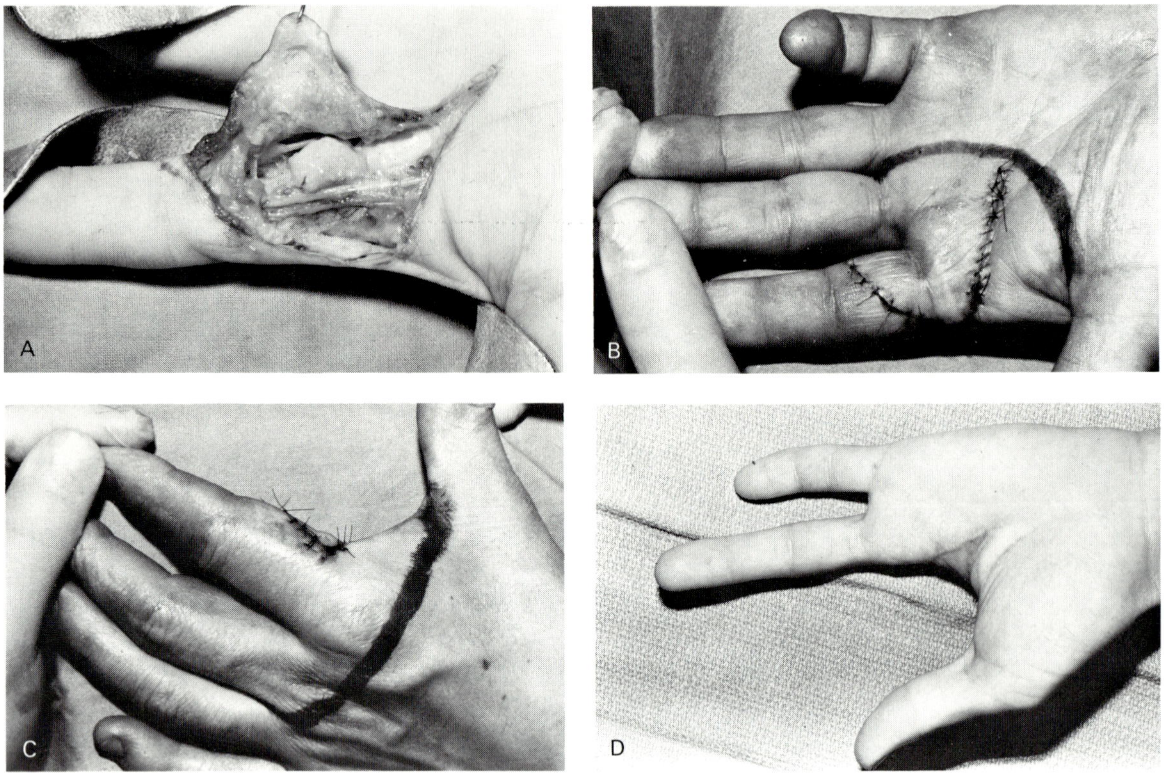

Figure 22-41. *This 28-year-old white male had had a previous fibrous lesion removed from between the index and long fingers. Recurrence of this lesion led to additional biopsies which revealed epithelioid sarcoma. A resection of the two involved digits was carried out with an accompanying Z-plasty of the web space.*

mended and should be done at least one joint proximal to the origin of the tumor.

Vessels

HEMANGIOENDOTHELIOMA AND HEMANGIOSARCOMA

These lesions differ in respect to their tissue of origin. When entirely of endothelial origin the tumor is called a hemangioendothelioma and when the origin involves fibroblastic tissue as well it is called hemangiosarcoma. The former vary in degree of malignancy and rapidity of growth. When slow growing, the resection may need to be radical only in the involved area of the hand. Radiation may have some palliative effect. Hemangiosarcoma is exceedingly malignant with rapid growth and early metastasis. Therefore, amputation should be done promptly. Radiation may be palliative.

LYMPHANGIOSARCOMA

This rare tumor arising within lymphedematous tissue usually occurs 20 to 30 years after radiation therapy and the onset of the lymphedema. It is lethal despite radical amputation to remove it.

KAPOSI'S SARCOMA

This rare malignant vascular tumor starts with small reddish-brown lesions which coalesce on the hands and feet. Some of these may involute spontaneously. The diagnosis is made by biopsy in which one of four stages may be identified: (1) dilatation of vessels and deposition of hemosiderin, (2) lymphocytic proliferation and infiltration of the dermis, (3) endothelial proliferation and (4) sarcomatous tumor with mitoses.

The treatment is repeated low-voltage roentgen therapy and occasionally wide excision and grafting. The prognosis is poor but variable. Systemic involvement is common, leading to the demise of the patient.

Nerve

Malignant neurilemmoma (malignant Schwannoma, neurogenic sarcoma) arises from preexisting

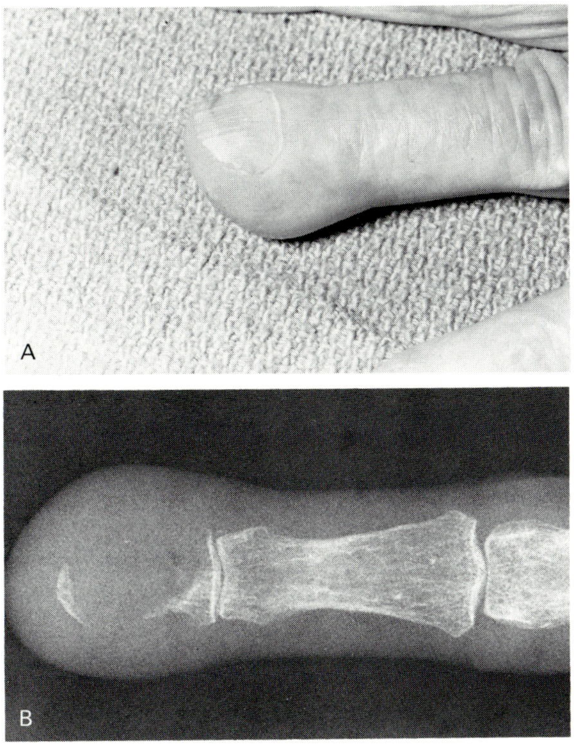

Figure 22-42. *This elderly white female showed a non-painful mass in the tip of her ring finger which precluded removal of her wedding ring. A roentgenogram revealed destruction of the distal phalanx and biopsy revealed squamous cell carcinoma; the primary tumor was later detected in the uterine cervix. (From Graham, W.P. et al.[7] Reprinted with permission of the publisher.)*

neurofibroma with almost half of those reported occurring in patients with von Recklinghausen's disease. Even though the tumor surrounds and spreads within the nerve of origin, function may still be normal. The early stage of the malignancy, in which the microscopic analysis shows large hyperchromatic nuclei, does not require amputation but can be adequately treated with wide local excision. Definitive surgery should await permanent histological sections because of the difficulty in interpreting frozen sections. It is important to note whether the lesion arises from a peripheral nerve if an accurate diagnosis is to be made.

The most malignant form shows microscopic loss of the palisading of the early stages of the tumor and develops much interlacing of cells. It is innocent in appearance and has a tendency to spread extensively along perineural spaces and vessels. Local recurrence is frequent but lymph node metastases are uncommon. Wide local excision and possible amputation are recommended.

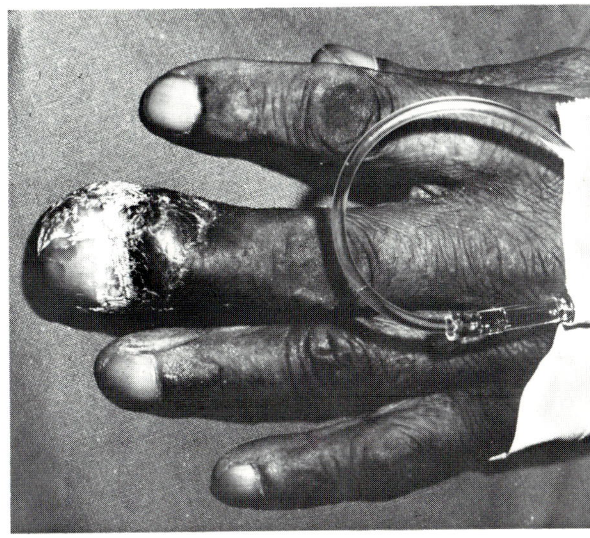

Figure 22-43. *This elderly black male had extensive carcinoma of the lung with isolated metastasis to the distal phalanx of a digit. (From Graham, W.P. et al.[7] Reprinted with permission of the publisher.)*

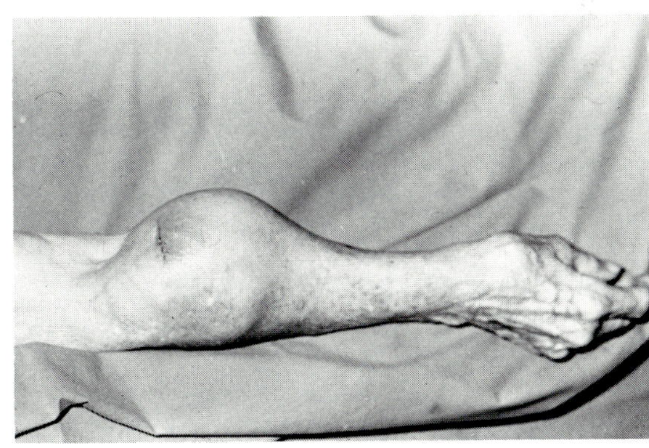

Figure 22-44. *This elderly white female had a proven biopsy of rhabdomyosarcoma of the forearm musculature. An amputation at the upper humeral level was carried out. She ultimately succumbed to a myocardial infarction three years later without evidence of recurrence of her primary tumor.*

References

1. Carroll, R.E.: Osteoid osteoma in the hand. J. Bone Joint Surg., 35A:888, 1953.
2. Clark, W.H., Jr., From, L., Bernardino, E.A. and Mihm, M.C.: The histogenesis and biologic behavior of primary human malignant melanomas of the skin. Cancer Res., 29:705, 1969.
3. Eaton, R.G., Dobranski, A.I. and Littler, J.W.: Marginal osteophyte excision in the treatment of mucus cysts. J. Bone Joint Surg., 54A:909, 1972.
4. Edgerton, M.T. and Turek, D.B. Macrodactyly digital gigantism, its nature and treatment. In: *Symposium on Re-*

constructive Hand Surgery (Littler, J.W., Cramer, L.M. and Smith, J.W., Eds.). C.V. Mosby, St. Louis, 1974.

5. Enzinger, F.M.: Epithelioid sarcoma, a sarcoma simulating a granuloma or a carcinoma. Cancer, 26:1929, 1970.
6. Franklin, J.D., Reynolds, V.H. and Page, D.L.: Cutaneous melanoma. A twenty-year retrospective study with clinico pathologic correlation. Plast. Reconstr. Surg., 56:277. 1975.
7. Graham, W.P., Kilgore, E.S., Gordon, S.L. and Williams E.H.: Metastatic tumors of the hand. Hand, 5:177, 1973.
8. Kilgore, E.S., Newmeyer, W.L. and Graham, W.P.: Mucus cysts. The dorsal distal interphalangeal joint ganglion. Plast. Reconstr. Surg., 53:313, 1974.
9. Lichenstein, L. and Sawyer, W.R.: Benign osteoblastoma. J. Bone Joint Surg., 46A:755, 1964.
10. McGovern, V.J., Mihm, M.C., Bailey, C., Booth, J.C., Clark, W.H., Cochran, A.J., Hardy, E.G., Hicks, D.J., Levene, A., Lewis, M.G., Little, J.H. and Milton, G.W.: The classification of malignant melanoma and its histologic reporting. Cancer, 32:1446, 1973.
11. Morris, W.J. and Owsley, J.Q.: Plastic surgery. In *Current Surgical Diagnosis and Treatment,* 2nd ed. (Dunphy, J.E. and Way, L.W., Eds.). Lange Publishers, Los Altos, 1975.
12. Potenza, A. and Winslow, D.: Rhabdomyosarcoma of the hand. J. Bone Joint Surg., 43A:700, 1961.
13. Smith, R.L., Miller, S.H. and Shochat, S.: Compression treatment of hemangiomas. Plast. Reconstr. Surg., 58:573, 1976.
14. Wanebo, H.J., Fortner, J.G., Woodruff, J., MacLean, B. and Binkowski, E.: Selection of the optimum surgical treatment of stage I melanoma by depth of microinvasion: Use of the combined microstage technique (Clark-Breslow). Ann. Surg., 182:3:302, 1975.

23 Congenital Deformities

In modern society where "survival of the fittest" has been modified to "survival at all costs" it has befallen surgeons to make all patients with major congenital anomalies fit for survival. In undertaking this, the surgeon becomes responsible not only for the long-range management of the patient's physical reconstruction but also for the psychological support of the parents and later of the child whose handicaps contrast him with his peers. To be effective, there must be a coordinated team effort of the surgeon, pediatrician, social worker, psychologist, prothetist, therapist and schoolteacher. The initial program must periodically be updated.

Congenital defects of the upper extremity present cosmetic and functional problems, and often the first exceed the second. The surgeon soon recognizes his limitations in improving cosmesis and function in many of these problems. Indeed, surgical scars are hardly less obvious than some derangements of development. Furthermore, a child will get the maximum function from the extremity "the way it is," and sometimes has to be taught to consider it a handicap. In such instances, the handicap is more that of the parents and the physician than of the child.

The dynamic forces of growth and differential development are often greater than the surgeon's capacity to modify them. This, together with the many anomalies of functionally essential structures, imposes great limitations and is ample reason in many instances for not interfering. Any plan of reconstruction on the congenitally deformed upper limb must be directed and integrated with (1) the functional needs, (2) the capacity of the patient to adapt to the benefits of surgery and (3) the cosmetic problem.

Embryology of the Upper Limb

A sperm unites with an ovum to form one cell called a zygote which weighs 0.005 mg. The single-cell zygote undergoes cellular division, referred to as cleavage, during the first week, as it passes down the fallopian tube to be embedded into the uterine wall. During the following seven weeks the embryo is changed to a fetus and marked cellular differentiation occurs, establishing the organ systems. This second period is called the organogenic phase; at its conclusion a shift from cellular differentiation to cellular growth takes place as the 8-week-old fetus enters a period of 32 weeks of enlarging its size.

The following sequence outlines the origin and development of the arm bud:

Two weeks: embryo 2.1 mm—no arm bud

Three weeks: embryo 4.2 mm—arm bud originates by a mesodermal swelling with an epithelial cap from the ventral body wall at the level of the fifth to seventh cervical somites

Four weeks: embryo 7 mm—the arm bud grows caudally and capillary networks with drainage channels are formed by mesoblast cells. The formation of the vascular networks stimulates cellular differentiation and growth. The limb develops in a proximodistal sequence and the most active cellular division is in the mesoderm just under the epithelial cap

Five weeks: embryo 11 mm—mesoderm condenses into precursors of muscle and bone which are indistinguishable at this stage. Constrictions appear, distinguishing the hand from the forearm

Six weeks: embryo 16 mm—nerves from the spinal cord invade the condensed mesenchyme and the muscle elements distinguish themselves. The mesenchyme destined to become the skeleton chrondrophies and the digital swellings are present in the hand disc

Seven weeks: fetus 20 mm—most specific arm structures are present, joints are present, specific muscle groups appear and individual muscles are recognizable

Eight weeks: fetus 26 mm—clefts between the digits develop and the thumb becomes distinguishable. The upper extremity has differentiated into its recognizable adult components at 8 weeks and the remaining 32 weeks are primarily concerned with their growth.

Incidence of Congenital Anomalies

The following is the list of some reports on the incidence of congenital defects. Some reports are concerned with congenital anomalies in general and others are concerned with a specific category of anomalies.

General Incidence

- Ivy:[11] 8.5 upper extremity defects/1,000 live births. His 5-year study found 703 cases of polydactyly and 85 cases of syndactyly. Polydactyly was more common among blacks.
- Birch-Jensen:[5] One upper extremity defect/6,438 living persons (he did not count polydactyly or syndactyly, the two most common defects)

Syndactyly

- Paletta:[22] Syndactyly was found 1/2,500 live births
- MacCollum:[15] Syndactyly was found 1/2,000 live births
- Nylen:[21] Syndactyly was found 1/3,000 live births.

Polydactyly

- Handforth:[9] Polydactylism was found 2.4/1,000 births in the southern Chinese. Polydactyly is the most common and syndactyly the next most common congenital anomaly occurring in the upper extremity.

Causes of Congenital Anomalies

Genetic

Heredity plays a role in the etiology of most congenital defects. Barsky[1] states that approximately 5 per cent of hand deformities are inherited. If both parents are normal but one child has a defect, there is a 25 times greater chance of subsequent children having a defect than in the normal population.[1] However, if a non-dominant defect is anticipated, it will not be more apt to occur in the first child than in any subsequent child. Furthermore, the age of the mother does not seem to have any bearing on upper extremity defects except in Down's syndrome (mongolism). Although the major anomalies of the upper extremity are sporadic, simple patterns of inheritance are frequently responsible for digital abnormalities. Upper extremity anomalies also occur with several known chromosomal syndromes.

Environmental

The environment of the embryonic cells in the critical phase of the first trimester influences the pattern of growth and development. Experimentally, it has been proven that maternal nutrition is a factor in creating congenital defects. Deficiencies in copper, iodine, vitamin A, riboflavin and vitamin D have been incriminated.[27-31] Similar deficiencies have not been proven to cause anomalies in man.

Environmental factors known to produce anomalies in man are several: (1) chemical factors—thalidomide, antivitamins and anoxia,[24] (2) irradiation—exposure of unborn children to the atom bomb,[1] (3) endocrine factors—5 to 7 times greater incidence of congenital malformations in offspring of diabetics,[1,3] (4) infections—40 to 80 per cent congenital malformation rate with maternal rubella in first trimester,[1,3] (5) mechanical factors—correlation with severe maternal trauma.[16] This may be coincidental and is not conclusive.

Classification of Congenital Anomalies*

International agreement on terminology for the classification of congenital limb deficiencies has

*This section on classification was graciously provided by Alfred B. Swanson, MD. and is based on the article: A classification for congenital limb malformations. J. Hand Surg., 1:8, 1976. Material used by permission.

long been sought without success, despite intermittent efforts of many scientists. This classification is a broad outline for the systematized categorization of congenital malformations. Further subclassification is possible for those who have a special interest in certain anatomical areas.

A workable classification must use simple, easily remembered terminology. It must be concise enough to receive clinical entities with minimal confusion, but at the same time broad enough to permit the full categorization of complex cases. An ideal classification could be made by grouping cases according to etiology, but unfortunately the etiology of many of these defects is still obscure. Enough basic evidence has been collected, nonetheless.

Most limb defects occur during the embryonic phase of differentiation. Environmental factors inhibit the rate of orderly differentiation of the part which is most rapidly changing. Certain common congenital defects can be predicted consistently by disturbing the embryo at precise stages of development. It is possible to observe clinical manifestations of arrest of development and of differentiation, and to determine at which time during the embryonic stage and at which site on the limb the defect occurred.

The degree of severity and the place at which the insult occurs on the fashioning limb bud can be compared to those of abscess formation in adult tissues. In the abscess there is an area of central destruction surrounded by an area of cellular infiltrate, with resulting scar tissue formation and structural deformity. The same destructive process occurring in embryological life before structural formation had occurred would certainly lead to disorganization of the developing tissue about the area of destruction. The various clinical pictures are felt to represent varying degrees of destruction within this organization of the limb mesenchyma. The time at which the insult occurs and the sequential development of the part are also important, as is the location of the destructive process, and will determine the type of ensuing deformity.

This classification takes note of the similarities in certain pathological entities. Subclassification of the groups recognizes the differences and expresses the mildness or the severity of the type. An example is clubhand (arrest of radial longitudinal development). In addition to the fact that the radius is either partially or totally absent, the condition can be associated with hypoplasia or aplasia of the thumb or carpal bones or of the musculature on the preaxial or radial side of the limb. Each group can be subclassified into its degrees of severity as desired for completeness.

Occasionally the insult to the limb may result in mixed involvement. As an example, the severe central longitudinal arrest of development (clefthand) may be manifested as an almost transverse arrest of the entire hand, with only rudimentary radial and ulnar digits. The judgment of the clinician will be required to categorize these relatively rare cases appropriately. In certain cases where mixed involvement prevents the examiner from establishing a specific classification, he may want to put it into a mixed-type category. This type of categorization should occur infrequently, however, and in the committee's experience has not been necessary.

A universally used classification for congenital malformations has many exciting benefits. Identifying prevalence and types of malformations on a continuing basis could serve to alert public health authorities to outbreaks of malformations within the population, e.g. the thalidomide tragedy. Other possibilities for comparison and evaluation are numerous. This system is being organized for computerization. It is hoped that the classification, which has international acceptance, can be the framework for further study of congenital defects. Primary and supplemental diagnoses may have separate but identifiable descriptors for computer retrieval within the system.

Categories

I. Failure of formation of parts
II. Failure of differentiation (separation) of parts
III. Duplication
IV. Overgrowth (gigantism)
V. Undergrowth (hypoplasia)
VI. Congenital constriction band syndrome
VII. Generalized skeletal abnormalities

Failure of Formation of Parts

Upon recommendation of the Subcommittee on Nomenclature and Classification in Congenital Limb Deficiency (International Society for Prosthetics and Orthotics), which met in Dundee, Scotland, in June 1973, and in Montreux, Switzerland, in October 1974, the following terminology was proposed. This subclassification is an enlargement and refinement of a portion of the broader classification of congenital anomalies, which has been accepted by the American Society for Surgery of the Hand and the International Federation of Hand Societies. The proposed new system for Category I deals only with congenital skeletal deficits.

The system establishes that all skeletal deficiencies fall either into transverse or longitudinal deficiencies.

Transverse deficiencies appear as amputation-type stumps and are classified by naming the level at which the remaining stump terminates, it being understood that all elements distal to the level named also are absent (Table 23-1). An application of this terminology to one of the most common types of transverse deficiency (the forearm, upper third, or short below-elbow defect) is shown in Figure 23-1.

The Task Force on Standardization of Prosthetic-Orthotic Terminology of the Committee on Prosthetic-Orthotic Education has accepted the "transverse deficits" category of the new terminology to identify amputation levels deriving from trauma or disease, and for the types of prostheses applicable to these levels.

All skeletal limb deficiencies other than the transverse type are arbitrarily placed in the longitudinal category. In identifying longitudinal deficiencies, all absent bones or portions of bones that are missing are named. Any bones not named as being absent are understood to be present (Figs. 23-2, 23-3) (Table 23-2)

Table 23-1. *Failure of Formation of Parts*

Transverse limb deficiencies (congenital amputations) with suggested abbreviations*

UPPER LIMB (UL)	
Shoulder (sh)	Total
Arm (Arm)	Total
	Upper $\frac{1}{3}$
	Middle $\frac{1}{3}$
	Lower $\frac{1}{3}$
Forearm (Fo)	Total
	Middle $\frac{1}{3}$
	Upper $\frac{1}{3}$
	Lower $\frac{1}{3}$
Carpal (Ca)	Total
	Partial
Metacarpal (MC)	Total
	Partial
Phalangeal (Ph)	Total
	Partial

*Attention is drawn to an oddity which apparently can occur. Total absence of the shoulder or hemipelvis (and all distal elements) would be a transverse defect. However, if only a portion of the shoulder is absent, the deficiency would be of the longitudinal type.

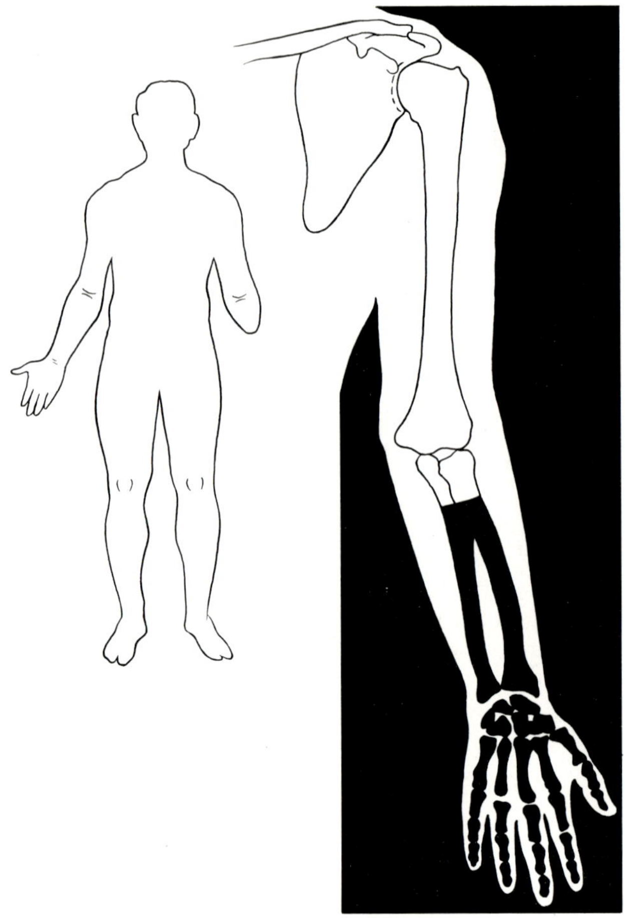

Figure 23-1. *T-L, Fo upper one-third.*

The rules of thumb which evolved as a result of this study are:

1. Supplemental conditions
   a. Always put absences first, followed by supplemental conditions, e.g. T-R, Ca partial; with hypoplasia of Ra and Ul.
   b. In hypoplasia associated with T- deficiencies as above, name hypoplastic forearm bones, since one may be affected but not the other.
2. Partial absence of long bones in L/deficiencies
   Identify the approximate amount of missing segment—e.g. L/L, Hu partial (prox. $\frac{3}{4}$)
3. Order of classification
   In classifying L/deficiencies always proceed from proximal to distal, e.g. L/R, Hu partial (prox. $\frac{3}{4}$); Ra total; Ca partial.
4. Abbreviations
   In anatomical description and classification the use of abbreviations and acronyms frequently provides a system of shorthand which is of value as long as the meanings of the terms employed are essentially self-evident. In applying the new international terminology for classification of congenital limb deficiencies, it is clear that:

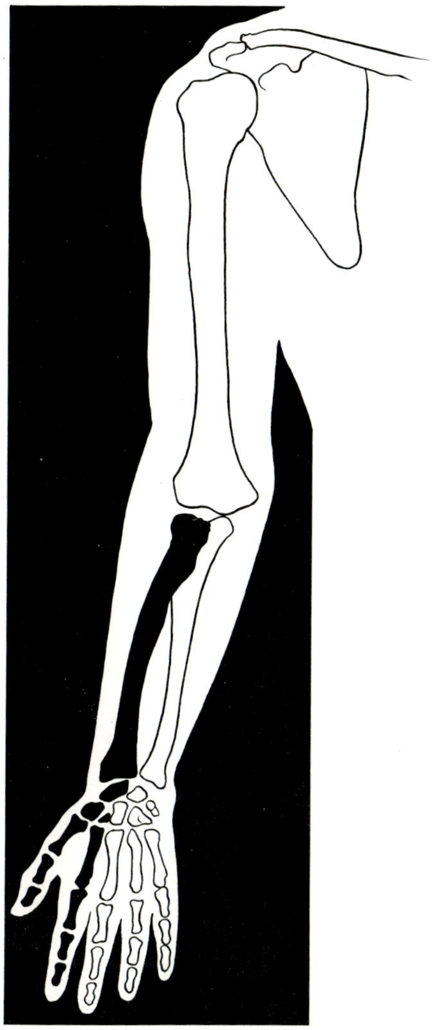

Figure 23-2. *L/R, Ra total; Ca partial, Rays 1, 2 total.*

a. Certain of the broad categories included in the system would be useful for data organization but do not have to be included for each limb classified, as these categories are self-evident from the bone(s) or limb segment(s) named, e.g. upper limb in both transverse and longitudinal deficiencies.
b. The terms "transverse" and "longitudinal" themselves can be abbreviated with little danger of confusion, e.g. T-L and T-R for transverse left and right respectively and L/L and L/R for longitudinal left and right.

When one or more metacarpals and the corresponding phalanges are completely absent, it seems unnecessary to spell out the two levels separately but simply refer to them as Rays. Similarly, when two sequent bones are affected to the same degree, they could be combined in the classification. Thus, a combined longitudinal deficiency of the right upper limb, humerus total, radius total, carpus partial, metacarpal 1,2 total, phalanges 1,2 total, could more simply be written L/R, Hu and Ra total, Ca partial, Rays 1,2 total.

5. Surgery

Although the surgical conversion of congenital deficiencies is not a basic classification item, information on such conversion may be included on the description-classification form as supplemental data, as follows:

a. In cases of surgical amputation to provide a better limb remnant for prosthetics fitting, a horizontal line (—) in red pencil or ink should be made on the form at the appropriate level.
b. In cases of joint fusion, the surgery should be indicated by an (X), again in red pencil or ink, through the joint fused.
c. An osteotomy would be shown by an appropriate marking, again in red pencil or ink.

A problem common to all classification systems is that roentgenograms taken when a child is very young may not reveal bones which are not yet ossified; thus early diagnosis should be considered

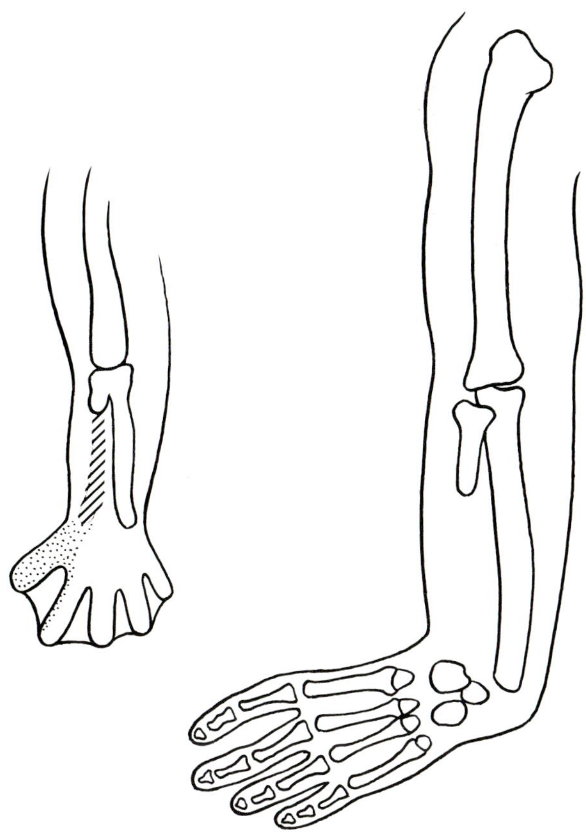

Figure 23-3. *L/R, Ra partial; Ca partial; Ray 1.*

Table 23-2. *Failure of Formation of Parts*

Longitudinal deficiencies—All bones named to be designated as partially or totally absent

UPPER LIMB (UL)

Scapular (Sc) Total or partial		Clavicle (Cl) Total or partial
	Humerus (Hu) Total or partial	
Radius (Ra) Total or partial		Ulna (Ul) Total or partial
	Carpal (Ca) Total or partial	

	Radial		Central		Ulnar	
Metacarpals (MC) Total or partial	1	2	3	4	5	Rays
Phalanges (Ph) Total or partial	1	2	3	4	5	

tentative and subject to revision when the child is restudied at a more mature age.

Another problem encountered is that some bone remnants are unidentifiable. It is recommended that the classifier use his best judgment as to what is present or missing, but indicate by a (?) that this is a presumption and not necessarily an exact identification. Figure 23-4 is an example of examination and classification forms that can be used to outline the necessary descriptive information about the patient's deformity.

Failure of Differentiation (separation) of Parts

A. Shoulder
   1. Undescended shoulder
   2. Absence of pectoral muscle(s)
B. Arm
   1. Elbow synostosis
C. Forearm
   1. Soft tissue
   2. Synostosis
      a. Proximal radius/ulna
      b. With/without radial head dislocation
D. Hand
   1. Carpal
      a. Deformities
      b. Synostosis
   2. Metacarpal
      a. Deformities
      b. Synostosis
   3. Digital
      a. Deformities
      b. Symphalangism
      c. Syndactyly
         1. Simple
         2. Complicated
            a) Soft tissue
               1) Synonychia
               2) Other
            b) Skeletal
               1) Fusions
                  (a) Phalanges (side to side)
                  (b) Acrosyndactyly
                  (c) Apert's syndrome
               2) Disarray
               3) Brachysyndactyly
      d. Contractures
         1. Soft tissue
            a) Thumb web space
            b) Arthrogryposis
            c) Camptodactyly
            d) Trigger digit
         2. Skeletal
            a) Clinodactyly

Duplication

Duplication of parts probably occurs as a result of a particular insult to the limb bud and ectoder-

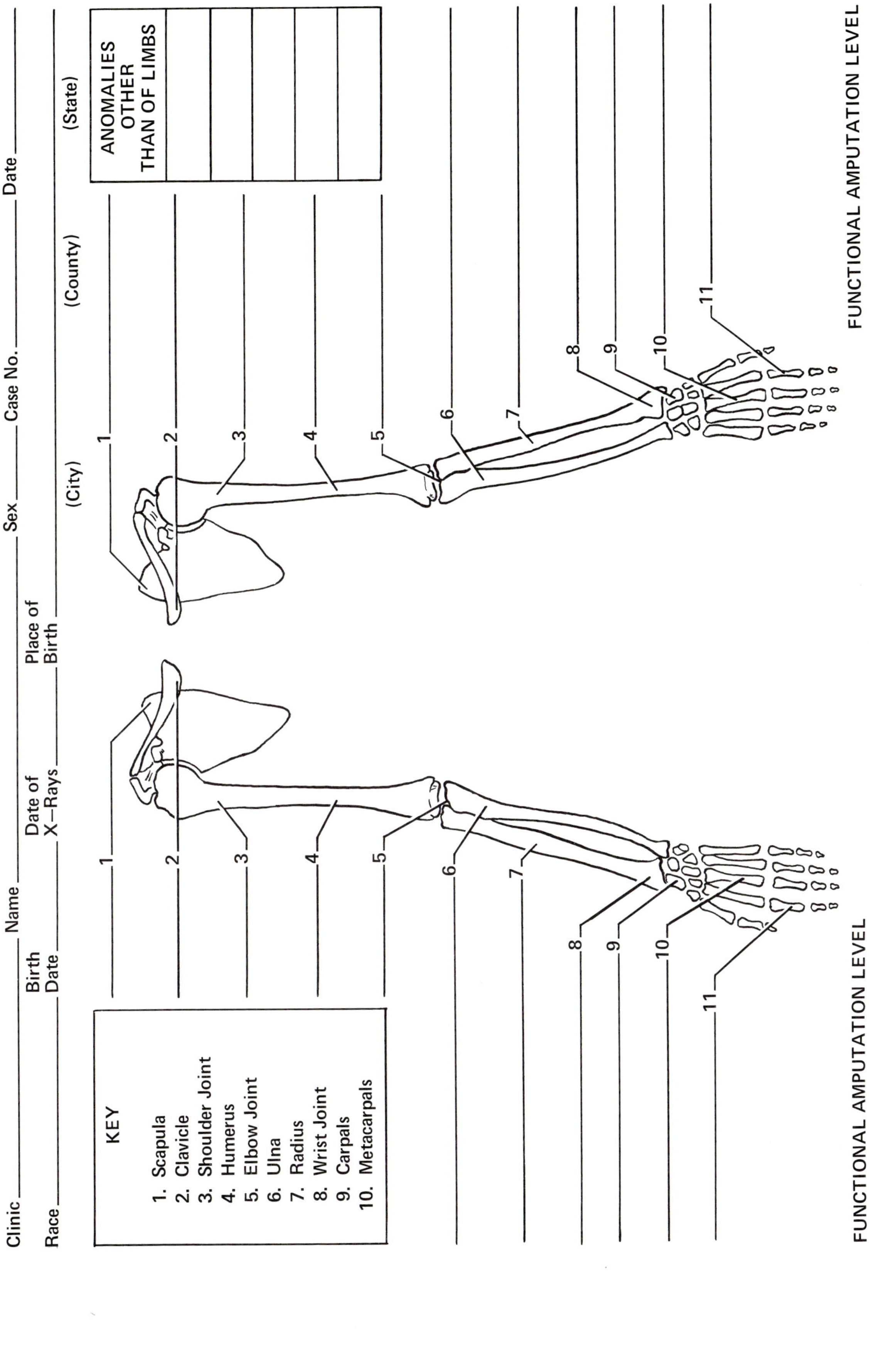

Figure 23-4. *Examination and classification form to record upper limb deformities.*

mal cap at very early stages of their development so that splinting of the original embryonic part occurs. These defects may range from polydactyly to twinning or mirror hands.

- A. Skeletal
  - 1. Humerus
  - 2. Radius
  - 3. Ulna
  - 4. Carpals
  - 5. Metacarpals
  - 6. Phalanges
- B. Skin and nails
- C. All tissues
  - 1. Whole limb
  - 2. Partial limb
  - 3. Polydactyly
    - a. Radial
    - b. Central
    - c. Ulnar
  - 4. Mirror hand

Overgrowth (gigantism)

In digital gigantism the abnormality usually is greatest at the periphery. The whole limb may be affected. Some cases appear due to skeletal overgrowth with normal-appearing soft parts. Others show excess fat; lymphangioma or angioma may be present. Deformities may increase secondarily because of asymmetrical growth of the part.

- A. Arm
- B. Forearm
- C. Hand
- D. Digit

Undergrowth (hypoplasia)

Undergrowth, or hypoplasia, denotes defective or incomplete development of the parts. This may be manifested in the entire extremity of its divisions. Hypoplasia may be used as a supplemental diagnosis for remaining skeletal elements in Category I. However, this category should be represented separately in this classification system because of the prevalence of the condition.

- A. Skin and nails
- B. Musculotendinous
- C. Neurovascular
- D. Extremity
  - 1. Arm
  - 2. Forearm
  - 3. Hand
    - a. Whole hand
    - b. Brachymetacarpia
    - c. Brachyphalangia

Congenital Constriction Band Syndromes

Focal faulty development along the course of the limb may be the result of necrosis of the developing mesenchymal tissue. Annular constriction bands or rings may represent an area of necrosis in the superficial tissues. When these constriction bands are severe, they may result in intrauterine gangrene and true fetal amputations may occur. The occasional associated syndactyly in these cases may be the end-result of the intrauterine healing process. The necrosis of tissue and its resultant fusion of parts are not unlike untreated third-degree burns with bridges of scar. The syndactyly and confused anatomical arrangements of parts found in these cases may be the result of a healing necrotic infarct occurring during the stage of separation of parts. Controversy has existed as to whether this is an intrinsic or extrinsic defect. Amniotic bands have been implicated as the cause of the defects; others feel that the amniotic bands are secondary to the healing limb injury.

Generalized Skeletal Abnormalities

Defects in the hand may be a manifestation of a generalized skeletal defect such as appears in dyschondroplasia, achondroplasia, arachnodactyly, etc.

Treatment of Congenital Anomalies

In undertaking treatment certain issues must be considered. There must be an understanding of: basic hand function, the existing adequacy of function, threats to this function by developing deformity, possibilities and techniques of improving function surgically and non-surgically, the timing of such treatment and its inherent risks.

The prime functions of the hand are prehension, release and percussion. Sensibility, mobility and adaptability are necessary for the execution of these functions. The hand is the instrument of sensibility and dexterity at the end of a mobile cantilevered system the base of which is the trunk.

Stability and the capacity of placement and much of the power of prehension lie in the musculoskeletal function proximal to the hand. There is an inordinant capacity to compensate for missing function somewhere along this complex system. The basic drives for food and protection automatically invoke compensatory mechanisms in the presence of any congenital defect.

To avoid meddlesome treatment, an evaluation of existing function must be carefully made in considering any need for treatment of the limb. Particular attention should be directed at the competence of placement of the hand, its capacity for grasp and pinch, and the range of motion in relationship to basic needs of independence and survival. This requires a study (even by movies) of function and action, showing the child's handling of toys and instruments. These should be chosen to demonstrate the competence of different actions. Instability, inadequacy of range, weakness, and failed coordination in the execution of function should be noted. The intelligence of the patient must be assayed, especially in considering any treatment program which is predicated upon learning and training.

The only spontaneous threat to existing function in congenital anomalies is a progression of the abnormality by virtue of differential growth. Therefore, the child must be evaluated periodically and function and form must be reassayed. Measurements of the range of motion and the size and angulation of parts must be made and often complemented with serial photographs and roentgenograms.

The surgeon must have the expertise required to handle tiny tissues and knowledge of the anomalous aberrations and techniques of correcting them. The reconstruction may necessitate a variety of procedures which include: arthrodesis, tenodesis, amputation, tendon grafts, lengthening or transfer, ostectomy, osteotomy or bone grafting, skin grafts, transfer of sensibility, pollicization, and dactylization and a host of alignment procedures. The surgeon must appreciate the limitations and risks inherent in all these procedures and be sensitive to committing the patient to an excessive number of operations. Finally, he should evaluate the applicability of prosthesis for given problems.

The timing of surgery must be individualized. Ideally, the surgery is undertaken when the tissues have reached adequate size for ease of identification but before the problems of fixed patterns of ineffective function and/or harassment by peers become insurmountable. Generally, the optimum time for reconstructive surgery is 2 to 4 years, by which time there has been good cortical maturation for function of the whole extremity. However, progressive deformities such as terminal syndactyly and the radial clubhand frequently force surgery at an earlier age. In the consideration of timing, the consequence of surgical interference with the epiphyseal plates must be considered.

Prostheses play an important role in restoring function in malformations of the upper extremity.[20] Both passive (cosmetic) and active (functional) devices are available. The usefulness of a prosthesis correlates with its adaptation to the needs of the patient. The patient's use of it depends upon his need for it and the timing of its fitting, and on the instruction which he has had. Children with one normal upper extremity are less inclined to maintain the need for a prosthesis than those with bilateral functional deficit. Furthermore, the simpler the mechanics of the prosthesis, the more likely it is to be accepted and used by the patient. The prosthesis should be able to operate commonplace devices and perform ordinary functions so that the patient will not need many special tools. This simplifies the training program so that the patient can readily appreciate the functional value of the prosthesis. If a child feels confident with his prosthesis, it will readily be accepted by his peers without ridicule. A simple explanation by the child's teacher of the problem and the workings of the prosthesis will often help.

At times it is necessary to accommodate a patient's hypersensitivity in public by fitting a prosthesis for cosmetic rather than functional needs. Such passive devices should, however, be discouraged whenever possible since they can never equal the value and psychological reward of an efficient, functional (active) prosthesis.

The prosthesis should be fitted in the first or second year of life after there has been sufficient maturation of cortical control of vision and its coordination with the musculoskeletal system.

Anomalies of the Arm

ABSENCE (AMELIA)

This condition of complete absence of the upper extremity is primarily a problem when it is bilateral. The patients are spontaneously very adept with their feet, which to a large extent can substitute for their hands, providing they are normal. Shoulder-disarticulation prostheses have been devised but, because of the lack of an upper-arm stump, fitting and control are difficult. Many patients use their feet in preference to a prosthesis. Electrical or carbon dioxide powered prostheses are available and are particularly applicable in cases of bilateral amelia.

DUPLICATION (POLYMELIA)

Duplication of the upper extremity is exceedingly rare. It involves complete or partial duplication of components of the arm, forearm, wrist and hand.[13]

STIFFNESS (ARTHROGRYPOSIS MULTIPLEX CONGENITA, FIG. 23-5)

The abnormality is occasionally transmitted as a hereditary dominant trait. One or all extremities may be involved. The dominant feature of the disorder is the absence of isolated or groups of muscles and stiffness of the joints they control. There may be webbing of the axilla and antecubital area and stiffness of the elbow in flexion or extension, dislocation of the radial head and stiffness of the forearm as well as the wrist and digits. At times there is spontaneous fusion of the stiff joints.

The treatment is surgical. It is hampered by the fact that muscles and tendons are absent or fibrotic even when there might otherwise be hope for joint mobilization or arthroplasty. In many instances the functional impairment is not great; however, it may be overwhelming, as in the case of bilateral elbow and forearm stiffness in a nonfunctional habitus. In such cases, osteotomy and fusion in a more functional position are undertaken.

Anomalies of the Forearm

ABSENCE (PHOCOMELIA)

In phocomelia the hand articulates with the humerus. Generally speaking, the same problems exist with amelia except that the patient does have a stump and may have a functioning hand. This introduces the need to individualize the prosthesis so that the hand, if it functions, can activate the terminal device and lock and unlock the elbow.

MADELUNG'S DEFORMITY

Madelung's deformity results from a deficiency of the ulnar half of the distal radial epiphysis. As a consequence, growth of the radial side of the radius creates bowing, forcing the articular surface to angle ulnarly at the carpus. The distal radioulnar joint is deranged. There is relatively excessive length of the ulna so that it may be subluxed dorsally at the carpus, impairing forearm rotation and wrist motion.

This condition is inherited as an autosomal dominant. It is four times more common in females than males and is twice as frequent bilaterally than unilaterally.

No treatment is necessary if there is no pain and adequate adjustment to the impairment is made in motion. Otherwise, treatment is considered at the end of the growth period. This consists of: (1) osteotomy of the distal radius to correct the angulation volarward and ulnarward, (2) shortening of the ulna by a Darrach resection[6] of the distal ulna or a Milch segmental osteotomy[17] more proximally.

The transverse osteotomy of the radius is done through a longitudinal incision on the radial border of the forearm 2 to 3 cm proximal to the articular surface. The radial nerve must be protected and the incision must be adequate for exposure. The osteotomy site is angled enough to correct the radial and volar angulation of the radius. Internal fixation is optional.

The ulna is shortened through an ulnar longitudinal incision. Injury to the dorsal branch of the ulnar nerve must be avoided. The Darrach procedure (Fig. 23-6) is done by osteotomizing the ulna transversely just proximal to the head (2 cm from the styloid). If the ulnar head is resected proximal to the pronator quadratus, the distal ulna can displace subcutaneously and become painful. The head is held in a bone clamp and dissected in retrograde fashion by hugging the bone with a #15 scalpel blade. The dead space is obliterated by closing the periosteum with nylon sutures.

The Milch procedure[17] (Fig. 23-7) is done similarly and more proximally by 2 to 3 cm. A 1.5- to 2-cm segment of bone is removed and the gap is closed and secured with a wire suture placed through drill holes. An alternative is to osteotomize in a step-cut (bayonet) fashion and hold the segments together with a screw.

The extremity is immobilized in a long-arm cast with the forearm in neutral rotation and the wrist extended for 3 weeks. A follow-up roentgenogram

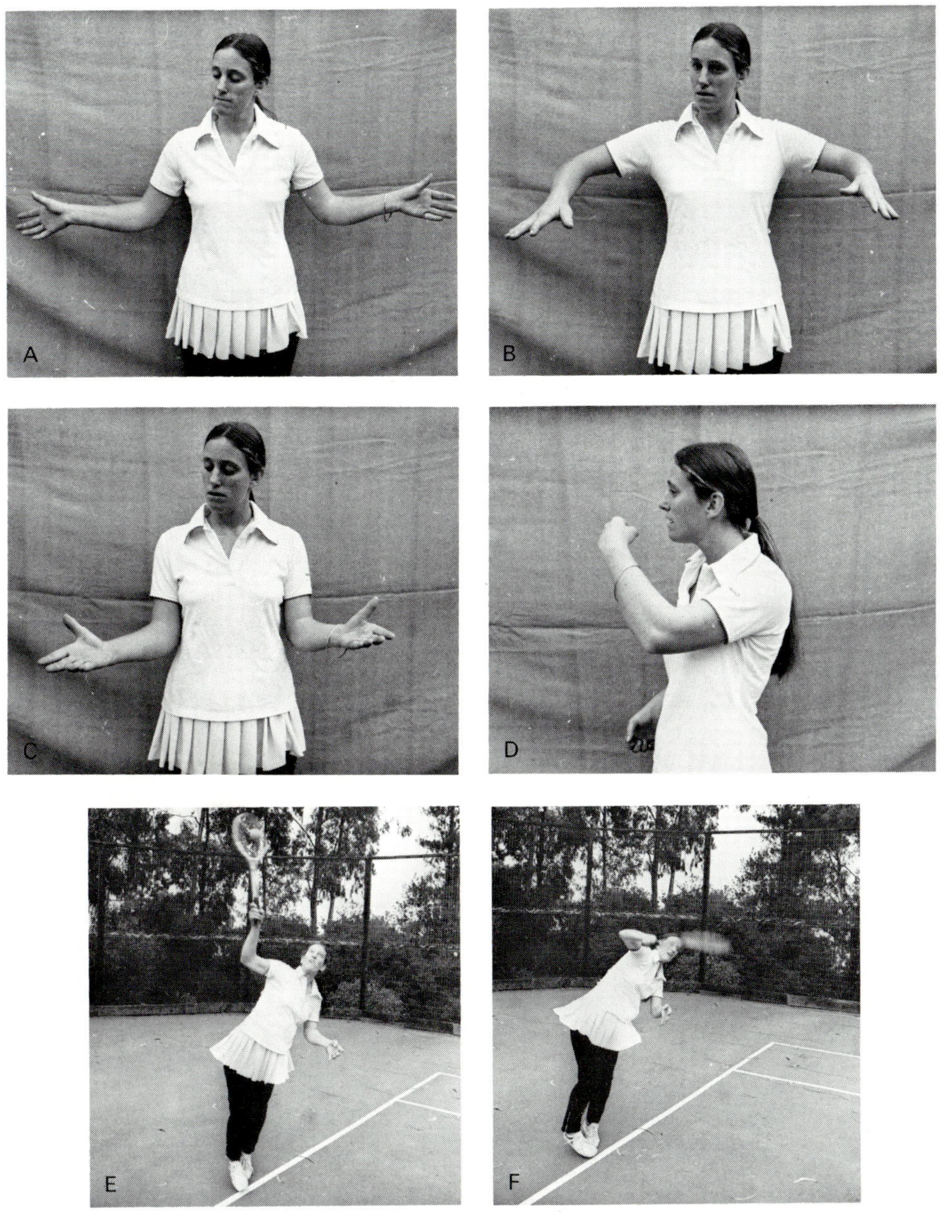

Figure 23-5. *Young girl with arthrogryposis who has virtually no problems with daily living, e.g., tennis, swimming and horseback riding.*

is taken and further immobilization elected on the basis of the findings.

CONGENITAL DISLOCATION OF THE RADIAL HEAD

This condition is rare and is manifested by limitation of rotation of the forearm. However, it does not need treatment unless there is pain or the limitation of motion is excessive. The diagnosis rests on the radiological findings. There is no fracture of the ulna, the radial head is dislocated (usually anteriorly) and the radial shaft appears longer than normal. The capitellum and the radial notch of the ulna which articulate with the head of the radius are underdeveloped, as may be the radial head. The dislocation is irreducible.

If treatment is required, resection of the radial head should be postponed until the epiphyses have closed. A slightly curved longitudinal 7-cm incision is made for excising the radial head; it starts over the lateral epicondyle and curves to the dorsum distally. The incision extends between the anconeus posteriorly and the extensor carpi ulnaris

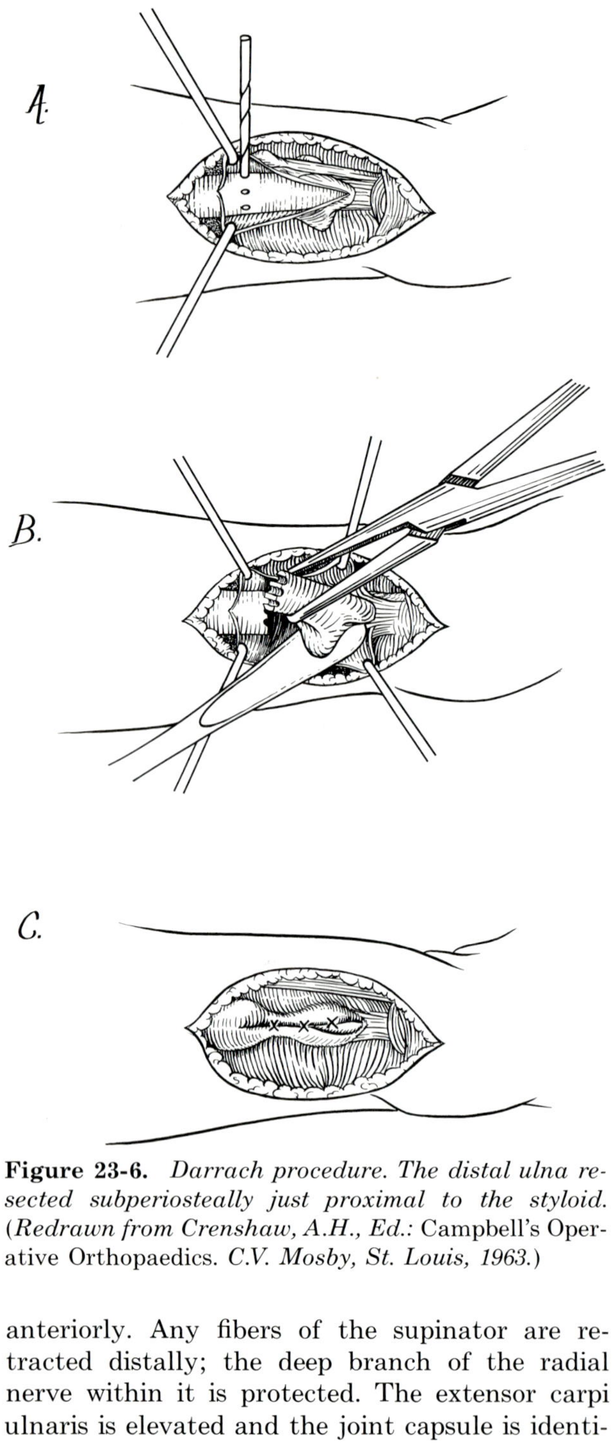

Figure 23-6. *Darrach procedure. The distal ulna resected subperiosteally just proximal to the styloid. (Redrawn from Crenshaw, A.H., Ed.:* Campbell's Operative Orthopaedics. *C.V. Mosby, St. Louis, 1963.)*

anteriorly. Any fibers of the supinator are retracted distally; the deep branch of the radial nerve within it is protected. The extensor carpi ulnaris is elevated and the joint capsule is identified and entered. The neck of the radius is then exposed, sectioned with an osteotome or side-cutting burr and removed. Any spicules of bone are smoothed off with a rongeur. If there is good alignment in relationship to the capitellum, a Silastic stem prosthesis of the radial head may be inserted after reaming out the medullary cavity. The capsule is closed with nylon sutures and the wound is similarly closed. A well-padded long-arm cast is applied with the elbow at a right angle and the forearm in neutral. Immobilization is maintained for 7 to 10 days and motion is then started cautiously.

CONGENITAL RADIOULNAR SYNOSTOSIS

This disorder is associated with a dominant phenotype that has variable expression, affecting males twice as often as females. Half of the cases are bilateral. The condition appears to be caused by failure of differential development between the proximal radius and ulna during the eighth to ninth week of embryonic life. At this stage there is a common cartilaginous investment of the radius and ulna which fails to separate, and the pronated fetal stance is perpetuated by the synostosis that ensues. The radial head may be present or absent and the synostosis broad or narrow.

No treatment is necessary unless the degree of pronation is a functional problem. It is difficult to

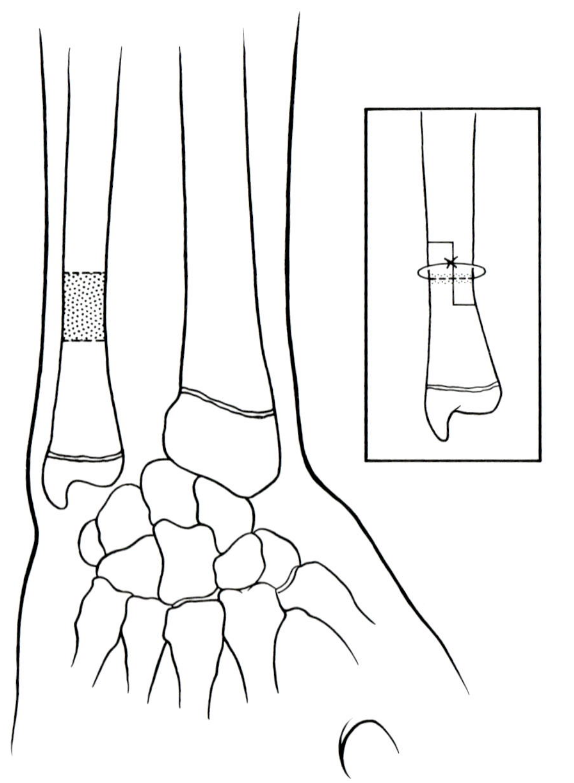

Figure 23-7. *Milch procedure. A segment of ulna removed from its distal third and the gap closed by wiring the fragments. This may be done by simple resection as a step cut in a bayonet configuration. (Redrawn from Crenshaw, A.H., Ed.:* Campbell's Operative Orthopaedics. *C.V. Mosby, St. Louis, 1963.)*

treat; even after sectioning the synostosis and the interosseous membrane completely, there may be no improvement. It is probably best to consider rotation osteotomy of the radius to correct a disabling pronation deformity.

Anomalies of the Forearm and Hand Units

RADIAL CLUBHAND (HEMIMELUS, FIG. 23-8)

This condition, consisting of complete or partial absence of the radius and often elements of the radial side of the humerus, wrist and hand, has various etiologies. Approximately 10 per cent of cases are hereditary, and others may be brought on by such circumstances as drugs (thalidomide) and infections (syphilis). The abnormality is frequently associated with a number of other major congenital anomalies of the heart, genitourinary and gastrointestinal tracts and the musculoskeletal system.

The deformity is principally one of radial deviation of the forearm and wrist with radial deviation of the ulna. The radial carpus and the thumb ray may be hypoplastic or absent, as may the capitellum. There is also soft tissue derangement, including hypoplasia or absence of extrinsic muscles on the radial side of the forearm. The fascia and the median nerve on the radial side are often shortened. Sometimes the median nerve has a dorsal sensory branch replacing the absent dorsal sensory branch of the radial nerve. The range of active motion and grip strength are limited. The metacarpophalangeal joints are extended and permit a limited degree of flexion. The proximal interphalangeal joints usually have a flexion contracture and limited active extension.

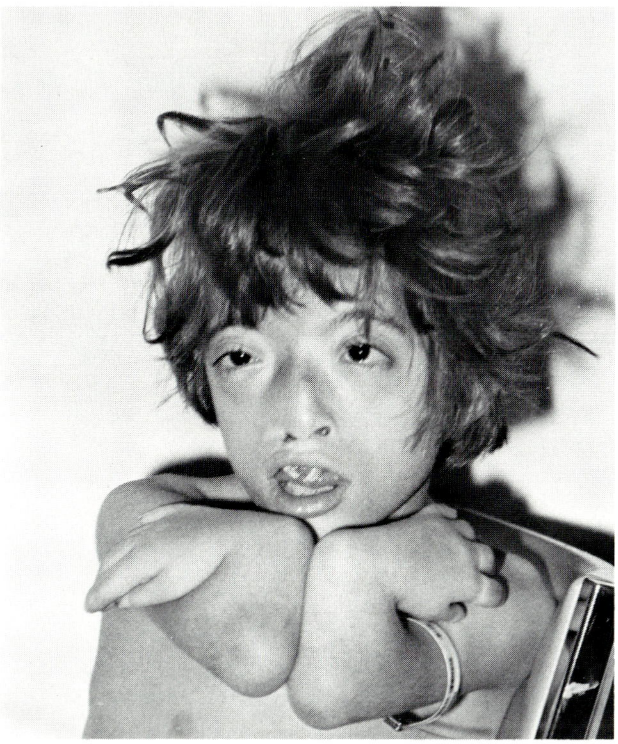

Figure 23-8. *11-year-old retarded child with bilateral radial clubhands previously untreated. This boy had also had a cleft lip.*

Treatment depends upon the age at which the patient is seen. If the individual is full grown, there is frequently no need for treatment since the patterns of satisfactory functional use have been well established and compensate for the deformity. However, if surgery is contemplated, it is essential that the patient have adequate elbow motion or functional decompensation may result.

When the patient is seen within the first 3 years of life, non-operative and operative treatment have been rewarding. Elbow function is important as a prerequisite in this circumstance also.

The objectives of treatment are the proper alignment of the forearm and wrist and restoration of prehension[4] (Fig. 23-9). Four procedures are involved: (1) overcoming the soft tissue contracture on the radial side of the wrist, (2) centralizing the carpus on the end of the ulna, (3) correcting the severe bowing of the ulna and (4) reconstructing the thumb. For the first few years of life (awaiting ulnar epiphyseal maturation) the wrist is maintained in a brace. This may be in the form of a clock spring or a static splint which is modified from time to time until the desired alignment is attained. Sometimes the tightness of skin and deep soft tissue precludes progress and early surgical release (section of fascia and Z-plasty of skin) is necessary. By 4 or 5 years of age the carpus is transferred so that it is centralized on the end of the ulna and held there with a Kirschner wire. The lunate and a portion of the capitate are resected. A large Kirschner wire is inserted along the third or fourth metacarpal and then redirected proximally into the ulna. The distal ulna and its epiphysis are disturbed as little as possible during the procedure by freeing only the necessary amount of surrounding soft tissue to relocate the hand. The wire is left as long as possible. If the fingers are pulled into flexion when the hand is centralized, the superficialis tendon will have to be lengthened. At all times care must be taken to avoid injury to the

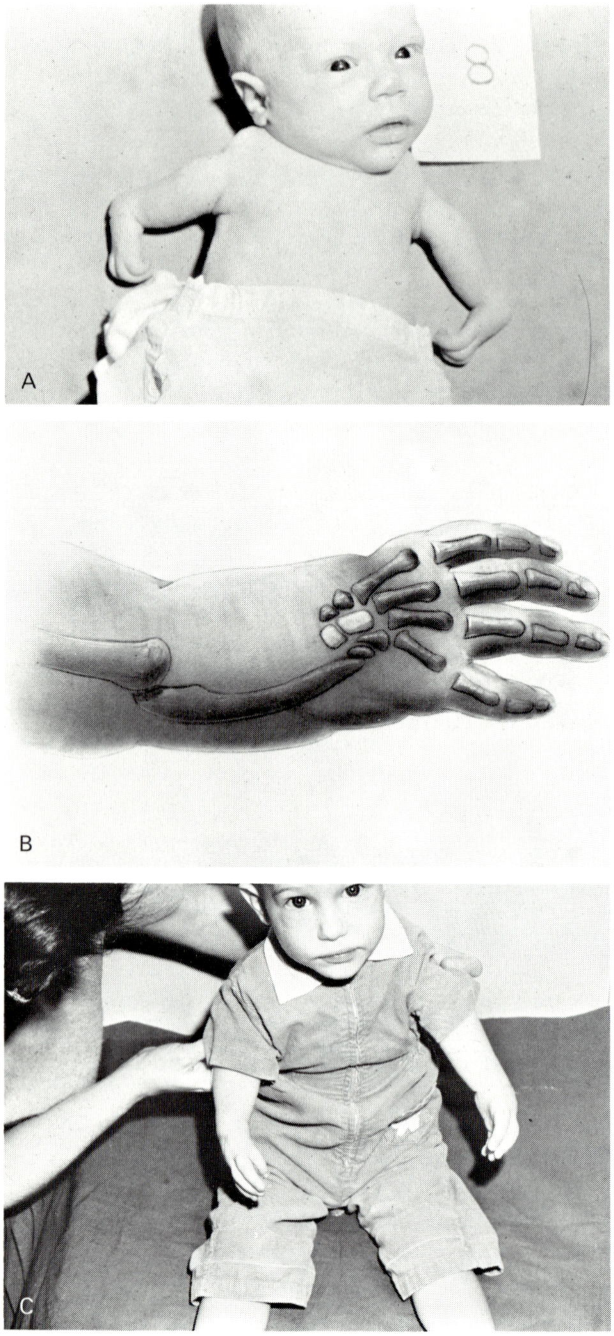

Figure 23-9. *Bilateral radial clubhands corrected by the technique described.* (**B** *from Bora, F.W. et al.*[4])

superficial median nerve. Flexion of the elbow will usually relieve any stretch upon this nerve. Once the hand has been centralized, pollicization can follow.

Pollicization may be done as the classic procedure (Chap. 17) or in modified form in stages.[15] The objectives of the latter method are to promote adaptive spreading of the space between the index and long fingers and pronation of the index finger. In the first 6 to 8 months of life the intervolar plate ligament and intermetacarpal fascia (interosseous) are divided. At a later time (about 2 years) the index metacarpal may be recessed and rotated to facilitate pinch. As the child ages (another 2 to 3 years) further recession and more rotation of the index metacarpal may be needed. As a rule, it is not necessary to shorten the tendons.

ULNAR CLUBHAND (HEMIMELUS)

This condition is far less common than the radial clubhand, and the etiologies are not quite as clear-cut. As with the radial clubhand, the patient may have associated congenital anomalies elsewhere. The longitudinal defect is expressed in various degrees of absence of structures on the ulnar side of the extremity. There may be total absence of the ulna and the ulnar carpus and ulnar rays distally. The absence may be more distal than proximal or vice versa. It may also be proximal and distal with the central portion present. There may be a synostosis between the radius and ulna and, when the ulna is completely absent proximally, there may be a synostosis between the radius and humerus. The hand deviates ulnarward. The radius may do the same. There are apt to be the same type of soft tissue deficiencies and malformations centered on the ulnar aspect of the forearm that characterized the radial clubhand. Bilateral defects occur but are seldom symmetrical.

Treatment is dictated by the nature and magnitude of the deformity and function that is lost. The derangement of the elbow joint is often the greatest problem. Fusion of the radius and humerus is common and may be in the extended position. In other instances there is a radioulnar synostosis or dislocation of the radial head. When the deformity is bilateral, an osteotomy of the radiohumeral synostosis and functional arthrodesis may be necessary. In other instances, it may be necessary to resect the head of the radius. If ulnar drift of the wrist is marked, early splinting is instituted and later soft tissue releases, tendon transfers and/or centralization of the carpus on the radius are carried out.

DUPLICATION OF THE ULNA (MIRROR HAND, DIMELIA)

This deformity is unilateral and is not hereditary. The normal radial aspect of the forearm and hand is absent and in its place is a duplication of the ulna and its carpal bones and fingers. Thus the elbow has 2 olecranons which are rotated so that the fossae of the olecranons face each other. The ulnar postaxial digits tend to be somewhat more normal than the ulnar preaxial digits. There are often 8 digits and no thumbs. The prime functional problems are limited elbow, forearm and wrist motion. In addition the hand lacks a thumb, and the intrinsic muscle function is weak. Syndactyly and flexion of the fingers are present also.

Surgical treatment is directed at improvement of pronation and supination by resection of one of the olecranons (usually the preaxial), and construction of a thumb and thumb web. This may be done by the method of Entin,[9] in which the first and third preaxial digital rays are resected and the skin flaps obtained from filleting these fingers used to form a new web between the second and fourth ray. A rotation osteotomy of the second metacarpal is then undertaken using a bone strut from one of the resected metacarpals as a graft. This is placed between the second and fourth metacarpals. Surplus tendons may be transferred to reinforce movement of the pollicized finger or other weak digits.

Anomalies of the Hand

ABSENCE (ACHERIA, FIG. 23-10)

Terminal transverse defects of the hand may involve the whole hand (acheria), digital rays (adactylia) or other phalanges (aphalangia). These defects are usually unilateral and, when there is a history suggesting inheritance, an autosomal recessive trait is indicated. Complete absence of the hand and carpal bones can be treated with a prosthesis fitted at 9 to 18 months of age. This is motored by a shoulder harness and has a terminal hook device. For cosmesis (to make the defect appear more like a traumatic injury) the tiny stubs of digits may be resected, rendering the stump smooth.

If there are remnants of mobile metacarpals, the surgical construction of a pinch mechanism by utilizing bone grafts and skin flaps may be considered.

LOBSTER-CLAW HAND (ECTRODACTYLY, FIG. 23-11)

This deformity, which is usually bilateral, may be inherited as an autosomal dominant trait. It consists of an absence of all or part of the central ray. Associated with this is a deepening of the web (cleft) at the site of the absence and at times a syndactyly of neighboring digits.

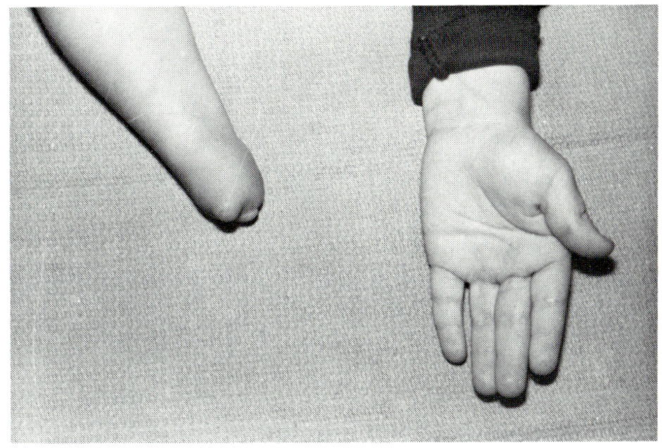

Figure 23-10. *Acheria.*

Treatment is dictated by whether or not the patient has a satisfactory pinch mechanism between existing fingers and the thumb. If he does, then the cleft may be closed by creating a surgical syndactyly for cosmetic reasons. The cleft is opened and the adjacent metacarpals are drawn together with sutures and the skin is then closed. This may be done as a W-plasty, raising flaps that will interdigitate upon closing the wound in a zigzag fashion. The procedure should be performed at 2 to 3 years of age.

Anomalies of the Thumb (ectrodactyly)

The thumb may be absent with or without coexisting longitudinal radial defects. The need for treatment is dictated by whether the problem is unilateral or bilateral and by the specific problems

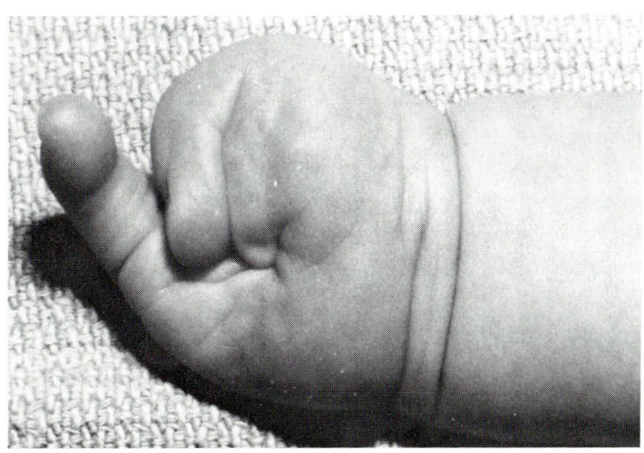

Figure 23-11. *Lobster-claw hand.*

of the patient. At age 2 to 4 years, a new thumb may be created by pollicization of an adjacent index finger.[14] Construction of a thumb by bone graft, tube pedicle and neurovascular island or by toe transfer is not recommended.

ABSENCE OF PHALANGES

When the thumb metacarpal is present and the hand is otherwise normal, function may be improved by deepening the web with a Z-plasty. This might be the preferred procedure if the opposite hand is totally normal.

HYPOPLASIA OF THE THUMB (POUCE FLOTTANT, FIG. 23-12)

The thumb metacarpal is hypoplastic or absent and the thumb literally floats on the radial side of the hand. Its position is usually far distal to its normal origin at its carpometacarpal joint. If the phalanges are of normal size and the extrinsic muscles are intact, the unstable thumb can be stabilized with an iliac bone graft between it and the index metacarpal. This will maintain the length of the thumb and position it in abduction and pronation.

In most cases, the thumb is too diminutive and lacks the needed motor units, so that pollicization of the index finger is the procedure of choice following amputation of the thumb. This should be undertaken particularly if the deformity is bilateral. This condition contrasts with a hypodactylia of the thumb (*Muscle deficiency,* below).

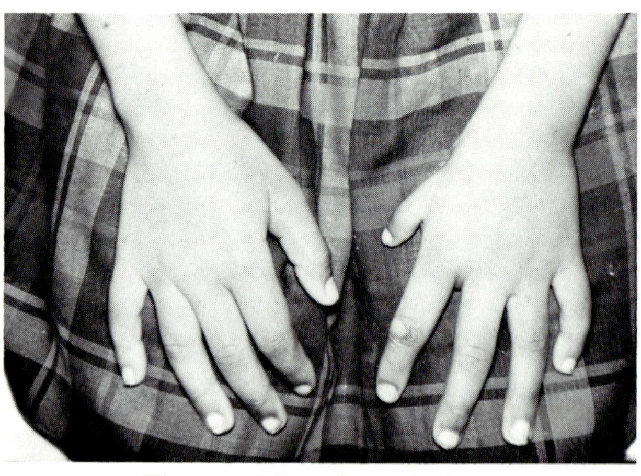

Figure 23-12. *Pouce flottant.*

DUPLICATION OF THE THUMB (POLYDACTYLY, FIG. 23-13)

This may be partial or complete. The need for treatment is cosmetic for the partial duplication and functional for the total duplication. Treatment consists of resecting the part that lacks motor control at about 2 years of age. This is usually that on the radial side. The radial collateral ligament of the metacarpophalangeal joint may have to be reconstructed and the tendon of the abductor pollicis brevis transferred from the amputated thumb to the base of the proximal phalanx of the remaining thumb. The metacarpal head may continue to grow more prominently than normal on the radial side, necessitating secondary reduction osteotomy for cosmesis.

The simplest form of thumb duplication is broadening of the distal phalanx. If this is unsightly, the thumb can be narrowed by a central wedge resection en bloc of the nail, nail bed, and phalanx distal to the epiphysis[1] (Fig. 23-14). The bone wound is closed by one horizontal mattress suture of nylon placed over a small gauze pledget on either side of the digit. The nail bed and nail are approximated with meticulously placed fine sutures mounted on a tiny cutting needle. The transverse mattress suture is removed after 4 weeks. This same technique is applicable to the bifid thumb, in which case it may be necessary to centrally resect half of each phalanx and approximate the lateral halves.[10]

DELTA PHALANX OF THE THUMB (FIG. 23-15)

Occasionally a delta phalanx, which is a triangulated phalanx associated with the takeoff point of a potential or actual supernumerary thumb, is seen. The deformed phalanx is osteotomized and the angulation corrected with a bone graft.[32]

TRIPHALANGEAL THUMB[2] (FIVE-FINGERED HAND)

In this rare condition there is no thumb. Instead, there is a radial finger with 3 phalanges, no thenar musculature and a typical "finger" metacarpal. This digit can be pollicized as described for pouce flottant.

MUSCLE DEFICIENCY

A variety of muscle deficiencies are seen about the thumb. These may occur with or without hy-

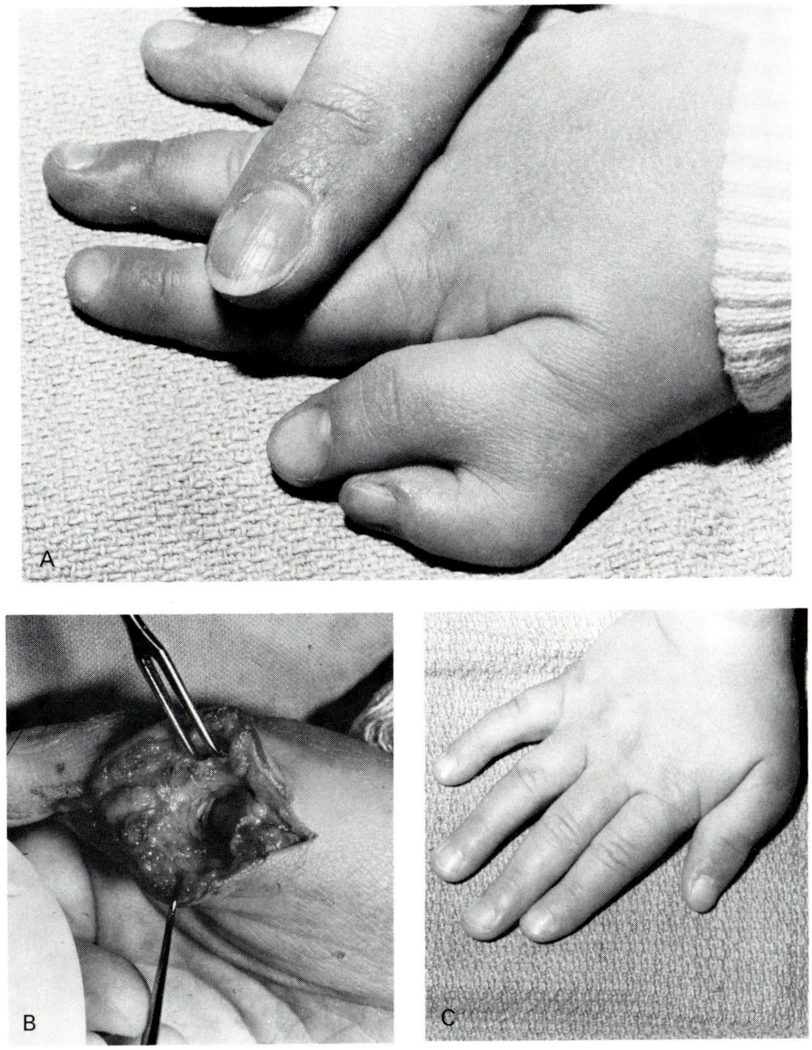

Figure 23-13. *Duplication of the thumb treated by resection and arthroplasty of the common metacarpophalangeal joint.*

poplasia of the skeletal elements. In hypodactylia[2] there are varying degrees of deficiency of musculotendinous units but both phalanges and the metacarpal are present in rudimentary form. In contrast to pouce flottant, the carpometacarpal junction is normally positioned. Depending on the size of the thumb and the muscles present, better motor control might be developed by tendon transfers than by amputation of the thumb and pollicization of the index finger.

Specific muscle deficiencies may include part or all of the thenar wad, the extensors or the flexors. Absence of the extensors has to be differentiated from the presence of the stenosing tenosynovitis or trigger thumb. The former is rare and the latter common. A tendon transfer, extensor indicis proprius, is the transfer choice for the absent extensor pollicis longus.

Tupper[26] has described maldevelopment and radial displacement of the flexor pollicis longus, which splits distally with one tendinous insertion to the volar aspect of the distal phalanx and the other into the normal extensor pollicis longus tendon; this causes an abduction stance and impaired pinch.

Correction of this deformity is accomplished by rerouting the flexor pollicis longus in young children and releasing the radial collateral ligament and reefing the one on the ulnar side at the metacarpophalangeal joint. Older patients who have adapted to the deformity may require capsuloplasty of the metacarpophalangeal joint and reattachment of the dorsal tendinous insertion to replace the deficient short abductor. Less satisfactory results may be anticipated in the older individual.

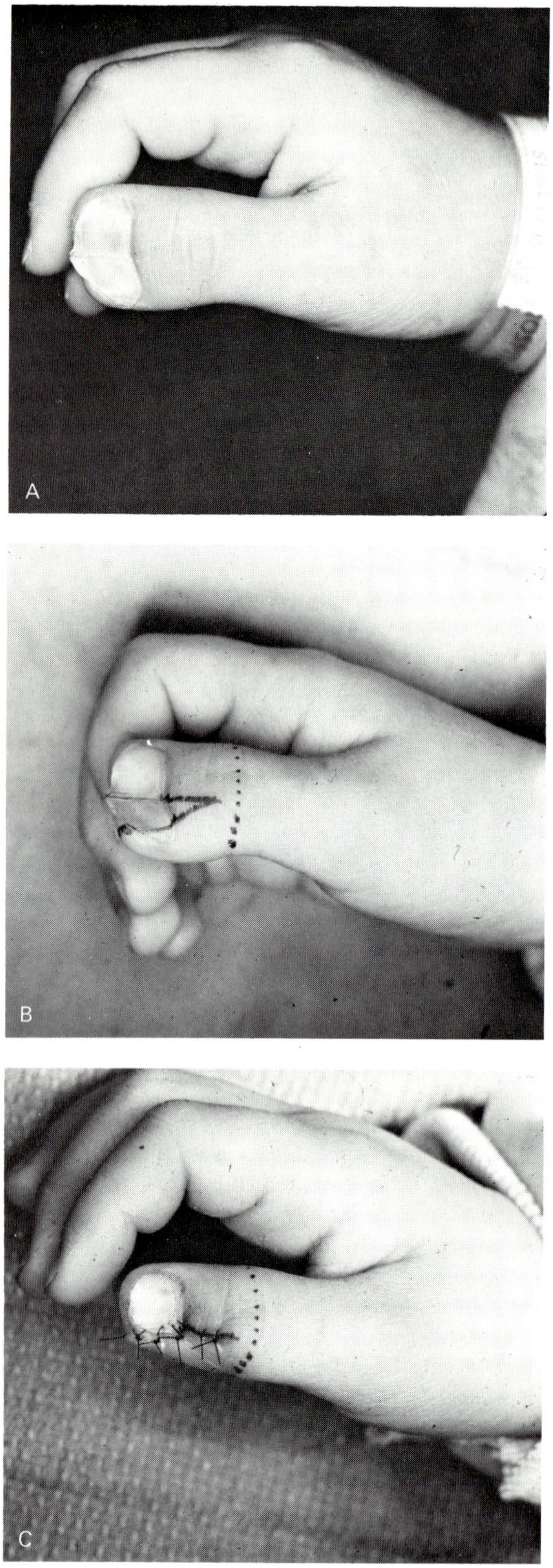

Figure 23-14. *Broad distal phalanx of the thumb treated by wedge resection.*

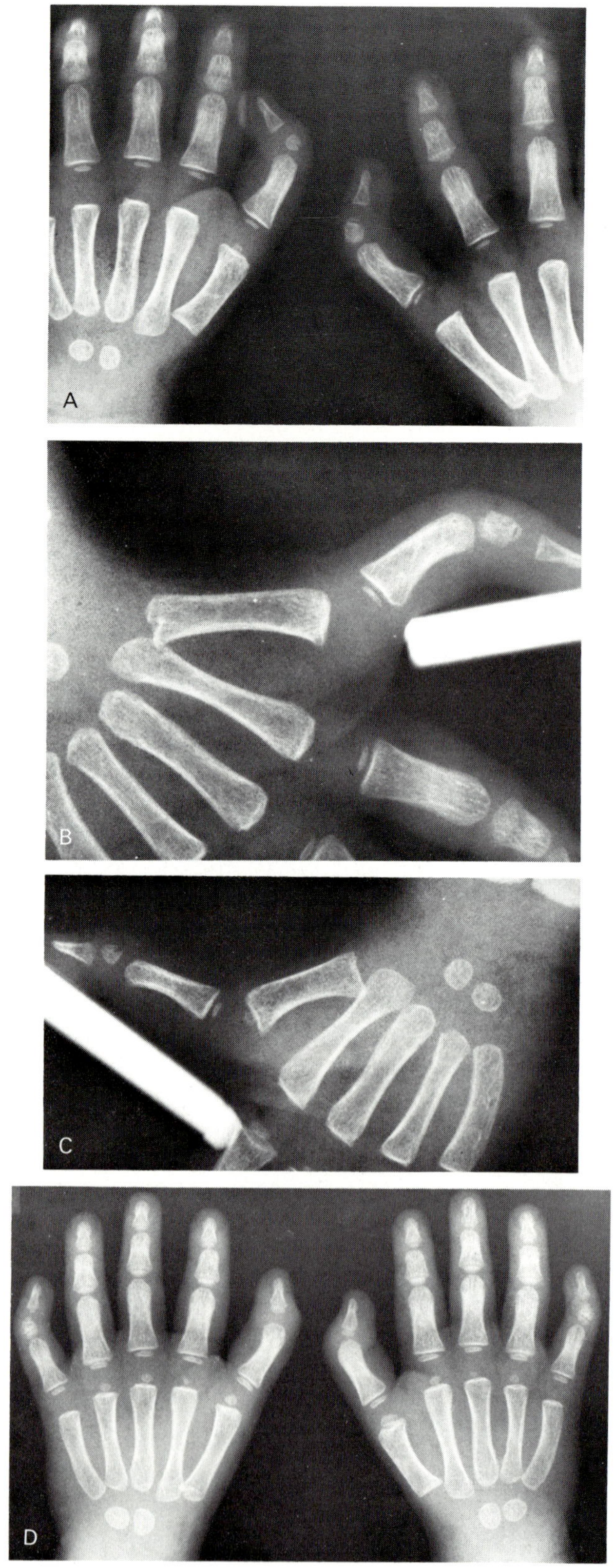

Figure 23-15. *Bilateral delta phalanges of thumb treated by excision of the extra phalanx and construction of a functioning distal joint.*

THUMB SYNDACTYLY

This soft tissue anomaly prevents thumb abduction from the digits and, therefore, eliminates normal pinch. Depending upon the tightness of the web, the following procedures may be considered to release the web contractures: (1) Z-plasty, (2) Z-plasty plus a split-thickness skin graft, or (3) a skin flap for treating the more difficult cases.

Anomalies of the Finger

POLYDACTYLY (FIG. 23-16)

Polydactyly can involve any digit or multiple digits. It is the most common congenital abnormality of the hand. When bilateral, it is usually on the ulnar border and a hereditary dominant (Fig. 23-17). If it is unilateral, it usually occurs on the radial side. Polydactyly may be manifest by a soft tissue nubbin, with or without a cartilaginous body, or range to a fully developed digit with "normal" articulations and neuromuscular function (Fig. 23-18). There may be varying degrees of

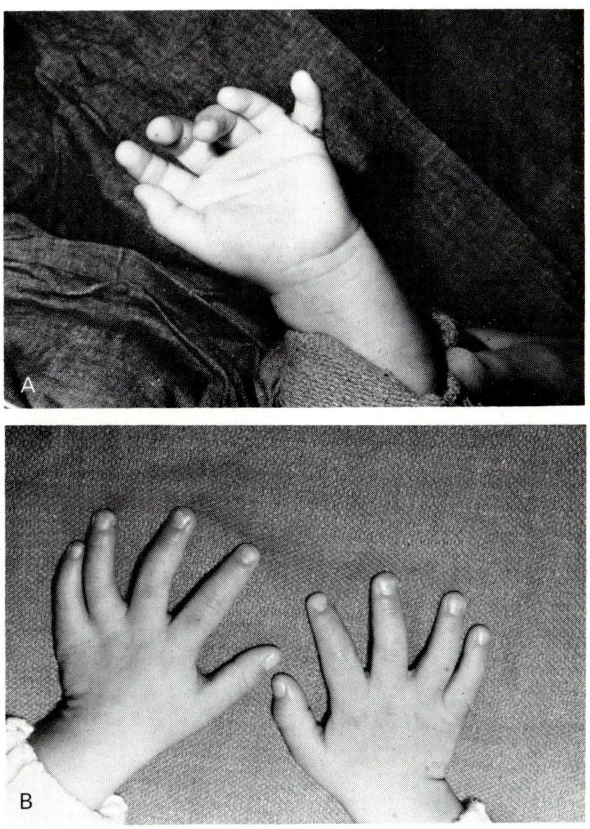

Figure 23-16. *Polydactyly of the right little finger treated by resection.*

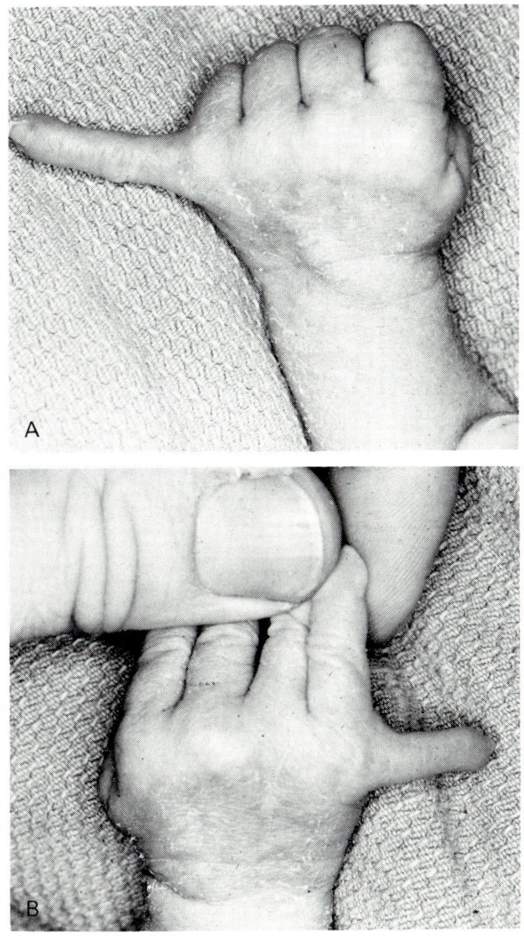

Figure 23-17. *Bilateral polydactyly and multiple other congenital anomalies.*

syndactyly, especially when the central digits are involved.

In order of frequency, polydactyly arises from ray I, ray V, ray III, ray IV, and ray II. There may be a supernumerary articular facet for the extra digit. Syndactyly of the central digits may obscure the polydactyly and the presence of a distorted (bifid) metacarpal.

Treatment is dictated by the degree of normalcy of the rest of the hand, the impact on function and the esthetic effect of the supernumerary element.

Most of these are insignificant appendages on the radial or ulnar side and ligated at birth. When the extent of the duplication does not lend itself to this simple treatment, a more formal evaluation of the hand for coexisting anomalies must be done.

The time of surgery is largely dictated by the rate of progression of a deformity, which influences the overall function and appearance of the hand. Required surgery should be undertaken prior to school age.

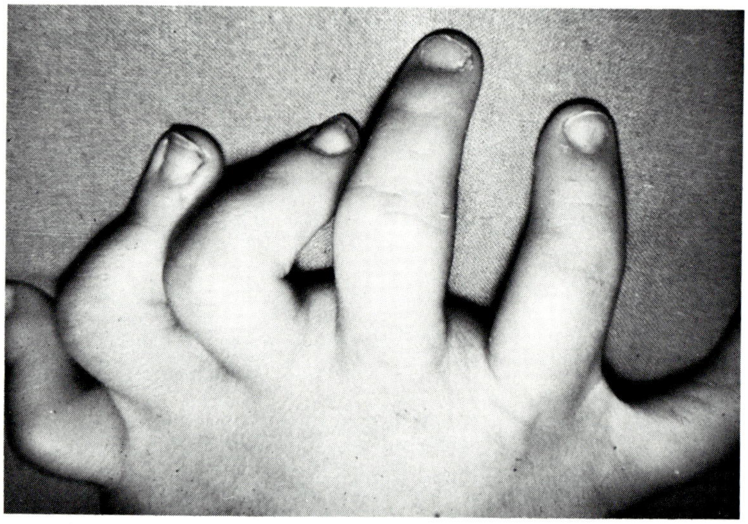

Figure 23-18. *A six-fingered hand with no thumb.*

SYNDACTYLY (FIG. 23-19)

This is the most common congenital anomaly of the hand which is referred for surgery and second to polydactyly in overall incidence. When it is hereditary, it is inherited as a dominant phenotype. It is an accompaniment of many syndromes: Apert's syndrome (acrocephalosyndactyly, craniosynostosis), Poland's anomaly (absence of ipsilateral sternocostal portion of the pectoralis major muscle and hypoplasia of the extremity), ectodermal dysplasia, oculodigital, orodigital complexes, focal dermal hypoplasia (Goltz-Gorlin syndrome), and Mobius syndrome[13] (Fig. 23-20).

Syndactyly occurs in simple and complex forms. The simple form is webbing between 2 digits, most commonly the ring and long fingers (Fig. 23-21). It may be basal, terminal, intercalated or complete and may involve skin alone or adjacent bone (synostosis). The tendinous components of the digits may be complete and independent. The innervation may be abnormal (abbreviated or fused) and the same is true of the vasculature. Progressive deformity is seen only when a long digit is tethered by the adjacent short one. This occurs most commonly in syndactyly between the ring and little finger. If deformity is progressive, early correction should be considered to facilitate proper longitudinal growth. Generally, the digits should be separated before school age if the deformity is obvious. The thumb and little finger should be liberated early to promote proper function of these marginal digits.

The objective of surgery is to separate the adjacent digits, creating a cosmetic web and avoiding contracture of either the web or the scar along the digit. Zigzagging the incision of the side of the digit and the web meets the objective in most instances. If distortion (bowing) subsequently occurs, it is more likely to be a function of differential growth than of scar contracture. A free skin graft is always necessary to cover the proximal bare areas of the proximal phalanges and sometimes is required further distally.

The apex desired for the web is marked by a small hypodermic needle passed through the base of the syndactyly. This should be slightly proximal to the normal crest of the web, allowing for the effects of wound contraction. The skin incision is marked carefully to have a liberal zigzag configuration with two sides (volar and dorsal) reciprocating (Fig. 23-22). This will allow the defect created by one flap to be filled by its reciprocating flap from the other side. The proximally based flaps for the web are pointed distally. The base of the smaller volar one lies just proximal to the crest of the new web. The larger and longer dorsal flap is based at the metacarpophalangeal joint. Once these flaps are raised and positioned, lateral bare areas will be left which require subsequent closure by skin grafts.

The flaps for this procedure should be raised with great caution using magnification to identify the volar neurovascular bundles and any possible anomaly that might be present. If the syndactyly is tight, the tips of the interdigitating flaps will extend to or beyond the midline of the axis of the digits. On raising the volar components of such flaps it is therefore essential to pay great heed to the location of the neurovascular bundles and to avoid carrying two bundles into one digit. Thus it is best that the deeper dissection proceed from

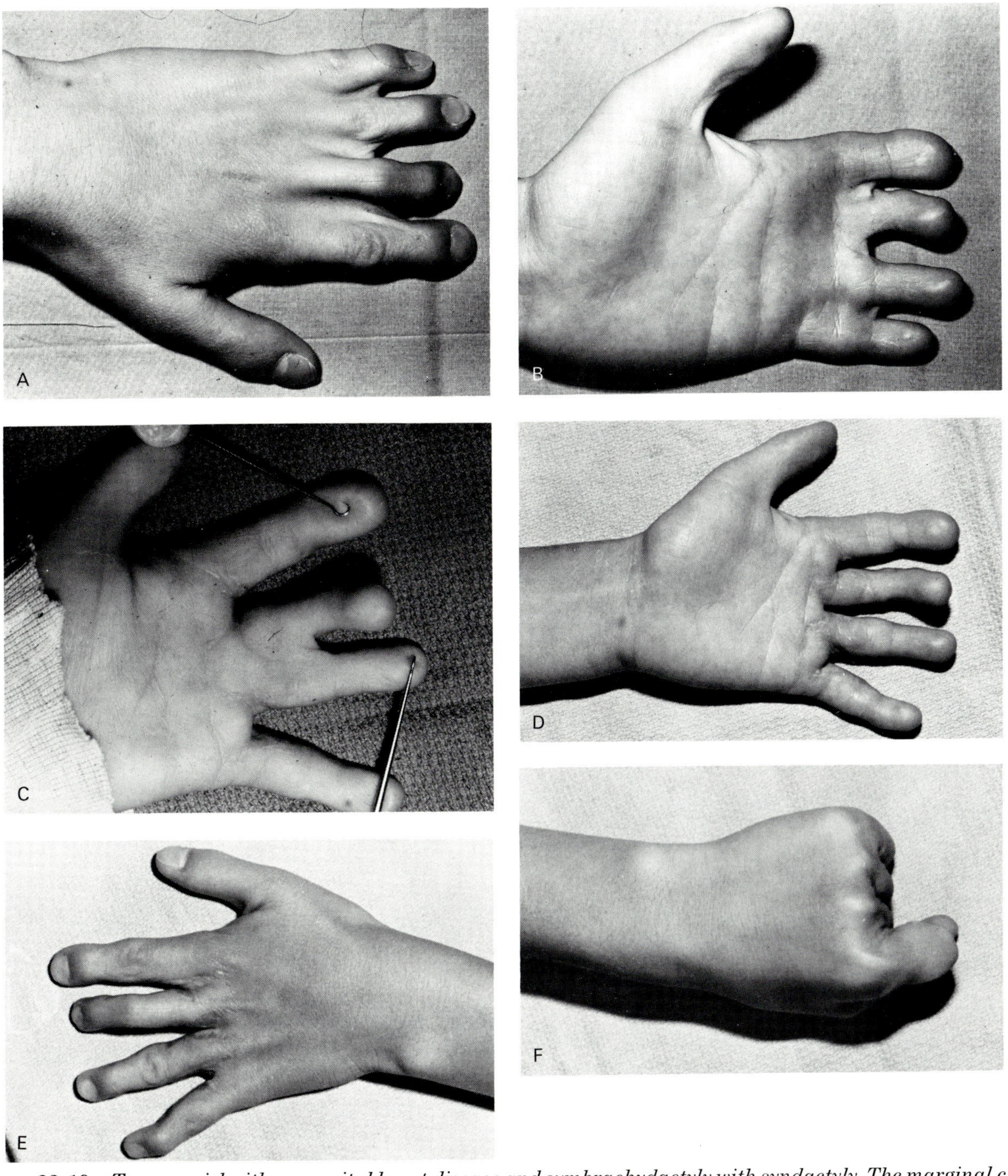

Figure 23-19. *Teenage girl with congenital heart disease and symbrachydactyly with syndactyly. The marginal clefts were constructed first and the central web last* **(C).** *The limited index flexion* **(F)** *resulted from the symbrachydactyly.*

proximal to distal so that these structures can be identified where they are largest. A synostosis can generally be cut with a knife. Hemostasis is assured by using needlepoint cautery at low voltage. Sutures are placed so that the flaps do not choke the fingers and, where loose approximation is not possible, a liberal-sized, thick split-thickness skin graft is applied. The grafts are sutured in place.

The dressing is a critical element for success. It is applied wet but without circumferential constriction. The web space must not be choked or stuffed. The fingers should be furled over a roll of soft gauze and a well-padded long-arm boxing-glove cast is applied which is removed at 7 to 14 days.

The prime pitfall of this operation is failure to ensure adequate blood supply and innervation of

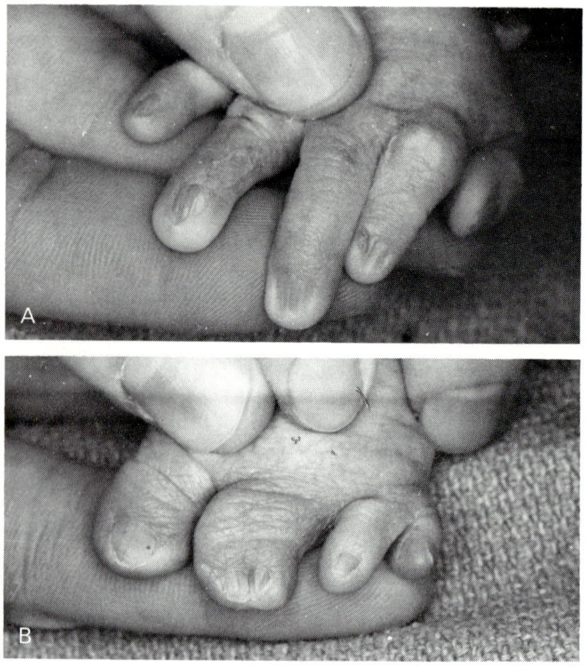

Figure 23-20. *The syndactyly, focal dermal hypoplasia and nail hypoplasia that occurs in children with Goltz-Gorlin syndrome.*[13]

the digits. For this reason, both sides of a digit should never be subjected to the release of syndactyly at the same time. Furthermore, a significant deficit of circulation noted during surgery on one side should guide the surgeon on the other side. Should it be impossible to preserve sensibility to the adjoining digits, the least functionally important side should be denervated.

Complex Syndactyly

In complex syndactyly, the skin bridge is often the least of the developmental, functional and cosmetic problems. A multitude of skeletal aberrations—brachydactyly (shortening), symphalangism (ankylosis) (Fig. 23-19), angulations and supernumerary parts, e.g. polydactyly—may be present. Therefore, the program of treatment must be primarily directed at skeletal alignment and function. The potential for progressive deformity, as well as impairment of motion and growth, must be evaluated.

In acrosyndactyly, the synostoses are the problem. The prime concerns are the determination of how many fingers to save and the early separation of these bony bridges of contained digits (Fig. 23-23). When congenital constricting rings coexist, they usually have to be released first. In the case of Apert's syndrome (acrocephalosyndactyly, mitten hand), the first concern following the separation of the digital tips is freeing of the border digits. The synostotic tips are sectioned at about 4 to 6 months of age and the separation is allowed to heal spontaneously. This is limited to the index-long fingertips and ring-little fingertips, since only 3 fingers are freed. If the thumb syndactyly is minimal, 3 web releases can be done at one time, with the central ray resection. When the ray to be deleted is determined, the skin from that finger is incorporated into the flaps used to cover the remaining digits. As the child grows, osteotomies may be needed to correct rotation or angulation deformities.

In symbrachydactyly, as seen in Poland's syndrome with hypoplasia of the extremity, the digits should be separated early (1 year) to encourage motion and growth.

All patients operated upon for syndactyly should be followed into adulthood and appropriate secondary procedures undertaken as function and cosmesis dictate. Parents must appreciate that surgery will not correct stunted growth or necessarily reduce the awareness of the defect.

ABSENCE OF FINGERS (ECTRODACTYLY, FIG. 23-24)

This condition may be partial or complete for any ray. The missing element may be at any level in the ray. When the defect is centrally located, a cleft or lobster-claw hand results. Ectrodactyly of the little finger is less common than that of the thumb. Occasionally this problem appears as a monodactyly in which there is only one ray in the whole hand.

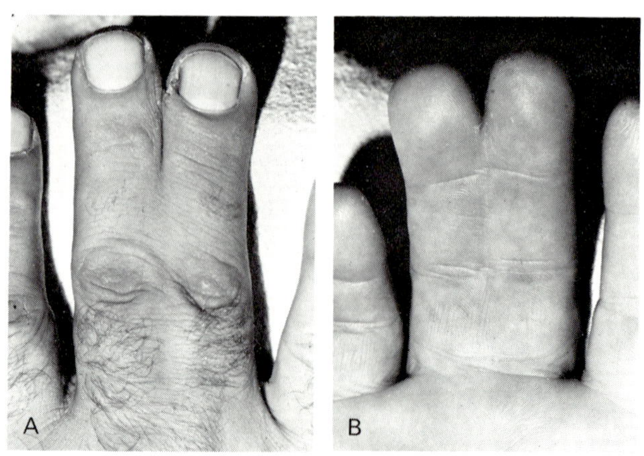

Figure 23-21. *Young male with an uncorrected syndactyly of the ring and middle fingers.*

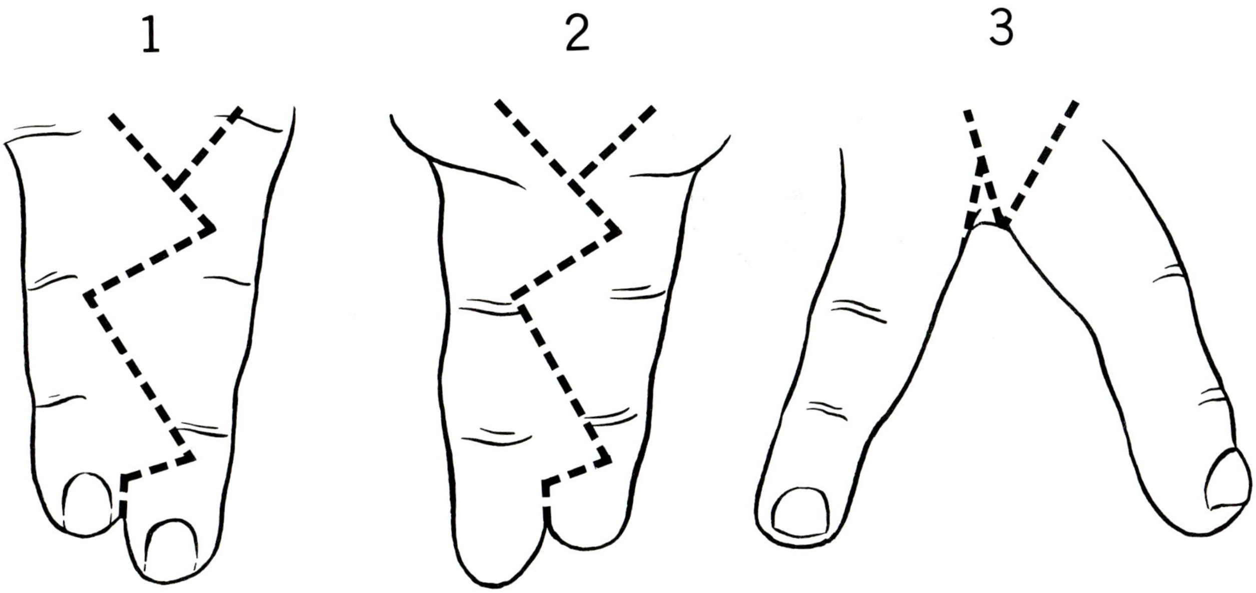

Figure 23-22. *Technique of syndactyly correction discussed in the text. All adequate procedures to correct syndactylism require some skin grafting of the web area.*

Treatment is directed at providing a pinch mechanism. This may be achieved by rotation osteotomy, dactylization of a metacarpal, resection of a metacarpal to develop a web, and expansion of the web by skin graft or Z-plasty.

SMALL FINGER

This deformity occurs as an isolated involvement of one bone or as an involvement of multiple bones and rays. It is an inherited anomaly of transverse segmentation. It occurs as a part of many complex syndromes and is generally transmitted as a dominant phenotype, e.g. dwarfism. Most cases require no treatment. However, when one digit is unduly dwarfed and the rest of the hand is "normal," resection may be appropriate. Difficult cases with limited function are candidates for more extensive procedures which include those listed for ectrodactyly above.

LARGE FINGER (MACRODACTYLY, GIGANTISM, FIG. 23-25)

It is conjectural whether this rare problem is truly a congenital anomaly or whether it is acquired. Seldom is it associated with other congenital abnormalities. Present opinion suggests that this hypertrophy is induced by the changes of neural elements in neurofibromatosis (possibly a variant of von Recklinghausen's disease). There is hypertrophy of all mesenchymal tissues except tendons and vessels. The phalanges are more often hypertrophied than the metacarpals except in advanced cases. The gigantism may develop insidiously or rapidly. Invariably, it is confined to the distribution of the median or ulnar nerve. Adjacent digits of the same innervation are involved, and no intervening digits of the same innervation are spared. In severe cases the degree of enlargement of the bones may seem to replace the surrounding soft tissue, with severe impairment of motion.[12] There may be bowing of the involved digit. Characteristic pathological changes are extensive periosteal fibrosis with scattered nodules of a mixture of primitive bone and cartilage cells. There are many tiny neurofibromata and the main nerves are infiltrated with fibrous tissue. An increase in fat is found everywhere, including the bone marrow. The distal portions of the digits are the most severely involved.

The treatment has to be individualized for each patient. The objectives are the preservation of sensibility and mobility and the reduction in volume of the digit. These digits have poor wound-healing properties. The longitudinal overgrowth of bone may be treated by epiphyseal destruction of the proximal and middle phalanges. Tsuge[25] has advocated excision of hypertrophic nerve with preservation of the digital vessels. This has been attempted soon after birth.[7] Resection of the distal phalanx or reduction of the length and breadth of the phalanx, particularly the thumb, has also been tried.[18] Amputation is resorted to after other

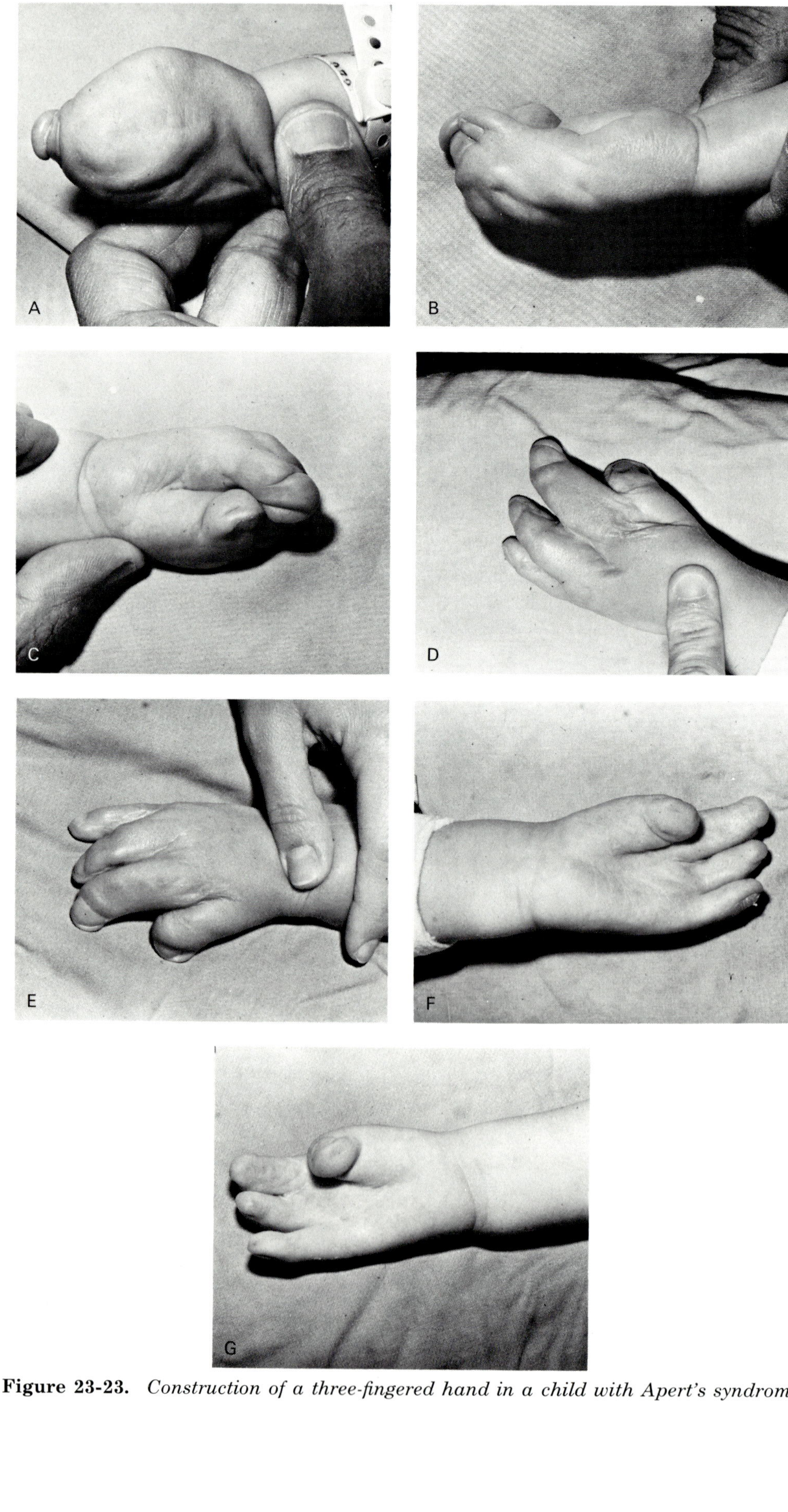

Figure 23-23. *Construction of a three-fingered hand in a child with Apert's syndrome.*

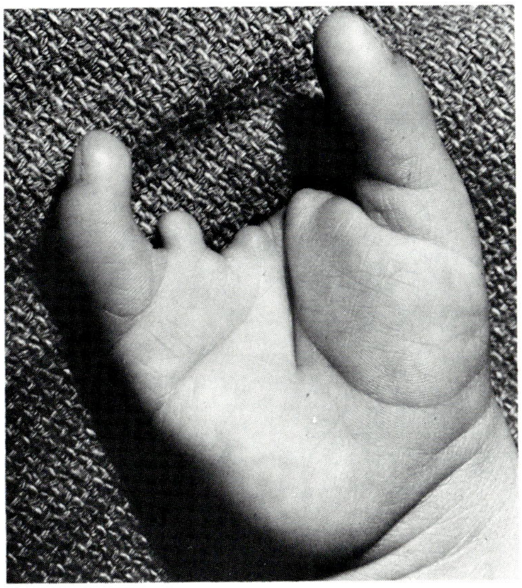

Figure 23-24. *Ectrodactyly. The nubbins were ultimately removed.*

measures have failed or if the growth period has passed and only one finger is enlarged. The involvement of the thumb may justify heroic measures if pollicization is not deemed appropriate.

LATERAL DEVIATION OF THE FINGER (CLINODACTYLY, CLINOARTHROSIS)

Clinodactyly is a deviation of the digit in the lateral plane. This is most often seen in the little finger as an isolated problem. The deviation is generally in the radial direction. It may be associated with a delta phalanx.

Treatment is indicated only if there is a major functional or cosmetic problem. Initially dynamic splinting may be tried and, if not successful, then surgery. This may involve resection of a deformed phalanx (delta phalanx) or wedge osteotomy. Occasionally, the angulation is at the metacarpophalangeal joint when all the fingers deviate ulnarward. This problem may have to be treated like post-traumatic ulnar drift or that associated with rheumatoid arthritis.

FLEXED FINGER (CAMPTODACTYLY, FIG. 23-26)

This congenital flexion contracture of one or more digits usually involves the proximal interphalangeal joint of the little finger. The pathomechanics have not been agreed upon. There may be a boutonniere stance. The contracture may be minimal, marked, static or progressive, and is usually familial.

There is no need for treatment in most instances. When the problem is progressing, splinting of the middle joint with simultaneous flexion of the wrist and metacarpophalangeal joints may be instituted. This may serve to overcome forces of contracture attributed to the superficialis, the volar skin and volar joint capsule. If the deformity progresses, surgery is indicated. Procedures which have been tried include tenotomy of the flexor superficialis, with or without Z-plasty, or grafting the released volar skin, and capsulotomy of the volar aspect of the joint.[23] An alternative procedure recommended by Millesi[18] is transfer of the flexor superficialis into the lateral extensor tendon to reinforce extension. No procedures known give uniformly predictable results in the treatment of this problem.

STIFF FINGERS (SYMPHALANGISM)

Symphalangism is usually bilateral and is transmitted as an autosomal dominant phenotype. It almost always involves the middle joint of the fingers and spares the thumb except in conditions such as Apert's syndrome and arthrogryposis. The stiffness is in extension. The incidence of involvement decreases progressively from the little finger to the radial side of the hand. Treatment is usually unnecessary unless there is impaired pinch or grasp or the digit hampers hand function.

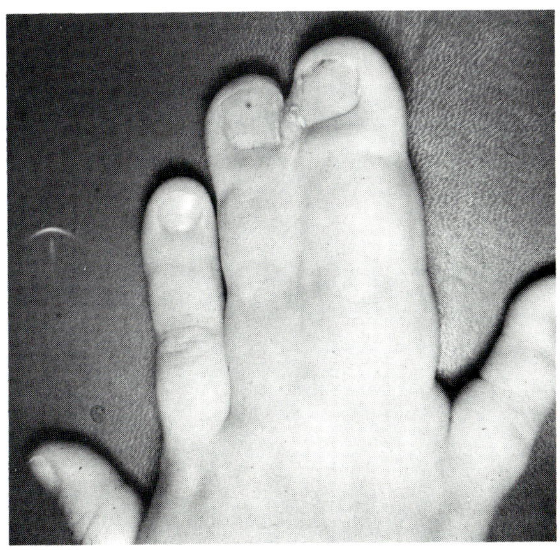

Figure 23-25. *Macrodactyly.*

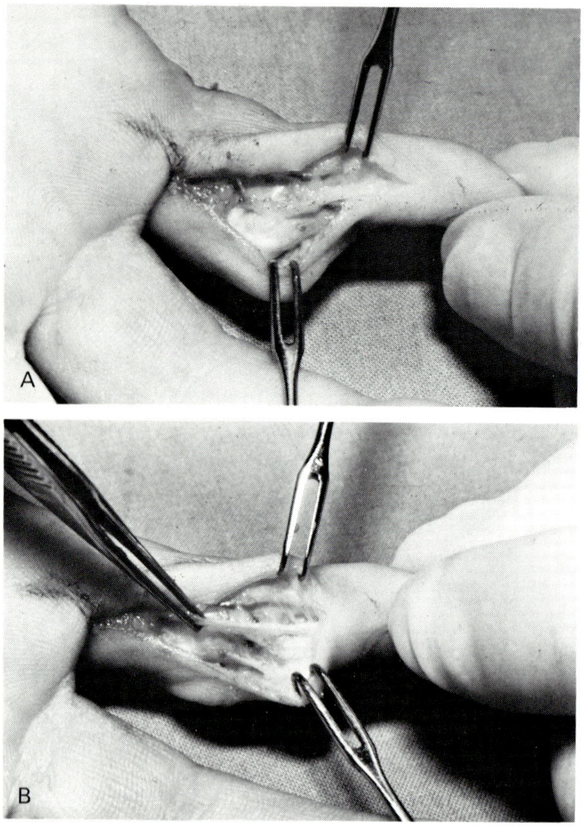

Figure 23-26. *Teenage girl with unilateral camptodactyly. Exploration of the finger revealed a stout band of fibrous tissue parallel to and in association with Landsmeer's ligament. Release of this corrected nearly all the flexion deformity.*

GROOVED FINGERS (ANNULAR BANDS, APHALANGIA)

Annular grooves may result from endogenous or exogenous influences.[12] The endogenous forces may represent focal necrosis and the exogenous type amniotic adhesions. They may occur with or without absences (spontaneous amputation, acral absence) of parts. Most cases are sporadic and few are familial.

They may be progressive and have been known to appear after birth. In the upper extremity, the fingers are most commonly involved. The involvement is unilateral and there may be distal lymphema secondary to the constriction.

If the grooves are shallow and static, no treatment is necessary. Deeper grooves should be corrected by multiple Z-plasties and occasionally by skin grafts. When the groove encircles a finger only, half the circumference should be operated upon at one time. If there is no function and salvage is hopeless in rudimentary digits (nubbins and bubbles), amputation is indicated.

References

1. Barsky, A.J.: *Congenital Deformities of the Hand and Their Surgical Treatment.* Charles C Thomas, Springfield, 1958.
2. Barsky, A.J.: Congenital anomalies of the thumb. Clin. Orthop., 15:96, 1959.
3. Behrman, S.: Genesis of fetal abnormalities. GP, 6:41, 1952.
4. Bora, F.W., Nicholson, J.T. and Cheema, H.M.: Radial meromeila: the deformity and its treatment. J. Bone Joint Surg., 52A:966, 1970.
5. Birck-Jensen, A.: *Congenital Deformities of the Upper Extremity.* Munksgard, Copenhagen, 1949.
6. Darrach, W. and Dwight, K.: Derangements of the inferior radioulnar articulation. Med. Rec., 87:708, 1915.
7. Edgerton, M.T. and Tuerk, D.B.: Macrodactyly (digital gigantism) nature and treatment. In: *Symposium on Reconstructive Hand Surgery* (Littler, J.W., Cramer, L.M. and Smith, J.W., Eds.). C.V. Mosby, St. Louis, 1974.
8. Entin, M.A.: Reconstruction of congenital abnormalities of the upper extremities. J. Bone Joint Surg., 41A:681, 1959.
9. Handforth, J.R.: Polydactylism of the hand in Southern Chinese. Anat. Rec., 106:119, 1950.
10. Hartrampf, C.R., Vasconez, L.O. and Mathes, S.: Construction of one good thumb from both parts of a congenitally bifid thumb. Plast. Reconstr. Surg., 54:148, 1974.
11. Ivy, R.H.: Congenital anomalies. Plast. Reconstr. Surg., 20:400, 1957.
12. Kelikian, H. and Doumanian A.: Congenital anomalies of the hand. J. Bone Joint Surg., Part I, 1002 and Part II, 1249, 1957.
13. Kelikian, H.: *Congenital Deformities of the Hand and Forearm.* W.B. Saunders, Philadelphia, 1974.
14. Littler, J.W.: The neurovascular pedicle method of digital transposition for reconstruction of the thumb. Plast. Reconstr. Surg., 12:303, 1953.
15. Littler, J.W.: Pollicization. Presented at the 30th Annual Meeting of the American Society for Surgery of the Hand. Members Day Program, February 26, 1975, San Francisco, California.
16. Meyer, H. and Cummins, H.: Severe maternal trauma in early pregnancy: Congenital amputations in infants at term. Am. J. Obstet. Gynecol., 42:150, 1941.
17. Milch, H.: Cuff resection of the ulna for malunited Colles' fracture. J. Bone Joint Surg., 23:311, 1941.
18. Millesi, H.: Camptodactyly. In: *Symposium on Reconstructive Hand Surgery* (Littler, J.W., Cramer, L.M. and Smith, J.W., Eds.). C.V. Mosby, St. Louis, 1974.
19. Millesi, H.: Macrodactyly: A case study. In: *Symposium on Reconstructive Hand Surgery* (Littler, J.W., Cramer, L.M. and Smith, J.W., Eds.). C.V. Mosby, St. Louis, 1974.
20. Murray, J.F., Shore, B. and Treffer, E.: Prosthesis for children with unilateral congenital absence of the hand. J. Bone Joint Surg., 54A:1658, 1972.
21. Nylen, B.: Repair of congenital finger syndactyly. Acta Chir. Scand., 113:310, 1957.
22. Paletta, F.X.: Congenital deformities of the hands and feet. Mo. Med., 50:19, 1953.
23. Smith, R.J. and Kaplan, E.B.: Camptodactyly and similar atraumatic flexion deformities of the proximal interphalangeal joints of the fingers. J. Bone Joint Surg., 50A:1187, 1968.
24. Swanson, A.B.: Severe congenital malformation of the upper limb—consideration for classification and treatment.

In: *Symposium on the Hand* (Cramer, L.M. and Chase, R.A., Eds.). C.V. Mosby, St. Louis, 1971.
25. Tsuge, K.: Treatment of megalodactyly. Plast. Reconstr. Surg., 39:590, 1967.
26. Tupper, J.W.: Pollex abductus due to congenital malposition of the flexor pollicis longus. J. Bone Joint Surg., 51A:1285, 1969.
27. Warkany, J. and Nelson, R.C.: Skeletal abnormalities in the offspring of rats reared on deficient diets. Anat. Rec., 79:83, 1941.
28. Warkany, J.: Congenital malformations induced by maternal nutritional deficiency. J. Pediatr., 25:476, 1944.
29. Warkany, J.: Factors in etiology of congenital malformations. Am. J. Ment. Defic., 50:231, 1945.
30. Warkany, J.: Factors of congenital malformations. Adv. Pediatr., 2:1, 1947.
31. Warkany, J. and Schroffenberger, F.: Congenital malformations induced in rats by roentgen rays. Am. J. Roentgenol., 57:455, 1947.
32. Watson, K. and Boyes, J.H.: Congenital angular deformities of the digits. J. Bone Joint Surg., 49A:333, 1967.

24 The Rheumatoid Hand*

Connective tissue diseases, especially rheumatoid arthritis, are common and profoundly alter hand function in a high percentage of cases. The functional disruption may be severe enough to preclude activities as simple as dressing, eating and tending to other personal needs.

Physicians involved with care of patients with rheumatoid hands must be knowledgeable in the connective tissue diseases and well versed in the many drugs available for effective treatment of specific disorders. The hand surgeon, as part of a team, has much to offer the rheumatoid patient with hand involvement.

The spectrum of connective tissue diseases includes rheumatoid arthritis, lupus erythematosus, dermatomyositis, progressive systemic sclerosis (scleroderma) and mixed combinations of these entities. Each of these will present specific diagnostic and therapeutic problems for which the reader should refer to the literature.

The diagnosis and treatment of specific hand deformities are quite similar for each of the collagen diseases, although there are some general differences. For example, patients with progressive systemic sclerosis are susceptible to problems of wound healing; patients with lupus erythematosus are not likely to have synovitis.

Rheumatoid arthritis is the most common of the collagen diseases. This chapter will deal only with rheumatoid arthritis, but the principles of management can, in most cases, be applied to the other connective tissue diseases.

Pathogenesis of Rheumatoid Synovitis

Rheumatoid arthritis is actually a misnomer. The disease is primarily a synovitis and not an arthritis. A pathological process in the synovium disrupts the joint and tendon systems of the hand and results in various subsequent pathological states.

The most characteristic serological feature of patients with rheumatoid arthritis is rheumatoid factor, which is defined as antibody directed against the heavy chain of IgG. Antiglobulins may occur in all five immunoglobulin classes (IgM, IgG, IgA, IgD and IgE), but are most characteristically found in the IgM class.

Rheumatoid factor, which is found in both serum and synovial fluid, binds IgG, forming macromolecular immune complexes. These complexes can deposit on any available membrane, the most pertinent being synovium. The complexes fix and activate complement, thus initiating the inflammatory process with resulting damage to the membrane and adjacent structures.

In the patient with rheumatoid arthritis, synovium is much more than an inert membrane for immune complex deposition. Immunoglobulins including rheumatoid factor are synthesized in

*The assistance of John Clough, M.D., Department of Rheumatology, Cleveland Clinic Foundation, in the preparation of the medical portion of this chapter is gratefully acknowledged.

lymphoctyes located there. Phagocytic cells (including polymorphonuclear leukocytes, monocytes and macrophages) congregate in synovium because of the chemotactic action of the C-5, -6, -7 complement complex. The deposited immune macromolecular complexes are opsonized by early-acting complement components (through C-3). The phagocytic cells, together with synovial phagocytes normally present there, attempt to ingest the large opsonized immune macromolecular complexes.

This results in the release of lysosomal contents and the activation of other inflammation-provoking materials such as kallikrein. Many lysosomal materials are released, but the ones which probably do the most damage to the joint or to the tendons are the cathepsins (active at low pH), collagenase (active at a pH of 7 to 9) and hydrochloric acid.

Thus the synovium in the patient with rheumatoid arthritis has several pathological roles: (1) It provides cells—polymorphonuclear cells, leukocytes and probably macrophages. (2) It is one source of so-called chemotactic factor (C-5, -6, -7 responsible for the attraction of the leukocytes). (3) It provides C-3 (opsonin) which stimulates the leukocytes to phagocytize the macromolecules. (4) It is the source of the damaging lysosomal enzymes. (5) The synovium may be disruptive from its bulk alone, and mechanically interfere with the excursion of tendon and movement of joints.

The role of the synovium in the creation of specific hand deformities will be discussed in conjunction with each deformity. In general, the inflamed joint synovium disrupts joints by mechanically stretching and enzymatically digesting the supporting tendon and ligament systems, and by destroying the cartilage and subchondral bone. Synovium may cause tendon rupture by several mechanisms, which may result in deformities as varied as loss of finger flexion or the boutonniere phenomenon.

The central role of synovium in rheumatoid arthritis must be emphasized. This synovium with its mechanical and enzymatic effects disrupts both tendon and joint systems. Within closed compartments such as the carpal tunnel or underneath the extensor retinaculum, the very bulk of the synovium may lead to ischemic tendon changes and thereby be a factor in tendon rupture. Also, the enzymes released may seriously weaken the tendon structure.

In the joint, the synovium has several effects. First, by its bulk, it stretches the collateral ligament and volar plate systems of the small joints of the hand and the ligamentous systems of the wrist. Secondly, its enzymes seriously weaken the strength of these ligaments and contribute thereby to its disruption. Musculotendinous tension across these joints then precipitates deformity. Obviously, any change in joint alignment will alter the vector of pull of flexor and extensor tendon systems and further increase the deformities.

Diagnosis

The diagnosis of rhematoid arthritis is usually made before the patient sees the hand surgeon. Occasionally, however, the patient with a synovitis of one or several joint or tendon systems in the hand without a previous diagnosis will be seen in the office of the hand surgeon. In this situation, the hand surgeon must be alert to the early signs of rheumatoid arthritis in the hands. At first glance, the patient may seem to have a common entity such as tennis elbow, De Quervain's disease or carpal tunnel syndrome.

When primarily involving tendon systems, rheumatoid arthritis may appear as a tenosynovitis at the wrist. If flexor, it often may be combined with a carpal or ulnar tunnel syndrome. If extensor, there will be swelling on the dorsum of the wrist. Note that with the extensor retinaculum this swelling may be just distal to the wrist and actually over the dorsum of the hand. Pain, tenderness, limited motion and extensor tendon rupture may occur.

The earliest joint symptoms are usually swelling and tenderness, with some increased warmth. The hand joints most commonly affected are the proximal interphalangeal (PIP) and metacarpophalangeal (MCP). Initially, the wrist or elbow may also be involved. These joints will demonstrate some loss of motion and usually pain. If only one joint is involved, it can mimic either septic arthritis or gout.

The patient with definite synovitis of any joint or tendon system in the hand, without obvious traumatic or infectious origin, should be considered as a possible rheumatoid arthritic, and the appropriate diagnostic tests should be ordered. Certain roentgenographic and laboratory tests will be discussed. For the details of the early diagnosis of rheumatoid arthritis, the reader is referred to a description of the classification system of the American Rheumatism Association and to the standard text by Hollander.[3]

The early roentgenographic changes in the hand include loss of soft tissue definition, usually related to soft tissue swelling about the joints. Later, early subchondral erosions appear. This is most commonly seen in the proximal interphalangeal joints, in the metacarpophalangeal joints and in the ulnar styloid (Fig. 24-1).

Laboratory studies that aid in the differential diagnosis of painful joints include: (1) acute phase reactants such as sedimentation rate, plasma fibrinogen, serum glycoproteins and serum protein electrophoresis for alpha II globulin level, (2) tests for rheumatoid factor such as latex fixation, bentonite flocculation and sensitized sheep cell agglutination, (3) tests for antibodies against nuclear components such as fluorescent antinuclear antibody, LE cell preparation, anti-DNA and anti-ENA and (4) serum uric acid.

The acute phase reactants are elevated in inflammatory diseases, including rheumatoid arthritis, other connective tissue diseases when active, infections and some malignancies. They are primarily useful in distinguishing organic from functional disease, and inflammatory from degenerative disease.

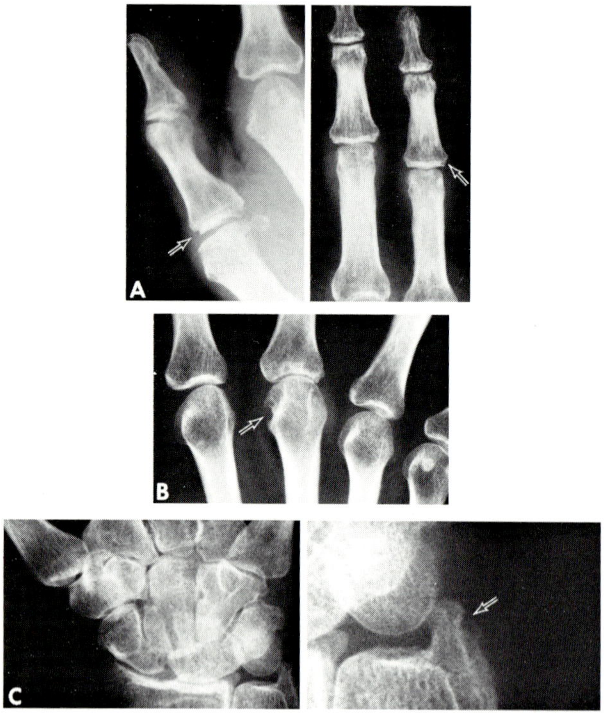

Figure 24-1. *The earliest roentgenographic findings of rheumatoid arthritis may be soft tissue swelling.* **A:** *The first bony changes are often small marginal joint erosions, seen here in the thumb MCP joint and the digital PIP joints.* **B:** *Another common site of marginal bony erosion is beneath the proximal attachment of the MCP collateral ligament, demonstrated here on the radial aspect of the long finger MCP joint.* **C:** *The wrist is often afflicted early in the disease process, with joint narrowing and erosions. These erosions commonly first involve the ulnar styloid.*

Tests for rheumatoid factor, all of which depend on agglutination of IgG-coated particles in its presence, are exquisitely sensitive only to IgM rheumatoid factor, and may be negative in the presence of rheumatoid factors of other immunoglobulin classes. This may explain why some patients with rheumatoid arthritis do not seem to have rheumatoid factor. Rheumatoid factors may be present in diseases other than rheumatoid arthritis—other connective tissue diseases, tuberculosis, subacute bacterial endocarditis, and in some normal persons, especially the elderly.

Differential Diagnosis

The differential diagnosis of the rheumatoid hand is that of any synovitis or arthritis. It includes the various collagen disorders, gout, pseudogout, degenerative arthritis, septic arthritis or tuberculosis arthritis and tendonitis. A most important differential to establish early is that of tuberculous tenosynovitis. Obviously, any of the anti-inflammatory drugs or steroids which are commonly used in rheumatoid arthritis are absolutely contraindicated in a tuberculous tenosynovitis. Occasionally, a patient is seen with tuberculous tenosynovitis which has been treated with steroids, with disastrous consequences.

In addition to the synovitis and tenosynovitis with resultant deformities, rheumatoid vasculitis and neuropathy occur. Obviously, treatment of these conditions does not fall within the province of the hand surgeon. Rheumatoid vasculitis can lead to gangrene (Fig. 24-2).

The least dramatic forms of vasculitis may be manifested only by small petechial lesions. However, these patients may have significant problems in postoperative wound healing or in digital perfusion. Patients with rheumatoid vasculitis should not be operated upon except in very unusual situations. These patients may have neuropathy, probably an ischemic phenomenon in the nerves, considerable pain and areas of sensory and motor deficit. Careful distinction must be made, however, between neuropathy and the carpal tunnel syndrome, ulnar tunnel syndrome and cervical radiculopathy. Obviously, with the increased flexor synovium, a carpal tunnel syndrome type of picture is common in the rheumatoid patient.

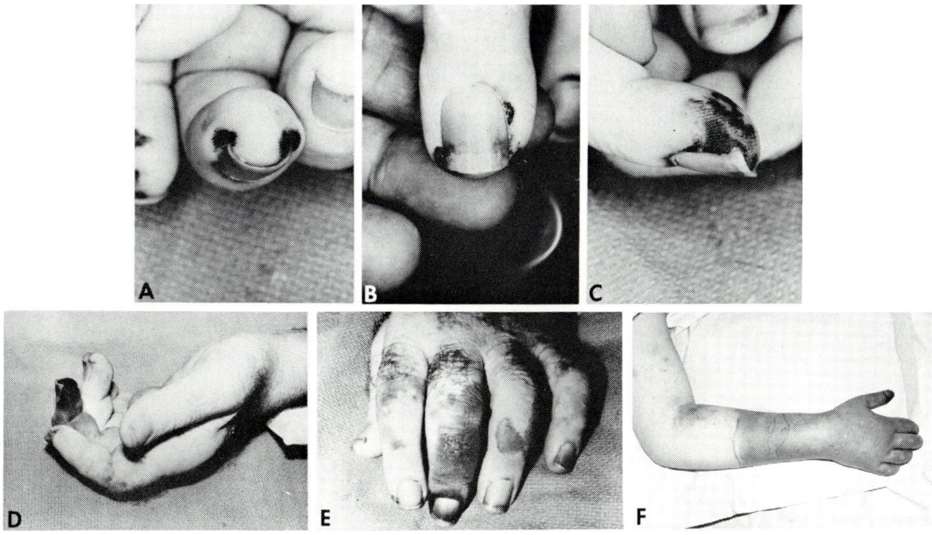

Figure 24-2. *Arterial and arteriolar inflammation is a basic pathological process seen in many rheumatoid lesions. There is a rare clinical syndrome of "rheumatoid arteritis" which includes not only areas of skin necrosis and digital gangrene but also peripheral neuropathy and visceral involvement with intestinal gangrene. Episcleritis, pleuritis, pericarditis and myocarditis may antedate or be concurrent with the digital changes. Renal and central nervous system involvement may occur. The underlying pathological process is not well understood. In severe cases, the prognosis is grave. Isolated digital lesions may occur. Patients need not have preexistent Raynaud's phenomenon. The digital changes may or may not be accompanied by the polyneuropathy and other systemic findings of the full clinical syndrome of rheumatoid vasculitis.* **A,B:** *Isolated areas of infarction may occur which may be sharply localized and heal without incident.* **C–F:** *The lesion may progress to gangrene of the distal phalanx, the entire digits or even the hand. (A-E courtesy of William P. Graham, III, M.D.)*

Medical Synovectomy

The surgeon who undertakes the care of the hand of a rheumatoid patient must be a member of a team. Care must include the active assistance of an internist well versed in the various medical problems of the rheumatoid patient and the various possible drug treatments and side effects.

Many drugs are commonly used in the treatment of rheumatoid arthritis. These include salicylates, antimalarials, steroids, gold, and cytotoxic or "immunosuppressant" drugs. Each of these drugs is effective in the appropriate patient, but the dosage of each must be carefully regulated, and all have significant side effects. Salicylates may cause gastrointestinal disturbances. Antimalarial drugs may combine with melanin and cause retinal damage. Steroids have serious side effects. Gold therapy may cause kidney or skin changes. Cytotoxic drugs may suppress the bone marrow, affect hepatic or gastrointestinal function and, in the case of cyclophosphamide, may produce severe bladder hemorrhage.

The therapeutic sites of action of these drugs are not known in detail at this time. Many theories have been advanced. Several drugs (especially steroids and antimalarials) probably act upon the lysosomal systems; some are thought to stabilize the lysosomal membrane, and others perhaps block the action of the enzymes once released.

General Surgical Considerations

When the hand surgeon evaluates the patient with rheumatoid arthritis, the general health and drug program must be carefully noted. The effect of the disease on all joints, lower extremity as well as upper, must be known. It is important to determine if the rheumatoid disease is early, "burned out," cyclical, or unremittingly progressive.

The patient's functional level must be accurately assessed. If a wage earner, is he able to continue his job and support his family? Can he drive, can he feed himself, can he dress and undress himself? If the patient is a housewife, can she do the housework, is she able to cook, can she lift pots and pans, can she peel potatoes? Which hand is dominant? What substitution patterns has the patient resorted to in order to continue to function? How rapidly is hand function deteriorating?

It is also important to examine the elbow and

shoulder carefully. Obviously, severe disabling elbow or shoulder pain which prevents positioning of the hand for function must be treated before considering surgery on the hand itself.

Furthermore, the lower extremities should be carefully evaluated. If the patient requires crutches for ambulation or is going to require surgery on the lower extremities which will necessitate crutches, platform crutches should be prescribed. If possible, rehabilitation of the lower extremities should be completed first, to minimize the use of crutches after hand and wrist reconstruction.

Anesthesia for the Rheumatoid Patient Requiring Hand Surgery

These patients present complex problems in hand reconstruction, and often require staged procedures. At the same time, they present difficult problems in medical management if their overall health is not good. They may have concurrent cardiac or renal disease. They are often receiving several drugs, including steroids, and therefore represent a significant risk for general anesthesia. If the patient has had steroids within the past year, and if general anesthesia is to be used, supplemental systemic steroids are advisable. Drug management is best done in cooperation with the rheumatologist and anesthesiologist.

Nearly all hand procedures can be performed with some form of regional anesthesia. The alternatives include axillary block, supraclavicular block and regional intravenous anesthesia. Many of the shorter procedures can be done with wrist block or digital block.

The regional block of choice is probably axillary. When properly performed, it has a high degree of reliability and will give approximately three hours of anesthesia. This may not be possible, however, if the patient has a significant adduction and internal rotation deformity of the shoulder. In these cases, either a supraclavicular block or intravenous regional anesthesia may be used.

A disadvantage of the intravenous regional anesthetic is that if the tourniquet has to be released because of prolonged tourniquet time, or should the surgeon choose to release it to obtain hemostasis prior to closure, the anesthesia is simultaneously lost. Also, should the procedure be relatively short, the anesthetic will not be fixed to the tissues and a sudden bolus of drug may be released into the general circulation.

The wrist block and digital block provide excellent anesthesia. They do not allow long periods of tourniquet ischemia, but do have a definite place in simple surgical procedures in the hand which are expected to take less than 25 minutes.

If general anesthesia is anticipated, a lateral roentgenogram of the neck in flexion and extension must be obtained to rule out C-1—C-2 instability, a common problem in the rheumatoid patient.

Synovectomy

The details of surgical synovectomy will be considered later under the individual joint or tendon systems. The following generalities are emphasized.

1. Surgical synovectomy should be done only as part of a combined medical-surgical approach. It is performed only for the patient with significant synovitis who has not responded to medical treatment after an adequate 6-month trial.
2. Surgical synovectomy is best done in the patient with early rheumatoid arthritis without fixed deformity, in the absence of roentgenographic changes, with a good coexistent medical program which has failed to control the synovium at that particular site.
3. No surgical synovectomy is complete.
4. The purpose of the surgical synovectomy is to remove both the chemical enzymatic element and the mechanical deforming force of the proliferating synovium.
5. At the time of synovectomy it is critically important to correct any coexisting dynamic imbalances. For example, should the synovectomy be performed at the metacarpophalangeal joint, it is important to do an intrinsic release if necessary, to release the ulnar collateral ligaments if indicated, and to rebalance the long extensor mechanism by reefing of the sagittal fibers.
6. There are certain definite contraindications to synovectomy. Synovectomy will not correct instability of joints. It will not correct a fixed deformity or extensor imbalance. It will not increase joint motion. It should never be done in the absence of a good medical program.
7. The results of synovectomy are difficult to evaluate. Because of the tremendous variation in the pattern of rheumatoid arthritis from patient to patient (be it the cyclical or unremitting type), age of onset, and variety of drug programs, it is difficult to define recurrence. Furthermore, synovitis at the same joint in a given patient may vary from day to day, with or without treatment. Function similarly will fluctuate. Accurate assessment of the results of synovectomy may be difficult. It is even more difficult to establish a meaningful control group.

Synovitis definitely recurs in some cases. However, several authors claim a decreased incidence of synovitis following synovectomy, and most will acknowledge a definite decrease in pain. Whether "prophylactic" synovectomy prevents deformity in rheumatoid arthritis is an unsettled question. It probably decreases the incidence of tendon rupture at the wrist level.

Systems Involved in the Hand of a Patient with Rheumatoid Arthritis

Usually several parts of the hand are simultaneously involved in rheumatoid arthritis. It is best to consider separately each of several components or systems of the rheumatoid hand. These include extensor tendon systems over the dorsum of the wrist and hand, the flexor tendon systems of the wrist, palm, and fingers, the wrist joint itself, including both the radial carpal and distal radial ulnar joint, the metacarpophalangeal joints, including extensor lag and ulnar drift, the proximal interphalangeal joint with either swan-neck or boutonniere deformity, the distal interphalangeal (DIP) joint and the thumb.

The Extensor Tendons of the Hand and Wrist

The extensor tendons over the dorsal aspect of the wrist and proximal hand are often involved (Fig. 24-3). This synovitis may or may not be associated with extensor tendon rupture or with synovitis of the wrist joint and distal radial ulnar joint.

In selecting patients for extensor tendon synovectomy, several factors must be considered. No patient should undergo dorsal extensor tenosynovectomy unless the synovium fails to respond to a vigorous, well-supervised trial of systemic drugs. Extensor synovectomy should be done if (1) after 4 months of drug therapy there has been no resolution of the dorsal synovium, (2) after a drug program there is only temporary resolution of the synovium, followed by its active return or (3) the patient already has had an extensor tendon rupture and requires tendon repair or transfer.

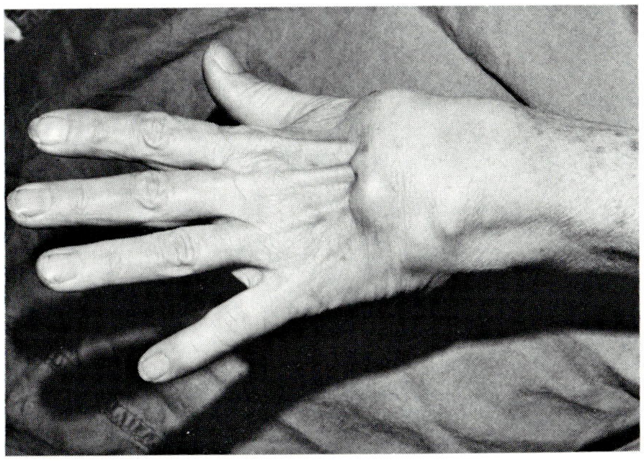

Figure 24-3. *Common appearance of extensor tenosynovitis. Note, in this patient, the absence of extensor rupture.*

OPERATIVE TECHNIQUE FOR WRIST DORSAL ARTHROTENOSYNOVECTOMY

A dorsal midline longitudinal incision is used, extending from the midmetacarpal level to 2 to 3 inches proximal to the wrist (Fig. 24-4). A dorsal bayonet incision should never be used in the rheumatoid patient. The distal flap raised in such an incision may slough at the proximal corner, jeopardizing the extrinsic extensor mechanism of the fingers. In an attempt to salvage the extrinsic extensor tendons, it may be necessary to perform an abdominal pedicle flap.

With the incision completed, the midline dissection is carried to the extensor retinaculum. Care must be taken to preserve as many of the dorsal veins as possible, for these veins supply the venous drainage for the hand. Dissection is then continued medially and laterally in a plane between the fat and the extensor retinaculum. Be mindful of the radial and ulnar sensory nerves.

The extensor retinaculum is then longitudinally incised either laterally or medially. An incision can be made through the extensor retinaculum overlying the extensor carpi radialis longus and the retinaculum raised as an ulnar-based flap as far as the ulnar margin of the extensor digitorum communis. As an alternative, the extensor retinaculum can be incised just to the ulnar side of the extensor digitorum communis and then raised as a radial-based flap. As dissection proceeds across Lister's tubercle, care must be taken not to buttonhole this retinacular flap and not to damage the extensor pollicis longus tendon which courses obliquely through this area.

A meticulous synovectomy of the extensor carpi radialis longus, extensor carpi radialis brevis, extensor pollicis longus, extensor indicis proprius and extensor digitorum communis can then be performed.

A simultaneous synovectomy of the wrist is often indicated for painful wrist motion, early signs of bony changes in the wrists or palpable wrist synovitis. A transverse incision is made in the dorsal wrist capsule and a meticulous synovectomy of the radiocarpal and intercarpal joints is done. A

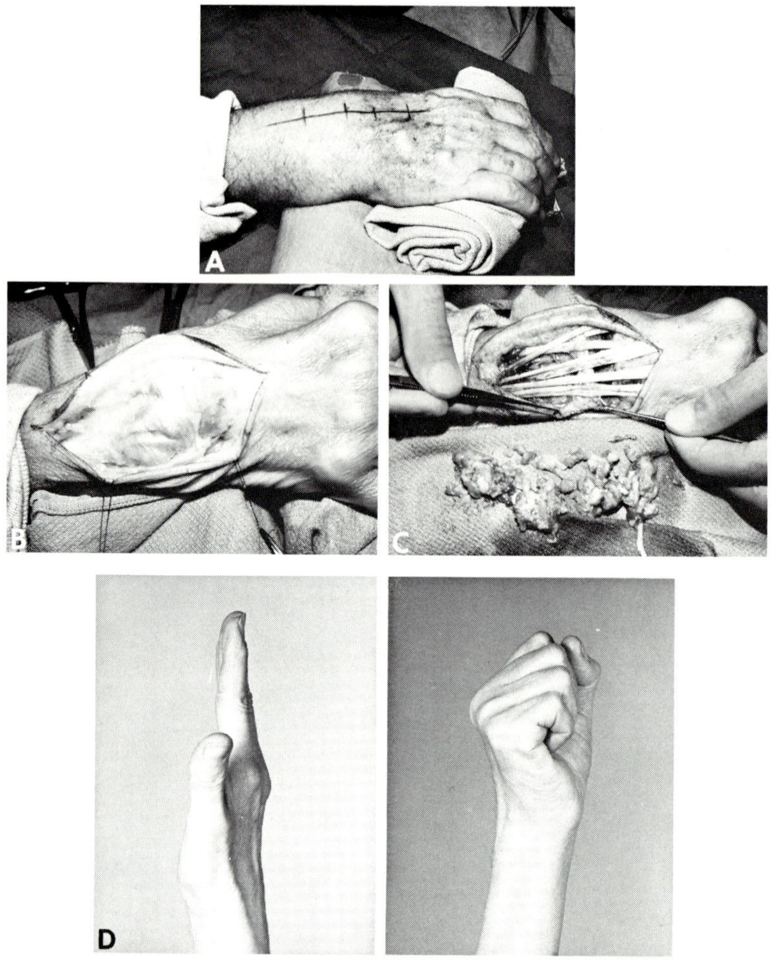

Figure 24-4. *Operative technique for dorsal arthrotenosynovectomy (see text).* **A:** *A dorsal midline longitudinal incision is recommended.* **B:** *Dissection is developed in a plane just superficial to the extensor retinaculum.* **C:** *After synovectomy of the extensor tendons and the radiocarpal joint, the wrist capsule is closed and the extensor retinaculum transposed deep to the extensor tendons. This provides a smooth, deep surface for extensor tendon excursion and places the extensor tendons in a subcutaneous plane.* **D:** *With proper surgical technique and exercise program, and in the absence of MCP and PIP joint disease or flexor synovitis, full finger extension and flexion should be maintained.*

small sharp rongeur is helpful for this procedure. The dorsal wrist capsule should then be closed. Lister's tubercle should be smoothed to the dorsum of the distal radius, as this dorsal bony prominence can contribute to extensor tendon rupture.

For synovectomy of the extensor digiti quinti, a separate incision is made in the extensor retinaculum of the fifth compartment. A synovectomy of the distal radioulnar joint and extensor carpi ulnaris is usually advisable.

Finally, the extensor retinacular flap should be transposed deep to the extensor tendons and repaired to the site of original division. This thus forms a smooth surface over which the extensor tendons glide. In effect, the extensor tendons are running through the subcutaneous fat. The wound should be meticulously closed. Either Penrose wick drains or Hemovac drains are advisable.

A supportive hand dressing must be applied and the hand elevated in the postoperative period to minimize swelling. Early, gentle active finger motion is encouraged in the initial dressing. The supportive dressing and sutures are removed at 3 weeks.

Certain complications may occur. First, hematoma is serious in this wound. If the patient has marginal blood supply to the flaps, a hematoma will cause flap necrosis. This is a disaster, because an abdominal pedicle flap is often required to salvage the situation. The first symptoms of hematoma are pain, often throbbing, and swelling of the fingers with some cyanosis and coolness. If a hematoma occurs, it should be promptly evacuated.

Second, in the rheumatoid patient, early gentle finger motion is important to prevent loss of metacarpophalangeal flexion from dorsal scarring and tethering. Obviously, simultaneous extensor tendon repairs or transfers must be protected during this period.

The incidence of recurrence of the dorsal synovium of the extensor tendon is low, and the incidence of rupture following dorsal tenosynovectomy is also low. A dorsal tenosynovectomy is one instance in which synovectomy seems to have a prophylactic role.

EXTENSOR TENDON RUPTURES

Extensor tendon ruptures are common. There are several probable causes related to the dorsal tenosynovium: (1) The actual invasion by the synovium into the tendon will result in structural tendon weakness. (2) The pressure of the synovial bulk under the fixed retinaculum may decrease the blood supply to the extensor tendons. (3) Lysosomal enzymatic digestion will soften the tendons. (4) An actual mechanical fraying of the tendons occurs as they pass back and forth over bone such as Lister's tubercle or the prominent ulnar head.

Any extensor tendon or combination of tendons may rupture (Fig. 24-5). The extensor digiti quinti and extensor communis commonly rupture at the wrist level, the extensor digitorum communis ruptures as it passes from beneath the extensor retinaculum, and the extensor digiti quinti ruptures over the ulnar head (Fig. 24-6).

The diagnosis of extensor rupture may not be straightforward, either for the fingers or for the thumb (Figs. 24-5, 24-7, 24-8). If the extensor indicis proprius and extensor digiti quinti remain, a ruptured extensor digitorum communis will cause a droop of only the long and ring fingers. Similarly, if the extensor digiti quinti ruptures but a strong communis to the fifth finger remains intact, the lag may be slight.

The intrinsics extend the finger interphalangeal joints, and it is finger metacarpophalangeal extension which is absent following long extensor rupture. Thus, in assessing extensor tendon ruptures, the examiner must be certain that the metacarpophalangeal joints are unsupported.

Two important conditions must be ruled out in considering the diagnosis of extensor rupture. First,

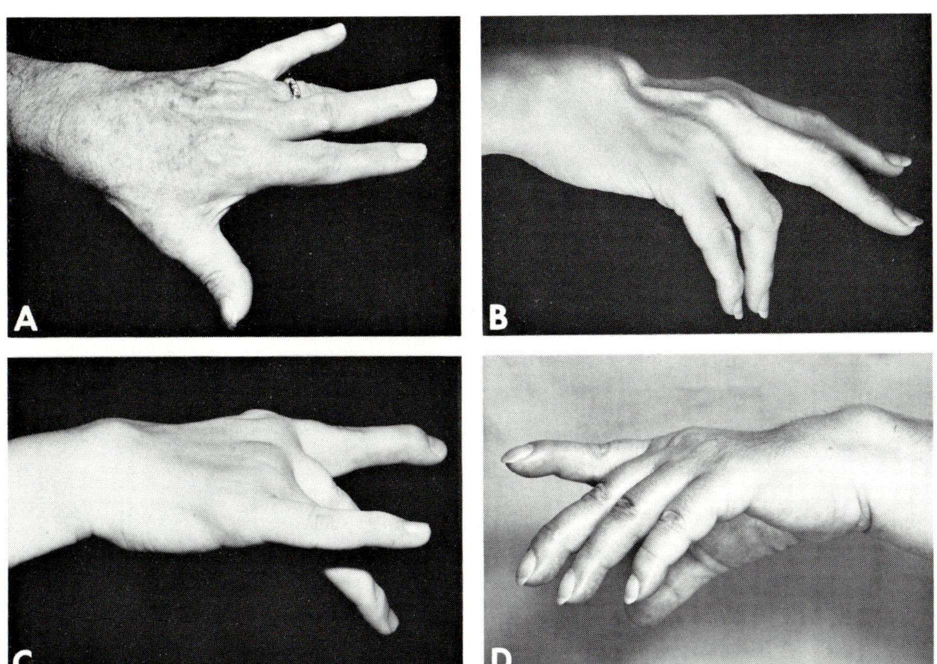

Figure 24-5. *Extrinsic extensor tendon ruptures (see text).* **A:** *Rupture of the extensor digitorum communis to the ring and little fingers may show only extensor lag of the ring finger if the extensor digiti quinti is intact. Furthermore, with the juncturae tendinum system, the lag may be incomplete.* **B:** *Rupture of the extensor digitorum communis to the ring and little fingers and the extensor digiti quinti will result in droop of the ring and fifth fingers.* **C:** *Extensor lag of the long and ring fingers occurs with rupture of the communis tendons with preservation of extensor proprius indicis and quinti.* **D:** *The so-called triple rupture is seen with loss of all extrinsic extensors except the extensor indicis proprius.*

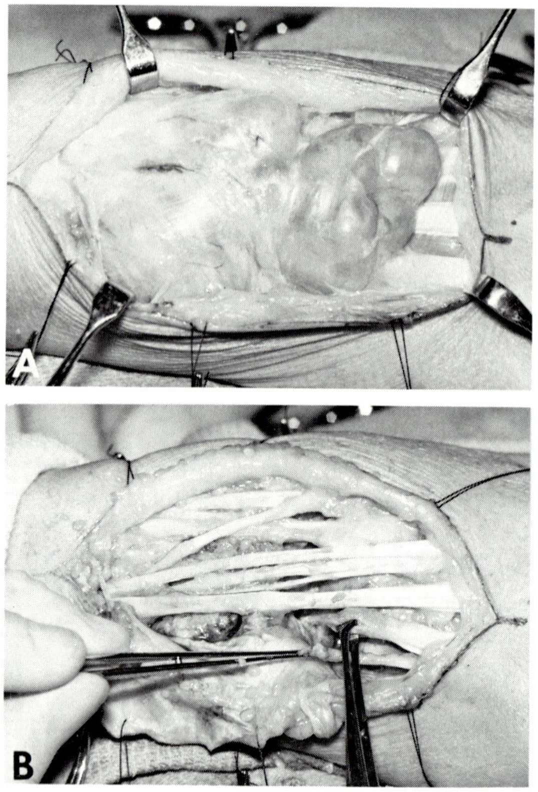

Figure 24-6. *Extensor tendon ruptures. A common finding is a proliferative dorsal tenosynovitis under the extensor retinaculum with a prominent ulnar head* **(A)**, *resulting in* **(B)** *the rupture of the extensor digitorum communis to the long and little digits and rupture of the extensor digiti quinti.*

dislocation of the extrinsic extensor mechanism to the ulnar side of the metacarpal head often occurs in rheumatoid arthritis. The long extensor rests at or near the axis of motion for the metacarpophalangeal joint. With the loss of mechanical advantage, metacarpophalangeal extensor lag occurs and may mimic extensor rupture. On careful examination, the tendon can be palpated just to the ulnar side of the metacarpal shaft with attempted active finger extension.

Second, it is important to recall that there may be simultaneous involvement of the elbow with significant synovitis. Millender et al.[31] have reported compression of the radial motor branch as it passes through the supinator. This radial neuropraxia may then result in loss of finger extensor function. Obviously, should this occur, the treatment is directed to the elbow.

Diagnosis of the ruptured extensor pollicis longus is simple, but requires careful examination. This common rupture usually entails weakness of thumb adduction and weakness but not absence of thumb interphalangeal extension. Note that the intrinsic system will extend the interphalangeal joint of the thumb, although with less than normal strength (Fig. 24-7). Thus, with rupture of the long thumb extensor proximal to the metacarpophalangeal joint (usually at Lister's tubercle), the patient may still have thumb extension. The diagnosis must be made by noting the inability of the patient to extend and adduct and lift the entire

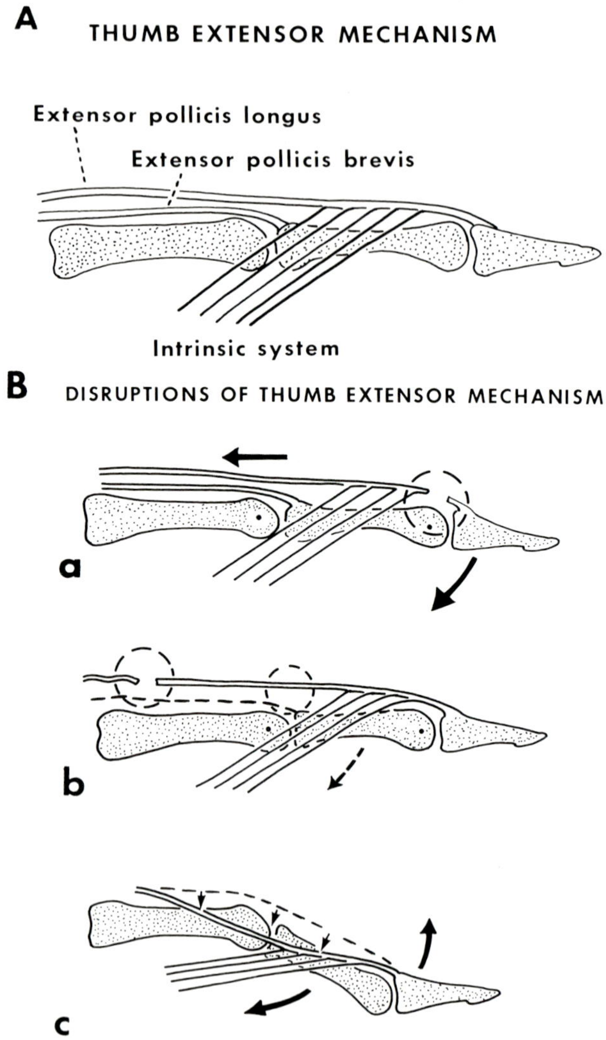

Figure 24-7. *The thumb extensor mechanism.* **A:** *Both the extensor pollicis longus and the intrinsic system can extend the IP joint, although the former has more power. The extensor brevis, when present, will extend the MCP joint.* **B:** *Therefore, only a disruption at the distal phalangeal insertion (a) will cause marked IP extensor lag. Most ruptures in the rheumatoid patient occur in the extensor pollicis longus at Lister's tubercle. With intrinsic muscle function and in the presence of an extensor pollicis brevis (b), surprisingly good thumb extension may remain (see text and Fig. 24-8). In the absence of an extensor pollicis brevis and with intact long extensor function (c), MCP synovitis and pathological changes may cause an extensor lag at the MCP joint, analogous to that seen in the fingers, resulting in the so-called Type I thumb of Nalebuff.*

thumb from a flat surface (Fig. 24-8). The most common functional deficit noted by the patient is weakness of thumb adduction and elevation.

Treatment of ruptured extensor tendons will vary from patient to patient and depend upon the findings at the time of dorsal tenosynovectomy. If a single common extensor has been lost, then the distal portion is best repaired in a side-to-side fashion to the adjacent common extensor. If the patient has a rupture of the communis to the little finger, this will not be detected clinically because of the extensor digiti quinti. If the extensor digiti quinti has been ruptured, its distal portion may be repaired in a side-to-side fashion to the common extensor of the ring finger, or the extensor indicis proprius may be transferred.

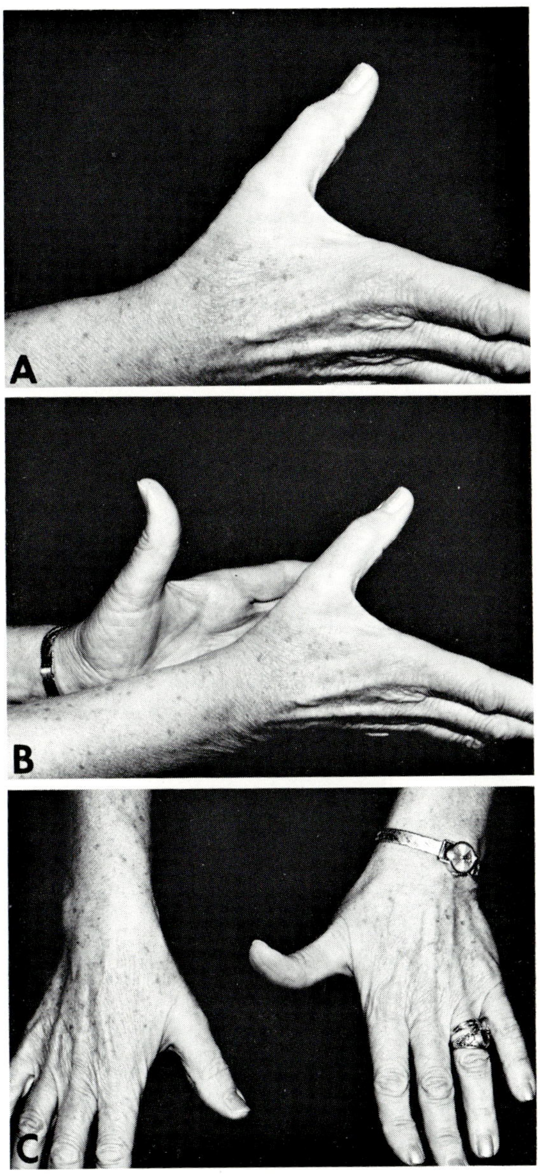

Figure 24-8. *Rupture of the extensor pollicis longus (see text and Fig. 24-7).* **A:** *Good thumb extension remains with function of the intrinsic system at the IP joint and the extensor pollicis brevis at the MCP joint.* **B:** *Only when contrasted with the opposite thumb is the extensor lag apparent.* **C:** *The best test on physical examination is attempted elevation of the thumb from a flat surface upon which the hand rests. The absence of the extensor pollicis longus in this patient's right hand is immediately obvious.*

If the patient has a double extensor rupture, most commonly occurring in the ring and little fingers, the following combination of transfers is recommended: The distal slip of the ring extensor is repaired in a side-to-side fashion to the common extensor to the long finger. The extensor indicis proprius is then transferred as an extensor for the little finger (Fig. 24-9).

If a triple extensor tendon rupture is present (long, ring and little fingers), then the extensor indicis proprius may be transferred for one, and the flexor digitorum superficialis of the ring finger routed about the radial subcutaneous part of the forearm, split at its distal portion and put in as an extensor for the remaining two fingers.

The traditional transfer for the rupture of the extensor pollicis longus at the wrist level utilizes the extensor indicis proprius. The path of this transfer should be through the subcutaneous tissues (i.e. rerouted from Lister's tubercle into the subcutaneous plane) with the repair just proximal to the metacarpophalangeal joint. The one exception to this is the patient who has a significant Type I thumb deformity (see text below). In these situations, the tendon transfer should be put into the base of the proximal phalanx to help correct the metacarpophalangeal extensor lag. If the extensor indicis proprius is not available for transfer to the thumb because it is needed for other extensor tendon transfers or because of simultaneous rupture, then the palmaris longus is an adequate substitute. It does not replace the adduction function of the extensor pollicis longus, but it does give excellent thumb abduction and extension.

For all extensor tendon transfers, note that the excursion is potentiated by wrist motion (Fig. 24-10). The function of extensor tendon transfers to the fingers will be less than satisfactory following wrist fusion. The patient with a fused wrist will be unable to flex the wrist to potentiate finger extension or, conversely, to extend the wrist to relax the extensor transfers and allow metacarpophalangeal joint flexion. This may be particularly important when the flexor digitorum superficialis of the ring finger is used as an extensor transfer.

There are reports of the transfer of the wrist extensors to reestablish finger extension. As a gen-

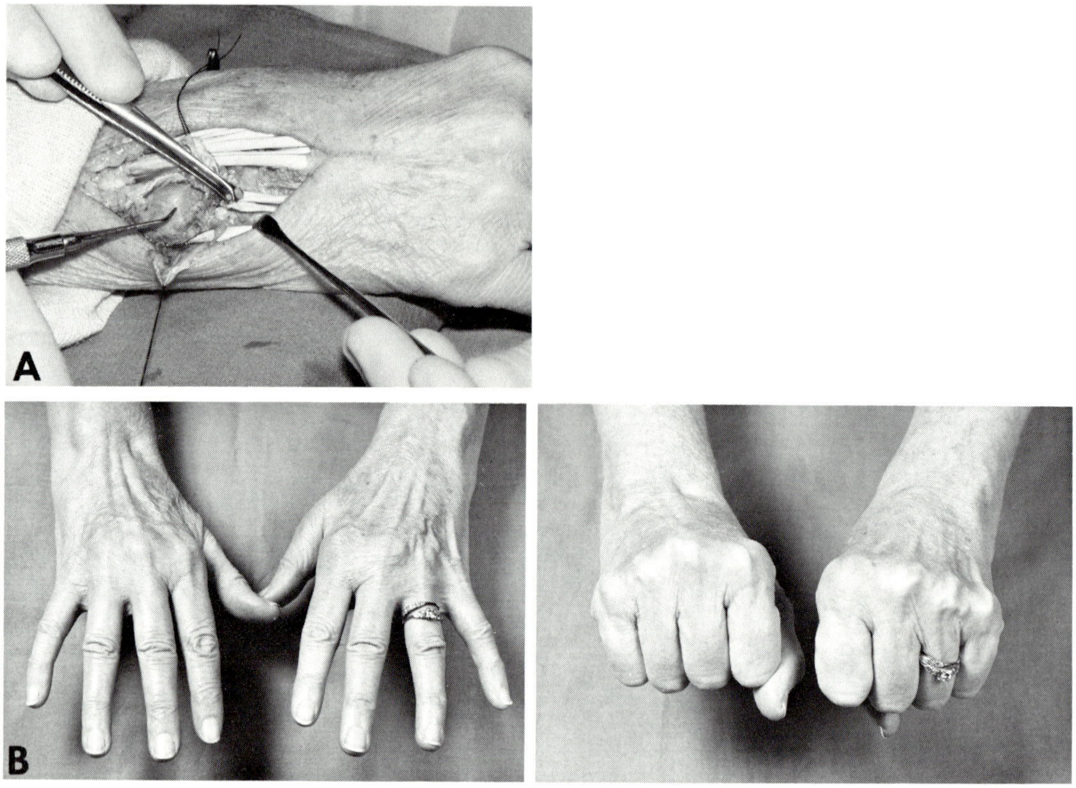

Figure 24-9. **A:** *"Double extensor tendon rupture" with loss of extension of ring and little fingers in the right hand, secondary to a prominent ulnar head (indicated by dental probe).* **B:** *After the appropriate transfers and therapy program, full extension and flexion are realistic goals if the flexor system and small joints are functional.*

eral rule this is not recommended (Fig. 24-10). If the patient has had a wrist fusion and the wrist extensors are used for transfers, their excursion will suffice to give adequate MCP extension, but will not allow full range of finger flexion and extension. If the wrist is not fused, the transfer is also not advised. To weaken wrist extension in a rheumatoid is contraindicated. Not only will it weaken the power of the hand but it may well contribute to the volar subluxation of the wrist. Furthermore, wrist extension is synergistic with finger flexion, and thus the transfer is out of phase.

Regardless of the transfer or repair selected, it should be placed under firm tension with the wrist in maximum extension and the fingers in full flexion. The repair should be protected for 6 weeks. If the wrist is mobile, it is supported in extension and some finger motion is allowed, but with an active dynamic extensor aid.

Flexor Tendons of the Wrist, Palm and Fingers

Synovitis of the extrinsic finger flexor system in the wrist, palm and fibro-osseous tunnel is common (Fig. 24-11). The symptoms vary.

One of the most common complaints is weakness of grasp, with or without some loss of finger flexion but often associated with pain on continued use. Morning finger stiffness may be troublesome.

Median nerve compression from the synovitis within the carpal tunnel often occurs, and may definitely contribute to the complaints of weakness and pain. These symptoms and the paresthesias and atrophy may be overlooked or attributed to the arthritis by both patient and physician unless specifically checked.

Loss of finger flexion is quite common, but may have one of several mechanisms: (1) A localized nodule present distal to a pulley will block flexion, just as one proximal to a pulley will trigger on extension. (2) At the other extreme, the sheer bulk of the synovium throughout the flexor system may limit finger flexion (Fig. 24-11). (3) Flexor tendon rupture does occur, most often at the level of the carpal canal or the distal edge of the transverse retinacular ligament. Note that the terminal phalangeal flexors pass through the narrow isthmus of the carpal canal and then diverge to pass to their respective digits. It is not surprising that the flexors to the thumb and fifth finger are in particular jeopardy.

The role of the intrinsic musculotendinous units

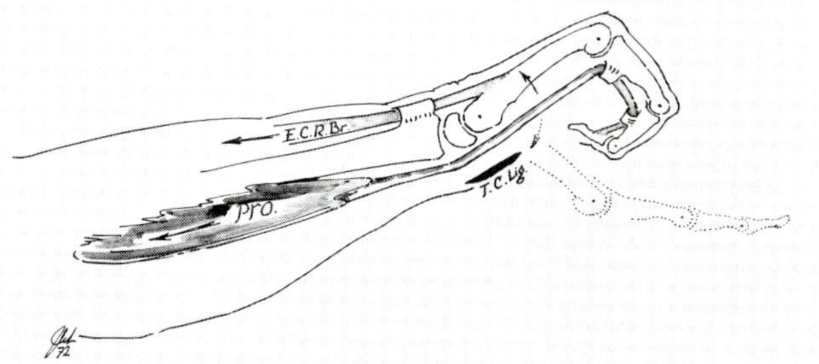

Figure 24-10. *For the normal wrist, the wrist extensors have an important role. By active wrist extension the amplitude of the finger flexor system is reinforced. Conversely, wrist flexion increases the effective amplitude of the extrinsic finger extensor system. Thus, active wrist mobility (if the wrist is stable and pain-free) will potentiate extensor tendon transfers. (From Burton, R.I., Littler, R.W., and Eaton, R.G.: The finger flexor system and its restoration by tendon grafting. American Academy of Orthopaedic Surgeons Sound-Slide Program #423, 424, 425, 1973.)*

in finger flexion must be distinguished from that of the long flexors (Fig. 24-12). Obviously, care must be taken to differentiate the loss of finger flexion due to other common causes. Other common causes of lost proximal interphalangeal flexion are intrinsic tightness or pathological conditions in the proximal interphalangeal joint (see section on swan-neck deformities).

The principal indications for flexor tendon synovectomy are two. First, the persistent carpal tunnel syndrome requires surgical relief, unless the condition is alleviated either by systemic treatment of the rheumatoid arthritis or injection of the carpal tunnel with steroids. (Note that such injection should not be done more than 3 times because of the weakening effect of the steroid injection on the tendon strength, with the risk of later flexor tendon rupture.) The second indication for flexor tendon tenosynovectomy is loss of finger flexion from triggering, synovitis or tendon rupture. In the latter situation, tendon grafts or transfers are necessary.

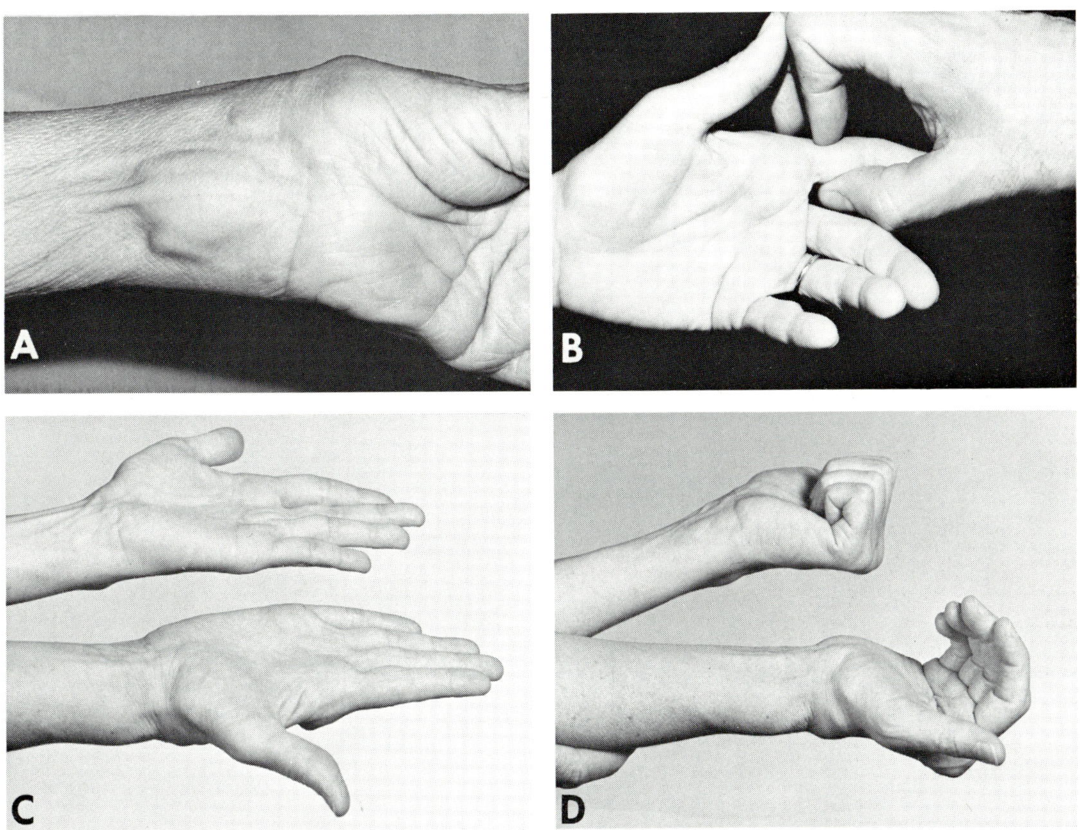

Figure 24-11. **A:** *Flexor tenosynovitis may cause visible swelling anterior to the wrist proximal to the transverse flexor retinaculum. The synovitis will extend through the carpal canal, but does not bulge because of the heavy fascia. Synovitis of the flexor system in the palm is detected as crepitus.* **B:** *Involvement within the fibro-osseous tunnel is best appreciated by palpating the bulk within the flexor sheath.* **C,D:** *This patient had a marked flexor tenosynovitis without rupture but with loss of digital IP flexion, symmetrical in the two hands. The left hand had a radical flexor tenosynovectomy. The pre- and postoperative hands in flexion and extension demonstrate the functional improvement.*

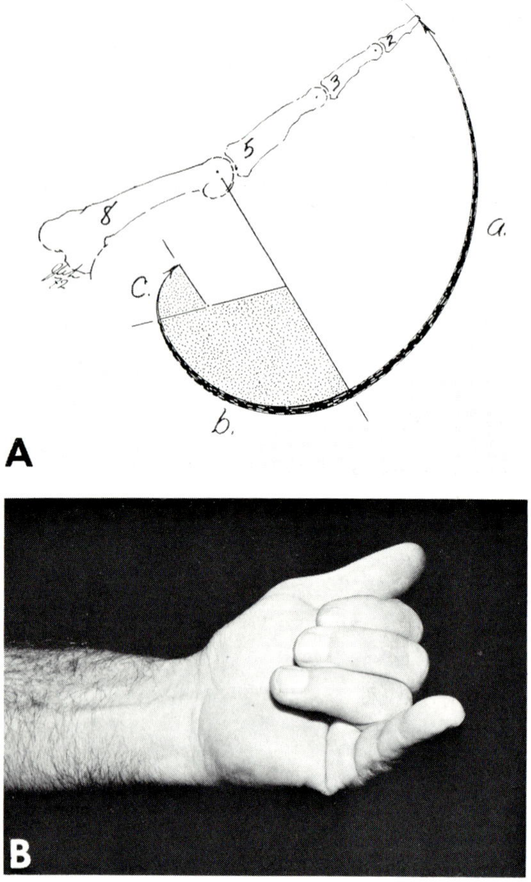

Figure 24-12. **A:** *The fingertip is swept through the arc a by the intrinsic muscle system. The stippled area (arcs b and c) is the function of the long finger flexor. Rupture of both the deep and superficial flexor will result in loss of IP flexion, but the intrinsic system will still pull finger through arc a. (From Burton, R.I., Littler, J.W. and Eaton, R.G.: The finger flexor system and its restoration by tendon grafting. American Academy of Orthopaedic Surgeons Sound-Slide Program #423, 424, 425, 1973.)* **B:** *Typical loss of interphalangeal flexion from rupture of both extrinsic flexors to the little finger.*

Operative Technique

A curved incision is made parallel to and just to the ulnar side of the base of the thenar eminence (Figs. 24-13, 24-14). At the level of the wrist it is carried gently proximally and ulnarward. In this exposure, care must be taken not to damage the palmar sensory branch of the median nerve as it enters the hand just to the radial side of the palmaris longus tendon. Dissection is then carried down to the flexor tendons by incising the palmar fascia (this should be preserved as an extension of the palmaris longus for opponens transfer in cases of marked thenar atrophy), the transverse carpal ligament, and the antebrachial fascia in the distal forearm. Great care must be taken to identify the median and ulnar nerves. With a marked synovial proliferation, the appearance of these nerves and the tendons covered with synovium may be similar. This is particularly true in the median nerve just distal to the carpal canal, as it branches to form the common digital nerves.

A meticulous tenosynovectomy should then be performed. Not infrequently, there is infiltration of the synovium into the substance of the tendons, particularly of the profundus. As possible, the intratendinous synovial nodules should be removed through fine longitudinal incisions in the tendon. In such cases, the margins of the excision should be carefully closed with 6-0 inverting sutures.

At this point in the surgical procedure, tendon excursion should be checked. A smooth blunt instrument is passed under the proximal tendon and traction is placed upon each tendon. If finger joints are supple, the finger should flex fully with the fingertip sweeping to the palm. Each terminal phalangeal flexor and each flexor digitorum sublimis is tested in sequence. Should any digit fail to sweep through its expected arc, the flexor mechanism to that digit must be explored in the fibro-osseous tunnel, first in the distal palm and then, if necessary, in the individual digits.

A transverse incision can be made in the distal palm and the proximal portion of the flexor sheath exposed. With the finger passively flexed, synovium will be extruded from the proximal end of the fibro-osseous tunnel. Often, if this is carefully removed, the proximal tendon traction will accomplish full finger flexion. Should this not be the case, the entire fibro-osseous tunnel must be exposed using, most conveniently, the anterior zigzag incision as described by Littler in 1952 and Bruner in 1960. Pulleys and annular restraints must be left at strategic locations, the base of the proximal phalanx and the midportion of the middle phalanx (Fig. 24-15).

In these cases, frequently one of the two long flexors is severely eroded by the rheumatoid synovium. The bulk which must pass through the pulleys can be reduced by removing not only the synovium but also one of the diseased tendons.[55] Preferably, the terminal phalangeal flexor is left in place and the superficial flexor excised. This will then allow a more nearly normal sweep of the two interphalangeal joints. However, should the patient have a tendency to recurvature at the proxi-

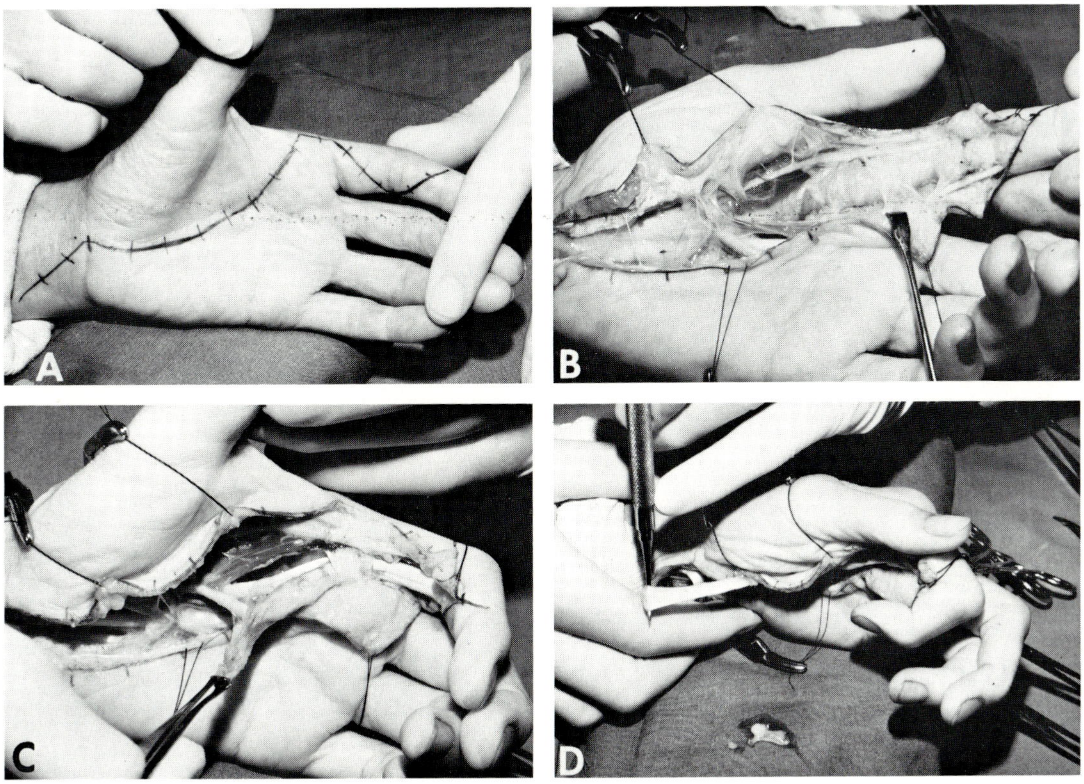

Figure 24-13. *Flexor tenosynovectomy of single ray, palm, and digit (see text).* **A:** *The incision conforms to the basic principles of hand exposure. Great care must be taken to identify and protect the digital nerves. If all four flexor systems are explored, a transverse incision at the distal palmar crease is advised.* **B:** *Wide exposure is obtained. Note the digital nerves. The synovitis at the wrist and proximal palm and the marked involvement throughout the fibro-osseous tunnel are apparent.* **C:** *A meticulous synovectomy is performed. To prevent tendon prolapse, pulleys must be preserved in the strategic areas at the base of the proximal phalanx and at the midportion of the middle phalanx (Fig. 24-15).* **D:** *Following flexor tendon synovectomy, gentle traction with a smooth instrument on the proximal profundus tendon should deliver the finger through the full range of passive flexion.*

mal interphalangeal joint and some flexion deformity of the terminal joint (swan-neck posture), it is better to leave the superficial flexor and remove the terminal phalangeal flexor. The slight flexion deformity of the distal joint will prevent recurvature at that joint, and the superficialis power to the proximal joint will help to safeguard against further swan-neck posture. Obviously, a normal flexor tendon is not excised.

Following this surgery, traction on the tendons at the wrist should accomplish full finger flexion, except as limited by other phenomena such as intrinsic tightness or joint contracture—both of which can be accurately tested for and ruled out preoperatively.

In the rheumatoid patient with flexor tenosynovitis, tendon ruptures may occur (Fig. 24-12). Primary repair is usually not possible. Frequently, the tendon ends are involved with the synovial process and are thus eroded, frayed, necrotic or include nodules. In old ruptures, the musculotendinous unit may have retracted proximally; the resultant myostatic contracture will not permit direct repair. Fortunately, these ruptures usually occur proximal to the fibro-osseous tunnel. Therefore, flexor tendon grafts may not be necessary. Often the distal finger flexor can be repaired to a transferred intact superficialis of an adjacent finger.

If the patient's only symptoms are those of a carpal tunnel syndrome, the customary treatment of that entity is carried out with the following addition. Once the exposure has been obtained, a synovectomy of the tendons in the wrist and palm should be performed. Occasionally carpal tunnel syndrome will be the presenting symptom in a patient in whom rheumatoid arthritis had not been previously diagnosed. In these cases, the pathological examination of the synovium will establish the diagnosis.

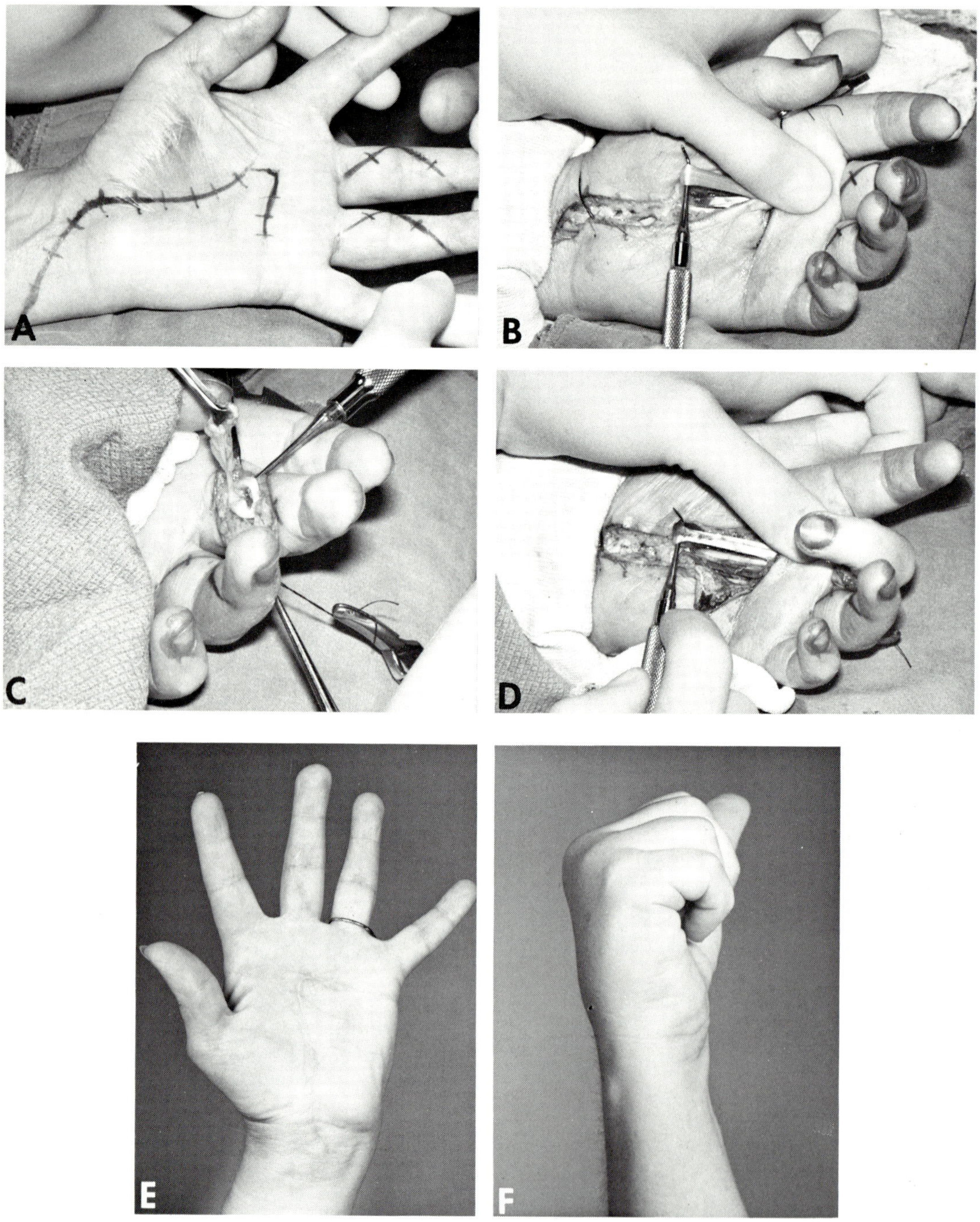

Figure 24-14. *Flexor tenosynovectomy of two rays.* **A:** *Typical combination of incisions which can be modified as needed.* **B:** *Proximal traction on the long finger profundus does not result in IP flexion.* **C:** *Digit exposed and synovium removed from flexor systems.* **D:** *Traction on the tendon now flexes finger* (*compare with* **B**). **E,F:** *Finger extension and flexion one year later.*

The Wrist

The rheumatoid wrist involves two separate components: (1) the radiocarpal and intercarpal joints and (2) the distal radioulnar joint. When evaluating the rheumatoid patient with hand involvement, the surgeon must remember that position, stability, mobility and amount of pain in the wrist have a profound effect on overall hand function. Two facts must be emphasized: (1) Anterior subluxation of the wrists lessens the strength of both wrist flexion and extension and thus weakens grasp. (2) Alignment and function of the metacarpophalangeal joints are directly related to wrist

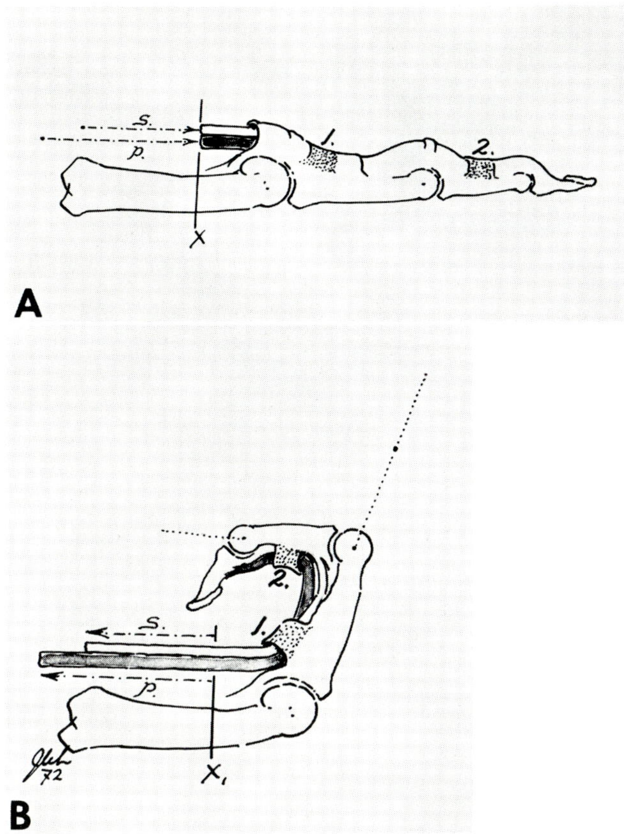

Figure 24-15. *The fibro-osseous tunnel extends from the MCP joint in the distal palm to the base of the terminal phalanx. The tendons have differential excursion within this retinacular system. Two annular restraints (1 and 2) are strategically located at the base of the proximal phalanx and at the midportion of the middle phalanx to prevent tendon prolapse and conserve efficiency of excursion. (From Burton, R.I., Littler, J.W. and Eaton, R.G.: The finger flexor system and its restoration by tendon grafting. American Academy of Orthopaedic Surgeons Sound-Slide Program #423, 424, 425, 1973.)*

position. As the wrist drops into radial deviation, the long flexors and extensors approach the metacarpophalangeal joint from an ulnar direction and potentiate the tendency for ulnar drift at those finger joints.

THE RADIOCARPAL JOINT

The radiocarpal and intercarpal joints are commonly involved in rheumatoid arthritis (Fig. 24-16). The initial symptoms are pain and swelling of the wrist with loss of motion. Usually, the patient will lose extension before flexion. Coincident with this loss of extension, there is a tendency for anterior subluxation of the wrist. This is markedly accentuated should the patient have a rupture of the wrist extensor tendons, or should erosions be present in the anterior lip of the distal radial articular surface.

Synovectomy. The techniques of wrist synovectomy have been described in the previous section under extensor tendon synovectomy. Quite commonly, the two procedures are combined. Following wrist surgery, it is important to close the wrist capsule carefully and to transpose the extensor retinaculum deep to the extensor tendons. This forms a smooth surface for the excursion of these long extensors, which then course subcutaneously.

Arthroplasty of the Wrist. There are three basic types of arthroplasty for the radiocarpal joint. The first involves the creation of a fibrous union with some motion. After the wrist synovectomy is performed, the wrist is stabilized in a neutral position with a longitudinal Kirschner wire or Steinmann pin. After 3 to 4 weeks, the internal stabilization is removed and the patient starts a gentle exercise program. This technique is helpful for patients with some anterior subluxation of the carpus on the radius if wrist extensors are functioning well. It allows the preservation of some wrist motion. It is not applicable in three types of patients: (1) patients with dislocation of the wrist, (2) patients with marked erosion of the anterior surface of the radius and some instability and (3) patients with ruptured wrist extensor tendons.

The second type of wrist arthroplasty involves resection of some of the bone from the distal radius with the creation of an anterior shelf.[60] The carpus is then reduced into this and the patient begins range of motion exercises at approximately one month.

The third technique for wrist arthroplasty involves the use of implants. Some of these involve 2 or 3 component parts and are actually articulated; some involve silicone spacers,[73] and some involve replacement of just the distal radial surface. All of these techniques are relatively new, and long-range results are as yet uncertain. The early results of Swanson's spacer implant are encouraging.

Wrist Fusion. In the rheumatoid patient with a painful subluxed or dislocated wrist, hand function is seriously compromised. Not only is the patient limited by pain and loss of motion but the volar subluxation and often dislocation of the wrist seriously weaken the finger flexor extensor mechanism. Certainly wrist arthrodesis has a very defi-

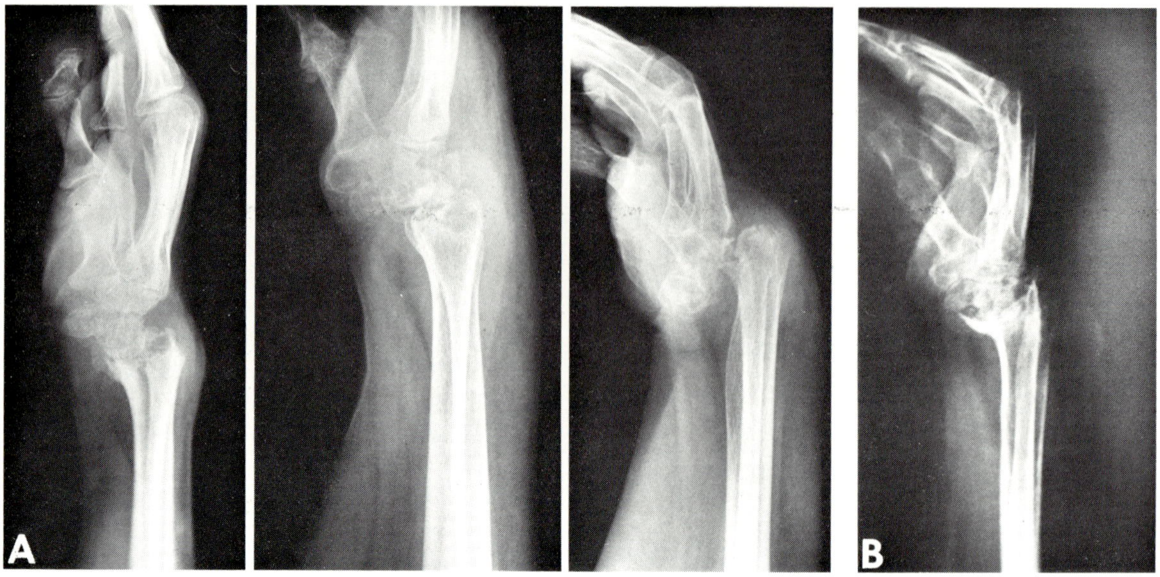

Figure 24-16. **A:** *With wrist synovitis and anterior radial erosions, the wrist tends to sublux anteriorly. With rupture of the wrist extensor tendons, actual anterior dislocation may occur.* **B:** *Occasionally, sufficient anterior radial bony stock is present to prevent dislocation. Patients may be surprisingly stable and maintain functional motion, although with pain and resultant loss of grip strength.*

nite place in the surgical treatment of the rheumatoid hand (Figs. 24-17, 24-18).

Wrist arthrodesis has one serious drawback. The stiff wrist decreases the effectiveness of subsequent finger extensor tendon transfers. It eliminates the ability of the patient to augment finger extension by wrist flexion or to potentiate the power of finger flexion by wrist extension.

The technique for wrist fusion preferred by the author is that recently popularized by Nalebuff and Millender.[66] The wrist joint is exposed as for a synovectomy. After the synovectomies of the extensor tendons and the wrist have been completed, the margins of the distal radius are carefully dissected from soft tissue attachments. Anteriorly, this must be done with great care. The entire articular surface of the distal radius is exposed. By using rongeurs, this is carefully decorticated and shaped to form a gentle concave surface which will match the convex residual of the carpal bones. The amount of carpal bone destruction differs from one rheumatoid patient to the next, and therefore the contour of the distal radius will vary from patient to patient. The carpal bones are then decorticated; with significant carpal destruction, this carpal decortication must be very carefully done. If carpal destruction has been extensive, an autogenous bone graft from the ulnar head or the ileum may be necessary. In all cases, the distal ulna must be resected to achieve pain-free pronation and supination.

The convex surface of the base of the carpal bones and the concave distal radius are coapted to check the fit. The wrist is then flexed and the Steinmann pin is driven longitudinally through the carpal bones and either between the second and third metacarpal or down the shaft of the second or third metacarpal. The wrist is accurately reduced and the Steinmann pin is tapped down the shaft of the radius. The finely ground bone graft is inserted and the fusion site coapted with some pressure. This coaptation may be maintained with an epiphyseal staple or with an oblique Kirschner wire. The wrist capsule, extensor retinaculum and wound are closed as for a dorsal arthrotenosynovectomy.

At 3 weeks, the external immobilization is removed and the patient is allowed to resume a program of gradually increasing activity. If he is on crutches, platform crutches are recommended. If he should subsequently require metacarpophalangeal joint implant arthroplasty, the longitudinal Steinmann pin can be removed at that time if necessary; otherwise it need not be removed.

THE RADIOULNAR JOINT

The radioulnar joint may be among the most symptomatic in the rheumatoid hand, what has been described by Backdahl as the *caput ulnae syndrome*[57] (Fig. 24-19). In this syndrome, the

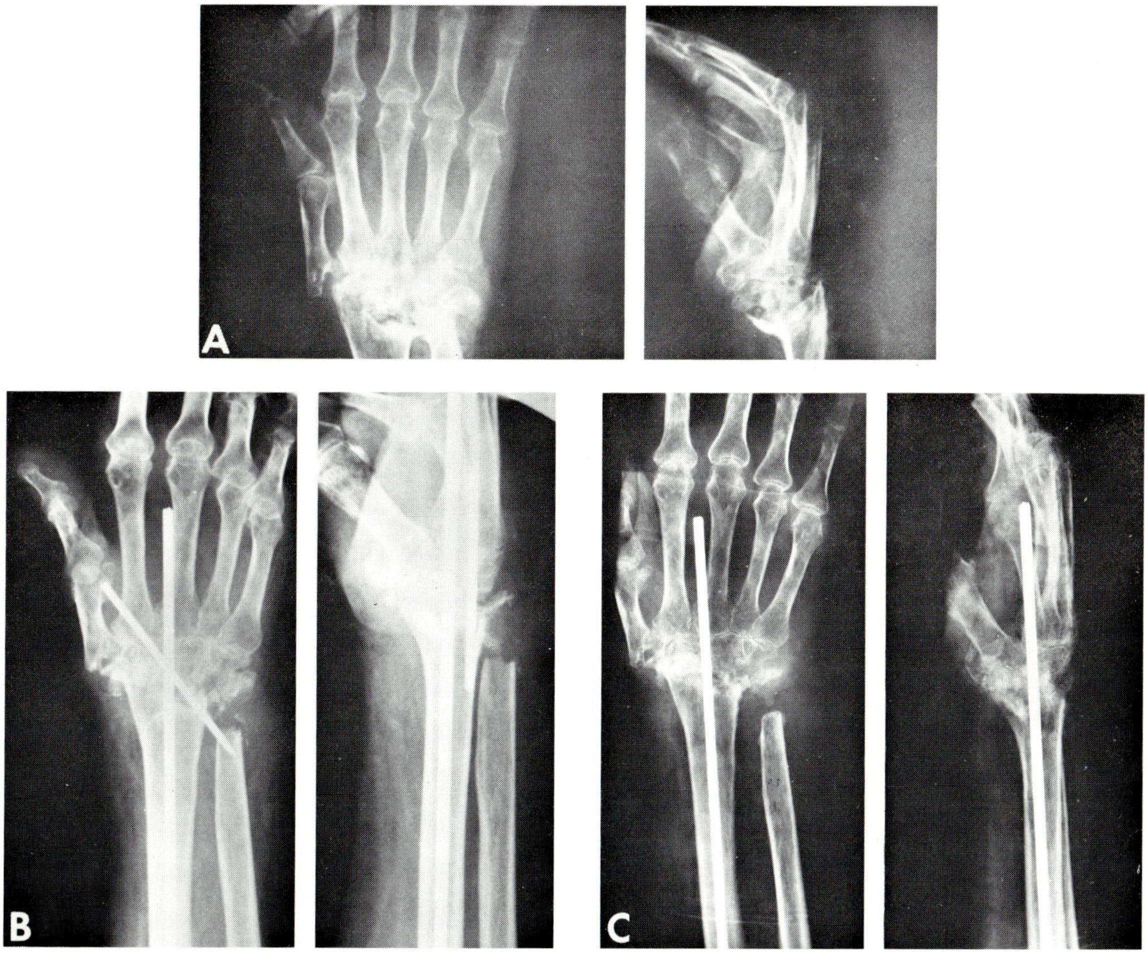

Figure 24-17. *Wrist arthrodesis (see text).* **A:** *Preoperative roentgenograms show carpal destruction. The wrist was stable but painful.* **B:** *Roentgenograms 3 weeks postoperatively. Note position of large Steinmann pin between second and third metacarpals, with a second smaller pin to control rotation and maintain coaptation. This second pin is removed at 4 to 6 weeks. As an alternative to this second pin, an epiphyseal staple is sometimes used.* **C:** *Roentgenograms one year later. Hand is well centralized on radius. Wrist is stable and pain-free, with healed fusion clinically and by roentgenography.*

ulnar head is dorsally subluxed and the carpus subluxed anteriorly and rotated in supination. With the loss of some radial length from the rheumatoid process and with the collapse of the carpal bones, there is a relative excess length of the distal ulna as well.

The patient's principal complaint is pain along the ulnar border of the wrist and distal forearm. This pain is aggravated by pronation and supination, rather than by wrist extension and flexion. Some synovial swelling is usually present about the ulnar head, most noticeable dorsally. Furthermore, the dorsal bony prominence and synovium contribute to extensor tendon rupture, particularly of the extensor digiti quinti and the extensor digitorum communis to the ring and little fingers (Figs. 24-6, 24-9).

At the time of distal radioulnar joint synovectomy, if there is no significant articular cartilage destruction, the dorsal capsule may be reconstructed and the flexor carpi ulnaris translocated without excision of the distal ulna.

Most commonly, however, there are significant bony erosions in the distal ulna. These changes cause painful crepitus in the distal radioulnar joint with forearm rotation and form a rough floor for the extensor tendons of the fourth and fifth compartments.

The distal ulna must then be excised. In the rheumatoid wrist there is a tendency to ulnar as well as volar subluxation of the carpus. Several techniques are available to avoid this excess ulnar subluxation of the carpus: (1) The surgeon should be conservative in the amount of ulna removed.

(2) The use of the ulna head implant spacer as designed by Swanson[72-74] has a definite place. (3) Tendon reroutings or transfers may be helpful. Swanson recommends rerouting of the extensor carpi ulnaris as is described below, and Clayton[60] recommends the use of the extensor carpi radialis longus brought obliquely across the dorsum of the wrist and sutured in the vicinity of the extensor carpi ulnaris insertion.

The implant technique recommended by Swanson will be described.[72-74] The implant not only provides some ulnar length but facilitates the reconstruction of the capsule of the inferior radioulnar joint to maintain a more normal carpoulnar relationship. The implant forms a smooth surface against which the distal radius may pass as the forearm is pronated and supinated, and over which the extensor tendon may glide. Great care must be taken in the exposure of the distal radioulnar joint. The initial approach is that for the dorsal tenosynovectomy. Two flaps are then raised in the capsule over the inferior radioulnar joint. The first and

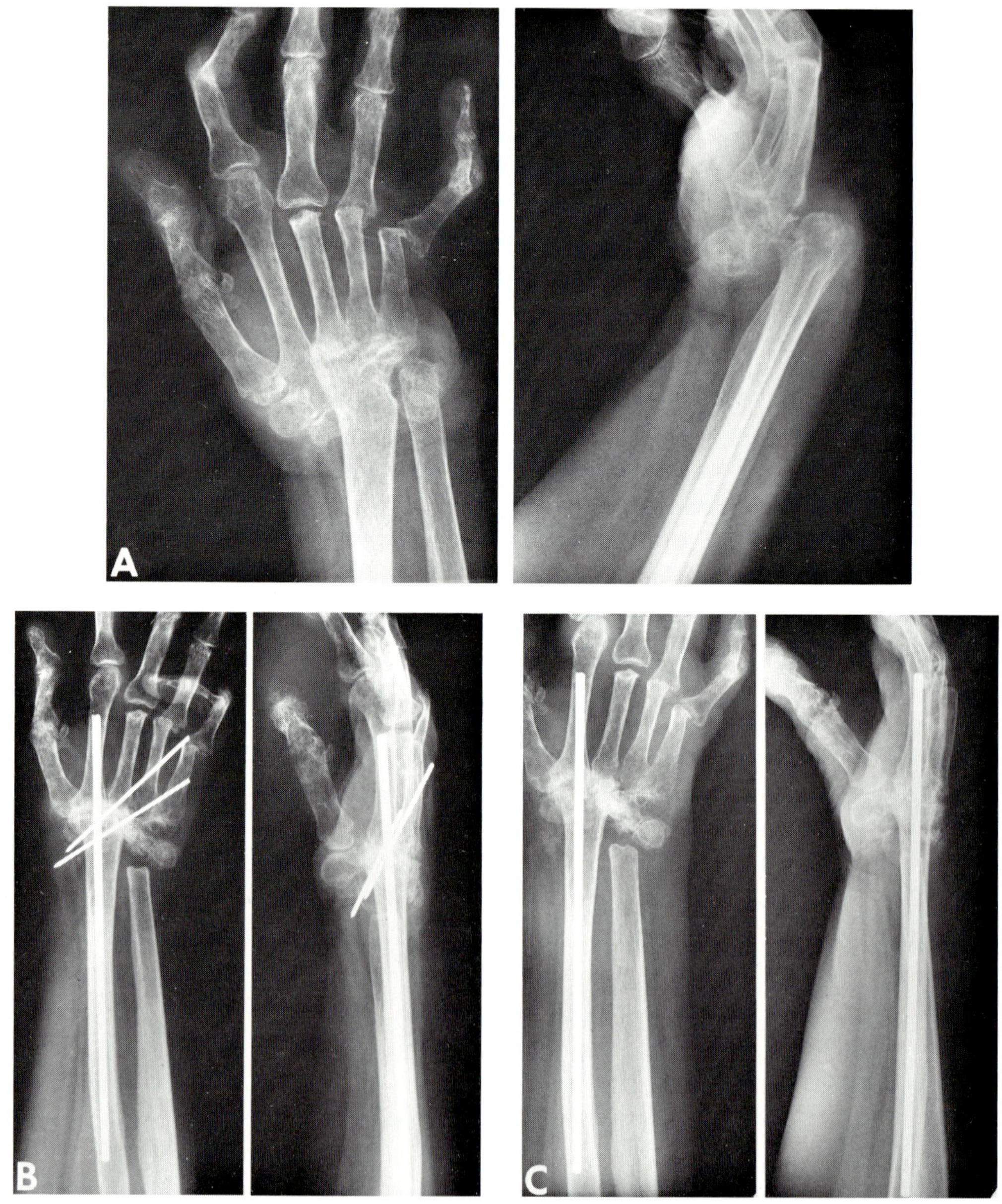

Figure 24-18. *Wrist arthrodesis (see text).* **A:** *Preoperative roentgenograms show dislocation of wrist and carpal destruction.* **B:** *Similar technique but with Steinmann pin in shaft of index finger metacarpal, because metacarpophalangeal resection arthroplasty many years previously had reduced the bony stock in the long finger metacarpal.* **C:** *One year later, the wrist remains stable, pain-free and clinically fused. Pain-free forearm rotation is present.*

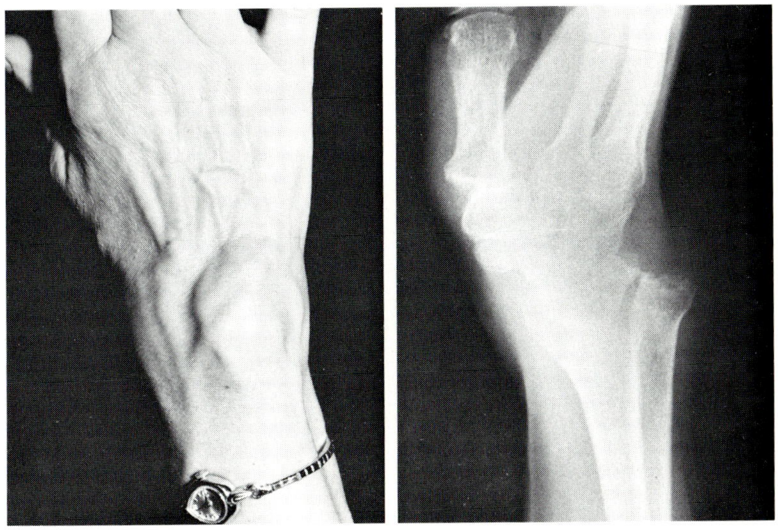

Figure 24-19. *The caput ulnae syndrome is common in rheumatoid arthritis. The distal radial ulnar joint is swollen and tender. The dorsal subluxation of the distal ulna and synovitis of the joint cause pain on forearm rotation and predispose to rupture of the tendons in the fourth and fifth extensor compartments (see text and Fig. 24-9)*

larger flap is proximal and ulnar based. The second flap is distal and radial based. The second flap is approximately 1 cm wide and 2 cm long. With these two flaps raised, a complete synovectomy of the distal radioulnar joint may be performed and the distal ulna excised. The medullary canal is reamed and the various implant sizers are tested. After wound irrigation, the implant is inserted with a no-touch technique. The tails of the suture about the stem are passed through drill holes in the dorsal cortex of the distal ulna to snugly hold the implant in place until the pseudocapsule forms. The distal ulna is reduced anteriorly and the carpus pushed dorsally and in pronation. The proximal large ulnar-based flap is imbricated and sutured either to the periosteum or through drill holes on the dorsal ulnar border of the distal radius. The extensor carpi ulnaris is transposed dorsally. The distal radial based flap is looped about this tendon and sutured back to itself, thus creating a sling which holds the extensor carpi ulnaris dorsally over the distal ulnar. This tends to hold the distal ulnar in a reduced position, decreases the ulnar deforming force of the extensor carpi ulnaris and helps to pronate the carpus. The wrist is immobilized in a supportive dressing and short-arm cast for 6 weeks.

Metacarpophalangeal and Proximal Interphalangeal Joints

Metacarpophalangeal joint involvement in the hand of the rheumatoid patient is very common. Just as the wrist is the key to the position of the metacarpophalangeal joints, any disruption at the metacarpophalangeal joint has a profound effect on the function of the rest of the finger, particularly the proximal interphalangeal joint.[44a]

Initially, with a synovial proliferation, the patient has pain and swelling across the metacarpophalangeal joints of the fingers. As the process evolves, the result is the characteristic deformity of the joints with extensor lag and ulnar drift.

There are many factors in the etiology of this deformity. Initially it probably involves a stretching out of the radial sagittal fibers which normally help to balance the long extensor tendon over the apex of the metacarpophalangeal joint. As these fibers become attenuated, particularly if the wrist is in radial deviation, the long extensor tendon tends to migrate toward the ulnar side of the metacarpophalangeal joint. Once this starts, it tends to potentiate itself, and usually in a relatively short time the extensor tendon will lie in the valley to the ulnar side of its metacarpal head. The extrinsic extensors thus lose the mechanical advantage for extension and become primarily ulnar deviators (Fig. 24-20). In the extreme, as is often seen in the little finger, the extensor may become entirely an ulnar deviator and flexor. Furthermore, this extrinsic extensor then acts directly upon the proximal interphalangeal joint, potentiating the tendency to recurvature.[44a]

The flexor mechanism contributes not only to ulnar drift but also to volar subluxation of the metacarpophalangeal joints. Because the proximal portion of the fibro-osseous tunnel and proximal

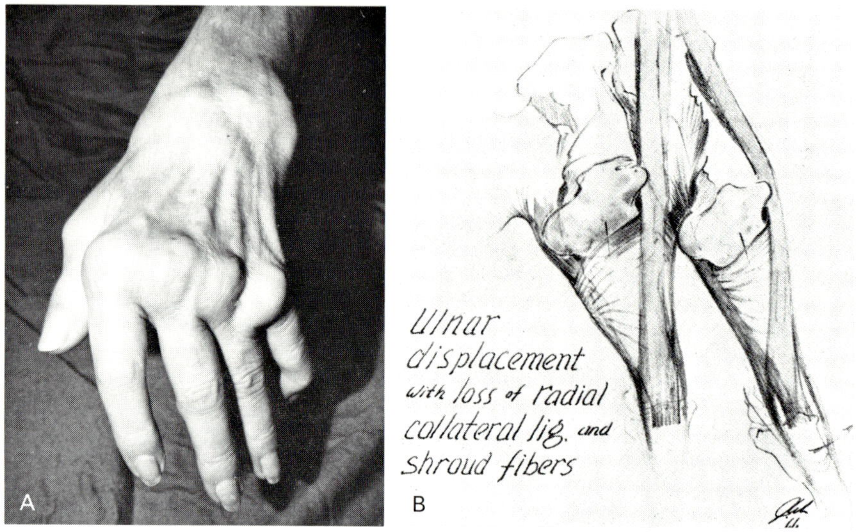

Figure 24-20. *The metacarpophalangeal joint in advanced rheumatoid arthritis characteristically has an extensor lag and ulnar drift.* **A:** *The extrinsic extensors can be seen to the ulnar side of the corresponding metacarpal shaft and passing into the valley between the metacarpal heads.* **B:** *The changes in the radial collateral ligaments and the ulnar shroud (sagittal) fibers are important in this deformity (see text). (From Littler, J.W.: The finger extensor mechanism. Surg. Clin. North Am., 47:415, 1967.)*

pulley system is suspended from the proximal phalanx via the volar plate and intervolar plate ligament assembly, the stretching out of the support systems about the metacarpophalangeal joint (radial collateral ligaments and capsule) results in the flexor tendons pulling directly upon the base of the proximal phalanx and contributing significantly to volar subluxation as well as ulnar drift.

The patient's habitual patterns of hand use also increase the tendency to ulnar drift at this joint. Activities of pinch, especially with an adducted thumb, the use of axillary crutches, and the use of hands to assist in pushing from the sitting position result in pressure on the fingers which increases ulnar deviation.

As the fingers droop into ulnar drift and extensor lag, the ulnar intrinsic mechanism tightens, further increasing and accelerating the deformity. Any attempt by the patient to voluntarily correct the malalignment at the metacarpophalangeal joint tightens the ulnar intrinsic and results in a restriction to proximal interphalangeal joint flexion (intrinsic tightness).

At the same time, as the patient strains to achieve finger extension, he uses the intrinsic system to extend the proximal interphalangeal joints maximally. The long extensor is pulling primarily at the base of the middle phalanx. The use of the hand with metacarpophalangeal joint fixed in flexion further strains the proximal interphalangeal joint into hyperextension, and thus is established the environment for the swan-neck deformity. These changes in the extrinsic and intrinsic extensor system thus have a definite effect in the creation of the swan-neck deformity commonly seen in association with the subluxed metacarpophalangeal joint with its extensor lag, ulnar drift and intrinsic tightness.

Any consideration of surgery on the metacarpophalangeal joint must also involve a careful assessment of the wrist and the proximal interphalangeal joints. Often the surgical approach must involve all of these joints.

The surgical treatment of the metacarpophalangeal joint in the rheumatoid hand involves two fundamental approaches: (1) synovectomy in the early stages of the disease and (2) techniques of arthroplasty when the joints have been destroyed by the process. Note that in both of these it is necessary to rebalance the extensor mechanism, both the intrinsic and the extrinsic components.

METACARPOPHALANGEAL SYNOVECTOMY

The indication for synovectomy is a marked synovial proliferation in the metacarpophalangeal joint which has not responded to systemic treatment and has persisted for 6 months. Definite contraindications exist: significant destruction of joint surfaces, instability, irreducible dislocation or fixed deformity. If these problems are present, implant arthroplasty is required.

Even if the synovectomy involves a single joint,

the incision should be transverse and not longitudinal. Although the longitudinal incision gives excellent exposure for the single joint, it will seriously compromise the choice of subsequent incisions should implant arthroplasty for multiple metacarpophalangeal joints eventually be required.

A transverse incision is made across the dorsal aspect of the metacarpophalangeal joint at the level of the metacarpal necks. Great care must be taken to preserve the dorsal veins which lie in the intervals between the metacarpal heads. Dissection is then carried down to the extensor mechanism. The ulnar sagittal fibers are divided from their attachments to the extensor mechanism. In an extracapsular plane, the long extensor mechanism is freed from the underlying joint capsule. The proximal portion of the wing tendon may be divided. At this point, it may be necessary to divide the juncturae tendinum to reduce the long extensor mechanism to the radial side of its metacarpal head. The capsule of this joint is incised and reflected as a separate layer. A complete synovectomy of the joint is performed. The synovial collections underneath the collateral ligaments and in the vicinity of the volar plate must be given particular attention. If there is a tendency for ulnar drift, do not hesitate to divide the ulnar collateral ligament.

If ulnar intrinsic tightness is present, an ulnar intrinsic release should be performed by dividing the wing tendon as it inserts into the extensor mechanism over the proximal phalanx. The bony insertion into the base of the proximal phalanx should also be released. This may be done through the main operative incision and does not require a separate incision on the dorsum of the finger. Some surgeons prefer to locate the musculotendinous junction of the ulnar intrinsic in the depths of the wound between the metacarpal heads and divide it at this level, rather than at the phalanx. In either approach, great care must be taken not to damage the digital nerve which lies just anterior to this tendon.

The joint capsule is then closed and the extensor mechanism is reduced to a normal position over the dorsal aspect of the metacarpophalangeal joint. It must be rebalanced if necessary. The stability of the extrinsic extensor at the dorsal apex of the metacarpal head must be checked through a full range of finger motion. Usually the radial sagittal fibers are attenuated and must be reefed with 4-0 nylon sutures. Preferably this material should be a light color, or the sutures should be inverted so that they will not show through the thin skin of the rheumatoid patient. The fingers should again be placed through full flexion and extension to make sure the long extensor mechanism remains balanced. A drain or small Hemovac should be placed in the wound. The dressing and postoperative program are the same as those for implant arthroplasty.

METACARPOPHALANGEAL JOINT ARTHROPLASTY

Arthroplasty of this joint in the proper situation will greatly improve finger function. It may be of two basic types, either the excisional arthroplasty[85,108,110] or implant arthroplasty[102-106,98] (Fig. 24-21). The excision arthroplasties all involve synovectomy of the joint, excision of the joint and a rebalancing of the extensor mechanisms. They differ primarily in the means used to obtain stability of the hand at the metacarpophalangeal joint level. The one most commonly favored at present is the Tupper arthroplasty.[108] Its main advantage over the other forms is that it better counteracts the tendency of the base of the proximal phalanx to sublux volarly. Tupper reports results comparable to implant arthroplasty.[108]

The two main types of implant arthroplasty now available are the Swanson and the Niebauer, which have a fundamental difference. The Niebauer prosthesis has a Dacron mesh on the outer surface of the stems. Thus tissue ingrowth stabilizes the implant. This prevents implant motion but concentrates all flexion and extension stress in a relatively small area of the implant, which is therefore more apt to fracture.

The metacarpophalangeal arthroplasty preferred by the author is the one developed by Swanson, who emphasizes that it is a refinement of excisional arthroplasty. Following joint excision and implant insertion a pseudocapsule forms around the implant. The arthroplasty is thus composed of the implant and its pseudocapsule. The implant should be inserted to be slightly loose and should indeed slide like a piston in each medullary canal. The postoperative exercise program is most important, as it molds the pseudocapsule to allow for mobility with stability in proper alignment.

The operative technique is important (Fig. 24-22). The exposure is the same as that used for synovectomy. A resection of the metacarpal heads through the distal neck is advised. The ulnar collateral ligaments should be released. If joint deformity is not fixed, it may be advantageous to preserve the radial collateral ligament as it will tend to give greater stability in pinch. An ulnar intrinsic release is performed, including the bony attachment to the proximal phalanx. Peripheral osteophytes are removed from the base of the proximal phalanx.

When the synovectomy has been completed, the bone resected, and the collateral ligaments released, the finger alignment and metacarpophalangeal space are inspected. The digit must be lax enough to place the base of the proximal phalanx dorsally to the distal metacarpal. If the finger is not loose enough, the volar plate should be divided transversely. This must be done with great care so as not to damage the underlying flexor tendons. If the volar plate is released, the amount of synovitis on the flexor tendons should be noted. A limited amount can be removed via the joint exposure.

The canals of both bones are then reamed. Various implant sizes are tested. The implant should be lax enough to move proximally and distally within the metacarpal and phalanx, yet snug enough to prevent undue rotation. The wound is irrigated. The implants are inserted, the capsule is closed, and the extrinsic extensor mechanism is rebalanced as in synovectomy.

If preoperatively the patient lacked proximal interphalangeal flexion, these joints are reexamined. With the releases at the metacarpophalangeal joints, the proximal interphalangeal joints may have gained significant flexion. If the patient still has a fixed swan-neck deformity without bony ankylosis, the proximal interphalangeal joint should be manipulated into flexion and transfixed with a Kirschner wire in this flexed position for approximately 3 weeks.

The postoperative exercise program is critical for arthroplasty of the metacarpophalangeal joint. As a general rule, the better the motion at the proximal interphalangeal joint the less motion is gained at the metacarpophalangeal joint arthroplasty, unless the proximal interphalangeal joint is stabilized during the exercise program. This may be done with a Kirschner wire placed across the joint or with external splints which support the proximal interphalangeal joint. The soft supportive hand dressing is removed in approximately 5 days, and then the exercise program is started. Active assisted metacarpophalangeal flexion and extension exercises are done 4 to 5 times a day. A dynamic brace is most helpful. The patient sleeps in some form of splint to prevent ulnar drift. This exercise program is continued for at least 3 months, although most of the motion gained will

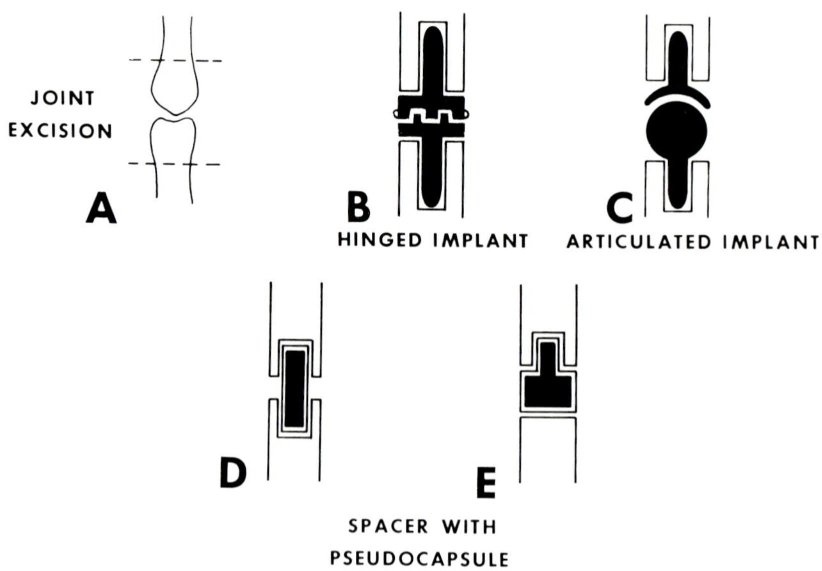

Figure 24-21. *Schematic representation of various types of arthroplasty.* **A:** *Joint excision, e.g. Fowler, Tupper (analogous to Girdlestone procedure for hip).* **B:** *Hinged implant, e.g. Flatt prosthesis (analogous to Waldius knee).* **C:** *Articulated implant. These are still in the clinical trial stage in the hand, but are well accepted in the hip (Charnley-Müller).* **D:** *Flexible dynamic spacer with pseudocapsule, with one stem in each bone, e.g. Swanson MCP and PIP implant.* **E:** *Spacer with pseudocapsule which maintains length and position, e.g. Swanson trapezium implant. In* **D** *and* **E,** *the pseudocapsule that forms around the implant and the tendon rebalancing are both integral parts of the arthroplasty (see text). (From Burton, R.*[16]*)*

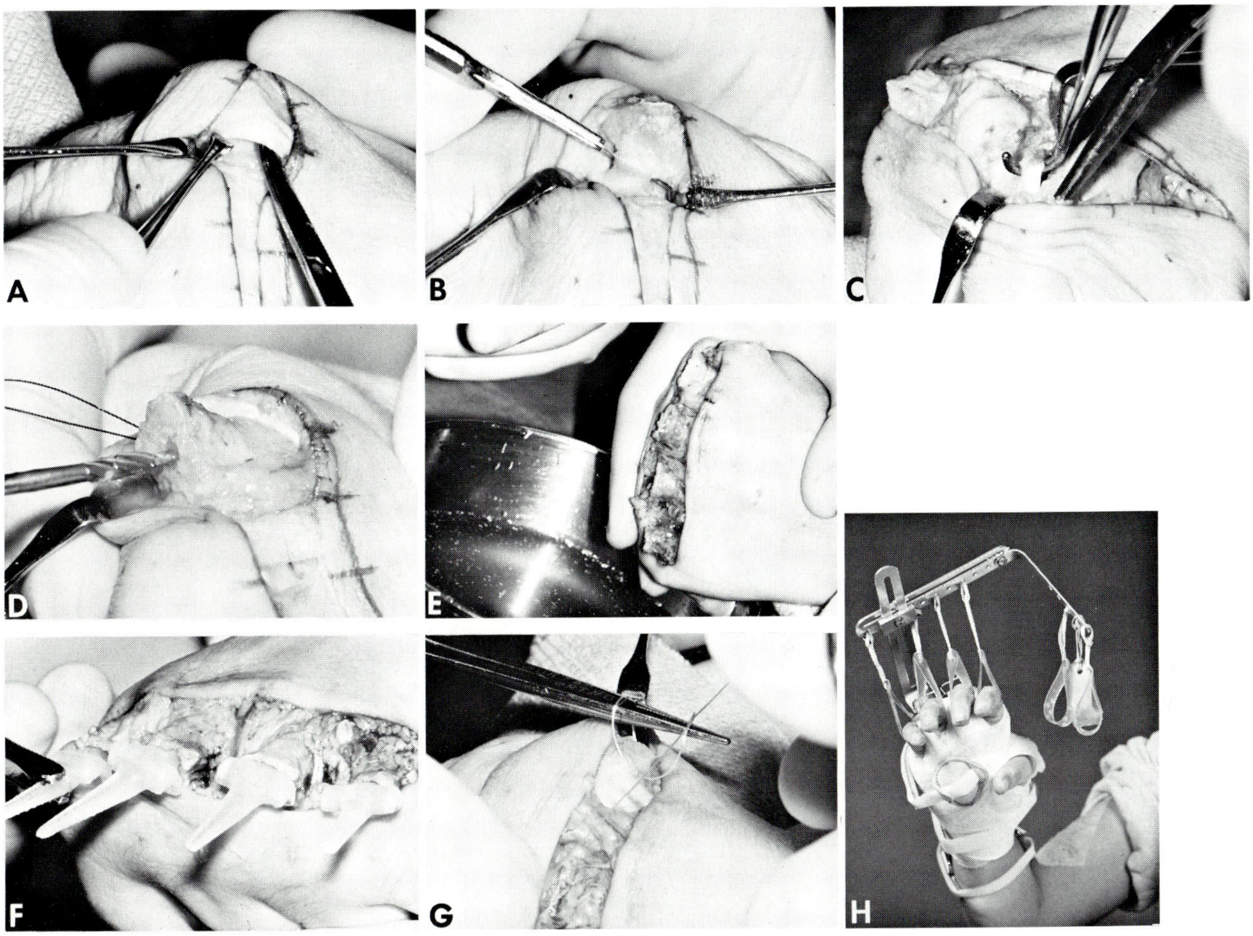

Figure 24-22. *Technique of Swanson MCP implant arthroplasty (see text). The hand is to the right and the fingers to the left.* **A:** *The ulnar sagittal fibers and proximal wing tendon are released and the extensor system separated from the joint capsule.* **B:** *The ulnar collateral ligament is released.* **C:** *The hook is under the tendon of the ulnar intrinsic. It may be released here, or at the bony insertion into the base of the proximal phalanx.* **D:** *After excision of the metacarpal head and bony irregularities from the base of the proximal phalanx, the medullary canals are reamed.* **E:** *The wound is irrigated. Note the amount of debris in the fluid in the basin.* **F:** *The implants are inserted with "no-touch" technique.* **G:** *The radial sagittal fibers are reefed to rebalance the extensor mechanism.* **H:** *The Pope-Swanson splint, or a similar dynamic splint, must be used to assist the postoperative exercise program.*

occur within the first 3 weeks. Note that the night splints may be needed for 6 months or longer. Sutures are not removed until the third or fourth week.

SWAN-NECK DEFORMITY

The swan-neck deformity, a posturing of the finger with the proximal interphalangeal joint hyperextended and the dorsal interphalangeal joint flexed, is common with rheumatoid arthritis (Fig. 24-23). It is often seen in association with metacarpophalangeal joint disease, particularly extensor lag and ulnar drift.[44a] The altered mechanics at the metacarpophalangeal joint have already been discussed.

The pathology of the swan-neck deformity includes changes in several structures at the proximal interphalangeal joint. First, for proximal interphalangeal motion to occur, lateral bands must have mobility. This mobility involves not only proximal distal motion but also dorsal volar. As the joint flexes, these lateral bands will pass distally and volarly. When they become adherent dorsally in the rheumatoid process, flexion of the joint will not be possible (Fig. 24-23). Subsequently, the dorsal portions of the collateral ligament systems may then adhere to the head of the proximal phalanx, and lack enough laxity in the dorsal portion to allow flexion. The central slip (with increased tone secondary to proximal changes) may scar to the underlying head of the

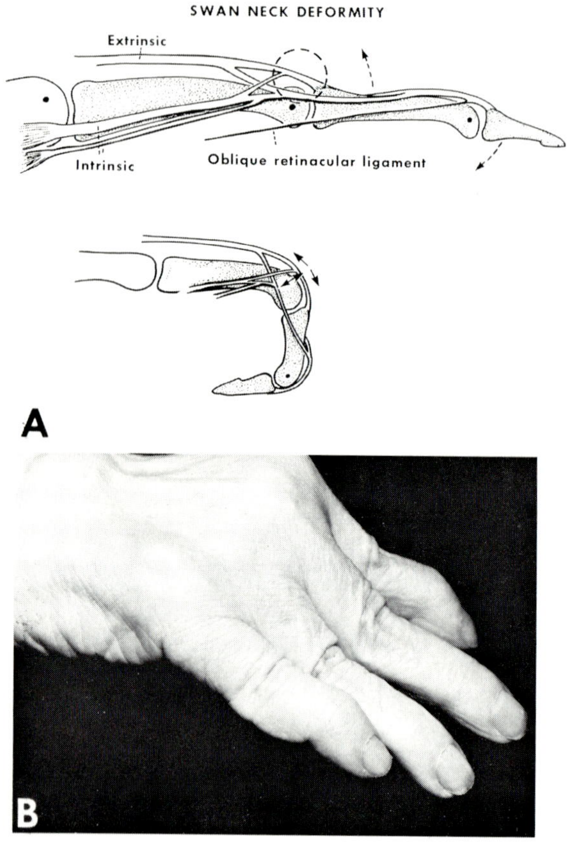

Figure 24-23. *Swan-neck deformity (see text).* **A:** *Normally, the lateral bands at the proximal interphalangeal joint move proximal-distal and dorsal-volar with joint motion. Dorsal scarring and tightness of these lateral bands preventing this mobility and combined with overpull of the extrinsic extensor (secondary to metacarpophalangeal changes) will tether flexion of the proximal interphalangeal joint. Reciprocal laxity of the distal extensor mechanism allows distal joint extensor lag.* **B:** *A typical deformity. Note the prominent lateral bands.*

proximal phalanx and joint capsule. Finally, the joint itself may progress to fibrous or bony ankylosis. Eventually the volar plate may scar, obliterating the anterior cul-de-sac necessary for middle phalangeal gliding motion anteriorly around the condyles of the head of the proximal phalanx.

Treatment of the swan-neck deformity is difficult, and varies with the stage.[96,96a] Regardless of the stage, however, the pathological changes at the metacarpophalangeal joint should be corrected first. There are three basic stages: (1) early, (2) middle and (3) late.

Early Swan-Neck. In the early swan-neck deformity, the joints are passively supple and the patient can actively flex the finger fully. However, on active extension there is posturing of the proximal interphalangeal joint in hyperextension with a droop of the distal interphalangeal joint. The finger must be carefully examined for intrinsic tightness. If it is present, an intrinsic release should be performed. However, proximal interphalangeal joint hyperextension must also be prevented. This may involve an anterior tenodesis of the sublimis as recommended by Swanson,[101] or a reconstruction of the oblique retinacular ligament as described by Littler.[93]

Mid-Stage Swan-Neck. In the mid-stages of the swan-neck deformity, the roentgenograms will show a normal or nearly normal joint and the finger will rest in its swan-neck posture. However, when the patient attempts proximal interphalangeal flexion, it is limited. Even passively, the joint flexion is lacking. In this situation, the lateral bands are adherent dorsally, the collateral ligaments are often tight, and the central slip is short and adherent. To gain proximal interphalangeal flexion, a release of the lateral bands as recommended by Nalebuff,[96] occasionally combined with selective release of the collateral ligaments, may be helpful. This procedure must be followed by early active flexion exercises. To prevent proximal interphalangeal recurvature, splinting may be required during the healing phase. If passive recurvature persists, then an anterior tenodesis or oblique retinacular ligament reconstruction may be needed. This may be too much surgery for many patients, especially rheumatoid patients with all eight fingers involved. At the mid-stage of the swan-neck deformity, it is therefore sometimes necessary to treat the situation conservatively.

Late-Stage Swan-Neck. In the late stages of a fixed swan-neck deformity, the roentgenograms usually show some significant loss of joint space and sometimes a bony union. Two alternatives are available for treatment: (1) an excision of the joint with the insertion of an implant, followed by reconstruction of the extensor mechanism, and (2) a fusion of the proximal interphalangeal joint in a more functional position.

The final decision depends upon several factors: age, handedness, occupation, condition of the extensor and flexor mechanisms, previous surgery, the finger involved, the number of digits deformed, and the condition of the metacarpophalangeal joint. If the patient has a normal metacarpophalangeal joint, then either procedure will give a satisfactory result. It should be recalled, however, that the index and long fingers function in pinch in a relatively extended position and require lateral stability. Therefore, fusion of these joints at approximately 30° will result in excellent function. However, the ulnar two fingers are involved in grasp. These joints, if fused in 30° of flexion, may not allow enough flexion of the digit to accomplish significant grasp, especially if the metacarpophalangeal joints lack flexion. In these fingers, therefore, an implant may be preferable. If arthrodesed, it is best in 45 to 60° of flexion.

The treatment of the swan-neck deformity when combined with metacarpophalangeal joint changes is more complex. Early, it may be treated by manipulation and Kirschner wire fixation as described above for implant arthroplasty for the metacarpophalangeal joint. In the middle and late stages, the alternatives are fusion or implant arthroplasty, as described below.

BOUTONNIERE DEFORMITY

The boutonniere deformity is the reciprocal of the swan-neck (Fig. 24-24).[44a,91] The central slip, instead of being tight, is lax. The transverse retinacular fibers stretch out and allow the lateral bands to drop anterior to the axis of motion at the proximal interphalangeal joint. With the transverse retinacular fibers stretched out dorsally and contracted volarly, the lateral bands lose their normal excursion and remain in the volar position. They may even function as flexors of the proximal interphalangeal joint. Combined with the shortened and thickened oblique retinacular ligaments, the lateral bands function as extensors of the distal joint. Thus, as the patient attempts to extend the proximal joint, a hyperextension deformity of this distal joint will occur. As in the swan-neck deformity, secondary changes occur in the collateral ligaments and volar plate. Eventual fibrous or bony ankylosis may result. The treatment of the boutonniere deformity is difficult and differs for the early, middle and late stages (Fig. 24-25).[91,96,96b]

In the early stage, the patient's finger will rest in the flexed position at the proximal joint with some distal joint hyperextension. Often with maximum active attempts the proximal joint will lack only a few degrees of extension. In this stage, the joint can be passively fully extended. A significant amount of synovitis may be present. At this time, a synovectomy of the joint may be indicated, although it should be combined with a Dolphin-Nalebuff boutonniere release of the central slip to rebalance the extensor mechanism.

In the mid-stage of boutonniere deformity, a 30 to 60° extensor lag is present, although passively the joint can be nearly fully extended. The oblique retinacular ligaments are usually quite tight. Before considering surgery at this stage, it is usually advisable to have the patient on an exercise program in an attempt to stretch out the oblique retinacular ligaments. If he is not, as the proximal joint is corrected these ligaments become so tight that they cause a fixed hyperextension deformity at the distal interphalangeal joint.

The late stage of boutonniere deformity is a fixed flexion deformity of the proximal interphalangeal joint, often measuring 90° or more. Roentgenograms will usually show a subluxation of the joint or even a fibrous or bony ankylosis.

In considering treatment at middle and late stages of boutonniere deformity, the patient's hand must be carefully examined and the functional status carefully evaluated and discussed with the patient. Although cosmetically poor, the boutonniere deformity does permit proximal interphalangeal flexion, and thus the patient can tightly grasp things in the hand. Hand function may be poorer postoperatively if the finger becomes stiff in extension. Most patients function better with loss of extension than with loss of flexion. This is particularly true if all four fingers are involved, or if there is significant involvement of the metacarpophalangeal joint as well.

As for the swan-neck deformity in the rheumatoid patient with the advanced boutonniere deformity, operative treatment is either arthroplasty or arthrodesis. For single finger involvement, especially the index or long digit, the mid- or late-stage boutonniere may be treated with fusion in the position described previously. For the ring and fifth fingers, the author prefers arthroplasty.

OPERATIVE TECHNIQUE OF PROXIMAL INTERPHALANGEAL JOINT SWANSON ARTHROPLASTY

The surgical technique of implant arthroplasty of the proximal interphalangeal joint preferred by the author is that of Swanson[39] (Fig. 24-26). The incision and exposure are the same for the swan-neck and boutonniere deformities. A dorsal midline or dorsal bayonet incision is made. The central slip is divided as a Z-step cut to gain length for the swan-neck correction. In the boutonniere, it is transected near its insertion. The lateral bands are dissected free and divided distal to the proximal

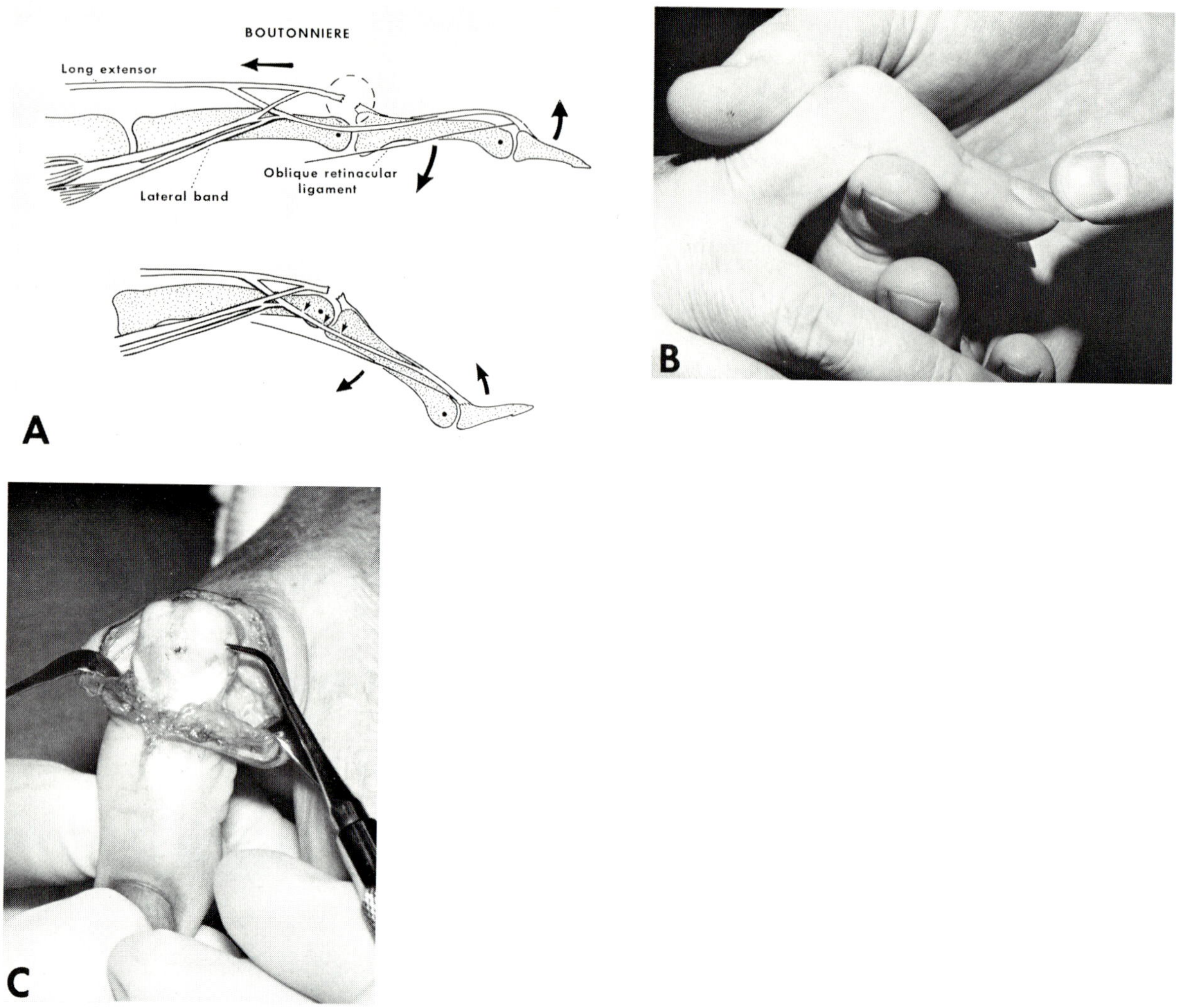

Figure 24-24. *Boutonniere deformity (see text).* **A:** *The pathology of this deformity involves attenuation or rupture of the central slip, volar dislocation of the lateral bands, changes in the transverse retinacular system and eventually shortening and hypertrophy of the lateral bands and oblique retinacular ligament with fixed hyperextension deformity of the distal interphalangeal joint. (From Burton, R.I. and Eaton, R.G.: Common hand injuries in the athlete. Orthop. Clin. North Am., 4:809, 1973.)* **B:** *Test for the tight oblique retinacular ligament. With passive proximal interphalangeal joint extension the* distal *joint develops a passive extension contracture.* **C:** *Operative findings with boutonniere deformity. The dental probe rests at the axis of joint motion. Note the volar dislocation of the lateral bands and the marked attenuation of the central slip.*

interphalangeal joint, leaving intact the leading margin of the radial lateral band to control the distal interphalangeal joint. This will contain fibers from the lumbrical and the oblique retinacular ligament. These tendons must not be handled and must be kept moist and protected throughout the dissection. Otherwise, scarring will result in severe limitation of motion.

The collateral ligaments are preserved if possible, to aid lateral stability. If necessary, in severe fixed deformity, they are released from their attachments to the head of the proximal phalanx, but not excised. A synovectomy of the joint is performed. The head of the phalanx is then excised. In the boutonniere deformity, the volar plate may need to be released. The canals of the two bones are reamed. The implant size is selected: it should be relatively loose if of the Swanson type. (If it is of the Niebauer type, it should fit more snugly.) A small drill hole is placed in the mid-dorsal base of the middle phalanx, the wound is irrigated, and the implant is inserted. The two lateral bands and the central slip are sutured against the dorsal base of the middle phalanx with 4-0 nylon or wire suture passed through the drill hole. It is important to judge accurately the ten-

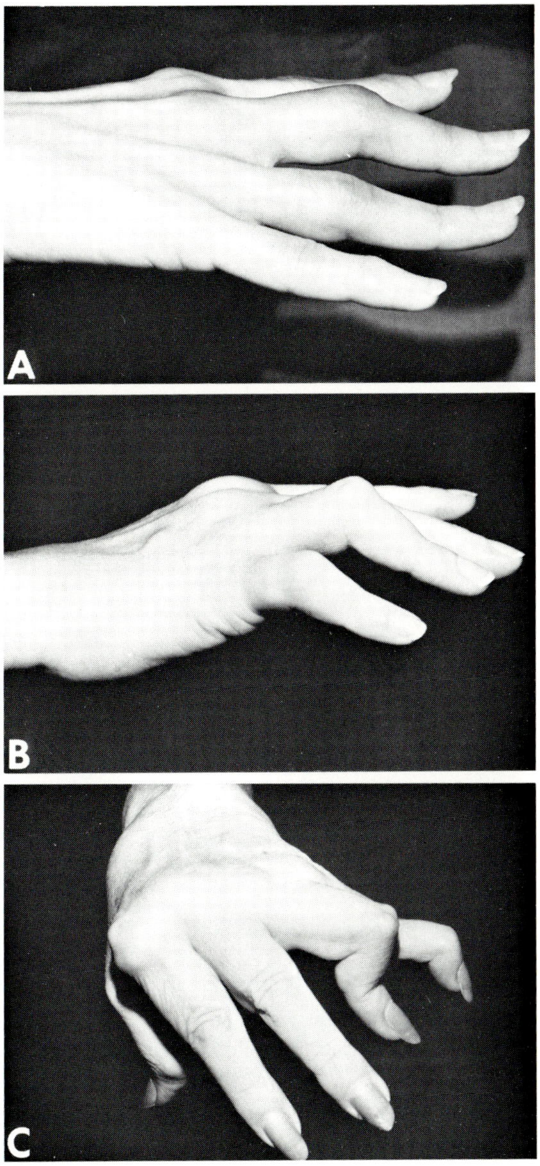

Figure 24-25. *Stages of boutonniere deformity (see text).* **A:** *Early, active extensor lag at the proximal joint, passively correctable.* **B:** *With increasing deformity, the extensor lag worsens and passive correction is not complete. The oblique retinacular ligaments start to tighten.* **C:** *Advanced fixed deformity of both interphalangeal joints.*

sion on these three tendon structures to avoid extensor lag and yet keep good flexion. Postoperatively the joint is supported in full extension for one week. Then the patient is started on a carefully supervised exercise program, involving gentle active flexion of the proximal interphalangeal joint 3 times a day. The proximal interphalangeal joint is splinted in 0° extension at all other times for 2 months. For 8 weeks the distal interphalangeal joint is splinted continuously in 0° extension (or a longitudinal Kirschner wire may be used) to prevent mallet deformity. Also, this distal interphalangeal splinting concentrates all flexion-extension at the proximal interphalangeal joint and aids the exercise regimen.

Distal Interphalangeal Joint

Before treating the distal interphalangeal joint in the rheumatoid hand, the proximal interphalangeal joint must be carefully examined. The treatment of the abnormal distal interphalangeal joint in the swan-neck or boutonniere deformity is done only in connection with correction of the primary pathological changes at the proximal joint.

In the absence of proximal interphalangeal deformity, a mallet posture of the distal interphalangeal joint often occurs in the rheumatoid patient. It is treated by arthrodesis of the distal joint in a few degrees of flexion (see right little finger of patient in Fig. 24-26).

The surgical technique involves a dorsal bayonet incision. Care must be taken not to damage the nail bed. The joint is excised. The two surfaces are then coapted to make sure the alignment is appropriate. A longitudinal Kirschner wire is driven down proximally into the middle phalanx. Fine cancellous bone chips should be placed into the gently distracted arthrodesis site. These may be obtained from the ulna, radius, metacarpal head (if simultaneous arthroplasty is being done) or head of the middle phalanx. The fusion site is compressed, and an oblique wire is introduced to maintain coaptation and control rotation. The oblique wire is removed at 3 weeks, and the longitudinal wire when bony union occurs (usually 6 to 8 weeks).

The Rheumatoid Thumb

The hand for its total functional adaptability depends upon the thumb. Without pain-free thumb mobility with stability, even some of the most routine tasks are impossible.

Six basic pathological states in the rheumatoid thumb will be discussed: (1) the unstable interphalangeal joint with an uninvolved metacarpophalangeal joint, (2) the ruptured extensor pollicis longus, (3) the Type I thumb (Nalebuff), (4) the Type II thumb (Nalebuff) (5) the Type III thumb (Nalebuff)[112,127] and (6) the adducted thumb metacarpal with secondary lateral instability of the metacarpophalangeal joint (Type IV).

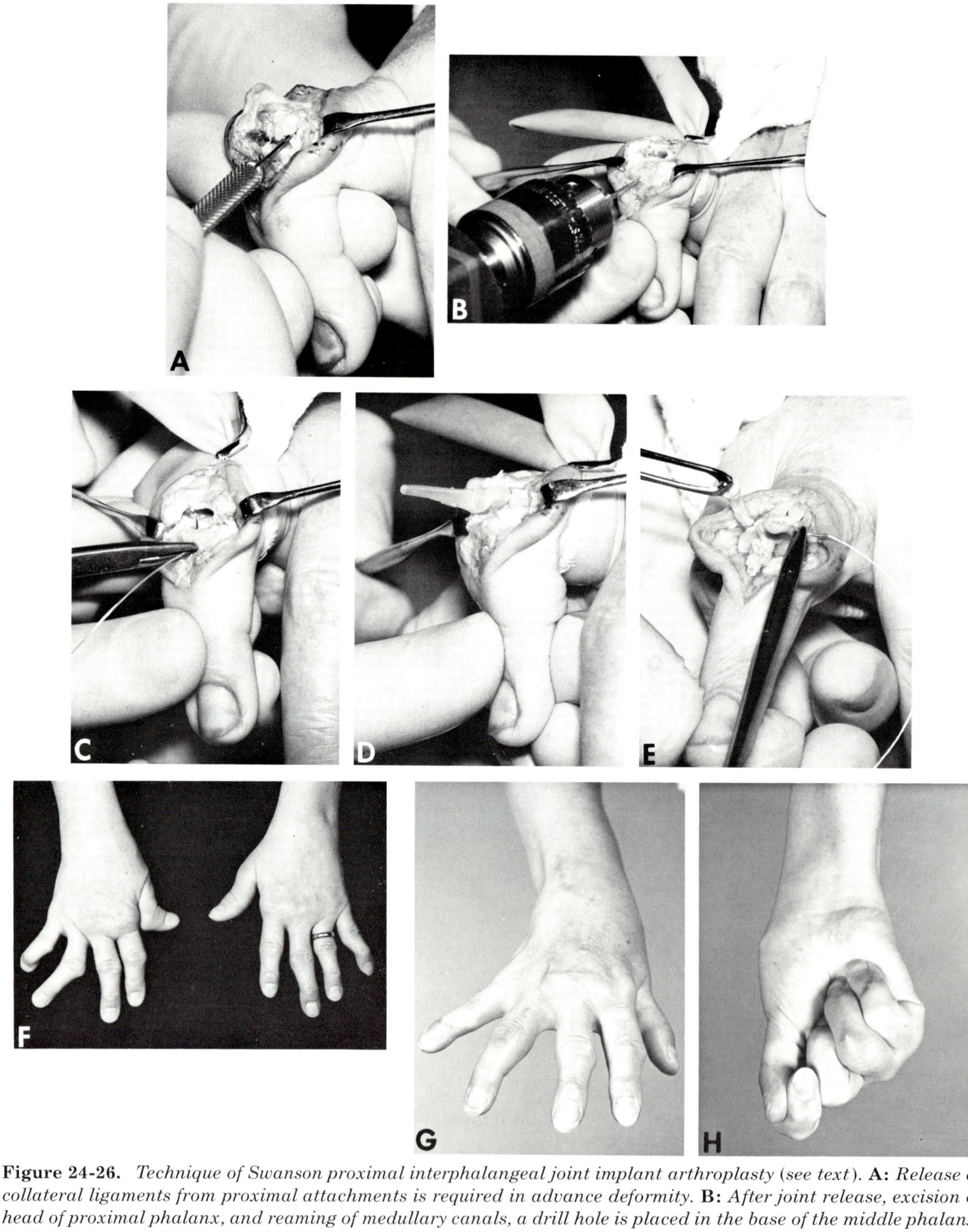

Figure 24-26. *Technique of Swanson proximal interphalangeal joint implant arthroplasty (see text).* **A:** *Release of collateral ligaments from proximal attachments is required in advance deformity.* **B:** *After joint release, excision of head of proximal phalanx, and reaming of medullary canals, a drill hole is placed in the base of the middle phalanx.* **C:** *Suture is passed through this hole.* **D:** *Implant is inserted.* **E:** *Extensor mechanism is repaired to base of middle phalanx with suture previously passed. The tension of this repair is critical.* **F:** *Preoperative deformity of ring finger.* **G,H:** *Function one year following surgery.*

THE UNSTABLE INTERPHALANGEAL JOINT

The unstable or hyperextended interphalangeal joint may be secondary to metacarpophalangeal or carpometacarpal disruption[112,127] (see Figs. 24-27, 24-28, 24-29). In such cases, the proximal joint is treated first. If these more proximal joints are uninvolved, then the primary treatment is directed to the interphalangeal joint (Fig. 24-27). Usually the roentgenograms will show significant bony changes. Arthrodesis will yield predictably good function. The techniques of interphalangeal joint fusion are identical to those of distal interphalangeal joint fusion in the finger. The joint should be fused in 10° flexion, in neutral adduction, and in 5° pronation.

THE RUPTURED EXTENSOR POLLICIS LONGUS

The extensor pollicis longus tendon commonly ruptures in the rheumatoid patient. The main functional deficit, however, may not be loss of thumb extension if the patient has an extensor pollicis brevis and a relatively normal metacarpophalangeal joint (Figs. 24-7, 24-8). The patient may notice primarily a weakness of thumb adduction.

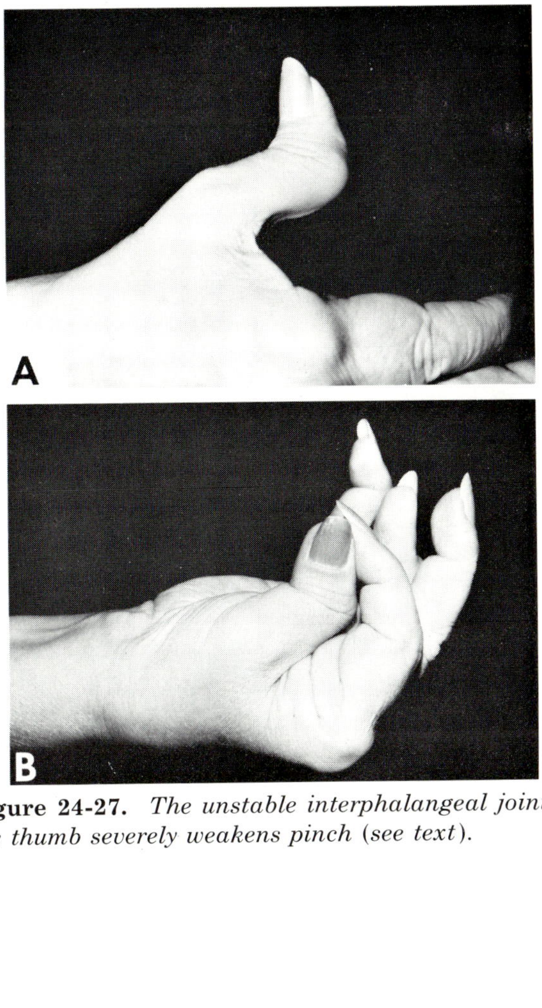

A

B

Figure 24-27. *The unstable interphalangeal joint of the thumb severely weakens pinch (see text).*

Reliable results are obtained by transfer of the extensor indicis proprius to the extensor pollicis longus. If no extensor indicis proprius is present the palmaris longus may be used. The transfer should be rerouted in the subcutaneous plane. The repair is best done with a Bunnell type of suture, and should be protected for 6 weeks.

TYPES I, II, III, AND IV THUMB (OF NALEBUFF)

Type I thumb is an extensor lag at the metacarpophalangeal joint, somewhat analogous to that at the metacarpophalangeal joints of the finger (Fig. 24-28). If seen early when the posture of the metacarpophalangeal joint in flexion is only an active extensor lag without permanent fixed flexion deformity, and if there is no lateral instability of the metacarpophalangeal joint, a rebalancing of the extensor mechanism combined with a synovectomy is good procedure. Essential to this operation is the redistribution of the extrinsic extensor power to the base of the proximal phalanx, using the intrinsic system to extend the interphalangeal joint of the thumb (Fig. 24-7). Thus, the long extensor power is placed into the base of the proximal phalanx and the intrinsic system is used to extend the interphalangeal joint. This technique of extensor pollicis longus rerouting is detailed by Nalebuff.[127] The exposure is essentially that used for a synovectomy or fusion. However, the extensor pollicis longus tendon is divided over the distal portion of the proximal phalanx and either sutured to the soft tissue cuff at the base of the proximal phalanx or passed through a drill hole. The transfer must be protected by 6 weeks of immobilization.

In the advanced Type I thumb, with gross instability, fixed flexion deformity or bony changes in the joint shown on roentgenograms, arthrodesis is recommended. If possible, it is best not to fuse both the metacarpophalangeal joint and the interphalangeal joint of the same thumb, because this will severely compromise the ability of the patient to adjust the pulp position of the thumb accurately against the tactile surface of the finger to which it is being opposed.

A dorsal ulnar, gently curved, longitudinal incision is made. The ulnar intrinsic wing tendon is divided from the long extensor tendon. The extensor pollicis longus and the extensor pollicis brevis are dissected away from the joint in an extra-

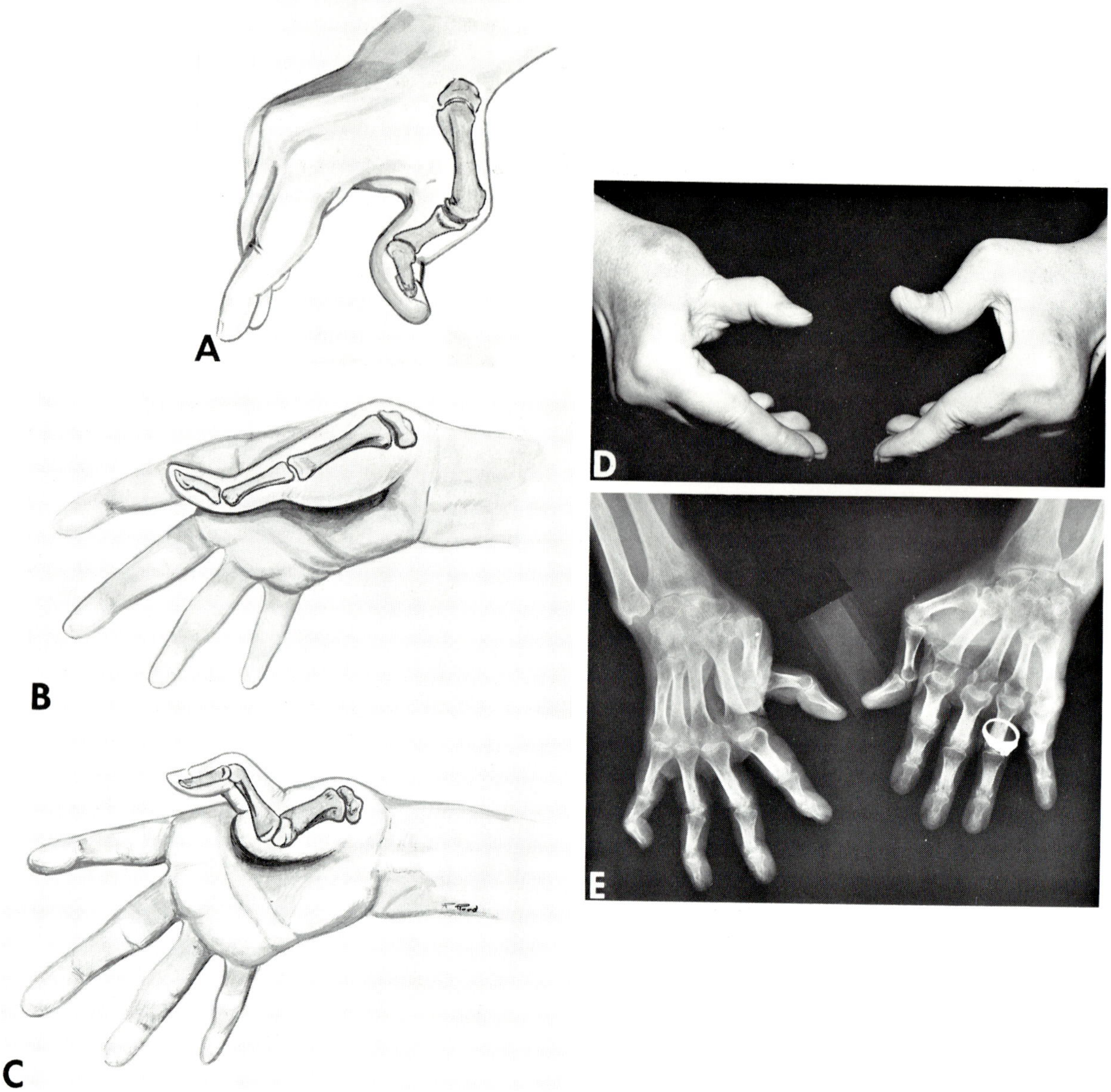

Figure 24-28. *Common thumb deformities in rheumatoid arthritis (see text).* **A:** *Posture seen with primary disruption of thumb arch at the metacarpophalangeal joint (Type I thumb of Nalebuff). Note the carpometacarpal joint may also be abnormal.* **B:** *Posture resulting from primary involvement of the basal joint of the thumb, with metacarpal adduction contracture and secondary hyperextension at the interphalangeal joint (Type II thumb of Nalebuff).* **C:** *Similar to* **B,** *except that distal compensatory hyperextension occurs at metacarpophalangeal joint (Nalebuff Type III thumb).* **D,E:** *Type I and III thumbs. (Modified from Burton, R.I.*[112]*)*

capsular plane. Capsulectomy and synovectomy of the joint are performed. The collateral ligaments often have to be divided from their proximal attachments in order to complete the synovectomy and reduce the deformity. With an osteotome or power equipment, a transverse cut is made in the metacarpal perpendicular to its long axis. A minimal amount of subperiosteal dissection is done. The cut is placed through the base of the proximal phalanx so that when the surfaces are coapted the arthrodesis rests in 10 to 15° flexion, 10° pronation, and neutral abduction.

The fusion site should be coapted under pressure and maintained either with two cross Kirschner wires or a longitudinal Kirschner wire and a single oblique wire. In closure, the wing tendon is repaired to the extensor pollicis longus. Immobilization is continued until bony union is demonstrated roentgenographically, usually 6 to 8 weeks.

The Type II and Type III deformities of the

thumb may appear as hyperextension deformities of the interphalangeal joint or the metacarpophalangeal joint respectively (Fig. 24-28). It is most important to recognize that the primary pathology is at the basal joint of the thumb, and not at the metacarpophalangeal or the interphalangeal joint. With basal joint disruption, the longitudinal arch of the thumb collapses. The metacarpal shaft will assume an adducted position with loss of web space. When this occurs, the patient's repeated attempts to grasp objects of significant size cause the thumb eventually to develop a hyperextension deformity of either the metacarpophalangeal or the interphalangeal joint.

In this Type II or Type III thumb, if the hyperextended metacarpophalangeal or interphalangeal joint is erroneously fused without treating the basal joint, the thumb will lie tightly adducted against the hand and be of little function. It is important therefore to treat the basal joint primarily. To do so will often rebalance the distal joints of the thumb, which may indeed then require no treatment at all.

In some patients with an adducted metacarpal shaft secondary to basal joint involvement, the thumb metacarpophalangeal joint develops a lateral instability (i.e. a chronic "gamekeeper" thumb) secondary to repeated valgus stress to the ulnar collateral ligament of that metacarpophalangeal joint. This has been called Type IV. This requires arthroplasty of the basal joint (often combined with release of the thumb web space) and fusion of the metacarpophalangeal joint.

The thumb carpometacarpal joint (Fig. 24-29) is a double saddle joint and thus works congruously in two planes. The interlocked reciprocally biconcave "saddle" surfaces permit palmar abduction-adduction and adduction flexion-abduction extension by gliding. With pronation or opposition, however, the longitudinal axis of the first metacarpal rotates, made possible by some normal ligament laxity at the carpometacarpal joint. With this torque, the ligaments tighten and the system is stable, although the joint surfaces are now no longer congruous. The most important ligament in this joint is the deep ulnar ligament or anterior oblique carpometacarpal ligament. Thus, although anatomically not an enarthrosis, the joint will allow flexion, extension, abduction, rotation and, when combined, wide circumduction and opposition.

Rotation, with the joints locked incongruously, causes pressure against the dorsal facets, especially if the volar ligament is abnormally lax (common in the rheumatoid patient).

In the early stages before deformity occurs, the primary symptoms of basal joint arthrosis are pain and weakness. Patients describe pain throughout the area of the base of the thumb. Initially the pain occurs with certain characteristic activities, but later progresses to the point of almost constant ache. Those hand functions which classically produce symptoms are of three main types: The first is tip-to-tip pinch with the thumb flexed and adducted across the palm, as in opposing the tip of the thumb to the fifth finger. Therefore activities such as threading a needle are symptomatic. In this regard, the symptoms of basal joint arthrosis of the thumb may closely mimic De Quervain's disease. Second, any function involving axial compression of the thumb is either painful or the thumb is too weak to perform. Many patients relate that they are unable to open a car door latch. When the fingers are clasped about the handle and the thumb is pushed to compress the door button the patient will experience pain or thumb weakness. Third, there is pain in wringing out rags, removing a lid from a large jar, or turning door knobs, or the necessary strength is lacking. Note that in all of these activities pressures in the joint are forcing the dorsal radial subluxation and putting pressure on the dorsal facets.

On physical examination in the stage before deformity occurs, tenderness and swelling are usually noted directly over the carpometacarpal joint, particularly along the radial border. There may be instability, crepitus and severe pain with stress of the carpometacarpal joint. Palmar abduction, extension, and opposition may be limited and painful. There are two helpful tests on examination, especially in differentiating basal joint arthrosis from De Quervain's disease (Fig. 24-30).

Arthrosis of the basal joint may be grouped into four stages. Stage I is ligamentous laxity. The carpometacarpal joint is unstable through ligament laxity. The joint is hypermobile, the metacarpal base riding dorsally and laterally, best seen on cineroentgenography as the thumb moves from extension abduction to flexion adduction. Pain is usually present only with the use of the thumb in heavy pinch or in a pinch in forced position. The axial compression test may be painful, but crepitus is absent. Roentgenograms may be normal or show a small spur. If the roentgenogram film is taken in pinch, some dorsal radial subluxation of the metacarpal base may be apparent. In Stage II, patients have progressed to definite arthritis at the carpometacarpal joint, with varying amounts of deterioration of the dorsal facet and with chronic subluxation. Weakness or painful instability with

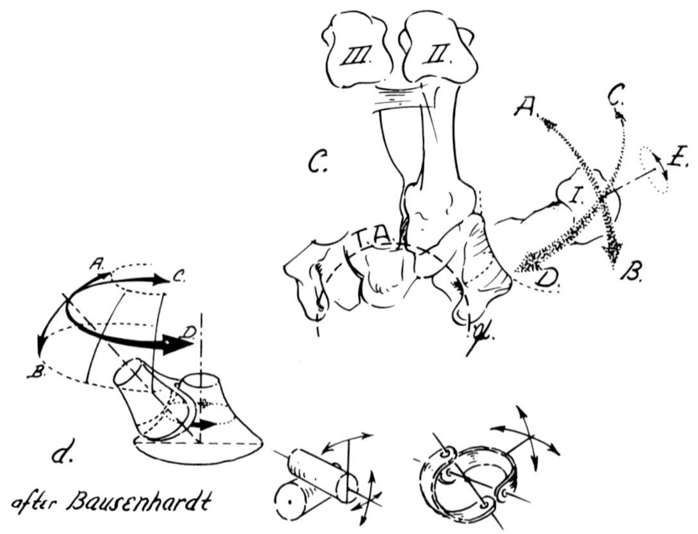

Figure 24-29. *The carpometacarpal joint of the thumb is unique. Three basic motions are achieved: palmar adduction to palmar abduction (A to B), extension abduction to flexion adduction (C to D) and rotation on metacarpal long axis (E). Rotation is permitted by some normal ligament laxity at the joint. The geometry of this articulation can be represented by a tapering cone with a curved surface upon which rests the saddle-shaped base of the metacarpal. The A, B, C and D designations correspond to those of the figure at the top.* (*From Littler, J.W.*[123])

crepitus is present on axial compression with the base of the thumb metacarpal riding laterally and dorsally. The patient will usually start to develop adduction contracture of the thumb metacarpal at this stage. By Stage III, a pantrapezial arthrosis is present, with involvement of all of the basal joints of the thumb. In Stage IV, the thumb metacarpal adduction deformity is marked, and the distal joint recurvature or lateral instability has occurred (Nalebuff Type II, Type III, or Type IV).

At any of the stages, conservative measures should first be tried. A decrease in activity or change in habit of thumb use may give relief, combined with an appropriate antirheumatoid drug regimen. Splinting or a leather gauntlet, although awkward, also may give some symptomatic relief; acceptance by the patient will vary depending on occupation and activity.

In the patient with severe involvement of the carpometacarpal joint without changes in the other trapezial joints and with a good metacarpophalangeal joint, arthrodesis of the carpometacarpal joint is the procedure of choice. The technique of Eaton and Littler[117] is preferred by the author (Figs. 24-31, 24-32). An incision is made along the subcutaneous border of the metacarpal and curved anteriorly at the base of the thumb. Care must be taken to avoid branches of the radial sensory nerve. The base of the thumb metacarpal is exposed in a subperiosteal plane and the joint surface removed with an osteotome. The thumb is placed in the fist position and a parallel resection is made of the joint surface of the trapezium, with bone carefully removed medially from the articulation with the second metacarpal. The fusion surfaces are coapted. One Kirschner wire is placed from the thumb metacarpal into the carpus. The second wire is driven from the thumb metacarpal into the index metacarpal. Plaster immobilization is used until bony union is seen on roentgenogram, usually in 2 to 4 months.

Because of compensatory motion at the other trapezial joints, the thumb has excellent mobility with stability and freedom from pain. The two main disadvantages are (1) time required for union and (2) increased stress to the metacarpophalangeal joint.

ARTHROPLASTY OF CARPOMETACARPAL JOINT

The concept of excisional arthroplasty of the basal joint is well established. The simple excisional arthroplasty (analogous to the Keller procedure on the great toe), although giving excellent motion, may result in weakness, instability and shortening. Froimson[118] recommends soft tissue interposition to replace the trapezium, perhaps best considered as an autogenous dynamic spacer, and he reports maintenance of better strength, stability and length.

The spacer developed by Swanson is an extension or refinement of the excisional arthroplasty for the basal joint of the thumb just as it is for the

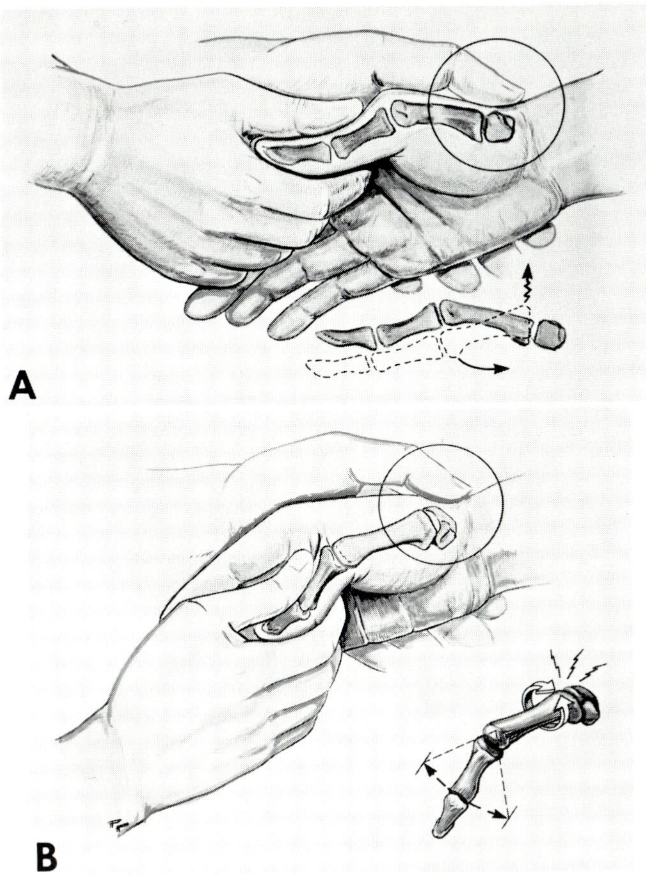

Figure 24-30. *Two helpful diagnostic tests to examine the basal joint of the thumb, described by Eaton and Littler and by Swanson (see text).* **A:** *Axial compression-adduction test. As the thumb is manipulated with simultaneous axial compression and adduction, the instability and crepitus are appreciated with the examining thumb. The base of the thumb metacarpal can be felt to ride laterally against the examiner's thumb. Painful crepitus and instability are usually present with this maneuver.* **B:** *Axial compression or rotation test is often painful. The proximal phalanx acts as a crank. In both tests the thumb is manipulated with one hand (right hand of examiner for right thumb of patient). The examiner's opposite thumb is used to palpate the joint, detecting the crepitus and instability.* (*From Burton, R.I.*[112])

finger metacarpophalangeal joint. The trapezium implant (Swanson or Niebauer type) is preferred to simple excision of the greater multangular. The implant maintains the excellent motion, while providing strength and stability in pinch. The implant developed by Swanson[129] is preferred by the author (Fig. 24-33).

The incision is of two types (Fig. 24-31). The straight one along the margin of the metacarpal shaft allows simultaneous decompression of the first extensor compartment, if necessary, and gives better exposure for the capsular repair.

The radial artery (Fig. 24-31) is retracted proximally and protected, while the capsule is carefully incised and the margins are tagged with black silk to facilitate identification for later meticulous closure. Particular attention must be given to the proximal capsular margin along the scaphoid. This cuff of capsule on the scaphoid can be developed only after the artery is mobilized, and is critical in postoperative stability.

Great care must be taken to keep the joint capsule intact, dissecting with a series of sharp, small knife strokes against the trapezium. It is seldom possible to remove the greater multangular as a single piece. Care must be taken to remove all of the trapezium, especially the portion directly adjacent to the index metacarpal in the depths of the wound. A hole may be inadvertently made in the capsule, particularly just anterior to the flexor carpi radialis, and must be repaired.

The subchondral plate at the base of the metacarpal shaft is debrided of osteophytes, the surface smoothed perpendicular to the axis of the shaft, and the canal of the bone reamed to receive the stem of the implant.

Five sizes of implant are available. In general, one smaller than the trapezium removed should be selected. The implant is inserted and the range of motion of the thumb and the stability of the implant are evaluated. Postoperative stability may be a problem unless particular attention is given to the capsular closure. The proximal capsular rim along the distal scaphoid is most important.

This capsular repair must then be reinforced. Initially, the abductor pollicis longus was used by Swanson as reinforcement, but this has proved less satisfactory than combining the repair with a flexor carpi radialis transfer. This latter technique of Swanson is similar to that developed by Eaton with two variations. First, the flexor carpi radialis is passed dorsally and radially around the metacarpal, rather than through the shaft. Second, the path of the transfer is more proximal, i.e. at the base of the metacarpal and in front of the implanted trapezium spacer. As the thumb is abducted and pronated in pinch, the tenodesis tightens and maintains stability.

Any one or several of four other procedures may be indicated with the implant arthroplasty: (1) Many patients have symptoms of entrapment in the first extensor compartment, which should be released. (2) Many will have symptoms of a carpal tunnel syndrome, and the nerve should be decom-

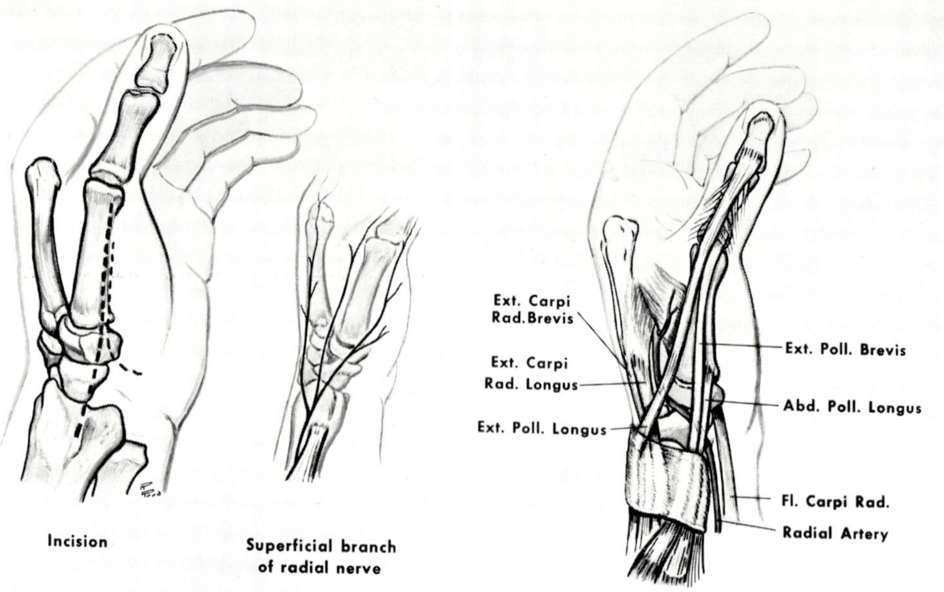

Figure 24-31. *Exposure of the basal joint of the thumb. The skin incision may be either of the two shown. Beware of the sensory branches of the radial nerves, and of the radial artery.* (*From Burton, R.I.*[112])

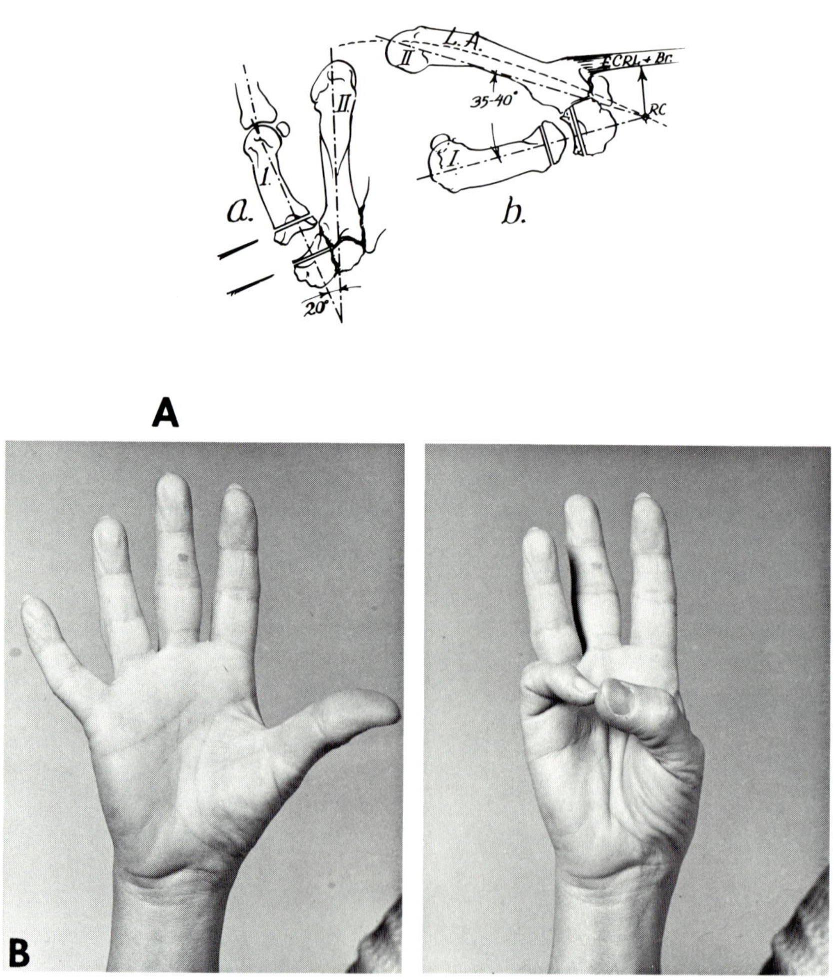

Figure 24-32. *Arthrodesis of the basal joint of the thumb* (*Eaton-Littler technique*). **A:** *The carpometacarpal joint is resected so that when the arthrodesis site is coapted the thumb metacarpal rests in the first position* (*see text*). (*From Eaton, R.G. and Littler, J.W.*[117]) **B:** *Excellent function results if the arthrodesis is properly done and the other trapezial joints and metacarpophalangeal joints are relatively uninvolved. Postoperative abduction-extension and opposition.*

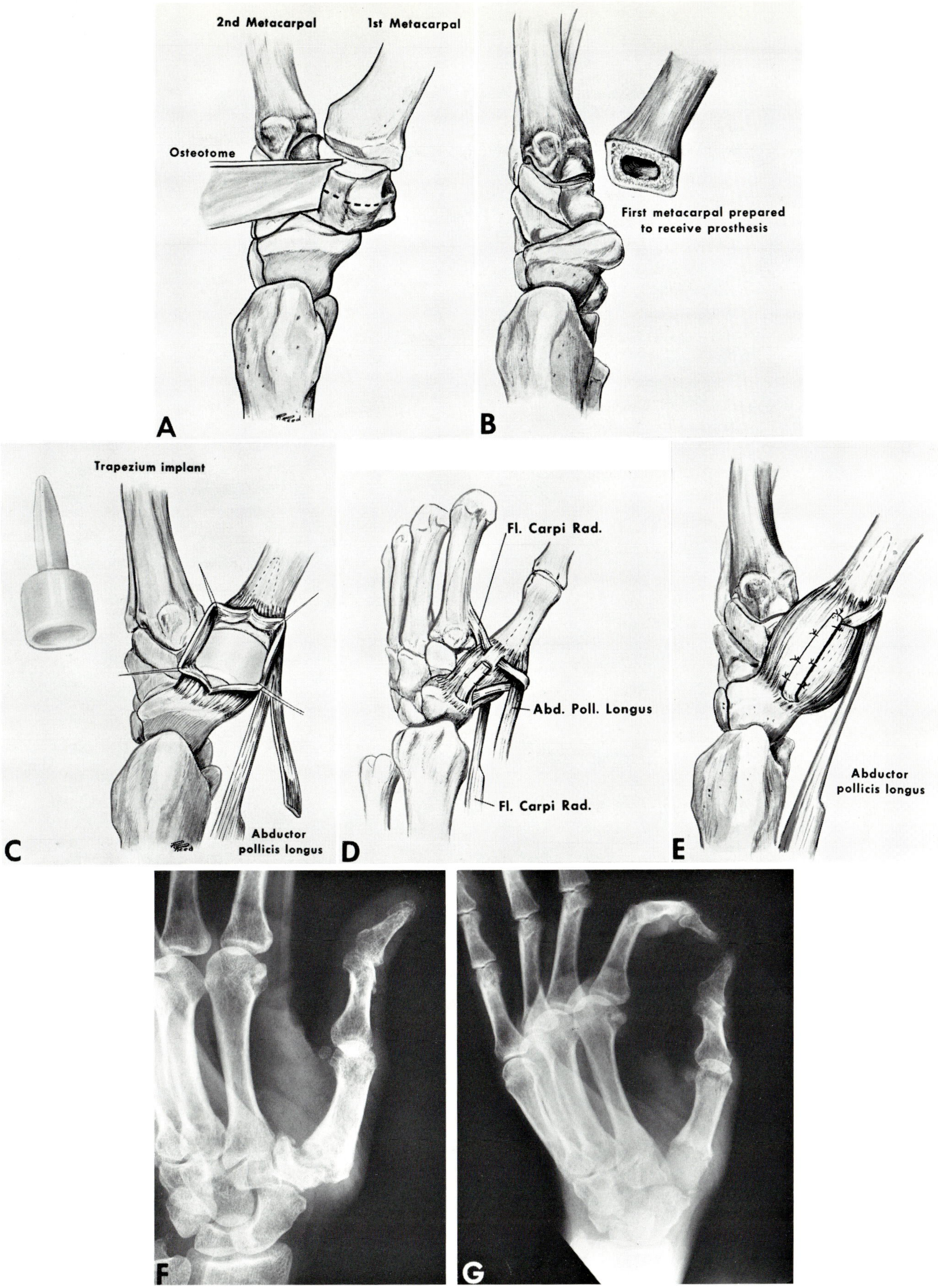

Figure 24-33. *Technique of Swanson implant arthroplasty of basal joint of thumb (see text).* **A:** *Trapezium fragmented in quadrants to facilitate removal without damaging the capsule. Maintenance of this capsule is important, especially along the scaphoid.* **B:** *Metacarpal prepared to receive implant.* **C:** *Implant inserted.* D: *Capsular closure with reinforcement by flexor carpi radialis tendon.* **E:** *Capsular closure with reinforcement by abductor pollicis longus tendon.* **F:** *Preoperative basal joint arthrosis, selected for implant rather than arthrodesis because of painful synovitis at MCP joint.* **G:** *Stability of implant in pinch one year later.*

pressed. (3) In long-standing cases with an adducted metacarpal shaft, an adductor muscle release is done through the incision for the median nerve decompression. (4) If the metacarpophalangeal joint hyperextends more than 30°, is unstable or has significant arthritic changes, it should be simultaneously fused or tenodesed. Otherwise, as it hyperextends the metacarpal shaft will adduct and a Type III thumb occur.

Postoperatively, the arthroplasty is immobilized for 6 weeks to allow the capsular repair to heal firmly. The thumb should be held in palmar abduction and modest pronation during this period, in the so-called fist position.

When the dressing and cast are removed, an active exercise program is begun and the patient is encouraged in progressive use of the hand. There is obviously no place for a passive exercise program.

Rheumatoid Nodules

Subcutaneous areas of fibrinous necrosis with surrounding fibroblastic and lymphocytic infiltrations occur commonly in rheumatoid patients, particularly over bony prominences and in areas where there is subcutaneous pressure. Thus, the hand surgeon often sees them over the olecranon, along the ulnar border of the forearm and on the dorsum of the metacarpophalangeal and proximal interphalangeal joints. They also are not infrequently seen on bony prominences over the flexor aspect of the hands, as over the proximal interphalangeal joint of the finger in a swan-neck deformity, or the hyperextended interphalangeal joint of the thumb. Occasionally they become infected and drainage or excision is necessary. As a general rule, however, if they are not infected excision is not worthwhile. They will tend to recur if they are located in an area that receives frequent pressure over a bony prominence, unless the underlying bony deformity is simultaneously corrected. They can be excised when the underlying problem is corrected, e.g. over the metacarpophalangeal joint at the time of synovectomy or arthroplasty.

References*

General Medical

1. Brewerton, D.A.: A tangential radiographic projection for demonstrating involvement of metacarpal heads in rheumatoid arthritis. Br. J. Radiol., 40:233, 1967.
2. Hammerman, D.: Cartilage changes in the rheumatoid joint. Clin. Orthop., 64:91, 1969.
3. Hollander, J.L. and McCarty, D.J., Jr., Eds. *Arthritis and Allied Conditions.* Lea & Febiger, Philadelphia, 1972.
4. Hollander, J.L., McCarty, D.J., Jr., Astoras, G. and Castro-Murillo, E.: Studies on the pathogenesis of rheumatoid joint inflammation. The "R.A. cell" and a working hypothesis. Ann. Intern. Med., 62:271, 1965.
5. Jacobs, H.H., Hess, E.V. and Beswick, I.P.: Rheumatoid arthritis presenting as tenosynovitis. J. Bone Joint Surg., 39B:288, 1957.
6. Kestler, O.C.: Histopathology of the intrinsic muscles of the hand in rheumatoid arthritis; clinico-pathological study. Ann. Rheum. Dis., 8:42, 1949.
7. McFarland, G., Jr. and Sherman, M.S.: The synovial reactions of rheumatoid arthritis. Clin. Orthop., 36:10, 1964.
8. Martel, W., Hayes, J.T. and Duff, I.F.: The pattern of bone erosion in the hand and wrist in rheumatoid arthritis. Radiology, 84:204, 1965.
9. Norgaard, F.: Earliest roentgenological changes in polyarthritis of the rheumatoid type: Rheumatoid arthritis. Radiology, 85:325, 1965.
10. Rheumatoid arthritis in nineteenth rheumatism review. Arthritis Rheum., 13:472, 1970.
11. Stage, D.E. and Mannik, M.: Rheumatoid factors in rheumatoid arthritis. Bull. Rheum. Dis., 23:720, 1973.
12. Steinberg, V.L. and Parry, C.B.W.: Electromyographic changes in rheumatoid arthritis. Br. Med. J., 1:630, 1961.
13. Townes, A.S. and Marcus, R.L.: Complement-fixing activity of rheumatoid synovial fluid. Ann. Rheum. Dis., 31:393, 1972.

General Surgical

14. Brewerton, D.A.: Hand deformities in rheumatoid disease. Ann. Rheum. Dis., 16:183, 1957.
15. Bunnell, S.: Surgery of the rheumatic hand. J. Bone Joint Surg., 37A:759, 1955.
16. Burton, R.I.: Introduction, arthroplasty in the hand. Orthop. Clin. North Am., 4:313, 1973.
17. Campbell, R.D., Jr. and Straub, L.R.: Surgical consideration for rheumatoid diseases in the forearm and wrist. Am. J. Surg., 109:361, 1965.
18. Clayton, M.L.: Surgery of the rheumatoid hand. Clin. Orthop., 36:47, 1964.
19. Cregan, J.C.F.: Indications for surgical intervention in rheumatoid arthritis of the wrist and hand. Ann. Rheum. Dis., 18:29, 1959.
20. Entin, M.A.: Surgical treatment of rheumatoid arthritis. Surg. Clin. North Am., 44:1081, 1964.
21. Eyler, D.L. and Markee, J.E.: The anatomy and function of the intrinsic musculature of the fingers. J. Bone Joint Surg., 36A:1, 18, 1954.
22. Flatt, A.E.: Surgical rehabilitation of arthritic hand. Arthritis Rheum., 2:278, 1959.
23. Flatt, A.E.: *The Care of the Rheumatoid Hand.* C.V. Mosby, St. Louis, 1963.
24. Flatt, A.E.: Reclamation of the rheumatoid hand. Lancet, 1:1136, 1961.
25. Garner, R.W., Mowat, A.G. and Hazelman, B.L.: Wound healing after operations on patients with rheumatoid arthritis. J. Bone Joint Surg., 55B:134, 1973.
26. Henderson, E.D. and Lipscomb, P.R.: Surgical treatment of the rheumatoid hand. J.A.M.A., 175:431, 1961.
27. Kampner, S.L. and Ferguson, A.B., Jr.: Efficacy of

*Recent and pertinent references. This bibliography is not intended to be a complete listing of all original articles.

synovectomy in juvenile rheumatoid arthritis. Clin. Orthop., 88:94, 1972.

28. Landsmeer, J.M.F.: A report of the coordination of the interphalangeal joints of the human finger and its disturbances. Acta Morphol. Neerl. Scand., 2:59, 1959.
29. Lipscomb, P.R.: Surgery of rheumatoid arthritis—timing and techniques: Summary. J. Bone Joint Surg., 50A:614, 1968.
30. McEwen, C.: Early synovectomy in the treatment of rheumatoid arthritis. N. Engl. J. Med., 279:420, 1968.
30a. Millender, L.H. and Nalebuff, E.A.: Evaluation and treatment of early rheumatoid hand involvement. Orthop. Clin. North Am., 6:697, 1975.
30b. Millender, L.H. and Nalebuff, E.A.: Reconstructive surgery in the rheumatoid hand. Orthop. Clin. North Am., 6:709, 1975.
31. Millender, L.H., Nalebuff, E.A. and Holdsworth, D.E.: Posterior interosseous nerve syndrome secondary to rheumatoid synovitis. J. Bone Joint Surg., 55A:753, 1973.
32. Moberg, E.: Cartilage lesions. In: *Symposium on Early Synovectomy in Rheumatoid Arthritis* (Hijmans, W., Paul, W.D. and Herschel, H., Eds.). Amsterdam, Excerpta Medica Foundation, 1969.
33. Pulkki, T.: Rheumatoid deformities of the hand. Acta Rheumatol. Scand., 7:85, 1961.
34. Riordan, D.C. and Fowler, S.B.: Surgical treatment of rheumatoid deformities of the hand. J. Bone Joint Surg., 40A:1431, 1958.
35. Sones, D.A.: Surgery for rheumatoid arthritis—timing and techniques: general and medical aspects. J. Bone Joint Surg., 50A:576, 1968.
36. Straub, L.R.: The rheumatoid hand. Clin. Orthop., 15:127, 1959.
37. Swanson, A.B.: The need for early treatment of the rheumatoid hand. J. Mich. State Med. Soc., 60:348, 1961.
38. Swanson, A.B.: Silicone rubber implants for replacement for arthritis or destroyed joints in the hand. Surg. Clin. North Am., 48:1113, 1968.
39. Swanson, A.B.: *Flexible Implant Resection Arthroplasty in the Hand and Extremities.* C.V. Mosby, St. Louis, 1973.
40. Vaughan-Jackson, O.J.: Rheumatoid hand deformities considered in the light of tendon imbalance. J. Bone Joint Surg., 44B:764, 1962.

Tendon Systems

41. Backhouse, K.M.: Rheumatoid tenosynovial involvement in the hand. Hand, 1:7, 1969.
42. Ehrlich, G.E., Peterson, L.T., Sokoloff, L. and Bunin, J.J.: Pathogenesis of rupture of the extensor tendons at the wrist in rheumatoid arthritis. Arthritis Rheum., 2:332, 1959.
43. Kellgren, J.H. and Ball, J.: Tendon lesions in rheumatoid arthritis: a clinico-pathological study. Ann. Rheum. Dis., 9:48, 1950.
44. Laine, V.A.I. and Vaino, K.J.: Spontaneous ruptures of tendons in rheumatoid arthritis. Acta Orthop. Scand., 24:250, 1955.
44a. Littler, J.W., Burton, R.I. and Eaton, R.G.: The dynamics of finger extension. Am. Acad. Orthop. Surg., Sound Slide Program #467, 468, 1976.
45. Mannerfelt, L. and Norman, O.: Attrition ruptures of flexor tendons in rheumatoid arthritis caused by bony spurs in the carpal tunnel; a clinical and radiological study. J. Bone Joint Surg., 51B:270, 1969.
45a. Millender, L.H. and Nalebuff, E.A.: Preventive surgery—tenosynovectomy and synovectomy. Orthop. Clin. North Am., 6:765, 1975.
46. Nalebuff, E.A. and Potter, T.A.: Rheumatoid involvement of tendon and tendon sheaths in the hand. Clin. Orthop., 59:147, 1968.
47. Nalebuff, E.A.: Surgical treatment of rheumatoid tenosynovitis in the hand. Surg. Clin. North Am., 49:799, 1969.
48. Nalebuff, E.A.: Surgical treatment of tendon rupture in the rheumatoid hand. Surg. Clin. North Am., 49:811, 1969.
49. Potter, T.A. and Kuhns, J.G.: Rheumatoid tenosynovitis. Diagnosis and treatment. J. Bone Joint Surg., 40A:1230, 1958.
50. Stellbrink, G.: Trigger finger syndrome in rheumatoid arthritis not caused by flexor tendon nodules. Hand, 3:76, 1971.
51. Straub, L.R. and Wilson, E.H.: Spontaneous rupture of extensor tendons in the hand associated with rheumatoid arthritis. J. Bone Joint Surg., 38A:1208, 1956.
52. Vainio, K.: Carpal canal syndrome caused by tenosynovitis. Acta Rheumatol. Scand., 4:22, 1957.
53. Vaughan-Jackson, O.J.: Rupture of extensor tendons by attrition at the inferior radio-ulnar joint. Report of two cases. J. Bone Joint Surg., 30B:528, 1948.
54. Vaughan-Jackson, O.J.: Attrition ruptures of tendons in the rheumatoid hand. J. Bone Joint Surg., 40A:1431, 1958.
55. Wissinger, A.: Digital flexor lag in rheumatoid arthritis. Plast. Reconstr. Surg., 47:465, 1971.

The Wrist

56. Albright, J.A. and Chase, R.A.: Palmar-shelf arthroplasty of the wrist in rheumatoid arthritis. A report of nine cases. J. Bone Joint Surg., 52A:896, 1970.
57. Backdahl, M.: The caput ulnae syndrome in rheumatoid arthritis. A study of the morphology, abnormal anatomy and clinical picture. Acta Rheumatol. Scand. (Suppl.), 5:1, 1963.
58. Campbell, C.J. and Keokarn, T.: Total and subtotal arthrodesis of the wrist. Inlay technique. J. Bone Joint Surg., 46A:1520, 1964.
59. Carroll, R.E. and Kick, H.M.: Arthodesis of the wrist for rheumatoid arthritis. J. Bone Joint Surg., 53A:1365, 1971.
60. Clayton, M.L.: Surgical treatment at the wrist in rheumatoid arthritis: a review of thirty-seven patients. J. Bone Joint Surg., 47A:741, 1965.
61. Dupont, M. and Vainio, K.: Arthrodesis of the wrist in rheumatoid arthritis. A study of 140 cases. Ann. Chir. Gynaecol. Fenn., 57:513, 1968.
62. Haddad, R.J., Jr. and Riordan, D.C.: Arthrodesis of the wrist. A surgical technique. J. Bone Joint Surg., 49A:950, 1967.
63. Hastings, D.E., Evans, J.A. and Hewitson, W.A.: Rheumatoid wrist deformities and their relation to ulnar drift. J. Bone Joint Surg., 54A:1797, 1972.
64. Kessler, I. and Vainio, K.: Posterior (dorsal) synovectomy for rheumatoid involvement of the hand and wrist. A follow-up study of sixty-six procedures. J. Bone Joint Surg., 48A:1085, 1966.
65. Mannerfelt, L. and Malmstem, M.: Arthrodesis of the wrist in rheumatoid arthritis. A technique without external fixation. Scand. J. Plast. Reconstr. Surg., 5:124, 1971.
66. Millender, L.H. and Nalebuff, E.A.: Arthrodesis of the rheumatoid wrist. An evaluation of sixty patients and a description of a different surgical technique. J. Bone Joint Surg., 55A:1026, 1973.

67. Pahle, J.A. and Raunio, P.: The influences of wrist position on finger deviation in the rheumatoid hand. A clinical and radiological study. J. Bone Joint Surg., 51B:664, 1969.
68. Shapiro, J.S.: The etiology of ulnar drift: a new factor. J. Bone Joint Surg., 50A:634, 1968.
69. Shapiro, J.S.: A new factor in the etiology of ulnar drift. Clin. Orthop., 68:32, 1970.
70. Stack, H.G. and Vaughan-Jackson, O.J.: The zig-zag deformity in the rheumatoid hand. Hand, 3:62, 1971.
71. Straub, L.R. and Ranawat, C.S.: The wrist in rheumatoid arthritis. Surgical treatment and results. J. Bone Joint Surg., 51A:1, 1969.
72. Swanson, A.B.: The ulnar head syndrome and its treatment by implant resection arthroplasty. J. Bone Joint Surg., 54A:906, 1972.
73. Swanson, A.B.: Flexible implant arthroplasty for arthritis disabilities of the radio-carpal joint. A silicone rubber intramedullary stemmed flexible hinge implant for the wrist joint. Orthop. Clin. North Am., 4:383, 1973.
74. Swanson, A.B.: Implant arthroplasty for disabilities of the distal radio-ulnar joint. Use of a silicone rubber capping implant following resection of the ulnar head. Orthop. Clin. North Am., 4:373, 1973.
75. Vesely, D.G.: The distal radio-ulnar joint. Clin. Orthop., 51:75, 1967.

Metacarpophalangeal and Proximal Interphalangeal Joints (including boutonniere and swan-neck deformities)

76. Brewerton, D.A.: Pathological anatomy of rheumatoid finger joints. Hand, 3:121, 1971.
77. Carroll, R.E. and Hill, N.A.: Small joint arthrodesis in hand reconstruction. J. Bone Joint Surg., 51A:1219, 1969.
78. Carroll, R.E. and Taber, T.H.: Digital arthroplasty of the proximal interphalangeal joint. J. Bone Joint Surg., 36A:912, 1954.
79. Dolphin, J.A.: Extensor tenotomy for chronic boutonniere deformity of the finger. J. Bone Joint Surg., 47A:161, 1965.
80. Flatt, A.E.: Restoration of rheumatoid finger-joint function. Interim report on trial of prosthetic replacement. J. Bone Joint Surg., 43A:753, 1961.
81. Flatt, A.E.: Prosthetic substitution for rheumatoid finger joints. Plast. Reconstr. Surg., 40:565, 1967.
82. Flatt, A.E.: Prosthetic replacement of joints in the rheumatoid hand. In: *La Main Rheumatoide* (Tubiana, R., Ed.). Expansion Scientifique Francaise, Paris, 1969.
83. Flatt, A.E. and Ellison, M.R.: Restoration of rheumatoid finger joint function. III. A follow up note after fourteen years of experience with a metallic-hinge implant. J. Bone Joint Surg., 54A:1317, 1972.
84. Flatt, A.E.: Studies in finger joint replacement. A review of the present position. Arch. Surg., 107:437, 1973.
85. Fowler, S.B.: Arthroplasty of the metacarpophalangeal joint in rheumatoid arthritis. J. Bone Joint Surg., 44A:1037, 1962.
86. Girzadas, D.V. and Clayton, M.D.: Limitations of the use of metallic prosthesis in the rheumatoid hand. Clin. Orthop., 67:127, 1969.
87. Granowitz, S. and Vainio, K.: Proximal interphalangeal joint arthrodesis in rheumatoid arthritis. A follow up study of 122 operations. Acta Orthop. Scand., 37:301, 1966.
88. Hakstian, R.W. and Tubiana, R.: Ulnar deviation of the fingers. The role of joint structure and function. J. Bone Joint Surg., 49A:299, 1967.
89. Kuczynski, K.: The synovial structures of the normal and rheumatoid digital joints. Hand, 3:41, 1971.
90. Laine, V.A.I., Sairanen, E. and Vainio, K.: Finger deformities caused by rheumatoid arthritis. J. Bone Joint Surg., 39A:527, 1957.
91. Littler, J.W. and Eaton, R.G.: Redistribution of forces in the correction of boutonniere deformity. J. Bone Joint Surg., 39A:1267, 1969.
92. Littler, J.W.: Quoted by Harris, C. and Riordan, D.C.: Intrinsic contracture in the hand and its surgical treatment. J. Bone Joint Surg., 36A:10, 1954.
93. Littler, J.W.: Restoration of the oblique retinacular ligament for correction of hyperextension-deformity of the proximal interphalangeal joint. In: *La Main Rheumatismale* (Fourniee, A., Ed.). Expansion Scientifique Francaise, Paris, 1966.
94. McMaster, M.: The natural history of the rheumatoid metacarpophalangeal joint. J. Bone Joint Surg., 54B:687, 1972.
95. Millender, L.H. and Nalebuff, E.A.: Metacarpophalangeal joint arthroplasty utilizing the silicone rubber prosthesis. Orthop. Clin. North Am., 4:349, 1973.
96. Nalebuff, E.A.: Surgical treatment of finger deformities in the rheumatoid hand. Surg. Clin. North Am., 49:833, 1969.
96a. Nalebuff, E.A. and Millender, L.H.: Surgical treatment of the swan-neck deformity in rheumatoid arthritis. Orthop. Clin. North Am., 6:733, 1975.
96b. Nalebuff, E.A. and Millender, L.H.: Surgical treatment of the boutonniere deformity in rheumatoid arthritis. Orthop. Clin. North Am., 6:753, 1975.
97. Niebauer, J.J., Shaw, J.L. and Doren, W.W.: The silicone-dacron hinge prosthesis: Design, evaluation and application. J. Bone Joint Surg., 50A:634, 1968.
98. Niebauer, J.J. and Landry, R.M.: Dacron-silicone prosthesis for the metacarpophalangeal joints. Hand, 3:55, 1971.
99. Shapiro, J.S.: The etiology of ulnar drift. J. Bone Joint Surg., 50A:634, 1968.
100. Smith, R.J. and Kaplan, E.B.: Rheumatoid deformities at the metacarpophalangeal joints of the fingers. A correlative study of anatomy and pathology. J. Bone Joint Surg., 49A:31, 1967.
101. Swanson, A.B.: Surgery of the hand in cerebral palsy and the swanneck deformity. J. Bone Joint Surg., 42A:951, 1960.
102. Swanson, A.B.: A flexible implant for replacement of arthritic or destroyed joints in the hand. New York Univ. Post-Grad. Med. Sch. Inter-Clin. Inform. Bull., 6:16, 1966.
103. Swanson, A.B.: Silicone rubber implants for replacement of arthritis or destroyed joints in the hand. Surg. Clin. North Am., 48:1113, 1968.
104. Swanson, A.B.: Finger joint replacement by silicone rubber implants and the concept of implant fixation by encapsulation. International Workshop on Artificial Finger Joints. Ann. Rheum. Dis. (Suppl.), 28:47, 1969.
105. Swanson, A.B.: Flexible implant arthroplasty for arthritic finger joints. Rationale, technique and results of treatment. J. Bone Joint Surg., 54A:435, 1972.
106. Swanson, A.B.: Flexible implant resection arthroplasty. Hand, 4:119, 1972.
107. Tubiana, R. and Valentin, P.: The physiology of the extension of the fingers. Surg. Clin. North Am., 44:909, 1964.
108. Tupper, J.: Talk presented at the Instructional Course Lectures, American Academy of Orthopedic Surgery, San Francisco, 1971.

109. Vainio, K. and Oka, M.: Ulnar deviation of the fingers. Ann. Rheum. Dis., 12:122, 1953.

110. Vainio, K., Reiman, I. and Pulkki, T.: Results of arthroplasty of the metacarpophalangeal joints in rheumatoid arthritis. Trauma, 9:1, 1967.

The Thumb

111. Aune, S.L.: Osteoarthritis in first carpo-metacarpal joint. An investigation of 22 cases. Acta Clin. Scand., 109:449, 1955.

112. Burton, R.I.: Basal joint arthrosis of the thumb. Orthop. Clin. North Am., 2:331, 1973.

113. Carroll, R.E. and Hill, N.A.: Carpo-metacarpal arthrodesis of the thumb: A clinical and cineroentgenographic study. Presented at 27th Annual Meeting of the American Society for Surgery of the Hand, Washington, January, 1972.

114. Carstam, N., Fiken, O. and Andren, L.: Osteoarthritis of the trapezio-scaphoid joint. Acta Orthop. Scand., 39:354, 1968.

115. Clayton, M.L.: Surgery of the thumb in rheumatoid arthritis. J. Bone Joint Surg., 44A:1376, 1962.

116. Eaton, R.G.: *Joint Injuries of the Hand.* Charles C Thomas, Springfield, 1971.

117. Eaton, R.G. and Littler, J.W.: A study of the basal joint of the thumb. Treatment of its disabilities by fusion. J. Bone Joint Surg., 51A:661, 1969.

118. Froimson, A.I.: Tendon arthroplasty of the trapeziometacarpal joint. Clin. Orthop., 70:191, 1970.

119. Gervis, W.H.: Excision of the trapezium for osteoarthritis of the trapeziometacarpal joint. J. Bone Joint Surg., 31B:537, 1949.

120. Goldner, J. L. and Clippinger, F.W.: Excision of the greater multangular bone as an adjunct to mobilization of the thumb. J. Bone Joint Surg., 41A:609, 1959.

121. Lasserre, C., Pauzat, D. and Derennes, R.: Osteoarthritis of the trapeziometacarpal joint. J. Bone Joint Surg., 31B:534, 1949.

122. Leach, R.E. and Bolton, P.E.: Arthritis of carpometacarpal joint of thumb: Results of arthrodesis. J. Bone Joint Surg., 50A:1171, 1968.

123. Littler, J.W.: The prevention and the correction of adduction contractures of the thumb. Clin. Orthop., 13:182, 1959.

124. McFarlane, R.M.: Observations on the functional anatomy of the intrinsic muscles of the thumb. J. Bone Joint Surg., 44A:1013, 1962.

125. Muller, G.M.: Arthrodesis of the trapezio-metacarpal joint for osteoarthritis, J. Bone Joint Surg., 31B:540, 1949.

126. Murley, A.H.G.: Excision of the trapezium in osteoarthritis of the first carpo-metacarpal joint. J. Bone Joint Surg., 42B:502, 1960.

127. Nalebuff, E.A.: Diagnosis, classification and management of rheumatoid thumb deformities. Bull. Hosp. Joint Dis., 29:119, 1968.

128. Napier, J.R.: The form and function of the carpometacarpal joint of the thumb. J. Anat., 89:362, 1955.

129. Swanson, A.B.: Disabling arthritis at the base of the thumb. Treatment by resection of the trapezium and flexible (silicone) implant arthroplasty. J. Bone Joint. Surg., 54A:456, 1972.

130. Thompson, T.C.: Discussion of paper by Goldner and Clippinger. J. Bone Joint Surg., 41A:625, 1959.

25 Other Arthritides

Although rheumatoid arthritis is perhaps the most devastating, many other types of arthroses strike the hand—osteoarthritis, traumatic arthritis, gout and pseudogout. This chapter deals with the generalities of these diseases. Insofar as possible to avoid duplication of material, the reader will be referred to other chapters for specifics such as operative techniques.

The Osteoarthritic Hand

Osteoarthritis is common in the United States, involving particularly the hip, knee and hand.[14] A survey in 1966 estimated that 40.5 million American adults have osteoarthritis in the hands and feet.[13,14] The joints in the hand most often involved are the distal and proximal interphalangeal of the fingers and the carpometacarpal of the thumb.

This type of arthritis is probably hereditary, tends to run in families, and is especially common in the postmenopausal female.[14] There is considerable variation in the onset of symptoms. For some patients the osteoarthritic process is slow and symptoms are minimal. In fact, marked roentgenographic changes may be seen in patients with relative freedom from pain. There is, however, a more malignant form, so-called erosive osteoarthritis, striking harshly and rapidly the proximal and distal interphalangeal joints. Those so afflicted have considerable functional loss from pain, stiffness and deformity.

For most patients the onset is usually gradual and without any specific antecedent trauma. The joints involved in the hand are often painful during the initial stages, when synovitis may be present, and during the later stages from joint incongruity. With cartilage degeneration, joint narrowing and marginal osteophyte formation occur. These are characteristic at the distal interphalangeal joint (Heberden's nodes) and also at the proximal interphalangeal joint (Bouchard's nodes) (Figs. 25-1, 25-2). Although such marginal osteophyte formation occurs at the carpometacarpal joint, it is detected primarily on roentgenogram.

The Distal Interphalangeal Joint

As the disease progresses at the distal interphalangeal joint, the synovitis may resolve. The joint is narrowed from loss of articular cartilage, becomes irregular from cyst formation, has dense subchondral bone and often shows angular deformity. It may spontaneously stiffen from a fibrous union at one extreme or become grossly unstable at the other (Figs. 25-1, 25-2).

Treatment of the distal interphalangeal joint involvement is nonoperative in the early stages. The acutely painful, swollen joint may be splinted. Salicylates and heat may give some relief. Persistent pain with activity and progressive deformity and/or instability are indications for arthrodesis (Chap. 13).

The so-called mucous cyst is a common accompanying condition (Chap. 22). It arises from the distal interphalangeal joint, adjacent to the extensor tendon and the underlying osteophyte (Fig.

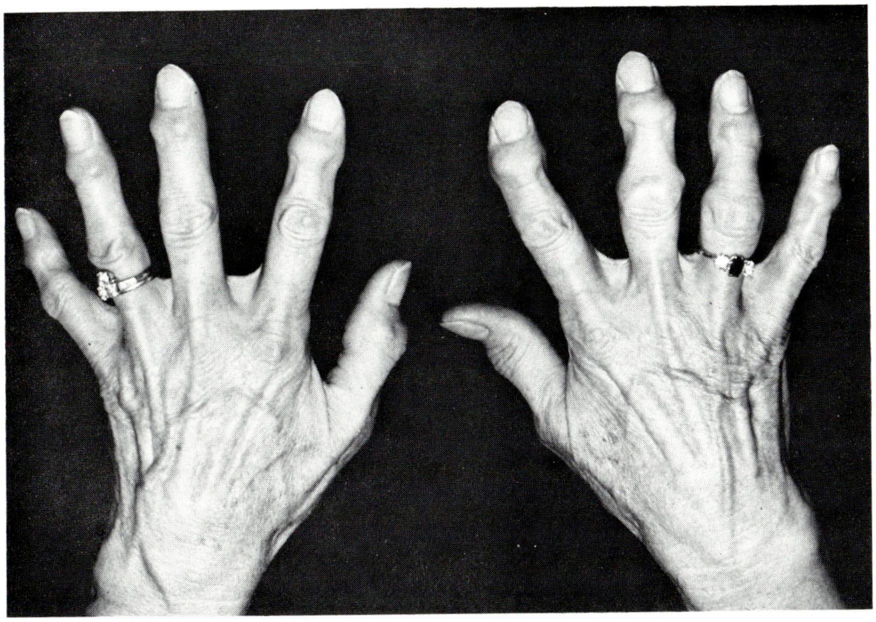

Figure 25-1. *The typical appearance of hands afflicted with erosive osteoarthritis. Note the involvement of the distal interphalangeal joints (Heberden's nodes) and the proximal interphalangeal joints (Bouchard's nodes), with relative sparing of the metacarpophalangeal joints. The distal interphalangeal joints may have significant angular deformities, and are often unstable (see text).*

25-3). The osteophyte plays an etiological role in the pathogenesis of this lesion, is usually visible only on the oblique roentgenogram and should be removed at the time of surgery.[3,10]

The indications for excision of a mucous cyst are (1) pain, (2) proximity to the cuticle, with risk of rupture and infection (as often seen from nail manicure) or (3) thin epidermal covering. Infection of the cyst may be serious, for it may follow the stalk to the distal interphalangeal joint. Severe joint involvement with osteoarthritis is an indication for arthrodesis at the time of cyst excision. However, with a history of previous cyst infection, it is advisable to do the arthrodesis as a second

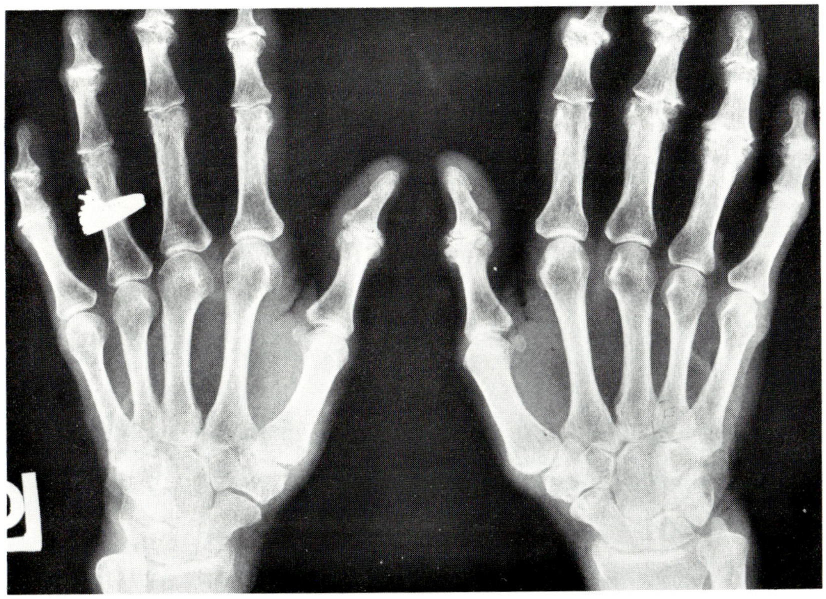

Figure 25-2. *Roentgenograms of patient from Figure 25-1. Note the joint narrowing, irregularity, cyst formation and marginal osteophytes, confined to the interphalangeal joints. Although not in this case, many patients have involvement of the basal joint of the thumb as well (see text).*

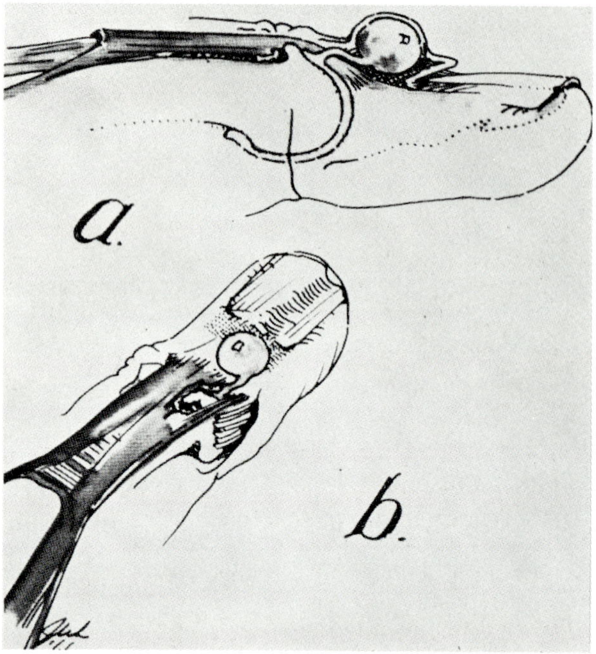

Figure 25-3. *Mucous cyst originating from the distal interphalangeal joint where the extensor tendon passes to and fro over a marginal osteophyte (see text). (From Eaton, R.G. et al.*[3])

stage, not entering the joint at the time of cyst removal.[11]

The Proximal Interphalangeal Joint

The proximal interphalangeal joint is often severely involved in erosive osteoarthritis (Fig. 25-1). Patients suffer from pain and loss of motion. The painful loss of flexion is particularly troublesome for the patient when it involves the ring and little fingers, as it markedly interferes with grasp. Angular deformity is not uncommon. The roentgenographic appearance is typical (Fig. 25-2).

Early treatment is conservative, with mild analgesias, anti-inflammatory agents, heat and advice regarding judicious patterns of hand use. Occasionally intra-articular steroids are temporarily helpful in decreasing the pain. Repeated injections (more than one or two) are definitely contraindicated because the degenerative process may be actually accelerated by the induction of a Charcot type of pattern.

Operative treatment is either arthroplasty (Chap. 24) or arthrodesis (Chap. 13). The index finger is usually best fused to provide stability in pinch; the ulnar three fingers are best treated by arthroplasty to give flexion for grasp.

The Carpometacarpal Joint

The carpometacarpal joint of the thumb is frequently afflicted with osteoarthritis, especially in the postmenopausal female.[1,4,16] The thumb has the mobility to reach the tip of any digit, and the power to oppose their combined strength. For this great mobility with stability, the thumb is indebted to the carpometacarpal joint. This is a double saddle joint; its stability depends upon both its bony configuration and its ligamentous support (especially the deep ulnar ligament).[1,2,4,9,12] As the essential dorsal facet erodes and the ligaments attenuate, the joint becomes unstable. With time, further joint degenerative changes occur with loss of cartilage, cyst formation and marginal osteophytes. The instability is usually painful. The pain, instability and crepitus are easily detected on physical examination (Chap. 24).

Several non-operative modes of treatment will often give appreciable, although temporary, relief. Heat and anti-inflammatory drugs may be useful. Intra-articular steroids may give definite but only temporary symptomatic relief, and should not be given repeatedly because of the risk of a Charcot-type joint. A laced leather gauntlet for external support will often relieve the symptoms by partially stabilizing the thumb, but acceptance by the patient will vary as the appliance is somewhat cumbersome.

Operative treatment, depending upon the stage, is ligamentous reconstruction, arthrodesis or arthroplasty.[1,2,4,5,6,16] Arthroplasty rather than fusion is indicated if the metacarpophalangeal joint is also involved or if the other joints of the trapezium are arthritic, a not uncommon finding.[16] The factors influencing the choice between arthroplasty and arthrodesis and the techniques preferred for each are discussed in Chapters 13 and 24.

Traumatic Arthritis

The hand's multarticulated system of joints is, by its very use, continuously in a position of jeopardy and is often injured. Fractures near or into joints and/or injuries to the ligamentous systems of these joints will frequently result in major disability with appreciable loss of hand function (Chaps. 11, 12). Four common sites will be discussed: (1) proximal interphalangeal joint, (2) finger metacarpophalangeal joint, (3) thumb metacarpophalangeal joint and (4) the carpometacarpal joint of the thumb.

The Proximal Interphalangeal Joint

The proximal interphalangeal joint is normally very stable to lateral stress and yet moves freely through an arc of 110°. Injuries near or into this joint may permanently alter this by either joint irregularity or ligamentous and tendinous scarring (Chaps. 11, 12).[2] Following injury, the joint is often swollen and tender for several months after the exercise program is commenced. During this interval, the patient must be encouraged with the active exercise program and occasionally aided with the use of anti-inflammatory drugs. These joints, following injury, usually retain an increased thickness from increased bulk of the collateral ligaments, even after full pain-free range of motion is restored.[2]

The long-term residual effects following proximal interphalangeal injury are apt to be stiffness and pain, not instability.[2] If, after several months of conscientious exercises, the joint remains stiff with loss of extension or limitation of flexion, and the joint surfaces are congruous, the appropriate soft tissue releases may be required (Chap. 21). If joint incongruity is present and is symptomatic, it is best treated by fusion or arthroplasty (Chaps. 13, 24). Usually arthrodesis is selected for the index and arthroplasty for the long, ring or little fingers (Chap. 24).

If the proximal interphalangeal joint, after 6 to 9 months of conservative treatment, continues with good motion but an unacceptable pain level, consideration can be given to arthroplasty (Chap. 24) or arthrodesis (Chap. 13). Such cases are uncommon, however, in the absence of roentgenographic changes or soft tissue contractures.

The Metacarpophalangeal Joint

The metacarpophalangeal joint, if disabled following trauma, is usually stiff in extension secondary to collateral ligament shortening and scarring (Chap. 21), dorsal capsular contracture, disruption of the joint itself by trauma or extrinsic tightness. Extrinsic tightness or soft tissue joint contracture not responding to a conscientious exercise program may demand selected tendon or ligament releases (Chap. 21). Secondary arthroplasty or arthrodesis has a definite role in the late reconstruction for the joint severely disrupted by trauma (Chaps. 13, 24). Note that fusion of a single metacarpophalangeal joint in the proper position, in the presence of a normal proximal interphalangeal joint, results in a functional digit and is preferable to implant arthroplasty for the single joint of an otherwise normal hand for which heavy use is anticipated.[11] Arthroplasty, if selected, is done essentially as for the rheumatoid hand but usually does not require intrinsic release or extrinsic rebalancing (Chap. 24).

The metacarpophalangeal joint of the thumb is often involved in trauma, most commonly resulting in tears of the ulnar collateral ligament with secondary valgus instability of the joint in pinch. Obviously, the best treatment is early diagnosis with primary ligament repair (Chap. 12).[2]

In late cases, the ligament can sometimes be reconstructed using the palmaris longus tendon.[2,11] In many people, the normal metacarpophalangeal joint of the thumb has limited motion. Whenever evaluating the patient with degenerative changes in the thumb metacarpophalangeal joint, always compare the opposite normal thumb. If the patient's normal thumb has a relatively immobile metacarpophalangeal joint, the disability from arthrodesis of the unstable, involved metacarpophalangeal joint is negligible and the result predictably excellent.

The Carpometacarpal Joint

The carpometacarpal joint of the thumb can have two severe traumatic residuals: instability following ligament injury or degenerative change following a remote Bennett's fracture.[2] The former is best treated by ligament reconstruction, using the flexor carpi radialis as described by Eaton,[2] and the latter by arthrodesis (Chaps. 12, 13).

Gout

Gout may be either primary or secondary.[8] The primary disease represents an inborn error of metabolism and is probably autosomal dominant.[8] The secondary cases are associated with increased nucleic acid turnover or decreased renal excretion of uric acid.[8]

Acute gout may initially manifest itself by the rapid onset of an acutely erythematous, warm tender joint in the hand or wrist, and is often associated with fever and leukocytosis.[7,8] One third of the patients do not have involvement of the joints of the foot in the primary presentation of the disease.[7] The differential diagnosis for the acute gouty attack includes cellulitis, septic joint and an acute rheumatoid process.

The treatment for the acute involvement is medical and systemic. In suspected cases, a physician familiar with the various serum and urine tests to substantiate the diagnosis and knowledgeable about the various medications should be consulted. The drugs used are of three main types: (1) the traditional colchicine, which has no serum or renal effect on uric acid levels, (2) the uricosuric drugs such as probenecid and (3) the xanthine oxidase inhibitors such as allopurinol.

The interval between acute attacks, the so-called interval phase of gouty arthritis, may be prolonged, ranging from months to years. During this time the joints are without symptoms and function is normal. As the attacks become more frequent, they are more apt to become polyarticular, may last longer, and may be associated with a more protracted febrile course. At this stage roentgenographic changes may develop, although the joints usually will recover normal function between attacks. The treatment at this stage also is medical and systemic.

Prior to the use of uricosurics and of the xanthine oxidase inhibitors, approximately 50 to 60 per cent of patients progressed to chronic gouty arthritis or tophaceous gout (Fig. 25-4). However, with the institution of these modern drugs, the incidence of the chronic form has decreased to an estimated 10 to 20 per cent.[7,8,15]

For those patients progressing to this chronic stage, the interval between the first attack and the tophaceous gout is usually 6 to 10 or more years.[7,8,15] In the chronic stages, in the absence of effective systemic therapy, monosodium urate monohydrate deposits accumulate in the tissues. This occurs primarily in relatively avascular areas such as cartilage, joint ligament and capsule, and tendon. Usually the tophaceous involvement is polyarticular. There is secondary joint destruction which leads to significant disability in the hand but may be painless. Tophi may ulcerate, drain a chalky material and become secondarily infected.

Microscopically, the tophus is a deposition of monosodium urate monohydrate crystals which are negatively birefringent with polarized light. These crystals can be seen intracellularly in the synovial fluid leukocytes. The mechanism whereby the crystals cause joint inflammation is unknown, although there are many theories.[8] The tophus itself, in relatively avascular tissues, is a deposition of urates interwoven with fibroblasts, polymorphonuclear cells, lymphoctyes, plasma cells and foreign-body giant cells. The adjacent soft tissue is compressed and forms a "capsule."

Any of the joints of the body may be involved, and in the hand the juxta-articular tophi are frequently located over the dorsum of the metacarpophalangeal joints. At this site they involve the tendons as well as the capsule and ligaments and will erode into the bone. A similar phenomenon may occur at the interphalangeal joints, particularly in the thumb. In the interphalangeal joints, the tophi may at first glance resemble Heberden's nodes or Bouchard's nodes. Hand joints are afflicted with cartilage degeneration, synovial proliferation with a pannus formation, subchondral bone destruction and then, secondarily, with advanced osteoarthritis with marginal osteophytes. This may progress to a fibrous or bony ankylosis, or to gross joint destruction with marked instability.

It bears emphasis that the joint involved in these processes will obviously undergo a marked secondarily superimposed osteoarthritis. The roentgenographic changes are usually first seen in the interval phase of the arthritis. These early changes are punched-out areas adjacent to the interphalangeal joints or metacarpophalangeal joints. Juxtacortical changes then occur with secondary osteoarthritis, which may progress to marked joint destruction.

Other areas of involvement in the hand are the finger pads, the palm and the flexor tendons at the wrist level. When occurring in the flexor tendons, the involvement varies from discrete fusiform or nodular infiltration to a massive tophaceous replacement of the tendons. These flexor tendon deposits may cause locking of the tendons at the wrist, preventing finger motion, or may result in a carpal tunnel syndrome.

Thus, gouty arthritis not infrequently involves the hand. When it does, it may appear in the acute phase as an acutely inflamed painful joint suggestive of sepsis or acute rheumatoid arthritis. In the chronic stages of tophaceous gout, large deposits involve the dorsal aspect of the metacarpophalangeal joints, juxta-articular sites at the interphalangeal joint level, the finger pulp or the palm and the flexor tendons at the wrist. It also may occur in the subcutaneous tissues over the extensor aspect of the forearm, particularly at the olecranon bursa.

The skin over these lesions may ulcerate and the lesions chronically drain their chalky contents, becoming secondarily infected and presenting a difficult therapeutic problem.

The treatment of gouty arthritis in the hand varies with the stage of involvement. In the acute or interval phase of the disease, the treatment is

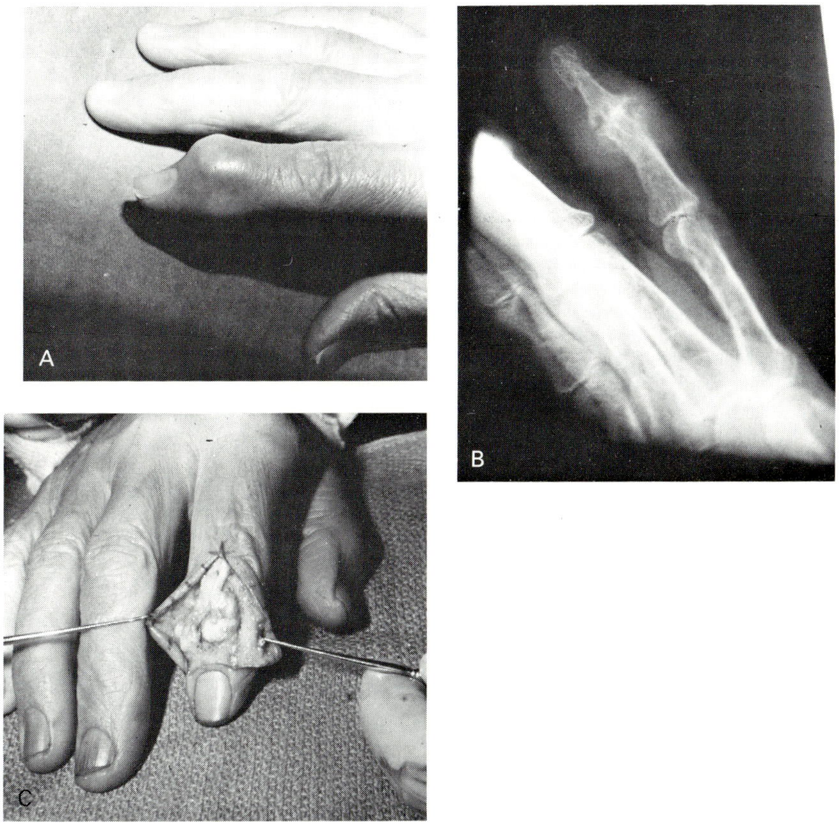

Figure 25-4. *Gout. This young woman had a large tophaceous deposit over the dorsal aspect of the distal phalanx of her index finger. Other than an elevated uric acid level, she had no manifestations of gout. She requested removal of the deposit for cosmetic reasons.*

systemic and involves the use of colchicine and uricosuric and xanthine oxidase inhibitor drugs. This must be managed by a physician familiar with the disease and the drugs. Note that a proper program may actually cause a loss of uric acid from the body and in the chronic stages may even result in some resolution of the tophi. Before the use of drugs, the chronic tophaceous stages required wide excision of the lesions with radical debridements and, not infrequently, amputations. With the introduction of the drugs, the indications for surgical intervention have become more specific and restricted.[15] In the early stages joint aspiration may provide significant relief. This obviously is in conjunction with systemic drug therapy.

Surgery can be subdivided into several categories. The first is the excision of large tophaceous deposits which do not resolve with drug therapy and which form a mechanical obstruction to joint function. These may be in relation to the metacarpophalangeal joint, where they block flexion and extension, or at the interphalangeal joints. At these joints there may be associated mallet, boutonniere, or swan-neck deformities.

Secondly, large tophaceous deposits should be excised if they are starting to drain their chalky contents before they become infected.

Thirdly, the carpal canal should be decompressed to relieve the symptoms in median nerve compression and any associated triggering of the long flexor tendons at that level. This dissection may be difficult, as the tophaceous granulomatous material may have completely infiltrated the tendons making excision difficult or impossible. Note that pain is a rare indication for surgery in this stage of gout, except as it might be associated with a carpal tunnel syndrome.

Major reconstruction of joints of the hand in advanced tophaceous gout is not advisable, as the tissue is usually infiltrated with the tophaceous material and the associated necessary reconstruction is difficult. In such cases, selective arthrodeses are preferable to arthroplasty.

Pseudogout

Pseudogout, which is most commonly described in the knee, may involve the hand. This entity involves a deposition of calcium pyrophosphate crystals which may be detectable on ordinary roentgenograms of the wrist and fingers as an opacity of the surface of the articular cartilage and/or of the fibrocartilaginous disc of the distal radioulnar joint. The diagnosis is based on the classic roentgenographic appearance and the identification of the calcium pyrophosphate crystals in the joint aspirate. The treatment of the condition is medical.[8]

Keinbock's Disease

Cystic necrosis of the lunate may occur as a direct consequence of fracture, not dislocation, but more often without any definitive relationship to a specific traumatic force. However, most of the latter cases exhibit minus ulnar variance (shortening of the ulnar in relation to the radius). This anatomical configuration may cause the lunate to receive the major compressive forces between the radius and the hand.

Following an injury, pain and swelling are localized to the lunate if a fracture exists. The fracture, however, may be very hard to demonstrate roentgenographically and sometimes tomography will be required. The early physical findings in cases that arise spontaneously are pain with extremes of motion, especially hyperextension, pain on impaction and direct tenderness. The physician is often mystified because of the absence of any radiological or laboratory abnormality, but the pain and tenderness may be severe enough to require immobilization of the wrist.

Radiographic changes of aseptic necrosis consist of a mixture of rarification and sclerosis and may take many months to appear at all. With progression of the process there is flattening of the lunate and secondary arthritic change in and about neighboring bones.

The treatment is adequate immobilization until pain and tenderness have subsided. If roentgenographic evidence confirms the diagnosis of aseptic necrosis, then shortening the radius by sectioning it transversely just proximal to the distal radioulnar joint may be considered. This shortening (about 3 mm) is designed to distribute compressive force against the carpus, relieving the lunate. The osteotomized radius can be approximated with a wire loop or fixed with a screw or Kirschner wire. Immobilization with a long-arm cast is maintained until there are signs of bony union.

The indication for resection of the lunate and implant arthoplasty with a Swanson Silastic prosthesis is painful aseptic necrosis intractable to other modes of treatment[17] with the arthritic involvement limited primarily to the lunate (Fig. 25-5**A**).

Implant arthroplasty is done through a longitudinal dorsal incision on the wrist, avoiding both the radial and ulnar sensory nerves. The wrist capsule is incised between the third and fourth compartments and carefully preserved. The extensor pollicis longus is retracted radially and the other digital extensors ulnarly. The lunate must be identified positively, roentgenographically if necessary, by marking it with a Kirschner wire. A threaded Kirschner wire is useful to provide traction on the lunate. The volar ligamentous support is tested after removal of the lunate and, if necessary, reefed with 3-0 or 4-0 nylon sutures.

An implant that fits comfortably is selected from the sizing set, and from this model the permanent implant is chosen (Fig. 25-5**B,C**). The stem of the prosthesis must fit into a hole properly directed into the triquetrum, which is usually created by a drill or curette. The insertion of the stem in this hole maintains the proper orientation to the adjacent bones. It may require repeated testing. Furthermore, for additional stability with the new high-performance silicone rubber, it is possible to stabilize the implant with a Kirschner wire for 4 weeks.

It is of utmost importance that the capsular integrity be established on the volar and dorsal aspect to hold the prosthesis in place. Closing the dorsal capsule securely may require the placement of two small drill holes in the radius to receive sutures and even reinforcement by the extensor retinaculum. If repair of the volar capsule is difficult, a second palmar incision may be necessary. Standard wound closure and dressing are followed by a forearm cast that is worn for 4 to 6 weeks. Full wrist activity is allowed after 12 weeks.

The results in general have been rewarding, with the relief of pain and good stability. There invariably is some limitation of wrist motion and, if there was preoperative arthritis of other carpal bones, this may not be arrested. Occasionally the prosthesis has dislocated volarward, necessitating decompression of the carpal canal and removal.

If arthritis is severe and involves most of the proximal carpal row, more extensive surgery has to be considered, e.g. proximal row carpectomy or wrist fusion.

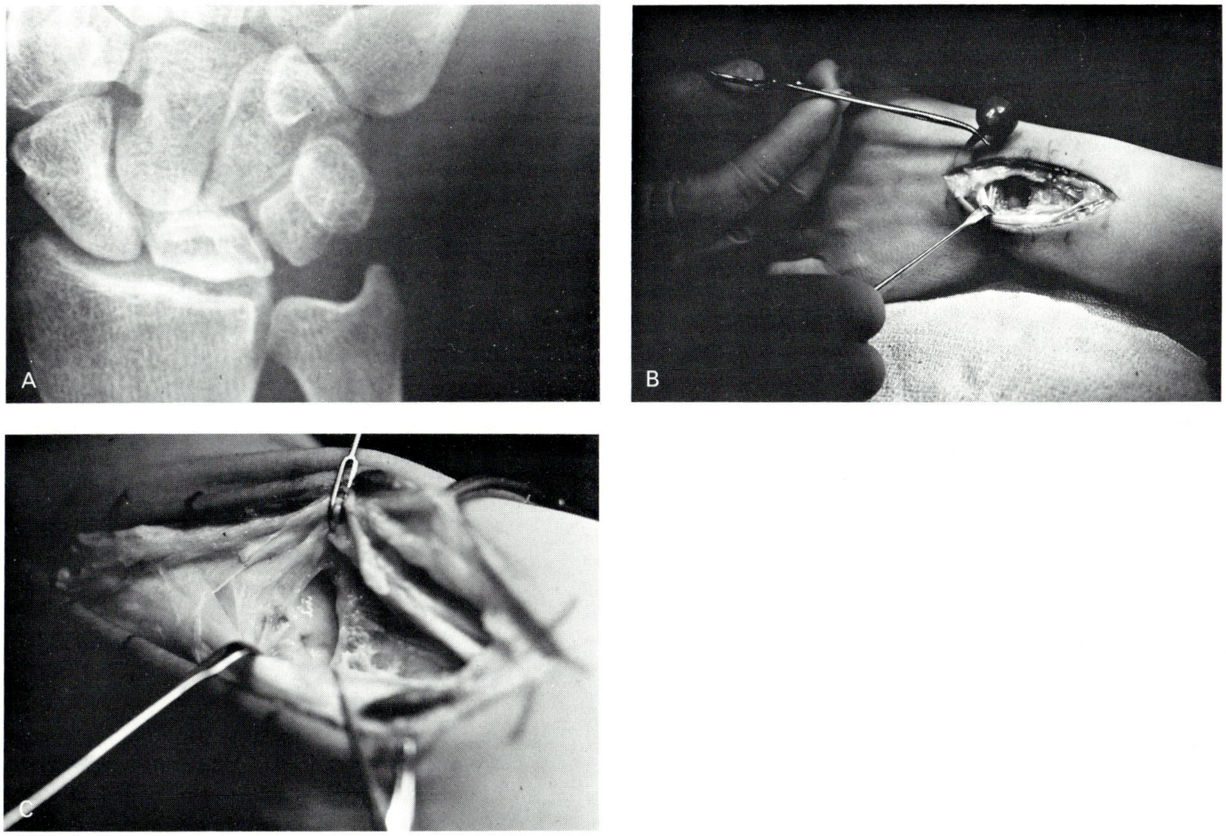

Figure 25-5. **A:** *Roentgenogram showing advanced aseptic necrosis of the lunate (Keinbock's disease).* **B:** *Operative view with lunate excised and wound prepared to receive implant.* **C:** *Close-up of cavity after removal of lunate prior to placement of the implant.*

Preiser's Disease

What has been said for the lunate also applies to aseptic necrosis of the scaphoid, most instances of which follow a recognizable fracture. The roentgenogram may not show the fracture for a week or two after the inciting trauma, and even then views in multiple planes and magnifications may be required. Identification of the fracture makes it easier to evaluate the effect of treatment than in the case of the lunate. Initially a long-arm cast should be applied until there is some evidence of healing of the fracture. When there are signs of aseptic necrosis, bone grafting (Chap. 11), implant arthroplasty or, in the young patient, prolonged immobilization of a year or more must be considered. Proximal row carpectomy and wrist fusion are procedures reserved for the intractably painful disabling state.

Resection of the scaphoid and implant arthroplasty with a Swanson Silastic implant in the presence of aseptic necrosis may be done when the arthritic process is limited to the articulations of the scaphoid[17] (Fig. 25-6**A**). There must be adequate support for the prosthesis, and therefore the procedure is not recommended if there has been a previous styloidectomy or the ligamentous support is absent and irreplaceable.

The surgical approach is through a dorsal lateral incision which protects all branches of the dorsal radial nerve. It passes between the first and second extensor compartments and the radial artery. The extensor pollicis longus is retracted radially and the extensor carpi radialis longus ulnarly. The joint capsule is preserved as the joint is entered. The scaphoid is identified radiologically. It is usually removed piecemeal with a rongeur while carefully protecting the volar ligamentous support. The correct implant size is chosen by fitting a sizer. The implants are left handed and right handed and are fabricated with a stem to fit a hole in the trapezium (Fig. 25-6**B**) made either by drilling or curetting. Precision and the testing of the stability of the implant in the defect are important. If the volar capsular ligamentous support is too loose, it must be reefed with 3-0 or 4-0 nylon sutures before

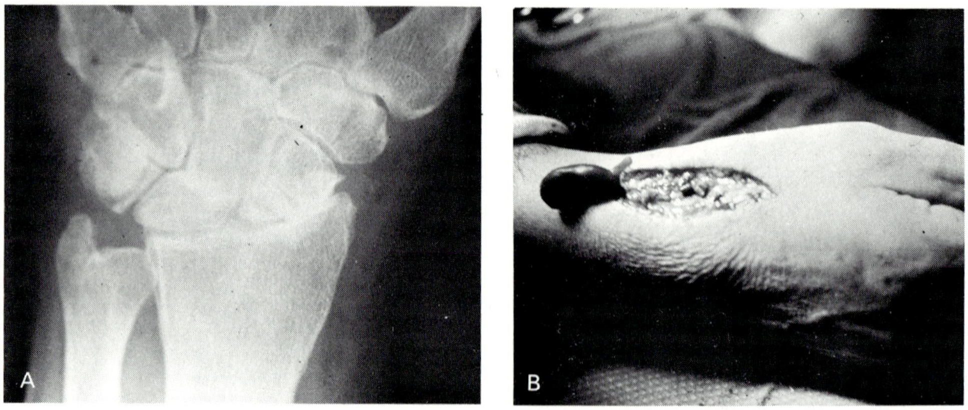

Figure 25-6. A: *Roentgenogram showing advanced aseptic necrosis of scaphoid (Preiser's disease).* **B:** *Operative view showing defect created by removal of the scaphoid and the sizing implant about to be positioned.*

the insertion of the permanent implant. Closure of the dorsal capsule is done to ensure secure containment of the implant when the wrist is moved passively in all planes. After closing and dressing the wound, a well-padded long-arm cast is applied for a week, followed by a forearm cast for 4 to 6 weeks. Full activity is resumed in 12 weeks.

The results have paralleled those previously described for the lunate.

References

1. Burton, R.I.: Basal joint arthrosis of the thumb. Orthop. Clin. North Am., 4:331, 1973.
2. Eaton, R.G.: *Joint Injuries of the Hand.* Charles C Thomas, Springfield, 1971.
3. Eaton, R.G., Dobransky, A.I. and Littler, J.W.: Marginal osteophyte excision in treatment of mucous cysts. J. Bone Joint Surg., 55A:570, 1973.
4. Eaton, R.G. and Littler, J.W.: A study of the basal joint of the thumb. J. Bone Joint Surg., 51A:661, 1969.
5. Froimson, A.I.: Tendon arthroplasty of the trapeziometacarpal joint. Clin. Orthop., 70:191, 1970.
6. Goldner, J.W. and Clippinger, T.W.: Excision of the greater multiangular as an adjuvant to mobilization of the thumb. J. Bone Joint Surg., 41A:609, 1959.
7. Hadler, N.M., Franck, W.A., Bress, N.M. and Robinson, D.R.: Acute polyarticular gout. Am. J. Med., 56:715, 1974.
8. Hollander, J.W. and McCarthy, D.J.: *Arthritis and Allied Conditions,* 8th ed. Lea & Febiger, Philadelphia, 1972.
9. Kaplan, E.B. *Functional and Surgical Anatomy of the Hand,* 2nd ed. J.B. Lippincott, Philadelphia, 1965.
10. Kleinert, H.E., Kutz, J.E., Fishman, J.H. and McGraw, L.H.: Etiology and treatment of the so-called mucous cyst of the finger. J. Bone Joint Surg., 54A:1455, 1972.
11. Littler, J.W.: Personal communication, 1970.
12. Napier, J.R.: The form and function of the carpometacarpal joint of the thumb. J. Anat., 89:362, 1955.
13. Roberts, J. and Burch, T.A.: Osteoarthritis prevalence in adults by age, sex, race and geographic areas: United States, 1960–62. Public Health Service Publ. No. 1000, Ser. 11, No. 15, Washington, 1966.
14. Sokoloff, L.: *The Biology of Degenerative Joint Disease.* University of Chicago Press, Chicago, 1969.
15. Straub, L.R., Smith, J.W., Carpenter, G.K. and Kietz, G.H.: The surgery of gout in the upper extremity. J. Bone Joint Surg., 43A:731, 1961.
16. Swanson, A.B.: Disabling arthritis at the base of the thumb. J. Bone Joint Surg., 54A:456, 1972.
17. Swanson, A.B.: *Flexible Implant Resection Arthroplasty in the Hand and Extremities.* C.V. Mosby, St. Louis, 1973.

26 Anesthesia

The successful choice and administration of anesthesia for operations upon the upper extremities demand close cooperation between surgeon and anesthesiologist. Surgical procedures in this area are some of the most delicate performed, and at times must be done in a patient who lacks the ideal preoperative preparation. An approximation of the duration of the operation, the need for a tourniquet, the possibility of using a pedicle flap or an extensive skin graft from a distant area, the need to use cautery, and the general condition of the patient must all be known. Frequently more than a single operation will be required to complete the reconstruction of a damaged hand.

Most operations upon the upper extremity can be done with the use of a regional anesthetic, but some conditions dictate the use of general anesthesia. Often in very young patients, individuals with neurological disorders, and mentally disturbed or emotionally distraught persons general anesthesia is selected. Certain surgical procedures which ordinarily would require general anesthesia are now being successfully performed with the aid of narcoleptic drugs.

General Anesthesia

When the surgeon anticipates an especially long procedure, or if multiple parts of the body are to be operated upon, general anesthesia is usually selected. For an elective procedure, the usual preparation that would attend any operation requiring general anesthesia can be made. For emergency surgery, the preferred conditions cannot always be met and appropriate safeguards should be taken at the time of the induction of anesthesia to avoid the aspiration of gastric contents.

For elective operations under general anesthesia, admission to the hospital is not mandatory, but often preferred. If a brief procedure is anticipated, the patient may be instructed ahead of time regarding fasting and the necessary preoperative evaluation and laboratory studies may be done immediately upon entering the hospital. The patient may be discharged from the recovery room or observation facility after full emergence from the anesthetic. Arrangements should be made to have someone accompany him home. The patient should be advised not to plan to drive or to operate machinery for 24 hours following the procedure.

Critical features often not appreciated in relation to anesthesia are the delirium during the emergence from anesthesia and its effect on the application of intricate dressings. Excitability and vigorous motions by the awaking patient can completely disrupt the entire surgical effort. Early emergence can also lead to activity which will preclude proper application of the dressing and limit its effectiveness in immobilizing the extremity. Bucking and straining as an endotracheal tube is removed can disrupt tendon and nerve repairs.

Regional Anesthesia

The unique innervation of the upper extremity makes regional anesthesia especially applicable for operations on the hand. Various techniques are available, and their use depends upon the experience of the surgeon or anesthesiologist and the problem being treated.

The virtues of regional anesthesia are multiple. A patient who has just eaten can be anesthetized with little risk of aspirating gastric contents, untoward reactions are minimized and less sophisticated monitoring equipment is required. The limitations are the possibility of an incomplete anesthetic, unexpected reactions to the local administration of these drugs, postanesthetic neuritis resulting from intraneural injection and insufficient duration of the anesthetic.

Guidelines for using regional anesthetics are listed below.

1. Acquisition of patient confidence
   Adequate, appropriate premedication
2. Gentleness
   a. Use of small-caliber needles
      (1) Slow injection to avoid pain from rapid overdistention of tissues
      (2) Careful easy advancement of needles, avoiding direct trauma to the nerves
   b. No intraneural injection
3. Patience
   a. In the performance of the block
   b. In waiting for the block to "take"
4. Reasonable expectations of the block's capabilities and the patient's tolerance
   Considerations for the patient's comfort during the performance of the block and the operative procedures

Ideally the preparation of the patient for a local block should be as thorough as that for a general anesthetic. The premedication should be carefully planned and the technique to be used discussed with the patient. Confidence must be obtained to ensure cooperation and to allay anxiety. It must be anticipated that a tourniquet will be used and the block must be planned to be of sufficient height and duration to obviate any ischemic pain. Both the anesthesiologist and the surgeon should be certain that the tourniquet is functioning properly and is of the proper size for the patient. The calibration of the inflating device of the tourniquet should be verified against the mercury manometer on the anesthetic machine before each operation. The padding under the tourniquet should be ample and, at the conclusion of the operation, the tourniquet and entire padding should be removed from the extremity immediately after deflating to avoid venous congestion. At this time the extremity is elevated by an assistant to eliminate congestion secondary to dependency.

Although most blocks are easily performed, diligent attention to detail ensures success and gentleness and patience ensure patient cooperation—enhancing the chance for a successful anesthetic.

Regional Anesthetic Agents

Although lidocaine is perhaps the most universally used local anesthesic in the United States today, other agents deserve mention. Mepivacaine hydrochloride (Carbocaine) has a slightly longer duration of action and is equally effective for regional and infusion anesthetics. Bupivacaine hydrochloride (Marcaine) is a newer agent which enjoys a longer duration of action than either lidocaine or mepivacaine. Its greatest use is for sympathetic blocks of the stellate ganglion where extended duration of action is desired or for reconstructive procedures of long duration for which a regional anesthesia is desired. Dosages for local anesthetics are:

	Maximum dose	
Lidocaine	300 mg	<4.5 mg/kg
Bupivacaine	175 mg	<2.5 mg/kg
Mepivacaine	400 mg	<6.0 mg/kg

The Use of a Tourniquet

Clinical experience has shown that $1\frac{1}{2}$ to $2\frac{1}{2}$ hours of ischemia by a tourniquet can be maintained with safety.[1] Studies by Wilgis indicate that PO_2 falls to undetectable levels with 2 hours of ischemia after inflating the tourniquet.[4] Recovery to a normal level of pH and PO_2 in the blood of the extremity may take 20 minutes.

Most important in the safe use of the tourniquet are proper calibration of the pressure manometer and precise and even padding beneath the tourniquet with cotton sheathing. Inadequate padding and inaccurate calibration risk nerve injury and a prolonged postoperative morbidity if neuropraxia results.

Brachial Plexus Block

SUPRACLAVICULAR APPROACH (FIG. 26-1)

This time-honored approach to the brachial plexus entails the risk of a pneumothorax if the

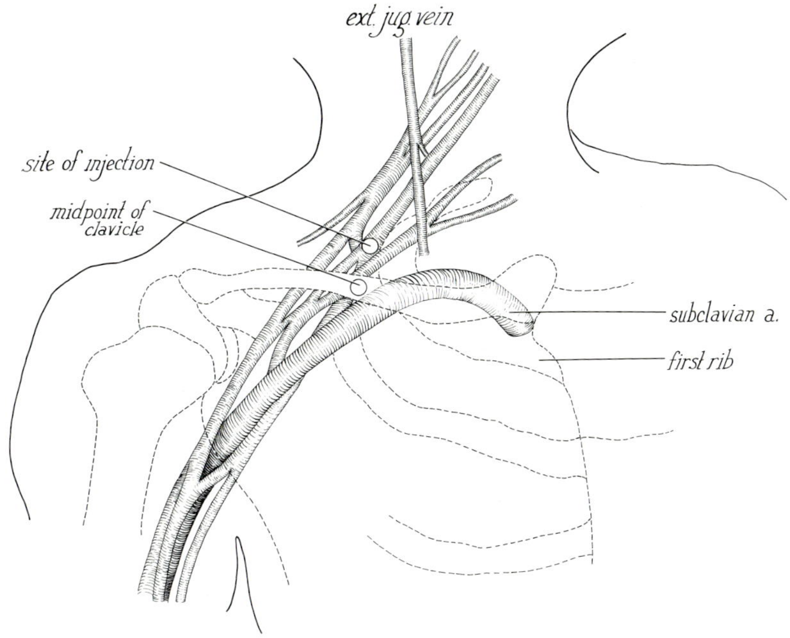

Figure 26-1. *Supraclavicular brachial plexus block. The midpoint of the clavicle is the superficial landmark and the upper surface of the first rib is the point of deepest penetration (not more than 2 to 2.5 cm in the average individual).*

pleura and lung are torn. The landmarks are the clavicle anteriorly, the first rib inferiorly, and the scalenus anticus muscle dorsally. The position of the patient is important. With the patient recumbent the head is turned to the opposite side and the shoulder is drawn down with the arm at the side. The midpoint of the clavicle marks the lateral margin of the first rib and, through a cutaneous wheal of anesthetic just posterior to this point on the clavicle, an 8-cm needle is directed medially, posteriorly and inferiorly until the first rib is struck (not more than 2 cm in the average patient) or paresthesias occur. Here, 15 cc of a 1.5 per cent lidocaine solution with 1 : 100,000 epinephrine is injected. If it is anticipated that the operation may be prolonged, a venous catheter may be inserted instead of the needle and left in place for additional injections.

The usual duration of anesthesia for this block is 2 to 2½ hours. The onset of the block may take 20 to 30 minutes and full anesthesia must be achieved before the procedure is started. Care must be taken not to injure the pleura or the subclavian vessels, or to inject directly into the plexus. Local infection precludes this type of block.

AXILLARY APPROACH[3] (FIG. 26-2)

This approach to the brachial plexus is often easier and more predictable than the supraclavicular technique. The axilla must be cleansed. The arm is abducted and the forearm flexed to 90°. The landmarks are the border of the pectoralis major anteriorly and the teres major and latissimus dorsi muscles posteriorly, plus the axillary artery. The artery is moved inferiorly with the operator's fingers and the 25-gauge 3.5-cm needle is placed through a skin wheal in a line perpendicular to the above muscular insertions. The tourniquet should

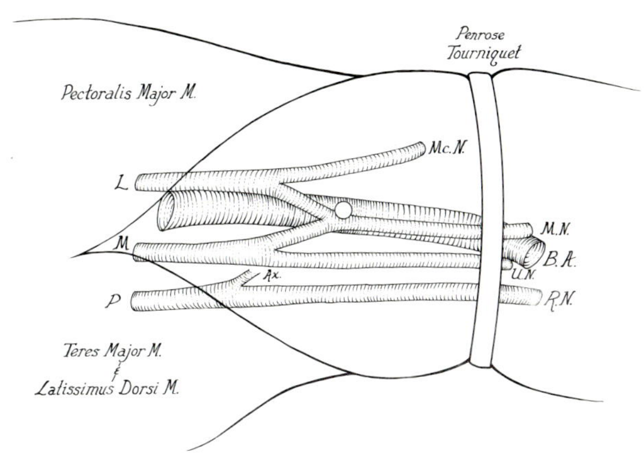

Figure 26-2. *Axillary brachial block. The arm must be abducted to 90° and the forearm flexed to 90°. The pectoralis major muscle anteriorly and the teres major and latissimus dorsi muscles are the guides to the neurovascular bundle. After the initial injection is made the needle must be redirected superiorly and inferiorly to the artery to block the musculocutaneous and radial nerves.*

be inflated or a snug Penrose drain placed below the level of injection to encourage movement of the solution up into the axilla. Paresthesias indicate the proper depth where 5 to 6 cc of a 1.5 per cent solution of lidocaine with 1 : 100,000 epinephrine should be injected. The needle must then be withdrawn and reintroduced at a 45° angle superiorly and inferiorly where the injection is repeated. This ensures the block about the radial (posterior) and musculocutaneous (superior) nerves. Since the axillary nerve has arisen high in the axilla, it is not usually blocked by this technique.

An alternate technique permits the prolongation of anesthesia by multiple injections. After the arm is prepared a fine polyethylene catheter on a needle is introduced parallel to the artery and directed toward the apex of the axilla. As soon as paresthesias have occurred the catheter is gently advanced while the needle is held stationary. The catheter can be indwelling and subsequent injections of approximately one half the usual amount of anesthetic agent given.

The axillary approach avoids the risk of pneumothorax and is usually a more predictable technique than the supraclavicular block. Intravenous or intra-arterial injection is avoided by aspiration before injection of the anesthetic agents. The needle should always be perpendicular to the humerus unless a catheter is being introduced.

Perfusion Anesthesia (Boer Block)[2] *(Fig. 26-3)*

For brief procedures on the upper and lower extremities, in which the tourniquet will not have to be released, intravenous lidocaine is often useful. The duration of anesthesia is approximately one hour and its effectiveness is quite predictable.

Two tourniquets (or a single dual tourniquet) are placed on the upper arm after the application of adequate padding. A small scalp vein needle (23- or 25-gauge) is placed in a forearm vein and the arm exsanguinated using an Esmarch bandage. The uppermost tourniquet is inflated to 300 mm Hg and a Penrose drain is placed about the forearm just proximal to the previously placed needle. Slowly 40 to 50 cc of 0.5 per cent lidocaine (3 mg/kg) is injected and the drain and needle are removed. The onset of anesthesia occurs within 3 to 5 minutes.

When the patient notes discomfort from the superior tourniquet, the lower cuff is inflated and the proximal one released. By this time anesthesia is present under the lower cuff and the operation can progress unimpeded for 45 to 60 minutes more. A circumferential subcutaneous ringing of the arm with 5 to 6 cc of 0.5 per cent lidocaine before the placement of the tourniquets will diminish most of the discomfort from the tourniquet.

Should it become necessary to deflate the tourniquet in the course of the operation, the skin margins can be infiltrated locally with lidocaine or procaine and sufficient anesthesia maintained to conclude the procedure. This technique is not suitable for prolonged procedures or operations requiring vascular repair.

Usually the tourniquet should not be deflated for a least 20 minutes after the introduction of the intravenous lidocaine, to avoid any untoward cardiac effects.

Perfusion anesthesia is extremely useful for draining the infected hand. Exsanguination is achieved by elevation of the limb before inflating the proximal tourniquet rather than compression of the arm with the Esmarch wrapping. This type of block, however, should not be used in the drug addict who has repeatedly injected irritating agents into his veins.[2]

Direct Nerve Block

RADIAL NERVE (FIG. 26-4)

Within the upper arm the radial nerve can be blocked at a point about 12 cm above the lateral humeral condyle, posterior and deep to the biceps muscle beneath the intermuscular septum between the brachioradialis and brachialis muscles. Figure 26-4 illustrates the technique for blocking the nerve just above the lateral humeral condyle, at which point it has divided into the superficial radial nerve and the posterior interosseous nerve.

If the pure sensory component of the radial nerve is to be blocked, it may be found by rolling the superficial radial nerve over the lateral border of the radius where it is subcutaneous. More distally, the dispersion of the nerve necessitates a block extending from the snuffbox to the ulnar side of the dorsum of the wrist.

MEDIAN NERVE (FIG. 26-5)

At the medial aspect of the biceps tendon the brachial artery can be felt and the median nerve

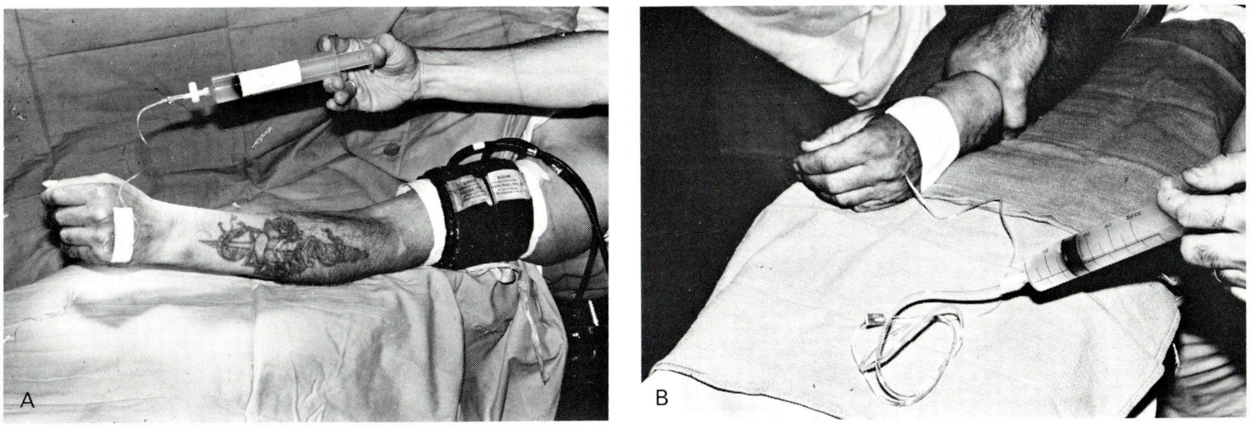

Figure 26-3. *Intravenous perfusion block. A padded double tourniquet is applied to the upper arm. After placement of a small scalp vein needle (25-gauge) the arm is exsanguinated by elevation or wrapping. The proximal tourniquet is inflated to 300 mm Hg and the anesthetic solution injected. The anesthetic may be held in the hand by pressure at the wrist or a small Penrose drain tourniquet.*

often palpated. A skin wheal is made midway between the tendon and the medial condyle of the humerus. At this point and with care to avoid the artery an injection of 6 to 8 cc of 1.5 per cent lidocaine should produce anesthesia within the median nerve distribution.

For short procedures on the radial side of the palm, a median nerve block at the wrist may be sufficient (Fig. 26-5**B**). The injection is within the carpal tunnel. The skin wheal is placed just radial to the palmaris longus tendon about 2 cm proximal to the wrist crease. The small needle (3.5-cm, 25-gauge) is slowly advanced at a 45° angle toward the palm until paresthesias are elicited. It is withdrawn 2 to 3 mm and the hub is depressed as it is advanced again beneath the transverse carpal ligament superficial to the medial nerve. If no further paresthesias occur, the slow injection of 5 cc of 1.5 per cent lidocaine is made. Usually the block becomes evident in 10 to 15 minutes. A small amount of anesthetic should be injected subcutaneously about the palmar cutaneous branch lying radial and superficial to the main nerve.

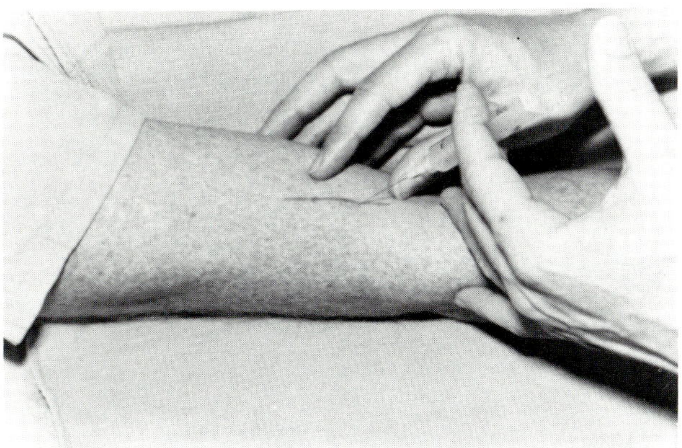

Figure 26-4. *Radial nerve block. An injection of 5 cc. of 1.5 per cent lidocaine is made 1.5 cm lateral to the biceps tendon and 2 cm proximal to the antecubital crease.*

ULNAR NERVE (FIGS. 26-5B, 26-6)

Anesthesia of the ulnar nerve is easily obtained at the elbow by injecting within the olecranon groove about the nerve. The injection should be carefully and slowly performed, avoiding injury to this superficial nerve.

At the wrist the nerve may be blocked as it enters the loge de Guyon at the pisiform bone (Fig. 26-5**B**). The injection is performed just dorsal to the flexor ulnaris tendon with the needle perpendicular to the tendon and between it and the ulna. A 1.5 per cent solution of lidocaine, 4 to 5 cc, is usually sufficient.

INTERMETACARPAL BLOCK OF THE COMMON VOLAR DIGITAL NERVES (FIG. 26-7)

To avoid the risk of damage to the digital vein and artery, an intermetacarpal block for individual digit anesthesia is preferable to injection within the digit itself.

The skin wheal is made between the metacarpal heads on the dorsum of the hand. The needle (2.5-cm, 25-gauge) is inclined proximally at 45° toward the wrist and is gently introduced until paresthesias occur or its tip is just felt beneath the palmar skin. It is withdrawn about 3 mm and very slowly

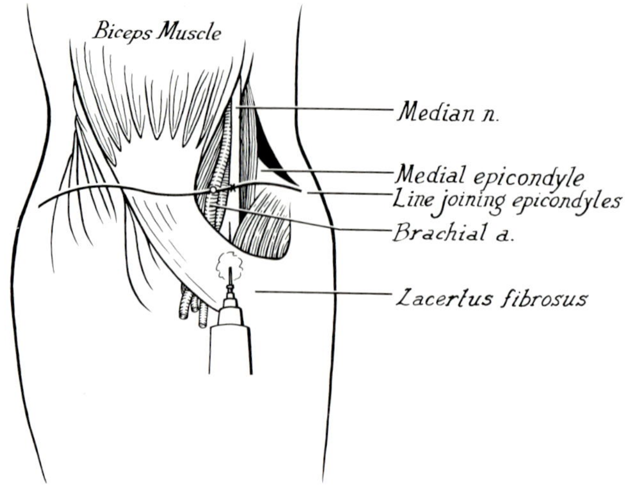

A

Figure 26-5. *Median nerve block. The median nerve can be blocked directly at the elbow midway between the biceps tendon and the medial epicondyle. Median nerve block at the wrist is done just radial to the palmaris longus tendon. A block of the ulnar nerve at the wrist is performed by inserting a 25-gauge needle beneath the flexor carpi ulnaris tendon, just volar to the ulna and perpendicular to the forearm.*

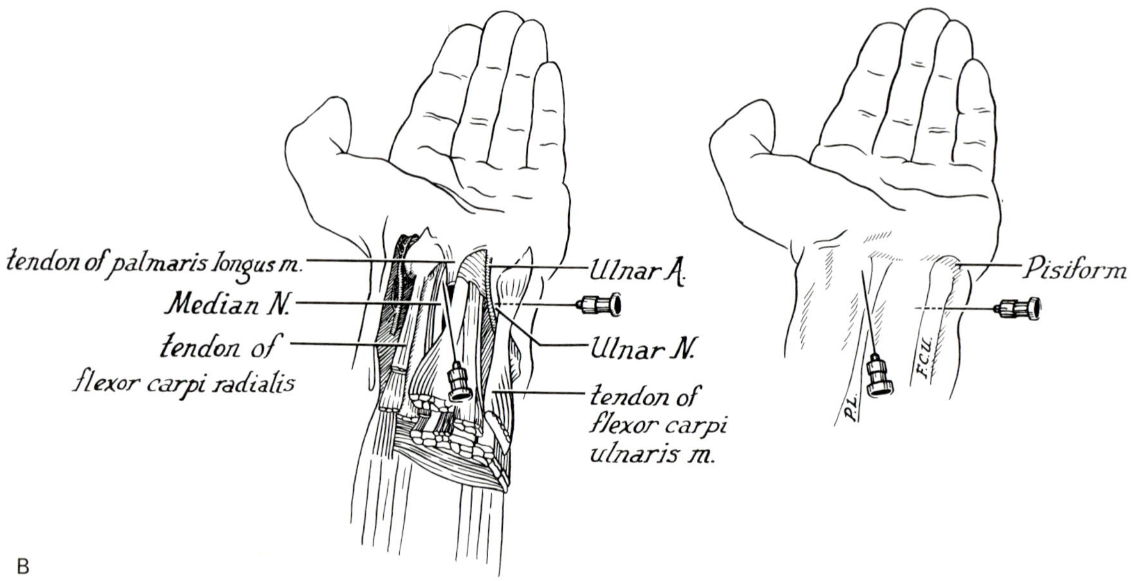

B

2 cc of 1.5 per cent lidocaine is injected. The procedure is repeated on the adjacent side of the metacarpal. If resistance is encountered on passage of the needle, it is inclined slightly to clear the intermetacarpal ligament.

If an injection is carried out within the finger itself, care must be taken not to overdistend the tissues and strangulate the digit. Vascular injury must be avoided.

Stellate Ganglion Block

Stellate block is useful for diagnosing and treating some vasospastic disorders and at times for the relief of pain. The stellate ganglion, a fusion of the lower cervical and first thoracic ganglia, lies between the transverse process of the seventh vetebral body and the first rib deep to the vertebral artery.

Commonly the patient is seated with his arms at his sides and facing the anesthetist. The important landmarks are the body of the seventh vertebra and the midpoint of the clavicle. An 8- to 10-cm needle is usually needed.

The skin wheal is made just above the clavicle at its midpoint. The injecting needle is inserted horizontal to the clavicle at an angle of 45° to the skin, and directed posteriorly and medially. It passes posterior to the carotid sheath. When the body of the seventh vertebra is encountered, 10 cc of 2 per cent lidocaine with or without epinephrine is injected. A Horner's syndrome indicates a successful block.

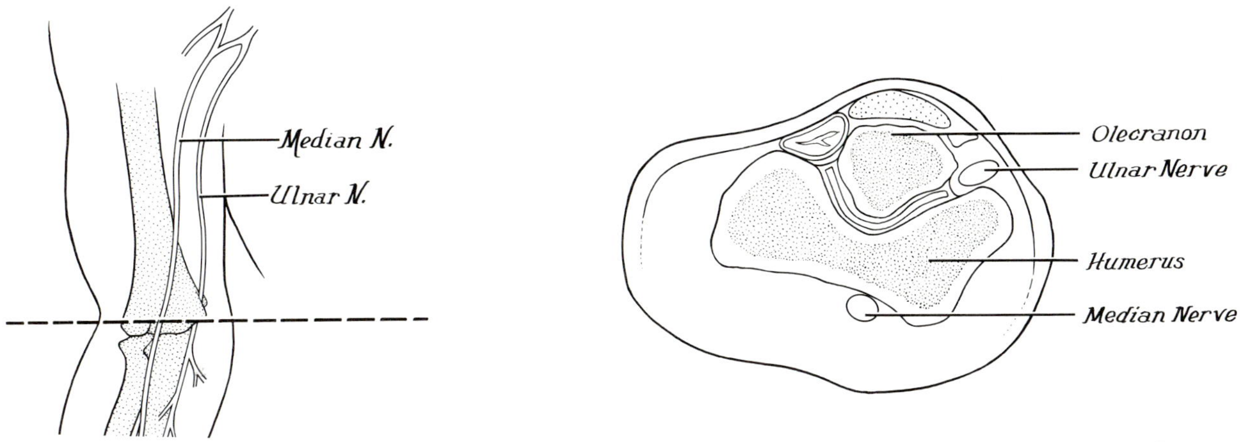

Figure 26-6. *Ulnar nerve block. The ulnar nerve is readily blocked at the elbow in the olecranon groove. Care must be taken to avoid traumatizing this sensitive nerve.*

Narcoleptic (Dissociative) Anesthesia

For many procedures, especially in children, narcoleptic anesthesia has proven effective. It can be given intramuscularly to induce anesthesia and then is maintained by serial intravenous injections. At times it causes unpleasant postanesthetic hallucinatory effects in the adult and should not be used in patients in whom there are upper respiratory infections. The pharyngeal reflexes are active under dissociative anesthesia and excessive upper airway secretions can produce laryngospasm. The patient must be well oxygenated and closely observed during the course of the anesthetic. Repeated use often produces the need for greater increments with succeeding anesthetics. Although it is ideal in the management of many burned patients, movements by the patient may preclude its use in nerve or tendon surgery. Also, occasional tonic-clonic movements occur in some patients.

The intravenous dose ranges from 1 to 4.5 mg/kg and the intramuscular dose from 6.5 to 13.0 mg/kg. Two mg/kg intravenously usually results in surgical anesthesia within 30 to 60 seconds for 5 to 10 minutes whereas it takes 3 to 4 minutes for the intramuscular dose to become effective.

Complications

Any anesthetic has complications associated with its use. The most hazardous problems that occur with general anesthesia are cardiac arrest, cardiac arrhythmia, hyperthermia and hypoxia or hypercarbia. Aspiration of nasopharyngeal secretions or regurgitated gastric contents may also occur. Unusually violent emergence from the

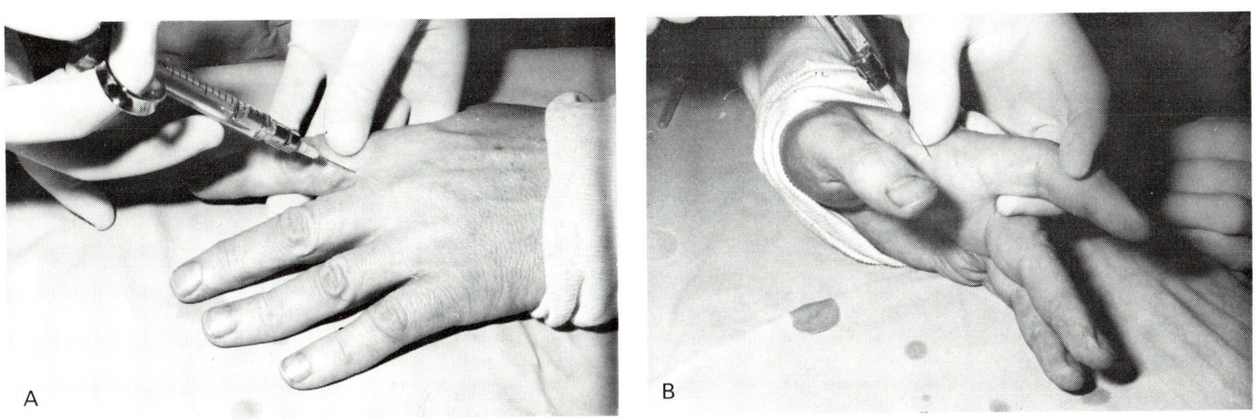

Figure 26-7. **A:** *Intermetacarpal digital nerve block. The needle is inclined at a 45° angle from the palm and gently inserted into the web space nearly to the palmar surface.* **B:** *The marginal digital nerves are approached from the radial side of the index finger or the ulnar side of the little finger.*

deeper planes of anesthesia may result in disruption of tendon or nerve repairs or even loss of fracture alignment. Movements during surgery, such as those which occur with an inadequate level of general anesthesia or with the use of dissociative anesthesia, may limit the surgeon in his reconstructive efforts.

Regional anesthesia is not without complications. The escape of intravenous lidocaine from an infusion block may cause myocardial depression, hypotension or even cardiac arrest. For this reason the surgeon and anesthesiologist must be certain of the efficacy of the tourniquet during such procedures.

Blocks which are performed by the direct injection of local anesthetic agents must be gently and carefully performed to avoid the production of pneumothorax from injury to the pleura or subclavian vessels. All blocks done near vessels have the potential of injuring the vessels, with local bleeding. Neuritis may occur even if the injection is not made into the nerve directly and can persist for an extended period of time (up to several months) with variable degrees of dysesthesia. Overdoses of an amide type of local anesthetic may be manifest by the cardiac effects noted above or their effects on the central nervous system: excitability or depression, drowsiness, visual disturbance and respiratory arrest. Fortunately allergic reactions to lidocaine are rare, but any foreign substance in a given patient may have an untoward response. Lidocaine, mepivacaine, bupivacaine are all contraindicated in patients who have a history of hypersensitivity to the amide type of local anesthetics.

A "caine reaction" can occur with any local anesthetic. Two effects may be produced involving either the cardiac or the central nervous systems. Initially the patient may note subjective disturbances: a metallic taste, headache, anxiety or nervousness. These can be followed by seizures and subsequently depression. Hyperventilation with oxygen and the administration of a short-acting barbiturate intravenously may abort the reaction. Ephedrine will counteract the cardiac depressive effects, diminish vasoconstriction and increase the effectiveness of the cardiac action. Intravenous Valium is often given with the appearance of the initial excitatory symptoms.

References

1. Flatt, A.E.: Tourniquet time in hand surgery. Arch. Surg., 104:190, 1972.
2. Graham W.P.: Intravenous regional anesthesia for outpatient operations on the upper extremity. Indust. Med., 39:37, 1970.
3. Kleinert, H.E., DeSimone, K., Gaspar, H.E., Arnold, R.E. and Kasdan, A.B.: Regional anesthesia for upper extremity surgery. J. Trauma, 3:3, 1963.
4. Wilgis, E.F.S.: Observations on the effects of tourniquet ischemia. J. Bone Joint Surg., 53A:1343, 1971.

27 Pain

Pain is the guardian of the hand against injury. An intact nervous system is essential for this protection. Neurological impairment can lead to disability by denervation or overactivity. With denervation the hand falls victim to noxious agents, stress and force; through neural overactivity excessive pain and inhibited use of the hand result.

The hand as one of the body's most sensitive structures readily succumbs to painful stimuli. Pain destroys function more easily than any other derangement of the hand. Its adverse influence can physically disable the whole extremity and psychologically disable the whole patient. Accordingly, the prevention, control and relief of pain are of paramount importance in treatment. By virtue of the exquisite sensibility of the hand, a painful stimulus readily conditions the patient to fear and the anticipation of more pain. Hence, every effort must be made to prevent pain and to relieve it promptly when it occurs.

Definition

Pain thresholds vary little from patient to patient but the interpretation and perception of pain are exceedingly variable. Different scientific disciplines have individual views of pain. The biologist regards pain as a stimulus that heralds imminent injury, the physiologist views it simply as a sensation and the sociologist as a motivating force in learning. The psychologist, however, sees pain as a dynamic interaction between cerebral interpretation and subjective expression.

To the patient pain is an unpleasant state that he wishes to avoid but occasionally aggrandizes for secondary gain. His awareness of pain and reaction to it will be influenced by the circumstances that brought it about and the environment in which it was initiated. Thus in victory an athlete will withstand pain far more readily than in defeat, as is reflected by his reaction to the stimulus. Swanson[13] has appropriately defined pain as "a disagreeable sensation which has as its basis a highly variable complex made up of afferent nerve stimuli interacting with the emotional state of the individual and modified by his past experience, motivation and state of mind."

Pain Appreciation

Hilgard[6] notes that any one stimulus increased to a sufficient intensity is capable of producing pain. Pain is no longer considered simply the summation of multiple stimuli. In certain areas it is the predominant sensation perceived by the stimulation of the tissue, e.g. the cornea. Hence it is considered a sensory modality unto itself.

Two varieties of peripheral pain are recognized: superficial and deep. Superficial pain is readily localized usually within the skin and provokes an immediate withdrawal of the stimulated part. It is often associated with tachycardia or palpitations. In contrast deep pain is poorly localized, dull and oppressive, invoking bradycardia, hypotension and syncope. Central pain follows peripheral pain and persists even after the peripheral stimuli have abated. Anxiety enhances and prolongs this component.[15]

Pain Reception and Transmission

Painful stimuli can be recognized at a variety of peripheral neuroreceptors which are not specific for pain.[1] Endogenous amines (histamine) and polypeptides (bradykinin) can stimulate pericapillary chemosensitive pain receptors.[5] These sensory nerves are not the same as the perivascular vasomotor nerves, which are not sensitive to bradykinin and are sympathetically innervated. The bradykinin-sensitive organs have their innervation from the dorsal roots. Salicylates are specific chemical antagonists for these electron-rich negatively charged sites. These receptors are probably the source of ischemic pain.

Pain originates from all other tissues through a variety of receptors which are especially notable about the origin and insertion of tendons and their sheaths and about the periosteum, ligaments and joint capsules. These receptors, the most perceptive of which are the cutaneous ones, aid in the localization of pain. There are vast intercommunications between the receptors and multiple axon cylinders which account for the diffusion of stimuli and referral of pain. This overlap also serves to inhibit pain.

Patterns of pain referral are illustrated in Figure 27-1. This clearly shows how stimuli from any receptor in the hand served by fibers from C-6, C-7 or C-8 roots can be referred to various areas along the entire upper extremity, shoulder or chest wall. Thus common problems within the hand, e.g. carpal tunnel syndrome, may appear predominantly as proximal pain, often exaggerated by anxiety and the fear of a "heart attack" or a "stroke."

Small unmyelinated C fibers (6 μ) and larger myelinated A fibers (5 to 10 μ) conduct painful stimuli, the larger size and myelination serving to expedite and localize the stimulus. C fibers are found throughout the nervous system both centrally and peripherally and in some sensory nerves are up to 12 times as common as myelinated ones. These C fibers also transmit the autonomic impulses which are exclusively sympathetic in the upper extremity. Mullan[10] claims that their effect "cannot be obliterated by localized surgical ablation." Neither A nor C fibers limit their conduction to painful stimuli. Pain conduction is not exclusive to any receptor, pathway, or cortical terminus. This accounts for the frequent impasse in the control of the unrelenting pain. According to Becker,[1] the variety of central pathways that can transmit painful stimuli account for the reactivation and "escape" of pain after an anatomical attempt at interruption (e.g. anterolateral cordotomy).

The sympathetic nervous system serves exclusively the adrenergic and cholinergic end-organs in the upper extremity. The adrenergic end-organs act in vasoconstriction and arrector pili activation while the cholinergic end-organs act in vasodilatation and hidrosis. In any state of pain, these organs are activated by the stimulation of this system. This in turn reinforces the painful problem and at worst leads to causalgia.

Anatomical Basis for Pain

Skin

As the shield of the body, skin is the most frequently injured tissue. Pain is produced by the compromise of circulation, the tension that leads to hypertrophic scars and specific injury to the skin.

Tense wound closures, poorly planned elective incisions, and focal pressure from improper splints and dressings are common preventable iatrogenic sources of pain. The loss of subcutaneous padding and the fixation of skin, e.g. to bone, also predispose to pain.

Fascia

Although fascia has its own pain receptors, its role in pain production is mostly a secondary one. Through its inelasticity it abets the congestion of tissues and the problems of stiffness which lead to pain. Unrelenting "throbbing" pain is the signal to consider fasciotomy as an emergency.

Musculotendinous Pain

Compression, contraction or stretching can invoke musculotendinous pain, as can acute or chronic repetitive action, examples of which are acute myositis crepitans, chronic myositis and peritendonitis (Chap. 8).

Vascular Pain

The vascular system generates pain through states of insufficiency, congestion, inflammation and rarely tumors (glomus). "Throbbing" pain signals venous and lymphatic congestion and diffuse burning pain connotes the generation of a decubitus. These are urgent signals which can be relied

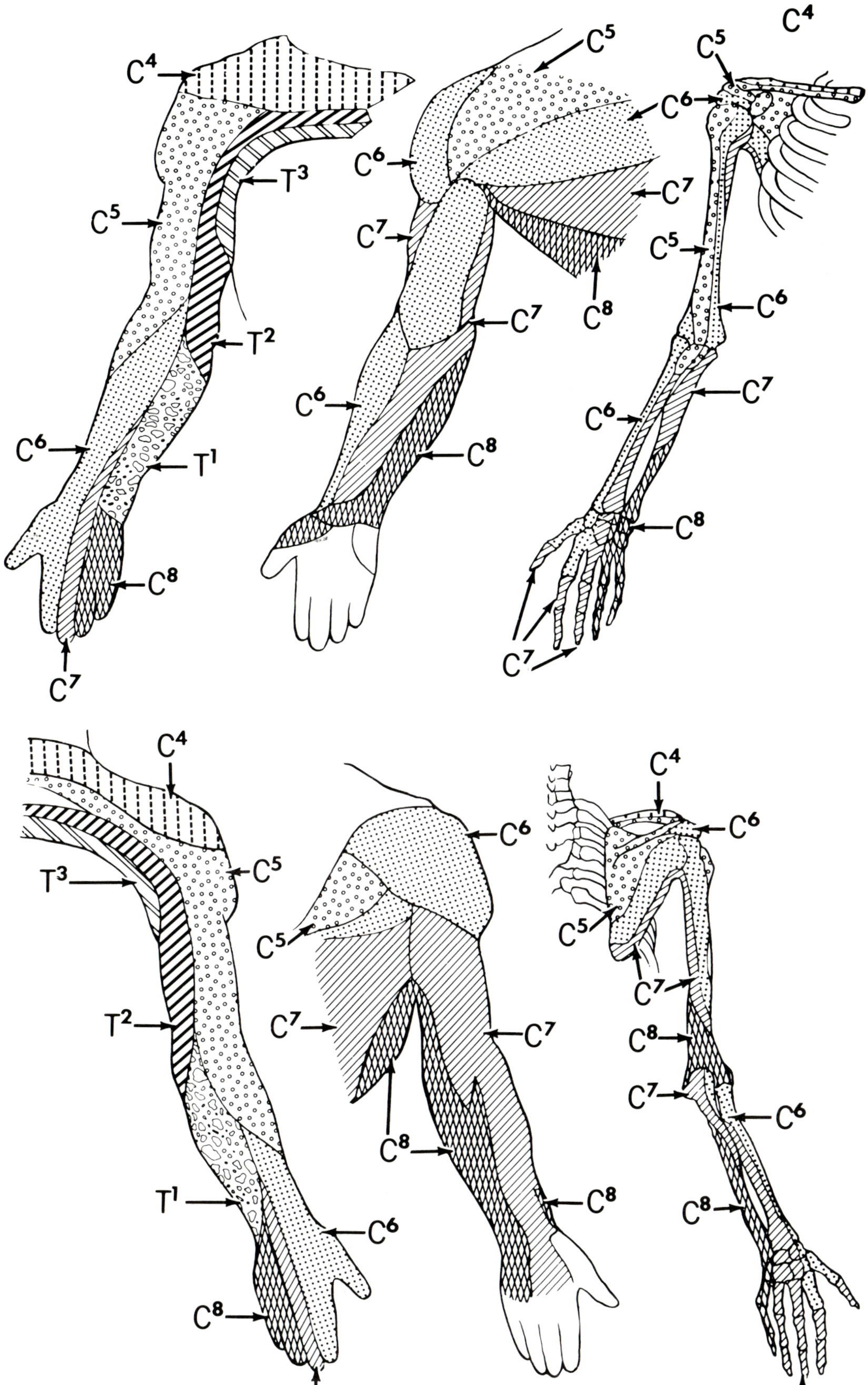

Figure 27-1. *The dermatomes and sclerotomes of the upper extremity, volar and posterior aspects.* **Left:** *Dermatomes.* **Center:** *Predominant segmental innervation of the superficial musculature.* **Right:** *Predominant segmental innervation of the skeleton and attachments of the deep musculature. The muscles, fascia and periosteum innervated by a single nerve root form a continuous series extending from the trunk distalward into the limb. The dermatomes overlie only a portion of the corresponding sclerotome.* (*Modified from Inman, V.T. and Saunders, J.B.*[8])

upon only in the presence of an intact nervous system.

Bone Pain

Fractures, periosteal contusion, inflammation and tension are causes of bony and periosteal pain. Examination under stress, compression and percussion are usually reliable methods of localization and diagnosis of pain from these sources. Unrelenting bony pain requires serial roentgenography and repeated examinations over days, weeks or months for proper clinical management.

Joint Pain

The mechanisms for initiating pain of joint origin are trauma, degenerative changes and inflammatory states. The distinction rests on the history, physical examination and roentgenographic findings. Occasionally the pain is referred from a distant source, e.g. palmar stenosing tenosynovitis manifesting itself as proximal interphalangeal joint pain (Fig. 8-4).

Stiffness is the basis for much joint pain when the shortened capsular and ligamentous tissues are stretched. Desmitis and synovitis are other common sources of pain. Painful crepitation upon joint motion indicates an irregular joint surface.

Neurogenic Pain

Organic neural disorders initiating pain are most commonly from peripheral trauma of an acute or chronic nature and less commonly from neuritis and central nervous system afflictions. A detailed history and neurological examination will usually pinpoint a peripheral organic cause for pain. Organic causes proximal to the brachial plexus, as well as functional states, can be diagnostically perplexing because of poor localization.

To properly evaluate the source of pain when it is severe (e.g. in causalgia) its intensity must be reduced to permit examination.

PAIN OF PERIPHERAL NEUROPATHY

At the moment of neural trauma pain varies in intensity from none to excruciating. Following the injury reactive anesthesia may occur, protecting the part for several minutes or hours. Subsequently anesthesia may persist or be replaced by a variety of painful sensations: hot, shooting, sharp, etc. (interim period). After 2 to 4 weeks the subjective awareness of neuroma formation and nerve regeneration manifested as dysesthesia begins (late period). An electric shock on percussion at the site of injury (Tinel's sign) characterizes this stage. The peripheral migration of this sign is a measure of the existence but not the quality or quantity of nerve regeneration. Its persistence causes volitional restraint in using the hand. Paul Brand has termed this the withdrawn "inhibited hand" in contrast to the insensitive "uninhibited hand" which is often traumatized by overuse.

Failing normal regeneration and with the persistence of pain, an indefinable period of fixed pain ensues. There are several varieties of fixed pain: the effects of irritative nerve lesions (neuromas or reflex sympathetic dystrophy), phantom pain and causalgia.

Irritative Nerve Lesions. The most common cause of fixed pain is a neuroma which may be within the substance of the intact nerve ("in continuity") or at the proximal nerve stump. The fixation of a neuroma against a rigid bed by scar tissue facilitates the initiation of pain by traction and compression.

The shoulder-hand syndrome, the classical example of reflex sympathetic dystrophy, is the product of overstimulation of the central nervous system affecting the peripheral neurovascular mechanism. However, any chronically congested, stiff painful hand is an expression of some measure of the problem. Although trauma is usually the initiating factor, it is commonly seen as a product of upper limb affection by non-traumatic illnesses such as coronary artery disease, stroke, cervical arthritis, peritendinitis, etc.

Failure to control pain of this nature leads to dystrophic changes affecting all structures under the influence of the sympathetic nervous system. Initial vasodilatation changes to vasoconstriction with diminished skin temperature and hyperhidrosis. The trophic changes of disuse affecting skin and muscles parallel the osteoporosis seen on roentgenography.

Nerve compression states cause diffuse pain which is distributed peripherally and proximally with diagnostic anatomical distribution (Fig. 27-1). This type of pain is frequently intermittent, depending upon the factors of edema and changes in external compression (Chap. 15). The most common entrapment is around the median and ulnar nerves in their respective tunnels at the wrist and elbow and less commonly within the proximal forearm.

Phantom Pain. Division of a peripheral nerve may precipitate phantom pain of a chronic and disabling nature. Most amputations are associated with a phantom awareness of the amputated part. The peripheral parts serving the greatest function (e.g. thumb and index finger) are highlighted in the phantom regardless of the level of amputation. Their representations in the phantom are the last to disappear. The degree of pain if present is generally tolerable, but may be excruciating and intractable. No single factor is responsible for the occurrence of phantom sensation and pain. "Neighboring painful impulses may increase the phantom sensations. They may make a previously painless phantom painful or may increase the pain. This is especially noticeable in pain of visceral origin."[11]

In the presence of a painful phantom, trigger points within the skin or at the nerve stump may exist, contributing to the complexity of the pain problem. According to Noordenbos,[11] the basic mechanism for pain production hinges on an amputation-induced deficiency of fast-fiber afferent impulses which normally inhibit the pain-producing summation of slow-fiber impulses within the multisynaptic afferent system of the spinal cord.

Causalgia. Causalgia is a rare severe pain (e.g. burning, bursting) which is not always disabling and by definition is relieved by sympathetic block. It emanates most often from high-velocity or traction injuries of the median nerve above the elbow. Its intensity is enhanced by physical and emotional stimuli.[12]

PAIN OF PROXIMAL NEUROPATHY

This is pain which arises from the brachial plexus or proximal thereto. It is commonly caused by compression. The cervical roots are compressed by hypertrophic osteoarthritic spurs or by intervertebral disc protrusion. Other components of the plexus are compressed by developmental or acquired abnormalities of the musculoskeletal structures about the neck and thoracic outlet. Compression with pain in this region can also be caused by a host of neoplastic and non-neoplastic masses. The diagnosis may be obscure. Intercommunications of nerve pathways within the brachial plexus produce manifold radiations of pain which may be either deep or hyperpathic. Other causes for pain from this region are blunt or penetrating injuries of the roots or plexus, clavicular fractures and traction injuries. Occasionally causalgia is seen after these injuries.

Roentgenograms are invaluable in the evaluation of these problems of pain. Routine cervical spine views with specific oblique and flexion and extension views reveal the existence of post-traumatic hypertrophic degenerative and intervertebral space changes. Any of these can be a source of hand pain which often is accentuated by extension of the neck and simultaneous rotation of the head to the contralateral side.

A meticulous neurological examination coupled with electromyographic studies is often essential for proper diagnosis. Special roentgenographic studies consisting of myelograms or arteriograms may be required.

Neuritic Pain. Dysesthesias are associated with a variety of inflammatory, metabolic and nutritional conditions. The dysesthesia may be a presenting symptom of an otherwise undiagnosed entity. For example, the pain of herpes zoster precedes the appearance of the diagnostic cutaneous lesions by a few days.

Pain of Central Nervous System Origin. Pain in the hand arising from the spinal cord and brain is rarely if ever the only manifestation of the basic pathological process. In these circumstances the routine history and physical examination will have to be augmented with neurodiagnostic techniques.

Referred Pain. Just as the peripheral origin of pain may radiate onto the shoulder and trunk, so may thoracic pain radiate to the extremity. This most commonly involves the cardiovascular system. Pain of cardiac origin must be considered in the differential diagnosis of diffuse pain of the upper extremity.

Functional Pain. Functional pain can be the result of various neuroses and psychopathies. Failing any or adequate organic evidence for pain, the services of a competent neuropsychiatrist skilled in the diagnosis and relief of these problems must be obtained before the illness becomes irreversible.

Inconsistencies are telltale signs of malingering and "pain for secondary gain." By repeated examination the astute clinician can detect and bring to light the inconsistencies in location, anatomical distribution, intensity and precipitating factors of the pain.

Treatment of Pain

Since most hand pain is initiated by trauma, a great deal can be done to prevent further pain and control that which already exists. This effort must be initiated with the first medical contact with the patient and be attended to throughout his care. Psychologically the freshly injured patient is highly receptive to favorable and unfavorable conditioning by environmental influences. He deserves reassurance and must be spared conversation which is going to generate fear, pessimism and despair. This compassionate support, however, must not detract from the patient's own most important responsibility for his own recovery.

Prompt treatment of the problem causing pain and prompt administration of adequate analgesia are the most influential steps in preventing the establishment of fixed pain.

Experts in hypnosis have clearly shown that words, manner of speech, subject matter and material factors in emergency rooms and operating rooms register with lasting influence on the patient even if he is semiconscious. In the reception of such influence, the patient is rarely discriminatory and more often than not personalizes whatever he hears, sees and smells even though it has no bearing on him. Hence the important factor of anxiety will be controlled and pain thereby reduced by efficient business-like management of the patient's problems without loose talk and disturbing sights and smells.

The most important preventive factors in the physical treatment of the patient are: (1) the deferring of manipulative evaluation of the injury until adequate anesthesia has been administered, (2) the maintenance of good circulation and particularly the control of congestion and (3) effective immobilization. Judicious prophylaxis against infection is also necessary.

Skin and Subcutaneous Tissue

Fresh wounds should be closed without tension and appropriately immobilized. Areas of painful granulation tissue should be curetted and grafted if necessary. Tight and sensitive scars should be revised and adherent or unpadded skin released or replaced by flaps when necessary. Painful dermatoses require accurate diagnosis and specific treatment (Chap. 7). The painful tension of skin over a developing nail horn on amputation stumps should be incised and the offending nail remnant removed with its bed. Dermal abscesses should be drained.

Musculotendinous Pain

Pain of musculotendinous origin requires splinting when acute and may respond dramatically to local or systemic steroids, salicylates or phenylbutazone. At times counterirritants, ultrasonic therapy, hot water and paraffin baths have an ameliorating effect.

Tenolysis and tenovaginotomy are effective pain-relieving procedures when specifically indicated. The subluxation of tendons under tension over natural or pathological bony prominences may be painful and require reefing of the tendon or ostectomy of the offending bony projection.

Pain of intrinsic musculotendinous origin may result from scar that straddles the intermetacarpal ligament between the dorsal and volar intrinsic tendons, described by Watson et al.[14] as intrinsic locking. This is relieved by section of the scar and partial resection of the ligament.

Vascular Pain

The throbbing pain of congestion and the burning pain of decubitis formation must be relieved immediately. For throbbing pain the skin and fascia may have to be slit if all other measures fail. The locus of burning pain must be inspected and if necessary a more suitably padded dressing applied.

Arterial blockage by embolus or thrombosis must be investigated and appropriately treated whenever there is an unexpected and progressive state of pain with diminution of the pulse and skin temperature (Chap. 10).

Vasospastic states, e.g. Raynaud's phenomenon and intra-arterial drug abuse, may be test-treated by a cervical sympathetic block. A good response may then justify a cervical-thoracic sympathectomy. Anticoagulation and antisludging substances (dextran) may be of value. Intra-arterial reserpine is also beneficial.

Bone and Joint Pain

The production of pain from most skeletal sources will be relieved by proper immobilization.

Beware of digital traction which can easily lead to painful joint stiffness and ulceration at the sites of counterpressure. Failure to respond suggests a misdiagnosis and necessitates further diagnostic efforts, including additional roentgenograms. Evidence of osteomyelitis or osteoid osteoma may in time present pathognomonic changes not noted on earlier roentgenographic examinations.

Immobilization is the key to the control of most sources of joint pain. However, injudiciously applied or prolonged it can become the source of joint pain secondary to stiffness. Hence the position of immobilization is of critical importance, as is the surgical judgment limiting or extending its duration.

Carefully governed active and passive motion is most effective and at times greatly aided by local steroid injections. Arthrolysis may be required to relieve persistent pain and stiffness.

Intra-articular fractures and dislocations require meticulous anatomical reduction. Painful arthritic joints which do not respond to anti-inflammatory medications may be candidates for arthroplasty or arthrodesis.

Antibacterial therapy and immobilization are needed for infected joints.

Neurogenic Pain

Attention to detail in the management of the injured nerve will go far in preventing neuromatous pain (Chap. 15). The prime issue is the reduction of scar by preserving the circulation and soft tissue padding around the nerve or its stump.

Once fixed pain has developed, non-operative treatment should consist of percussion of the nerve and sometimes local steroid injection plus mobilization. A protective glove or cushioned pad may be devised if surgery is not feasible.

Fixed pain in most instances responds well to operative and non-operative treatment. The limited number of patients that do not respond become enigmas by their intractability to the host of different techniques which may be tried, and are listed as follows:

- Relocation of neuroma
- Resection of neuroma in continuity and neurorrhaphy
- Proximal nerve section and relocation, silicone capping or triamcinolone injection, ligation with or without absolute alcohol injection
- Sympathetic block
- Sympathectomy
- Transcutaneous electrical stimulation
- Central nervous system procedures*
  - Cordotomy—anterior-lateral spinothalamic percutaneous cordotomy
  - Dorsal column stimulator implantation
  - Prefrontal lobotomy

The operative management of a symptomatic neuroma is discussed in Chapter 14.

The treatment of reflex sympathetic dystrophy requires first the treatment of the precipitating factor in the extremity or elsewhere. The specific treatment of the reflex dystrophy consists of sympathetic blocks integrated with a program of effective somatic and psychological activity.

Prevention must be stressed. All patients with acute coronary artery occlusion should be required to pass all the joints of the upper extremity through a full active range of motion many times daily, beginning with the onset of illness. When active effort is impossible or contraindicated, the range of motion should be carried out passively.

PERIPHERAL COMPRESSION SYNDROMES OF THE MEDIAN AND ULNAR NERVES

When the onset of the nerve compression is rapid, secondary to recent trauma, emergency surgical decompression is necessary. In chronic cases, night splinting and the local injection of dilute triamcinolone (5 to 10 mg/cc), around, *but not into,* the nerve, may relieve the problem. If not, a surgical decompression is necessary (Chap. 15).

Phantom Pain. Most phantom pain is mild and transient, requiring only the reassurance of the patient and his involvement in useful activity. At times analgesia is necessary. If the pain becomes fixed, the predictability of any treatment succeeding is guarded. Beware of committing the patient to unrewarding revisions of stump scars and neuromas by the mistaken conviction that these are the prime sources of the problem.

Admixture of sensory impulses from the affected limb and neighboring truncal areas through synapses within the central nervous system may induce reciprocal referral of adverse sensations and pain. Blocking the afferent impulses from either area (brachial plexus, sympathetic chain or interspinous ligaments) may invoke relief.[11]

When serial sympathetic blocks give definite

*These should be considered only with competent psychiatric consultation.

temporary relief of phantom pain, sympathectomy is indicated.

If the phantom pain is measureably accentuated by touching or pressing the stump, cordotomy may be of particular value for its relief. When stimulation of the stump does not invoke the phantom pain, cordotomy will not help.[10]

Causalgia. The treatment of causalgia is complete cervical sympathetic block (Chap. 26) followed in time if necessary by sympathectomy. Genuine causalgia is relieved almost immediately by sympathetic block. The relief may last for hours or indefinitely. There may be spontaneous regression. Sympatholytic drugs (reserpine) may have some benefit but sympathetic block or sympathectomy is more dependable.

PROXIMAL NERVE INJURIES

The initial treatment for nerve root compression problems is usually cervical traction (5 to 15 pounds adjusted for comfort with a slight flexion tilt). This is maintained to tolerance daily for 2 to 3 weeks before myelography is considered. If the myelogram reveals discogenic disease or compression from intervertebral osteophytes, surgical decompression may be undertaken.

The infrequent neurovascular compression state of the thoracic outlet (scalenus anticus) syndrome may be responsive to conservative measures consisting of weight loss, shoulder girdle exercises, postural correction and bracing. With the persistence of disabling symptoms surgical decompression may be necessary (Chap. 10).

Tumors about the brachial plexus can cause compression with radiation of pain to the hand. Some of these are resectable, e.g. lipoma, aneurysm, and even on occasion neurofibroma, while others may be inoperable, e.g. Pancoast's tumor.

A fracture of the clavicle with displacement or excessive callus formation may compress the plexus and be amenable to reduction or resection for relief of pain. Although total clavicular resection is not necessarily associated with any disability, only that portion of the clavicle responsible for the deformity need be resected.

A penetrating cervical injury may have to be explored for the control of hemorrhage and for debridement. It may be difficult or impossible to visualize or repair injured nerve tissue in a sea of blood. The persistence of pain after a penetrating injury of the brachial plexus requires exploration and the appropriate surgical correction, e.g. neurolysis, resection of neuroma, and neurorrhaphy or triamicinolone injections. Space-consuming and irritative foreign bodies need to be removed.

When traction injuries have occurred myelography may demonstrate extravasation of dye about the roots. These injuries are not amenable to direct surgical repair and management is usually medical.

Pain secondary to neuritis is treated medically by correcting the basic metabolic or inflammatory cause.

Herpes zoster may be aborted by the use of hyperimmune serum if the diagnosis is made before the emergence of the vesicles. Once the vesicles have erupted and crust formation has occurred, treatment is directed toward the prevention of secondary bacterial infection by topical and/or systemic antibiotics and appropriate dressings. Cytosine arabinoside and adenine arabinoside may be used in severe cases for their antiviral effects.[9]

The pain associated with the initial eruption is burning in character, whereas the postherpetic pain is sharp, shooting, intermittent and at times extremely disabling. Analgesics are usually effective for relief of pain in the initial and postherpetic states, but if the pain becomes intractable neurosurgical treatment may be undertaken.

The treatment of organic central nervous system disorders causing pain in the hand must be tailored to the specific diagnosis by the medical discipline involved. The role of the hand surgeon is to direct the preservation of sensory and motor function if these are threatened. Paralytic states may require dynamic splinting to avoid skeletal and musculotendinous stretching and contractures. A program of active and passive movement must also be prescribed.

Conclusions

Confidence and rest play a vital role in the management of pain. Self-confidence is bestowed by motivation and induced confidence by effective communication with the physician and attention to the details of the patient's environment. In the presence of trauma, rest is the greatest single factor of importance. As John Hilton in his classic work *Rest and Pain* has said, "Rest is the necessary antecedent to the healthy accomplishment of both repair and growth (which) bear an exact relation to due physiological rest, local and general."[7]

No single mode of rest is applicable to all cases;

it must be adaptive to both the hand and the total patient (e.g. splinting the hand and a "good night's rest").

Analgesics, tranquilizers and sedatives must be judiciously utilized in the control of anxiety, the insurance of rest and the relief of pain. The demand for these drugs by the patient at the dawn of the pain problem is a measure of his anxiety, which can perpetuate the pain well beyond the time required for physiological recovery.[3]

In order to minimize the need for drugs, psychological and physical activity must be maintained at all times, consistent with the requirements for immobilization.

The roots of fixed pain should not be driven deeper into the patient's psyche by unrelenting surgery. The failure of one well-planned and executed surgical procedure all too often predicts the failure of any subsequent operative procedure for a given problem. It is therefore to everyone's advantage that the patient be brought to grips with this reality and as much as possible helped to live with his own misery and adjust to it.

As shown by Blitz and Lowenthal,[2] pain thrives on inactivity and is thwarted by activity. Physical and sociological stimuli raise the threshold of pain and anxiety and aid the patient in concentrating in constructive activities. Failing proprioceptive input from physical activity of the upper extremity, the patient's pain is maintained and enhanced. Input of stimuli must be specifically designed to fit the patient's educational, sociological and physical aptitudes. Intractability then requires a detailed study to determine a psychoneurotic demand for the perpetuation of this pain.

Once pain is recognized as part of the facade of a malingerer there is no need for specific medical treatment. The patient should be dismissed from further care and any disability settlement rendered. Rating pain for disability evaluation is discussed in Chapter 28.

References

1. Becker, D.P., Gluck, H., Nelsen, E.F. and Jane, J.A.: An inquiry into the neurophysiological basis for pain. J. Neurosurg., 30:1, 1969.
2. Blitz, B. and Lowenthal, M.: The role of sensory restriction in problems with chronic pain. J. Chronic Dis., 19:119, 1966.
3. Drew, F.L., Moriarty, R.W. and Shapiro, A.P.: An approach to the measurement of pain and anxiety responses of surgical patients. Psychosom. Med., 30:826, 1968.
4. Guyton, A.C.: *Textbook of Medical Physiology.* W.B. Saunders, Philadelphia, 1968.
5. Guzman, F. and Lim, R.K.S.: The mechanism of action of the non-narcotic analgesics. Med. Clin. North Am., 52:3, 1968.
6. Hilgard, E.R.: Pain as a puzzle for psychology and physiology. Am. Psychol., 24:103, 1969.
7. Hilton, J.: *Rest and Pain.* J.B. Lippincott, Philadelphia, 1950.
8. Inman, V.T. and Saunders, J.B.: B.C.M. Referred pain from skeletal structures. J. Nerv. Ment. Dis., 99:660, 1944.
9. Krupp, M.A. and Chatton, M.J.: *Current Diagnosis and Treatment.* Lange Medical Publishers, Los Altos, 1973.
10. Mullan, S.: The transmission and central projection of pain. Med. Clin. North Am., 52:15, 1968.
11. Noordenbos, W.: *Pain.* Elsevier, Houston, 1959.
12. Seddon, H.: *Surgical Disorders of the Peripheral Nerves.* Williams and Wilkins, Baltimore, 1972.
13. Swanson, A.B.: Evaluation of impairment of function in the hand. Surg. Clin. North Am., 44:925, 1964.
14. Watson, H.K., Ritland, G.D., Belman, D.A.J. and McDonough, J.M.: Intrinsic locking over the transverse metacarpal ligament. J. Bone Joint Surg., 54A:900, 1972.
15. Wolff, H.G. and Wolff, S.: *Pain.* Charles C Thomas, Springfield, 1958.

28 Reports and Methods to Evaluate Impairment

Reports

The largest part of the cost of hand injury in our society is that of disability settlement. The dollar basis of settlement varies from one state to another and with the nature of liability in a given case.

Rating a case for permanent disability is an administrative matter and not in the purview of the physician. It is affected not only by the physical impairment of the case but also by the patient's age, sex, occupation, education and economic and social background. The physician's responsibility is to estimate anticipated physical impairment and, at the end of treatment, to record such impairment in subjective and objective terms. The American Medical Association's *Guides to the Evaluation of Permanent Impairment*[2] has tables which serve to convert the physician's findings into percentages of impairment.

Disability is a reduction or total loss of actual or expected ability to be gainfully active. It is either temporary or permanent, and always involves administrative and fiscal action and compliance by insurance companies whenever a workman's compensation injury is involved (in approximately 50 per cent of all injured hands). The timeliness and competence of initial and follow-up medical reports on impairment are the prime basis for fulfilling the fiscal responsibilities required by law (e.g. setting aside actuarial reserves, paying weekly compensation, etc.). Delinquency in this matter by the physician leads to confusion, ire, compensation mindedness, unnecessary prolongation of temporary disability and litigation for permanent disability. It is the intent of the Workmen's Compensation Law that the injured working man shall be sustained financially and given the best of care during his convalescence, and that a fair settlement will be rendered in the event of permanent disability.

The nomenclature used to describe the hand must avoid ambiguity. The surfaces and directions of motions referred to about the digits and body of the hand should never be "lateral" and "medial," but rather "radial" and "ulnar," not "anterior" and "posterior" but "volar" and "dorsal." The digits should be named as thumb, index, long (or middle), ring and little and the corresponding digital rays numbered I, II, III, IV and V. Proximal, middle and distal finger joints are referred to as MP (metacarpophalangeal), PIP (proximal interphalangeal) and DIP (distal interphalangeal). The two joints of the thumb are referred to as the proximal (MP) and distal (IP) joints.

Initial Reports

Initially it is often impossible—and unwise—to pass judgment regarding future permanent impairment. However, the existence of injury, the mechanisms and events pertaining to its origin, the physical and biological results and the treatment program must be passed on succinctly and promptly (within days of onset) by the physician to the insurance carrier. This initial report of injury (Table 28-1) should specify the working diagnosis and an estimate of duration of treatment and medical observation and of temporary disability. The novice invariably underestimates the amount of time this involves.

Table 28-1. *Initial (preliminary) Report of Injury (a cryptic report)*

1. Patient's name, address, telephone and social security number, age, sex, occupation and tenure of present job
2. Employer's name and address
3. Insurance carrier's name and address and telephone number
4. Date, location, time of injury
5. History and mechanism of injury
6. Preexisting impairment or disorder
7. Examination and diagnosis
8. X-rays and tests
9. Ambulatory or in-hospital treatment (including location)
10. Treatment
11. Estimate of duration of treatment and observation
12. Estimate of duration of temporary disability
13. Permanent disability (only if irrefutable)

It is urgent to determine at the time of injury, and to record in the initial report, the existence or non-existence of any previous injury or disorder causing functional impairment that antedates the new injury. Such factors are easy to obtain at the time of injury and hard to have acknowledged later, yet at the time of a permanent disability settlement, apportionment to preexisting and new factors must, in all fairness, be made.

Preexisting work-related impairments of function are commonly found among some categories of workers, particularly older ones who have worked around heavy and high-speed equipment. Many patients also have impairments which are not necessarily work related, e.g. Dupuytren's contracture, rheumatoid arthritis, osteoarthritis, carpal tunnel syndrome, trigger finger, etc. The examiner must meticulously evaluate such states to determine the age, circumstances, rapidity of onset and time, type and results of any previous treatment. He must attempt to find out how this preexistent problem affected the patient's job prior to the current injury and decide how, if at all, the job might have aggravated the preexisting condition. The examiner must determine to what extent the natural evolution of the problem would, by itself (without aggravation by his work), bring about some or all of the impairment under question.

Commitments by the physician regarding permanent impairment should be made in initial reports only when the permanency of the impairment is totally obvious, e.g. amputation, complex injuries, etc. To do so routinely, however, may unnecessarily prejudice the patient and others in seeking awards later, when it turns out there is no foundation for impairment.

Table 28-2A. *First Detailed Formal Report of Injury*

REFERENCE:

Patient's name, employer, date of injury, claim #

PARAGRAPH 1:

Introduction (patient's age, occupation, handedness, diagnoses re present and preexisting hand problems, major surgical procedures and dates thereof)

PARAGRAPH 2:

Working Status (type of work when he was injured, how long he has been doing it, *and* if and when he stopped work or started again after injury. If he stopped working, when he was or will be able to return to work. If work is modified, in what way is it so)

PARAGRAPH 3:

Past History (preexisting impairment or problems with the hand and general health)

PARAGRAPH 4:

History (mechanism of injury and complaints)

PARAGRAPH 5:

Examination (physical examination, including pertinent measurements [Table 28-2B], and results of roentgenograms and laboratory tests)

PARAGRAPH 6:

Treatment and Course (original and follow-up treatment, changes in measurements, tests and results of same. New problems. Copies of operative and other reports may be sent as enclosures)

PARAGRAPH 7:

Discussion (opinion re progress and prognosis, or need for other forms of treatment, consultations, referral, etc.)

Follow-up Reports

Any workman's compensation case involving a period of treatment or evaluation over 1 month's time requires a follow-up report of the status of progress, need for further treatment and prognosis. Such reports should generally be written at 1- to 2-month intervals, and the first of these is usually more detailed in its summary of the case than subsequent reports.

The first formal follow-up report of injury (Table 28-2**A**), to complement the initial (preliminary) report (Table 28-1), is generally submitted within 3 to 4 weeks when enough time has passed for the surgeon to have a mature feeling for the nature and ramifications of the problem. A system of reporting aids the surgeon in being thorough, and helps all readers to extract needed information. The report must not be wordy and repetitious.

The "Reference" should stipulate the patient's name, employer, date of injury and any known insurance claim number. The introductory paragraph should stipulate the patient's age, occupation, handedness and diagnoses regarding his hand (both preexisting and new). It should also stipulate any major surgical treatment procedure by name and date.

The second paragraph should be entitled "Working Status" and detail what his job is and how long he has been employed where he was injured; whether, since injury, he has continued at his regular or modified work; and the dates of any temporary disability. If he has had a sporadic work record, that should be indicated and explained. The report should also indicate if he had, at the time of injury, recently started some kind of new physical work which is different from that to which he is accustomed, and if he is performing modified work after injury its nature should be explained.

Table 28-2B. *Measurements taken as baseline to determine existence or non-existence of functional impairment.*

MEASUREMENTS	Side Side	
Circumference:		
Biceps	_____/_____	
Forearm	_____/_____	
__________ (Other)	_____/_____	
Grip: Trial 1	_____/_____	
Trial 2	_____/_____	
Trial 3	_____/_____	
Pinch: Trial 1	_____/_____	
Trial 2	_____/_____	
Trial 3	_____/_____	
Length of __________ (Part)	lost ____ cm	
Neck:		
Extension	__________)	
Flexion	__________)	% of normal
Lateral bend	_____/_____)	
Rotation	_____/_____)	
Shoulder:		
Abduction	_____/_____)	
Adduction	_____/_____)	. . . .ROM _____/_____)
Forward flexion	_____/_____)	)
Extension	_____/_____)	. . . .ROM _____/_____)
External rotation	_____/_____)	)
Internal rotation	_____/_____)	. . . .ROM _____/_____)
Elbow:		
Extension	_____/_____)	)
Flexion	_____/_____)	. . . .ROM _____/_____)
Forearm:		
Pronation	_____/_____)	)
Supination	_____/_____)	. . . .ROM _____/_____)
Wrist:		
Extension	_____/_____)	)
Flexion	_____/_____)	. . . .ROM _____/_____)
Ulnar deviation	_____/_____)	)
Radial deviation	_____/_____)	. . . .ROM _____/_____)

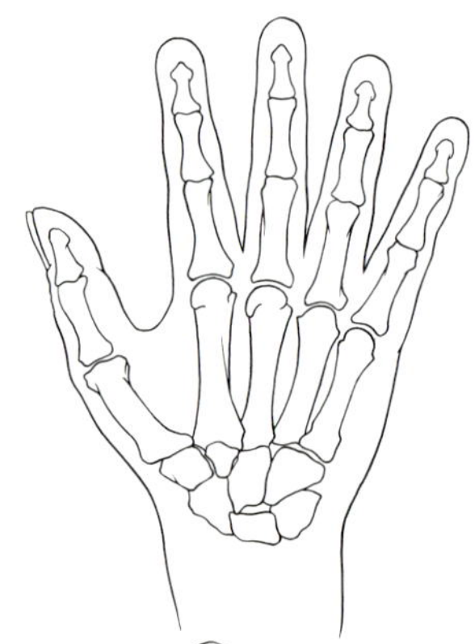

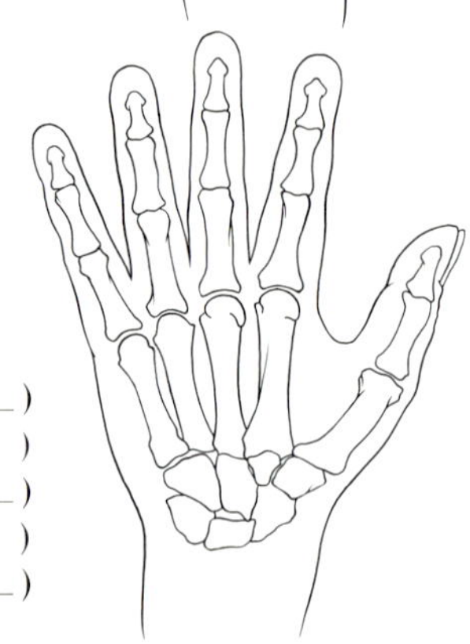

Measured in degrees

Thumb:

Abduction angle _____/_____ in degrees

Tip misses base V _____/_____ in mm

Joint measurements in degrees:

	Extension	Flexion	ROM	Difference in ROM
MP joint	_____/_____	_____/_____	_____/_____	_____/_____
IP joint	_____/_____	_____/_____	_____/_____	_____/_____
		AAROM	_____/_____	_____/_____

Finger:

Tips fail the following points in mm: (Note: normal = touch, abbreviated "T")

	SL	PP	MP	DP
Index:	_____/_____	_____/_____	_____/_____	_____/_____
Long:	_____/_____	_____/_____	_____/_____	_____/_____
Ring:	_____/_____	_____/_____	_____/_____	_____/_____
Little:	_____/_____	_____/_____	_____/_____	_____/_____

Joint measurements in degrees:

	Joint	Extension	Flexion	ROM	Difference in ROM
Index:	MP	_____/_____	_____/_____	_____/_____	_____/_____
	PIP	_____/_____	_____/_____	_____/_____	_____/_____
	DIP	_____/_____	_____/_____	_____/_____	_____/_____
			AAROM	_____/_____	_____/_____
Long:	MP	_____/_____	_____/_____	_____/_____	_____/_____
	PIP	_____/_____	_____/_____	_____/_____	_____/_____
	DIP	_____/_____	_____/_____	_____/_____	_____/_____
			AAROM	_____/_____	_____/_____
Ring:	MP	_____/_____	_____/_____	_____/_____	_____/_____
	PIP	_____/_____	_____/_____	_____/_____	_____/_____
	DIP	_____/_____	_____/_____	_____/_____	_____/_____
			AAROM	_____/_____	_____/_____
Little:	MP	_____/_____	_____/_____	_____/_____	_____/_____
	PIP	_____/_____	_____/_____	_____/_____	_____/_____
	DIP	_____/_____	_____/_____	_____/_____	_____/_____
			AAROM	_____/_____	_____/_____

Conclusion re impairment: Further treatment advised ____________________

(accepted) ____________________ (refused) ____________________

More time needed for improvement ____________________

Static and ratable ____________________

Factors of apportionment:

Preexisting condition ____________________%

Current condition ____________________%

The third paragraph should be entitled "Past History" and include all pertinent information concerning preexisting problems with the neck or upper extremities and with his health in general.

The fourth paragraph should be entitled "History" and give in detail the mechanisms and events surrounding the injury, integrating all sources of information. It should include the patient's specific complaints and distinguish new ones from preexisting ones.

The fifth paragraph is entitled "Examination" and must give a detailed account of all initial physical findings at the time of the first treatment for the injury. Included are the results of roentgenograms and laboratory work. Depending upon the nature of the case, this may or may not include pertinent measurements (Table 28-2**A**) taken as a baseline to document the existence or non-existence of functional impairment.

The sixth paragraph is entitled "Treatment and Course" and gives an account of the treatment measures initially undertaken and their results. Copies of operative reports and reports of special procedures (e.g. EMG) may be submitted as enclosures rather than in the body of the report. The amelioration or aggravation of the original condition or the development of new symptoms or objective problems should be described and the conclusions of any consultations or tests specified. Major changes in measurements (Table 28-2**A**) may be cited here.

The seventh and last paragraph should be entitled "Discussion" and contain any remarks or explanation about what was previously written, as well as an opinion about progress (satisfactory versus unsatisfactory) and prognosis.

Subsequent progress reports should follow a similar form. The introductory paragraph should repeat the previous one and add by name any additional diagnoses and significant surgical procedures and dates thereof. The second paragraph is entitled "Working Status" and summarizes when the patient stopped or started working or is expected to return to work. The third paragraph is entitled "Treatment and Course" and summarizes the subjective and objective status since the last report, giving details of tests, treatments and response to same. Such reports generally include in this paragraph the results of measurements (Table 28-2**B**) taken to determine existing impairment. These include circumferential measurements of the arm and forearm, grip-meter and pinch-meter readings and measurements of motion of joints affected by the patient's problem (see Examination and Measurements of Impairment in this chapter). The fourth paragraph is entitled "Discussion" and serves to elucidate the need for further treatment, problems in recovery, prognosis, and the time at which maximal recovery might be reached.

Final Reports (Table 28-3)

The condition of the patient should be considered static and ready for final evaluation of permanent impairment for disability rating purposes when all reasonable treatment has been rendered, and there is no sign of subjective or objective improvement in a period of 2 to 3 months. This assumes that there has been adequate motivation on the part of the patient, that he has applied the appropriate degree of physical effort to gain improvement, and that there have been adequate facilities for implementing his efforts. Such are the circumstances in most cases at the time of disability rating. The hand surgeon must be scrupulously fair to both patient and insurance company in assessing impairment. The concept *res ipsa loquitur* generally prevails.

The impairment should be judged primarily in relation to the patient's functional capacity at his occupation, not his avocations. This requires a careful analysis of the type of function required of a given hand for a given occupation. Relevant questions to appraise this include: how important is pinch? what special motions or activity are involved? how important is grip strength or unfatiguing repetitive muscular effort? is exposure to sun, heat or cold a problem? are there any known factors which precipitate pain?

The nature and degree of impairment cause disabilities of vastly different magnitude, depending on the character of functional demands on the hand. If a production line worker has been restored to full functional capacity, but can no longer play the guitar to his satisfaction and has no record of gainful guitar playing, then he has no residual impairment justifying disability. The loss of sensibility of the thumb and index finger in a mechanic is grounds for significant disability because he can no longer feel hidden nuts and bolts. Some artisans are affected by impairment in peculiar and less obvious ways. For instance, a dentist lacking the superficialis tendon to his dominant ring finger is handicapped by the loss of "independent" flexion of that digit. He cannot effectively hold a tool, the tip of which he must manipulate with his radial digits.

Two circumstances warrant rating and settlement before maximum treatment has taken place and maximum recovery achieved: (1) the patient refuses further treatment, (2) the patient desires a settlement with the intention of seeking further treatment as symptoms and objective impairment require at some undetermined future time. Under such circumstances, the settlement can allow for further treatment by keeping the claim file open with an actuarial reserve on the case, or, by giving

Table 28-3 *Follow-up Progress Reports (also Final Report of Impairment)**

REFERENCE:

Patient's name, employer, date of injury, claim #

PARAGRAPH 1:

Introduction (Recapitulation of "Introduction" on previous reports, adding any further diagnoses and major surgical procedures by date)

PARAGRAPH 2:

Working Status (recapitulation of "Working Status on previous reports, and any new changes reported)

PARAGRAPH 3:

Treatment and Course (subjective and objective status since last report with details of any new treatments, tests and results thereof. Includes pertinent measurements of sensibility, atrophy, loss of length, grip, pinch and motion)

PARAGRAPH 4:

Discussion (prognosis, needs for further treatment, rebuttal or comment on other opinions, answers to questions asked, estimate when maximal treatment will be reached, potential factors of impairment when maximum recovery is reached)

*The form for the Final Report of Impairment, when made by the treating physician, varies only as to "Discussion." Here all factors of impairment must be discussed. When such a report is made by a physician consultant seeing the patient for the first time, paragraph 3 would be "History, Treatment, and Course" and include current complaints, paragraph 4 would be "Examination" and include measurements (Fig. 28-2B), and paragraph 5 would be "Discussion."

the patient an amount estimated to cover all his potential future medical needs, it can close out the insurance claim.

The "Final Report of Impairment for Purposes of Disability Rating" should be prepared in the same form as the "Follow-up Reports" of the status of progress (Table 28-3), providing the patient has been under continuous treatment by the physician making the final report. If, however, the physician making the final report is seeing the patient for the first time, then the report should be more like the "First Detailed Formal Report of Injury" (Table 28-2**A**).

In the first instance, the only difference from previous "Follow-up Reports" which the treating physician has submitted would be his "Discussion" which would contain a summation of factors relating to permanent impairment. This would include estimates of subjective and objective impairment, such as the per cent of impairment of given digits calculated from Tables 28-4, -5, and -6, need for further treatment, and capacity to work.

In the second instance, where the examiner is seeing the patient for the first time, the "History" and "Treatment and Course" (including current complaints) are all combined in one paragraph before "Examination," and the "Discussion" includes any rebuttal or confirmation of other opinions gleaned from the medical records, as well as a summation of the factors relating to permanent impairment.

Four specific factors dealing with impairment to be considered in the patient's final disability rating must be covered by the physician's summation under "Discussion" in this final report. These consist of:

1. *Subjective Factors:* This should state "none," or, when present, should specify the magnitude of any pain or sensory loss. Included here would be any mention of limited endurance or loss of dexterity.
2. *Objective Factors:* Here the factors of impairment taken from Table 28-4, including their magnitude, are cited. They include amputation, atrophy, loss of grip and pinch, limitation of active motion of any parts (including ankylosis) and the per cent of impairment of any digit (Table 28-6).
3. *Treatment:* This should indicate the treatment which is still, or might reasonably be, needed, specified as to type, duration and, where indicated, cost (e.g. replacement of a prosthesis). If it includes the possibility of surgery, details, length of hospitalization, need for help by other medical (e.g. anesthesiologists) or paramedical (e.g. physiotherapists) personnel, and duration of subsequent temporary disability should all be specified, including an estimate of prognosis.
4. *Capacity for Work:* This part of the report should clarify the patient's capacity or his limitations in performing his usual occupation. If he has a limitation it should be expressed in the following terms and the per cent of impairment indicated:

Minimal—merely annoying (0 to 25 per cent)
Slight—interferes with some activity (25 to 50 per cent)
Moderate—prevents some activity (50 to 75 per cent)
Severe—prevents most or all activity (75 to 100 per cent)

Table 28-4. *Chart for Recording Results of Evaluation*

Date: ______________ Name: ______________________ Age: ____
Sex: ____

Occupation: ______________ Working: Yes ____ No ____ Major hand: ________

Preexisting functional problem: Yes ____ No ____ Side: Right ____ Left ____

Present problem:

Nature: ________________________________

Complex: Yes ____ No ____

Location(s): ________________________________

Status: Untreated: ________ Under treatment: ________ Status p̄ treatment: ________
Nature of treatment: Surgical ______ Medical ______ P.T. ______

Checklist of problems:

____1. Communication barrier
____2. General health
____3. Overall neuromuscular function
____4. Overall skeletal function

____5. Head
____6. Neck
____7. Shoulders
____8. Arms
____9. Elbows
____10. Forearms
____11. Wrists

____12. Hands
____13. Thumbs
____14. Fingers (II, III, IV, V)

____15. Deformity
____16. Tumor
____17. Atrophy

____18. Color
____19. Temperature
____20. Pulses
____21. Sweat

____22. Skin
____23. Wound
____24. Amputation
____25. Loss of substance
____26. Fingertip

____27. Nail
____28. Scar
____29. Contracture

____30. Synovium
____31. Ligament
____32. Joint
____33. Bone
____34. Muscle
____35. Tendon
____36. Tendon sheath

____33. Nerve (M,U,R)
____38. Pain (magnitude)
____39. Tenderness
____40. Anesthesia
____two-point
____pick up
____41. Motor loss

____42. Stiffness
____43. Loss of endurance or dexterity

____44. Irresponsible
____45. Poor motivation
____46. Low pain thresh-hold
____47. Psychosis
____488 Malingering
____49. Positive roent-genogram
____50. Positive lab test

Comments:

Table 28-5. *The Point System for Assessment of Digital Movement Function*

THUMB	1 POINT	2 POINTS	3 POINTS	POINTS AWARDED
A. Angle of maximum abduction between thumb and index digits (normal 85 to 90°)	30°–50°	50°–70°	70°–90°	
B. Distance tip of trimmed thumbnail fails to touch base of V in mm (normal = touch [zero mm])	38 mm–64 mm	12 mm–38 mm	12 mm or less	
C. Aggregate active range of motion of proximal (MP) and distal (IP) joints (normal 120 to 220°)	25°–50°	50°–100°	100°–220°	
			Total points for thumb	
FINGER				
A. Limitation of active extension. (Distance in mm tip of trimmed nail fails to touch the plane of the dorsum of the hand (normal = 0 mm = touch)	25 mm–50 mm	12 mm–25 mm	<12 mm	
B. Limitation of active flexion. (Distance in mm tip of distal fat pad fails to touch mid palmar crease.) (normal = 0 mm = touch)	25 mm–50 mm	12 mm–25 mm	<12 mm	
C. Aggregate active range of motion of proximal (MP), middle (PIP), and distal (DIP) joints (normal = 235 to 300°)	150°–175°	175°–250°	>250°	
			Total points for finger	

It is often necessary to add to this some explanation of what the physician feels the patient might be able to do, and whether or not rehabilitation should be undertaken. If so, its nature should be specified.

Examination and Measurements of Impairment

The examination for impairment will be thorough if it is systematized. The injured side is always compared with the uninjured side and recorded first (e.g. left-injured/right-uninjured). If both hands are injured, the dominant side is recorded first (e.g. right (major) injured/left (minor) injured). The following examination sequence is efficient and complete for evaluation and comparison of both upper extremities.

1. *Overall Survey:* As an organ of prehension and sensibility, the hand and its sensory function may be critically influenced by disorders of the skeletal and neuromuscular elements proximal to the hand (e.g. about the elbow, shoulder and neck). Furthermore, a hand problem may be secondary to, or a reflection of, a disorder which is more apparent elsewhere. For example, the patient with lower limb disability may be using crutches incorrectly

and acquire a crutch palsy of his radial, ulnar or median nerves by compression in the axilla or the heel of the hand. Likewise, advanced arthritis elsewhere may be the needed clue to a problem related to early arthritis in the hand. Therefore, the overall musculoskeletal function of the total patient must be surveyed and related to any problem that is about to be studied in the upper extremity.

Particular attention is paid to competence of motion of the head and neck and both upper extremities as the patient removes his jacket, shirt and jewelry and is then asked to reach for the ceiling and open and close both fists. Dexterity, awkwardness, weakness and evidence of pain are carefully noted.

2. *Study of Entire Upper Extremity:* Specific attention is paid to anatomical stance and skeletal alignment, color of skin and nail beds, pulses, temperature and the presence of sweat. The adequacy of fat padding and skin cover, the existence and character of any scars and the presence of any consistently painful area are noted.

Pain is considered genuine when the patient consistently withdraws the part after the same magnitude of painful stimulus (e.g. percussion, pressure or stretch) is applied. The amount of pain should be estimated as 1+ (minimal), 2+ (slight), 3+ (moderate) or 4+ (severe). These levels of magnitude are defined for purposes of functional impairment as follows: minimal (0 to 25 per cent of impairment)—is merely annoying, slight (25 to 50 per cent of impairment)—interferes with some activity, moderate (50 to 75 per cent of impairment)—prevents some activity, severe (75 to 100 per cent of impairment)—prevents most or all activity.

When pain is present, its nature, focus, distribution and cause should be identified. The examiner should, if possible, diagnose such conditions as a painful desmitis, synovitis, arthritis or scar, painful neuroma, nerve compression syndrome, sympathetic dystrophy, causalgia, etc. (Chap. 27).

3. Sensibility is tested by pinprick (Chap. 3). When a deficit exists, it should be quantitated on the volar aspect of digits by the test for two-point discrimination (Weber's test). This is expressed as the minimum distance apart in millimeters that the blindfolded patient can determine simultaneous stimulation by two ends of a paper clip.

The normal range on the volar skin of the digits is 2 to 4 mm. When the distance is 20 mm or more, it is equivalent to complete loss of tactile gnosis, even though protective sensibility is still intact. Sensory loss on the dorsum is not usually considered disabling.

If the median nerve is involved in sensory loss, an additional test, evaluating capacity and accuracy in picking up and identifying different sized common coins without looking, should be done.

Malingering is manifested by a claim of anesthesia in the presence of normal sweating and by appreciable inconsistencies in patterns of sensory distribution and claims of abnormality of response to careful testing.

Palmar sensibility is valued at 50 per cent of the functional capacity of the hand. Full loss is equal to 50 per cent of the value of amputation. The sides of loss of a digit are functionally different in value, the sides meeting between thumb and fingers in pinch being higher. The values set for the various digits are seen in Figure 28-1, and are a percentage of total hand function.

Table 28-6. *Conversion Table of Points for Digital Motion to Percentage of Normal Motion Retained and Lost and Per Cent Impairment of the Digit*

POINTS AWARDED FOR MOTION	PER CENT OF NORMAL MOTION RETAINED	PER CENT OF NORMAL MOTION LOST	PER CENT IMPAIRMENT OF DIGIT*
0	0	100	90
1	10	90	81
2	20	80	72
3	30	70	63
4	40	60	54
5	50	50	45
6	60	40	36
7	70	30	27
8	80	20	18
9	90–100	0–10	0–9

*By reference of these values to Figure 28-2, per cent impairment of the whole hand, whole extremity or whole man can be calculated.

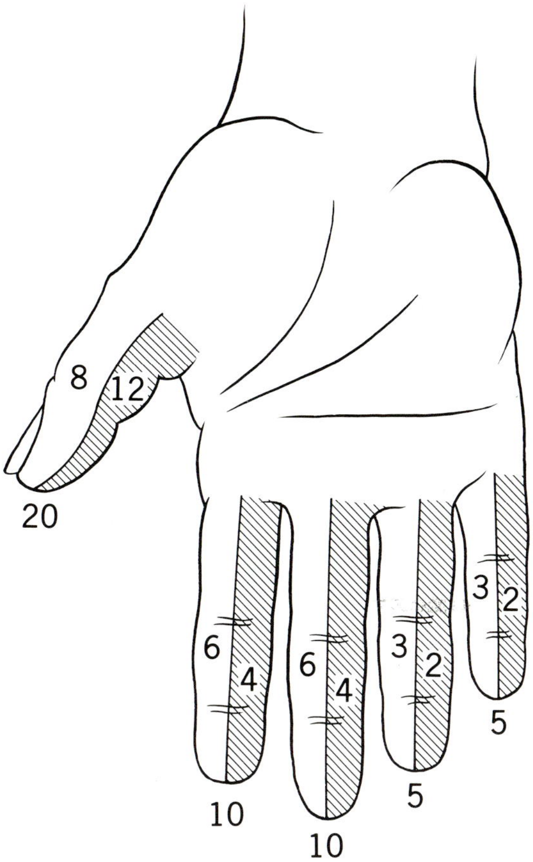

Figure 28-1. *Values of percentage impairment to the whole hand by complete loss of sensibility about the volar aspect of the digits are indicated opposite the tips of the digits. Comparative values of radial and ulnar sides are also indicated. Note that values for sensory loss are 50 per cent that for loss by amputation.*

4. The components of various muscle groups are systematically tested for function and power (Chaps. 2, 3). There are six categories of strength, defined as follows:
   a. Normal—complete active range of motion against full resistance
   b. Good (5 to 25 per cent impairment of strength)—full active range of motion against gravity and limited resistance
   c. Fair (25 to 50 per cent impairment of strength)—full active range of motion against gravity but not with added resistance
   d. Poor (50 to 75 per cent impairment of strength)—full active range of motion only when gravity is eliminated.
   e. Trace (75 to 99 per cent impairment of strength)—a trace of muscle contraction but no joint motion
   f. Zero—no muscle contractility at all
5. Joints are tested for stability, crepitation, and pain by manipulation. They are also tested in all planes (including spreading and adducting the digits) for active and passive range of motion, both of which should be equal. Significant enlargement is documented as a circumferential measurement in centimeters of the injured joint compared with the corresponding uninjured joint of the opposite extremity. Ankylosis and extensor or flexion contractures and lateral and torque deviations are noted.
6. Atrophy is noted as existing or not existing, and is documented by appropriate measurement. As a rule, this is limited to circumferential measurements in centimeters over muscle wads of the arm and forearm at a consistent distance from the lateral epicondyle (e.g. 10 cm proximal and distal thereto in the average adult male). The dominant arm and forearm tends to be larger than the nondominant, and certainly is not normally the smaller of the two.
7. Grip and pinch strength are recorded for three successive squeezes of grip and pinch dynamometers by each hand. The values obtained by a cooperative patient, exerting maximum power, should not vary more than 20 per cent at any given period of testing. However, a number of factors reduce the values obtained by these tests: faulty equipment, failure of the patient to hold the device properly, pain, fatigue and intentional withholding. Hence, the values obtained at different times should be compared whenever possible.
8. The level of any amputation must be accurately described and measured. The loss is most clearly conveyed in diagram form (Fig. 28-2). The amputation is described as transverse or oblique, and the obliquity is specified as dorsal, volar, radial or ulnar. If bone is involved, the precise level is determined at surgery or by roentgenography. The level of amputation of a digital ray should be specified as to tuft of the distal phalanx or the head, neck, midshaft or base of a given bone, or a given joint. The length lost is accurately determined by matching creases of the injured and uninjured hands and digits palm-to-palm or side-to-side and measuring the length of the missing part in centimeters. Impairment caused by the amputation can then be estimated.

For purposes of rating impairment, any loss by amputation is related to the percentage of functional value assigned the normal part (Fig. 28-2). The entire upper extremity has a 60 per cent functional value of the whole man, and 90 per cent of that value (54 per cent of the whole man) is assigned to the function of the five intact digits of a hand. This means that amputation of the five digits of one hand through their metacarpophalangeal joints results in a 54 per cent impairment of the whole man and 100 per cent impairment of the hand. The two phalanges of the thumb have a 40 per cent value of the whole hand and a 22 per cent value of the whole man. The three phalanges

LEVEL	a. % whole man	b. % whole upper extremity	c. % whole hand	d. % whole digit
A (Shoulder)	60	100	—	—
B (Elbow)	57	95	—	—
C (MP joint)				
All digits	54	90	100	—
Thumb	21.6	36	40	100
Index or long	10.8	18	20	100
Ring or little	5.4	9	10	100
D (PIP joint)				
Thumb	10.8	18	20	50
Index or long	8.6	14.4	16	80
Ring or little	4.3	7.2	8	80
E (DIP joint)				
Index or long	4.9	8.1	9	45
Ring or little	2.4	4	4.5	45

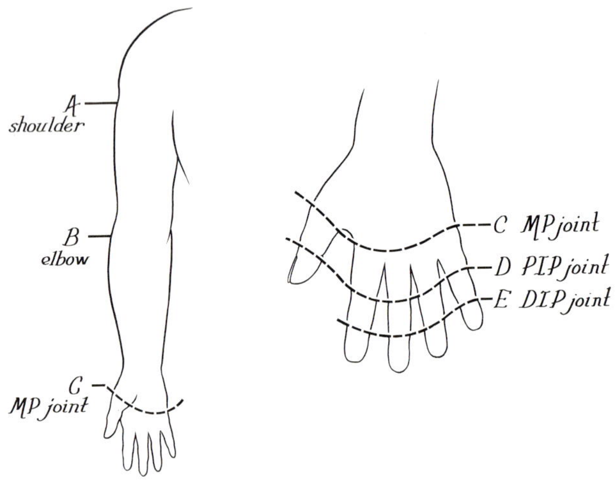

Figure 28-2. *Scale of functional values of parts of the upper extremity. These are the same as the impairment values that result from amputation. The values are expressed in per cent to (a) the whole man, (b) the whole upper extremity, (c) the whole hand and (d) the whole digit. Five amputation levels determine the per cent impairment: (A) shoulder, (B) elbow, (C) MP joint, (D) PIP joint and (E) DIP joint.*

of each index and long finger have a 20 per cent value of the whole hand and an 11 per cent value of the whole man. The three phalanges of each ring and little finger have a 10 per cent value of the whole hand and a 5 per cent value of the whole man.

9. The last objective evaluation is the determination of range of motion of the multiple joints from head and neck to the distal interphalangeal joints.
   a. *Head and Neck:* Motions are estimated as a per cent of normal. The motions observed are extension (chin up), flexion (chin to sternum), lateral bending to the right and left (ear to shoulder), rotation to the right and left.
   b. *Shoulders:* The base position from which the various motions in the anterior-posterior and lateral planes are measured is with the arm against the lateral wall of the trunk. The measurements are then made between the two radii consisting of the lateral wall of the trunk and the arm to get the angle after motion (range of motion) of any given movement. For abduction, the arm is carried laterally away from the trunk and overhead (normally 150 to 180°). For adduction, it is carried across the front of the trunk (normally 30°). The abduction-adduction range of motion is 180 to 210°.

      For forward flexion, the arm is carried forward of the trunk and overhead (normally 150°). For extension, it is carried backward of the trunk (normally 40°). The forward-backward range of motion is 190°.

      The base position for measurement of external and internal rotation is with the elbow flexed to a right angle and, if possible, the arm abducted 90°. The starting and ending positions of the forearm become the two radii for measuring the angle after motion (range of motion). For external rotation, the forearm is carried from horizontal to vertical and the angle from the starting point measured (normally 90°). For the internal rotation, the forearm is dropped from the horizontal and the angle from the starting point measured (normally 40°). The range of motion is 130°.

c. *Elbows:* Extension and flexion are recorded. The base position for taking the measurement is elbow extension. Normally this is a straight line (180° between humerus and forearm). In full flexion, the angle is normally 30 to 40°. The range of motion is normally 140 to 150°.

d. *Forearms:* Pronation and supination are the motions measured against a neutral base position in which the elbows are flexed to 90° and held against the lateral trunk wall, and the radial styloid is up. Each motion is normally through an arc of 70 to 90°, and the forearm rotation range of motion (degrees of supination added to pronation) is 140 to 180°. If stiffness prevents the assumption of the neutral position, the stance will reflect a lack of supination and pronation. This is then recorded in "minus degrees" for the deficit motion. Thus, a forearm in supination and failing the neutral position by 20°, but supinating 70°, would measure: supination −70°, pronation −20°, and range of motion −50°.

e. *Wrists:* The motions measured are extension, flexion, ulnar deviation and radial deviation against a neutral position in which the dorsum of the hand is level with the forearm and metacarpal III is aligned with the radius. The goniometer readings are made with radii consisting of metacarpal III and the radius; the patient may hold his elbows in 90° of flexion against the lateral walls of his trunk or may have his hands and forearms against a flat surface during the measurements.

Normally, extension and flexion are through an arc of 70 to 90°, for an extension-flexion range of motion of 140 to 180°. The arc of ulnar deviation is 30 to 40° and of radial deviation 20 to 30°, for an ulnar-radial range of motion of 50 to 70°. Failure to reach the neutral position should be expressed in minus degrees of a given motion as previously described under forearm motion, and then the range of motion in said plane of movement calculated by adding the positive (+) and negative (−) values.

f. *Digits:* Loss of active digital motion is assessed by three separate measurements for each digit and the result is computed as a percentage loss. The plane of movement assessed for fingers is simply that of extension-flexion. In the case of the thumb, the prime movement function is opposition (pronation), which is considered 60 per cent of its overall movement value. Therefore, for the thumb, rotation as well as extension and flexion must be assessed.

The composite assessment of each digit is simplified by using a point system (Table 28-6). The data base for this system is taken from the evaluation measurements (Fig. 28-2). The total number of points awarded any given digit becomes a measure of its overall movement function. The total will range from zero to 9, zero being equivalent to 100 per cent loss of movement function. Each point has a value of 10 per cent. A value of 9 points is equivalent to 90 to 100 per cent normal function. Thus, the conversion from points to percentage of retained and lost movement function is rapid (Table 28-6).

The functional value assigned to total digital movement is only 90 per cent of the overall functional value of the digit. Total ankylosis is therefore only 90 per cent of the value of amputation of the digit through the metacarpophalangeal joint (Fig. 28-2). The interpolation of per cent of normal motion lost into per cent impairment of the digit is found in the fourth column of Table 28-6.

g. *Thumbs:* The active motions to observe and measure for each thumb are the following:

1) The angle of maximum abduction between thumb and index digits
2) The distance the tip of the trimmed thumb nail fails to touch the distal fat pad of the palm over the base of the proximal phalanx of the little finger
3) The angles of extension and flexion of the metacarpophalangeal (MP) and interphalangeal (IP) joints. The range of motion (ROM) of each joint is then calculated and the difference between the two thumbs shown. Finally, the aggregate active range of motion (AAROM) of both joints is added up for use in computing the impairment of motion by the point system (Tables 28-4, -5, and -6).

The abduction angle, which is normally 85 to 90°, is measured by placing the limb of the goniometer in alignment with the phalanges of the index finger and thumb when the thumb web is spread maximally as the thumb moves volarly, perpendicular to the plane of the palm.

The second measurement is made with maximal adduction and flexion of the thumb and pronation of the ulnar border of the hand. Normally, this measurement is 0 mm, signifying that the tip of the thumbnail touches the base of the little finger.

The third measurement consists of goniometric readings of the MP and IP joints in full extension and flexion. When either joint is at a straight line, the reading is 180°, from which degrees are added for the amount of hyperextension and subtracted for the degrees of flexion. Normally there is great variation in motion of these joints. From a straight line (180°), flexion may bring either joint to an angle ranging from 165 to 90°. Hyperextension of either joint may produce angles up to 220°, signifying a range of hyperextension of 40° (the difference between 180 and 220°).

Calculations of range of motion (ROM) of each joint are necessary to determine the amount of movement that exists. This is made by taking the difference between the angle of maximal active extension (e.g. 180°) and the angle of maximal active flexion (e.g. 120°), which in this hypothetical case would be a ROM of 60°. The ROM of joints of the injured thumb are then compared with those for the uninjured thumb, and the difference recorded as a plus or minus value for the injured thumb. The aggregate active range of motion (AAROM) is the addition of the values of the ROM for both the MP and IP joints.

An example of how to record such measurements in the case of an injured left (minor) thumb with stiffness follows:

Thumb measurements (left minor injured/right major uninjured):

Abduction angle: 60°/90° (−30° on the left)

Tip of the thumbnail fails base of the little finger (V): 20 mm/touch

Thumb:	Extension	Flexion	Range	Difference in ROM
MP joint	160°/180°	160°/120°	0°/60°	−60° left
IP joint	190°/210°	150°/90°	40°/100°	−60° left
		AAROM	40°/160°	−120° left

Points awarded for assessment of active motion (Table 28-5): A—2, B—2, C—1

Total—5 (signifies 50 per cent normal movement function retained and 50 per cent lost)

Per cent impairment of thumb—45 per cent

h. *Fingers:* Two series of measurements are made bilaterally to document extension and flexion of the finger joints. The first is the distance in mm by which the tips of the fingers fail to reach the straight-line plane of the back of the hand (SL) in extension and the proximal palm (PP), midpalm (MP) and distal palm (DP) in flexion. When the tips reach these points they may be recorded as "touch."

The second series is the measurement of angles formed by the joints at extremes of extension and flexion. From this the range of motion (ROM) and the difference in ROM between the injured and uninjured hands to highlight the loss can be calculated.

Finally, the aggregate active range of motion (AAROM) of the fingers is calculated. The point system of assessment (Table 28-5) and percentage conversion for functional impairment (Table 28-6) can then be executed.

Normally, the metacarpophalangeal (MP) joint of any finger extends to 180° (a straight line) and flexes to angles varying between 100 and 90°, for a ROM of 80 to 90°. The proximal interphalangeal (DIP) joint extends to 180° and flexes to angles varying between 80 and 75°, for a ROM of 100 to 105°. The distal interphalangeal (DIP) joint extends to 180° and flexes to angles varying between 120 and 90°, for a ROM of 60 to 90°.

The following is an example of recording measurements in the case of an injury to the right (major) hand causing stiffness in all four proximal interphalangeal joints:

Finger measurements (right major injured/left minor uninjured)

The tips of the fingers fail the following points in mm:

	SL	PP	MP	DP
Index	10/touch	5/touch	15/touch	25/touch
Long	10/touch	5/touch	15/touch	25/touch
Ring	10/touch	5/touch	15/touch	25/touch
Little	10/touch	5/touch	15/touch	25/touch

Joint measurements in degrees:

	Joint	Extension	Flexion	ROM	Difference in ROM
Index:	MP	180/180	100/100	80/80	0
	PIP	160/180	110/75	50/105	−55 right
	DIP	180/180	135/100	45/80	−35 right
			AAROM	175/262	−90 right
Long:	MP	180/180	100/100	80/80	0
	PIP	160/180	120/75	40/105	−65 right
	DIP	180/180	125/100	55/80	−25 right
			AAROM	175/265	−90 right
Ring:	MP	180/180	100/100	80/80	0
	PIP	160/180	110/80	50/100	−50 right
	DIP	180/180	130/95	50/85	−35 right
			AAROM	180/265	−85 right
Little:	MP	180/180	100/100	80/80	0
	PIP	160/180	110/75	50/105	−55 right
	DIP	180/180	135/100	45/80	−35 right
			AAROM	175/265	−90 right

Points awarded for assessment of active motion (Table 28-5).

	Points A	B	C	Total	% Motion retained	% Motion lost	% Impairment of the digits
Index:	3	2	2	7	70	30	27
Long:	3	2	2	7	70	30	27
Ring:	3	2	2	7	70	30	27
Little:	3	2	2	7	70	30	27

Per cent motion retained and lost and per cent impairment of the digits (Table 28-6).

Estimation (Rating) of Impairment

The physician's role in establishing that there is permanent disability is the determination of impairment, that is, the existence and the extent of functional abnormality or loss about the upper extremity. The functional value of the hand is 90 per cent that of the entire upper extremity. The functional value of the upper extremity is 60 per cent that of the whole man. Impairment is considered permanent when maximal treatment has been rendered and maximal recovery and functional rehabilitation have been achieved.

As described in the section on Examination and Measurement of Impairment, relatively accurate objective and subjective determinations can be made, particularly when results of examinations are consistent. The functional abnormality or loss caused by injury or disease may be limited to one or more loci of the upper extremity, or it may be widespread. As indicated in Figures 28-1 and 28-2, the functional value assigned the various parts of the upper extremity vary. The orderly appraisal of function and completion of Table 28-4 gives the basis for computing impairment. When multiple impairments exist there must be an additive calculation which usually involves starting with the smaller parts (e.g. digits) first and working up to the whole upper extremity, both upper extremities, and the whole man.

By referring to the tables given in the American Medical Association's *Guides to the Evaluation of Permanent Impairment*[2], the recommended percentage values assigned specific functional impairments can be determined. There are tables of percentage impairment for amputation, loss of motion, ankylosis, pain, sensory deficit and loss of strength. The tables specify the percentage impairment of a given anatomical unit of the upper extremity (e.g. thumb, finger or hand), and they give conversion figures of that unit value to the percentage impairment of the whole upper extremity and the whole man.

When two or more objective or subjective impairments of a given anatomical unit exist, it is necessary to "combine" the values of the multiple impairments (e.g. partial amputation + sensory deficit of the tumb) by use of the last table in the text called the Combined Values Chart. On this chart, the higher of any two impairment values is located on the vertical coordinate and the lower on the horizontal and vertical columns. This value, in turn, is plotted against a third to calculate the combined value of three separate impairment values. Such a chain of calculations can be repeated indefinitely, and the ultimate value then represents the combination (total impairment) expressed in percentage.

When there is impairment of multiple anatomical units and multiple functions (e.g. amputation of multiple digits, loss of motion in multiple areas of the extremity, loss of strength and sensory deficits), the overall percentage impairment of the whole upper extremity or the whole man is determined. The combined percentage impairment of each unit (starting with the smallest unit) is determined first, and then the impairment to the whole upper extremity and whole man is calculated. Impairment of the whole man must be calculated whenever a given injury has caused impairment of both upper extremities.

The method of combining the multiple impairments into a common denominator, using the Combined Values Chart, is based on the concept that each successive impairment acts on that part of function that remains *after* that preceding impairment has acted. The order and chronology of the computations in combining impairments are immaterial. The ultimate common denominator impairment value, be it derived from just one or multiple impairments, is expressed as the nearest 5 per cent.

References

1. Boyes, J.H.: Evaluation of the results of digital flexor tendon grafts. Am. J. Surg., 89:1116, 1955.
2. *Guides to the Evaluation of Permanent Impairment.* American Medical Association, Chicago, 1971.
3. McBride, E.D.: *Disability Evaluation,* 6th ed. J.B. Lippincott, Philadelphia, 1963.
4. Moberg, E.: Objective methods for determining the functional value of sensibility of the hand. J. Bone Joint Surg., 40B:454, 1958.
5. Slocum, D.B. and Pratt, D.R.: Disability evaluation for the hand. J. Bone Joint Surg., 28:491, 1946.
6. Smith, W.C.: *Principles of Disability Evaluation.* J.B. Lippincott, Philadelphia, 1959.
7. Swanson, A.B.: Evaluation of impairment of function of the hand. Surg. Clin. North Am., 44:925, 1964.

29 Psychosocial Aspects of Hand Disabilities

Historically it has been stated many times that what separates man from other animals is his intelligence, his brains. Nevertheless, Charles Sherrington[21] wrote ". . . all man can do is to move things and his muscular contraction is his sole means thereto." Ivan Mikhaflovich Schenov[20] stated ". . . All the endless diversity of the external manifestations of the activity of the brain can be finally regarded as one phenomenon—that of muscular movement." Both authors seem to stress that in carrying man's will the brain's main function is to subserve movement. Although the brain has been generally credited for all of man's achievements, it has not been sufficiently recognized that without his hands he would have achieved nothing. Although other body parts have muscles and as a result move, no organ in the body has the capacity for motion that the hands have, and this makes man as dependent upon his hands as upon his brain.

The hands have a number of discrete structures which underlie their potential for movement and thereby their functional value. They can execute a number of basic patterned motions facilitated by their many bones, some of which are almost universal joints, moved by numerous muscles, some of which are small and yet powerful. Based on exquisite combination and coordination—through the brain—of those basic motions, the hands can execute an infinite variety of actions. It is this capacity for highly versatile and skilled movements which makes the hands in many ways unique. To perform movement, they require a large representation in the brain, to the extent that the representational cortical portion for the hands is almost equal to the total area for the body, legs and remaining portions of the arms.[22] The individual does not have to learn or be conscious of the thousands of possible variations of motions performed, since the brain is programmed to see that they are carried out from beginning to end with remarkable ease. The person can automatically and often without conscious awareness of intermediary or even final steps carry out his intended goals with a surprising degree of accuracy. Although other portions of the arms—i.e. upper arms, elbows and forearms, shoulders—participate in the execution of hand actions, they only subserve the latter functions. Although other body parts such as the feet may or may not have movements which facilitate man's goals and purposes, the hands as a rule are the ultimate executors of his intentions.

From the above it can be readily recognized that man's adaptability is markedly dependent on the hand's capacity to perform an infinite number of tasks. Here we are referring to the most important aspects of the hand, its generalized[3] quality, its use for carrying out many possible things. Campbell[3] believes that such capacity phylogenetically enhanced the development of perception and locomotion in primates, including man. Furthermore, the evolutionary lengthening and strengthening of the thumb permitted early man to carry food and weapons, which increased his potential for survival. Man has achieved because of his ability to reach, grasp and examine objects. These capacities are heightened and supplemented by man either availing himself of tools or manufacturing them. A probe, a stick or a cane is used as an extension of the hands as sense organs to enhance man's perception of the world around him. Other tools such as a stone, a pen or a crowbar are used as effector organs, executing man's intentions and thereby aiding and extending the hand's functions beyond its inherent capacities. The function as effector organs also enhances the function as organs of perception, in that man learns through execution. By obtaining through his senses feedback of his actions and performance he can monitor them, increasing his chances of attaining his goals and thereby becoming a more effective master of his environment. The hands function as sense organs through touch and proprioception and in particular through stereognosis. Physiologically, the primary function of touch is to register contacts and collisions,[2] while movements and position sense are continuously monitored through proprioception; length, shape and texture are sensed through stereognosis.

Specialized organs of touch exist close to the surface of the skin. They are most numerous on the fingertips, palms of the hands and soles of the feet, the back of the hands and the tip of the tongue. The minimum two-point discrimination is 32 mm on the back of the hand, 11 mm on the palm of the hand and only 2 mm on the fingertips.[2] Since the fingertips are most discriminative, they play an important role not only in touch but also in stereognosis. However, these modalities fatigue quite rapidly and thus, in sensing an object, the individual automatically feels with different fingertips, alternating them. As one fingertip becomes fatigued the next becomes more sensitive. It may therefore be concluded that the individual needs all or almost all of his fingertips if he is to maintain a normal degree of perception through his hands.

The hands execute many actions which free vision, which in turn is used to obtain and monitor information from distant objects and events which are not accessible to touch and close examination.[15] Emphasizing the importance of the hand in the organization of man's perceptual world, Piaget[18] concluded that the infant child comes to comprehend his environment by integrating all sensory modalities through the use of the grasp of his hands. Harlow's[11] research demonstrated the importance of touch in the emotional and physical development of infant monkeys. Through touch the animals had a greater sense of security and were able to thrive. It is quite likely that for the normal development of the human infant, particularly in learning to master his environment, the hands, through touch, play at least as important a role.

The hands serve a major role in communication, both for reception and for transmission of messages. After the face, the hands are the most important instrument in these functions.[7] In a newborn infant hand touch is possibly the earliest sense to become functional. As he grows he develops a whole set of motions or gestures by which to communicate. Those are later progressively replaced by words, though never completely, as they come to play a significant part in body language, i.e. non-verbal communication. Hand motions are used as postural kinesic markers during speaking and they may precede, accompany or follow speech.[19] Often such motions are the only messages sent as representational language. Gestures which are symbolic of emotions, events or ideas are used to replace or to substitute for emotions, acts and ideas which have expressive meaning. The emotions most commonly expressed through various gestures readily interpreted are anxiety, fear, anger and warmth.[4,8]

Examples of the expressive and social use of the hands in non-verbal communication are the tactile exchanges that occur in greeting (hand shaking), pointing (guiding and directing), expressing emphasis (striking one's open hand with the other) and demonstrating affection and support (embracing, stroking). It has been reported[1] that when the hands are used in therapeutic fashion, by touching, the patient becomes more verbally communicative and more receptive to the staff. Thus it is clear that hand disabilities may impair a person's capacities to interrelate and non-verbally communicate with others, and thereby foster a degree of social isolation.

The face and hands are the only body parts which are customarily exposed to the eyes of the observer. They are thus an important part of man's body image and self concept. Generally, they are considered organs of personal and interpersonal communication and are viewed as expression and representation of the self in social situations, and as such they have social and esthetic value.

Hands give many meaningful cues in presentational communication—such as the appearance of the hands, their positional presentation, the modes and purpose of their use, their relevance and propriety to speech content and the like. Given the high social value placed on youthfulness and vigor, and on appearance and performance in particular, an impairment in any of these areas caused by a hand disability will be treated by society with a considerable degree of intolerance. Often a negative social response is manifested by magnifying an individual's disability and extending it to other areas of his body, to his personal life and in particular to his character and personality, attributing shortcomings or imperfections which he does not have.[10] He may be treated as more disabled, dysfunctional and different than he really is. In sum, he is stigmatized.

In stigmatizing an individual society implicitly expects him not to display his disabilities, to keep out of sight and in his own place. Attempts to mingle are viewed as intrusions into society's territory and privacy. The individual is viewed as entitled to social intercourse only with those similar to himself. Society's feelings are often those of pity, fear and anger. The foregoing might be a possible explanation of why many private and public buildings have physical barriers which impede or make difficult the entrance of persons with severe ambulatory disabilities.

Because a disability of the hand is an individual matter, the afflicted person may view it as a personal and purely private affair. However, its visibility and his being a social animal make it also a public matter, a fact that many patients refute, resent or attempt to deny. An individual cannot help but be cognizant of the responses and cues that those about him knowingly and unknowingly exhibit as they encounter him, and experiences those responses as unfair incursions into his personal life. Even though initially he may reject or deny those incursions and may not view himself as different or impaired, if he is to advance toward a satisfactory adjustment he must contend with the social realities in which he lives, altered because of his disability.

One of those changed realities is that not only has he lost some control over hand movement and his physical environment but also he has lost some control over his social milieu. His privacy can be interfered with at any time and whenever others wish—not only friends and acquaintances but also strangers who, by staring and acting condescendingly, impose their feelings and attitudes upon him by reminding him of his disabilities and differences. As a consequence, the afflicted person may experience helplessness to alter those responses. This is true particularly when he is unsure of the impression he makes. In social situations a person with a hand disability is often uncertain as to the responses he will receive, even when there are indications they will be favorable. Therefore, even under the most auspicious conditions, his attitude is often one of apprehension and fear of rejection; in extreme cases he fails to assert himself and his performance is either severely impaired or inhibited.

Reactions of a person to the attitudes of others will elicit in them new responses. Timidity, submissiveness or fear will produce condescension, whereas arrogance and pseudosecurity will elicit contempt. However, displaying trust in oneself in a forceful and assertive fashion according to the needs of situations, although initially possibly causing contempt, may soon lead to admiration and respect. In sum, in the encounters that occur between the individual with a hand disability and society, both come to interpret the behavior of the other as intrusive and both at least initially feel tense and apprehensive. "Society" feels that the individual should keep to his place, while he feels that his freedom is being infringed upon.

A significant number of persons initially fail to use their impaired hands and may even conceal them in their pockets.[17] This behavior is usually transient but it may become permanent. One important precipitating factor is appearance, as stressed above. Another frequently important factor is the experience of unpleasant sensations or the lack of it. Often, even after a reconstructive surgical procedure has been carried out, the individual will unconsciously avoid the use of his painful hand. The same behavior may be displayed by individuals who, enduring sensory changes, describe their hands as feeling "funny," "creepy," "like cardboard," and the like.

Every individual has his value systems and beliefs which are commonly shared with members of his social group. Among them are stereotyped beliefs called prejudices. A patient's reaction to the social disapproval he might be subject to depends on (1) his personal assets and emotional strength, including his remaining physical resources, friends and family and ability to manage with decreased social approval, and (2) the degree to which he shares societal prejudice toward disabilities. He may feel discriminated against by others or think he is being stared at or treated with derision. Feelings such as these are at times nothing more than distortions produced by the individual in an attempt to deny his own repressed prejudices which he directs against himself. In his attempt he projects his feelings of low self-worth and prejudices by unconsciously disowning them and attributing them to others.

Typically a person who suffers a sudden hand disability from illness or trauma experiences real and threatened losses. In response, he goes through the phases of grief well described by Lindeman[16] and Engel[9]—an initial phase of denial or disbelief, a second phase of increased conscious awareness of the losses and a third phase of restitution. In the first phase the individual unconsciously avoids facing up to his disabilities and potential losses. His disavowal of reality may last from a few seconds or minutes to hours or days. It is followed by the second phase of increased conscious awareness, with all the attendant emotional upheaval characterized by intense sadness, apprehension, helplessness,[13] despair and anger. This second phase may last from a few weeks to many months during which he is almost totally absorbed by his losses and their detrimental consequences. At one point the individual no longer attempts to hold onto his former body image and self-concept and begins to devalue what he lost. He then gradually enters the third phase of resolution during which he not only devalues his loss but also upgrades his assets and potential until eventually he comes to feel comfortable with himself and society. This phase may also last from a few weeks to a few months.

Patients with hand impairments are of course confronted with psychosocial difficulties similar to those of patients with other types of physical disabilities. Nevertheless, a hand disability is more difficult to deny than most others, such as those internally located, i.e. a lung abscess or a mitral stenosis or those peripherally located, such as scoliosis of the spine or a facial nerve palsy. It is this writer's opinion that no other disability, regardless of its location, combines as potently factors that undermine the ability to deny as does the disabled hand because of its visibility, its capacity to interfere with functioning, and because it feels.

In reconstructive hand surgery the surgeon's goal is to restore hand function and cosmesis. Factors significant to treatment results are severity and type of disability, viability of remaining tissues and surgeon's skills. However, important as these are, often they are outweighed by psychosocial issues in determining treatment outcome. The practice of reconstructive hand surgery requires that the surgeon have a more thorough knowledge of his patient than at one time was felt necessary. This need for a more intimate knowledge of the patient has become more pressing in recent times with the rising expectations (all too often unrealistic) of modern society and the increasing tendency of patients to express their grievances and dissatisfactions with treatment outcome by resorting to legal means to obtain reparation.

Variables such as socioeconomic status, work, and particularly personality[6] factors such as intelligence, cognitive style, motivation and mechanisms of defense may have an inordinate influence on the choices and decisions made in the rehabilitation of the patient with a disabled hand. Surgery must be tailored to the patient's needs, job, hobbies, sports activities and other pursuits. Since such activities and occupations vary from person to person, when a reconstructive procedure is to be carried out and choices must be made as to the functions retained and sacrificed, those that the affected individual values most in facilitating and supporting his major activities, interests and life-style must be retained.

The same considerations apply where the trade-off to be made is not between activities, or functions, but between appearance and function. Obviously in making these choices the patient should be well informed of the alternatives available and, together with his family and surgeon, should actively participate in the decision in which his value system, beliefs and idiosyncracies will be reflected. The information given must be tailored to each particular patient, taking into account his defensive maneuvers and cognitive style, for what may be fitting for one person may not be for another with similar disabilities and circumstances. An unsophisticated individual will grasp clear yet simple explanations, whereas a more informed person may require a detailed and complete report on his hand disability, its severity, prognosis, appropriateness of possible goals and plan of treatment. In this manner his understanding is augmented, and in turn leads to his increased participation and cooperation.

Although in the management of any illness or disability it is important to gain a patient's cooperation, it is particularly significant in the management of an impaired hand. The treatment of a hand disability is typically slow, boring, tedious and painful, requiring considerable stamina and staying power on the part of the patient. Yet sometimes in spite of the best efforts of all those concerned, the result falls short of expectations. In consequence the hand surgeon must involve himself to a greater extent than he normally would in motivating, supporting and actively seeking his patient's cooperation.[20] Often he will be compelled to ensure that his client follow home exercises, make office visits regularly and not get unduly discouraged if he is to effect the best possible results of the reconstructive procedure. Needless to say the closer the patient, his family and attending staff are in their assessment of the existing degree of disability, its potential disruptive consequences and the goals to be achieved, the more favorable the prospects are for cooperative, trusting and reasonable behavior on the part of the patient, and for a satisfactory outcome from surgery. Such an outcome is facilitated by the team approach in which, led by the hand surgeon, skilled physiotherapists, occupational therapists, nurses, social workers and psychiatrists or psychologists work harmoniously, providing guidance, sympathetic support and recognition for the patient's efforts and minor gains in the face of the conflicts and frustrations arising from the disability.

The second phase of grief is the most critical as far as the adaptational outcome is concerned, since it commonly determines the success or failure of rehabilitative activities regardless of the excellence of the surgical procedure utilized and efforts employed. Where a person emerges from his emotional turmoil in a bitter, paranoid or regressed state, it is likely that this behavior will become firmly established, particularly if years have elapsed since the intense internal turmoil receded. Individuals with hand disabilities who settle into coping with their conflicts by resorting to maladaptive behavior are difficult to motivate and steer toward potentially beneficial vocational goals and social ventures. It is only when the individual is in a state of emotional upheaval, when his defensive and adaptive processes are in a state of flux, that he is amenable to external influence, receptive to guidance and to the potential goals and solutions offered. Consequently, the surgeon and staff must weigh carefully any decision to postpone surgical, vocational (returning to work or seeking a new job) or social (visiting friends or public places) goals until the individual's grief has receded, for then it may be too late to bring about the psychological changes in attitude needed for good adaptation. Therefore, even more than with many physical disabilities, timing in introducing new ideas and goals in a patient with a hand disability is of utmost importance if optimal results are to be achieved.

The accurate assessment along the course of treatment of the patient's capacity to assimilate and effectively utilize new information and therapeutic efforts, in spite of the pain involved, is critical. This is best gauged by observing the amount of sadness, anxiety and regression shown when new information is gradually and gently introduced. Janis[14] ably demonstrated that a moderate amount of anxiety before a surgical procedure prepares and facilitates a better postoperative performance by patients. The surgeon and staff must introduce anxiety-producing facts along the course of treatment to the extent that they mobilize the patient into effective rehabilitative action. Too little anxiety may permit him to avoid dealing with important issues concerning his care and too much anxiety may lead to his feeling overwhelmed, disrupting his coping capacities and the learning of new ways and skills.

The individual must be assisted in becoming increasingly cognizant that not only have changes in the appearance and functioning of his hand occurred but also that because of those changes he has deviated from standards set by society and will therefore be treated differently than heretofore. Compelled by the loss of his impaired hand and its consequences, the individual must reassess his views of himself, his world and his mode of relating to it. Not only the disability itself but also any new appendages, such as prosthetic devices, that facilitate functioning or improve cosmesis must be integrated into the new body image and self-construct. The patient must recognize that to achieve vocational goals and satisfy social needs he may have to use alternate means and strategies than those used until the onset of disability.[5]

The fact that a person has to publicly expose his disabled hand may hamper his adaptation in that he may feel self-conscious and his performance may be impaired. However he may come to gain security and satisfaction if supported and encouraged to increasingly expose himself to social situations in which he not only faces whatever scorn is directed to him but in addition makes increasing use of his affected hand in his interaction with others, e.g. shaking hands. Thus, if he neither indiscriminately yields to all social demands and rejections nor attempts in a global fashion to repudiate them, he will more readily act according to his assets, skills and social opportunities. In this manner he comes to accept that he is different and his social milieu comes to accept his being different also. In developing new means to cope he comes to integrate and accept his physical and functional changes into his body image, and adjusts his self-concept to the new realities by making the required changes in his life-style.

References

1. Agulera, D.C.: Relationship between physical contact and verbal interaction between nurses and patients. J. Psychiatr. Nurs., 5:5, 1967.
2. Burton, M.: *The Sixth Sense of Animals.* Ballantine Books, New York, 1974.
3. Campbell, B.: The evolution of the human hand. In: *Man in Adaptation: The Biosocial Background* (Cohen Y.A., Ed.). Aldine Publishing Co., Chicago, 1974.
4. Carmichael, L., Robert, S. and Wessel, J.: A study of the judgement of manual expressions as presented in still and motion pictures. Soc. Psychol., 8:115, 1937.

5. Coelho, B.V., Hamburg, D.A. and Adams, J.E.: *Coping and Adaptation.* Basic Books, New York, 1974.
6. Cone, J. and Hueston, J.T.: Psychological aspects of hand injury. Med. J. Aust., 1:04, 1974.
7. Ekman, P.: Nonverbal leakage and clues to deception. Psychiatry, 32:88, 1969.
8. Ekman, P. and Friesen, W.V.: *Unmasking the Face: A Guide to Recognizing Emotions from Facial Expressions.* Prentice Hall, Englewood Cliffs, 1975.
9. Engel, G.L.: *Psychological Development in Health and Disease.* W.B. Saunders, Philadelphia, 1967.
10. Goffman, E.: *Stigma: Notes on the Management of Spoiled Identity.* Prentice Hall, Englewood Cliffs, 1963.
11. Harlow, H.F.: The nature of love. Am. Psychol., 13:673, 1958.
12. Kahn, S. and Mithalal, H.: Nonsurgical aspects of surgery of hand. N.Y. State J. Med., 72:2201, 1972.
13. Knorr, N.J. and Edgerton, M.T.: Hand injuries: Psychiatric considerations. South Med. J., 64:1328, 1971.
14. Janis, I.L.: *Psychological Stress.* John Wiley & Sons, New York, 1958.
15. Legge, D., Ed.: *Skills.* Penguin Books, Baltimore, 1970.
16. Lindemann, E.: Symptomatology and management of acute grief. Am. J. Psychiatr., 101:141, 1944.
17. McCash, C.R.: Cosmetic aspects of hand surgery. Hand, 1:67, 1969.
18. Piaget, J.: *The Origins of Intelligence in Children* (Cook, M., Trans.). Basic Books, New York, 1952.
19. Scheflen, A.E. and Scheflen, A.: *Body Language and Social Order: Communication as Behavioral Control.* Prentice-Hall, Englewood Cliffs, 1972.
20. Schenov, I.M.: Cited in Ruch, C., and Patton, H.D.: *Psysiology and Biophysics* 19th ed. W.B. Saunders, Philadelphia, 1965.
21. Sherrington, C.: *Man and his Nature,* 2nd ed. Doubleday, Garden City, 1953.
22. Stoner, E.K.: Functional evaluation of the upper extremity. In: *Handbook of Physical Medicine and Rehabilitation* (Krusen, F.H., Ed.), W.B. Saunders, Philadelphia, 1968.

30 Considerations in Wound Healing

Trauma to an organism results in tissue disruption and the creation of a wound which initiates in an undefined manner a series of complex processes collectively known as wound healing. Ideally the end-result of healing should be regeneration, that is, the repaired tissue should duplicate in form, substance, and function similiar uninjured tissue. Regeneration of tissue following wounding occurs in lower animal forms. Unfortunately, with the evolution of man into a complex organism, regeneration is confined to simple tissues such as epithelium, fat and connective tissues. Compound tissues in humans heal not by regeneration but by repair. The major component of this repair is a rigid scar which unites wound edges but is otherwise nonfunctional and in many instances actually inhibits the normal function of the tissue it binds.

Processes of Wound Healing

Wound healing can be divided for convenience into three major processes: epithelialization, repair and regeneration of non-epithelial tissue and wound contraction. These processes occur to some extent in all compound wounds, though obviously not to the same degree in a wound closed primarily as in one allowed to close by granulation and contraction. Epithelialization occurs only when an epithelial surface has been injured.

Epithelialization

Normal epithelium regenerates at a slow rate in order continually to replace those cells which mature, keratinize and are shed. Mitotic activity required for regeneration seems to be under the control of a hormone which acts as an inhibitor. It appears to be a glycoprotein synthesized in the epithelium and complexed to epinephrine. It has not been isolated and purified. Larger amounts are present in the superficial layers of the epidermis than in the basal layers where mitosis ordinarily occurs.

After wounding, the inhibitory effect of the hormone is lost, and basal cells within 1 to 2 mm of the wound begin to undergo mitosis. A thin, single layer of newly created epithelial cells migrates as a syncytium over the wound edges. Even if a wound has been carefully repaired with sutures, migrating epithelial cells can be seen to enter the incision from each edge and continue to advance until they reach like cells. Epithelial cells secrete fibrinolysins which allow them to dissolve fibrin and advance beneath the dehydrated clot or scab. Once the syncytium ceases to move and epithelialization is complete, the new epithelium undergoes mitotic activity and thickens. The thickness approximates that of uninjured epithelium; however, normal rete pegs do not develop nor is a firm bond to the underlying dermis formed.

Wound epithelium, while histologically resembling its normal counterpart, is not as serviceable to the organism as the latter. If the newly created epithelium covers only scar tissue, its functional integrity is in constant jeopardy. Even minor injuries result in significant epithelial loss and the creation of more scar. Of greater importance is that this recurring stimulus for epithelialization over the course of time may cause uncontrollable mitotic activity and even result in the development of squamous cell carcinomas.

Repair and Regeneration of Non-epithelial Tissue

The second major component of wound healing, repair and regeneration of the connective tissue, has, by custom, been divided into three phases, each with several descriptive names; they are (1) substrate or inflammatory, (2) proliferative or fibroblastic and (3) maturation or absorptive. While the events which occur in each of these phases have been elucidated, their division into phases is somewhat arbitrary and temporally imprecise. Events in the repair stage are comparable for all types of tissue. Certain tissues such as bone and nerve will then undergo modifications which are necessary for them to perform their specialized functions. A discussion of these modifications is beyond the scope of this chapter.

SUBSTRATE PHASE

The substrate or inflammatory phase begins immediately after wounding and lasts for 3 to 5 days. Vascular channels which have been interrupted by the injury thrombose to limit loss of intravascular volume, also causing local wound ischemia. Surrounding vessels and lymphatics in proximity to the wound dilate. Protein-rich fluid containing albumin and fibrinogen enters the wound. Tissue oncotic pressure increases because of the increased protein content and fluid shifts into the wound, promoting edema and causing even more ischemia. The end-result of this ischemia is to produce a hypoxic, hypercarbic and acidotic wound environment which continues for approximately 7 to 10 days. The fibrinogen which enters develops into a clot which soon becomes dehydrated and forms a scab.

Cellular elements, neutrophils, lymphocytes, and monocytes enter the wound at the same time and in proportion to their intravascular concentrations. Thus, granulocytes are the most numerous type and, although lymphocytes and monocytes are present, they are difficult to discern until the granulocytes undergo lysis.

The primary function of neutrophils in wound healing appears to be the release of lysozymes which contain proteolytic enzymes including collagenases. These enzymes lyse debris in preparation for phagocytosis by mononuclear cells, macrophages, which also phagocytize lysed fibrin and necrotic neutrophils. Lymphocytes have not yet been found to play an active role in acute inflammation. In chronic inflammatory situations, when a foreign body is retained, the lymphocytes probably have an immunological function.

PROLIFERATIVE PHASE

The second phase of connective tissue repair usually begins 2 to 3 days after wounding, and lasts for 2 to 3 weeks. Its onset is heralded by the appearance of fibroblasts in the wound. Most investigators are of the opinion that wound fibroblasts develop from adult cells indigenous to the local area which dedifferentiate into fibroblasts as a response to tissue injury. Their number increases rapidly by mitosis and they become organized into a syncytium. The syncytium migrates in ameba-like fashion across the surface of the wound using the fibrin scaffolding as a guide. Fibroblasts exhibit contact inhibition. Upon contacting a like cell, they change direction and migrate to areas devoid of fibroblasts until the wound has been covered.

Capillary buds develop behind the fibroblast syncytium and follow it to the center of the wound. These buds bring to the wound not only a source of nutrition but also fibrinolysins which help digest and lyse the fibrin clot. Capillary buds are a prominent feature of healthy granulation tissue and account for its red color.

Fibroblasts synthesize and secrete collagen and ground substance, the major components of scar tissue. Collagens are a class of glycoproteins. Four types have been identified and each is tissue specific. Differences between them are due to the type of amino acids present, their concentration, and/or the configuration of the helical chain created. In an attempt to illustrate collagen synthesis, production of Type I will be discussed.

The synthesis of collagen begins when the nuclear DNA of the fibroblasts passes on a coded sequential amino acid message to messenger RNA. The messenger RNA leaves the nucleus and enters the cytoplasm, migrating toward the endoplasmic reticulum. The coded message is then passed to a soluble RNA molecule, and a polypeptide chain, the basic subunit of collagen, is formed, which consists of approximately 1,000 amino acids. Many different amino acids are present in the polypeptide chain and repetition of several of these is characteristic of the collagen molecule. Those amino acids which are repetitive and common to the collagen subunit are glycine, proline, hydroxyproline, alanine and lysine. The amino acids are arranged into variable sequences; however, repetition of two of these sequences, glycine-proline-hydroxyproline and glycine-proline-alanine, is another characteristic of the collagen molecule. Cystine, formerly thought to be absent from the collagen molecule, is present in Type III and Type IV collagen.

A vital step in the production of mature collagen is the hydroxylation of proline and lysine. Without hydroxyproline, the collagen molecule cannot be extruded from the fibroblast. It has been observed that hydroxylation of proline occurs when an amino acid subunit, glycine-proline-proline, undergoes a chemical reaction with the enzyme protocollagen hydroxylase in the presence of the necessary cofactors; molecular oxygen, alpha-ketoglutarate, ascorbic acid and molecular iron. Hydroxylation of proline occurs after the formation of the polypeptide chain. Incorporation of exogenously administered hydroxyproline into the polypeptide chain does not occur. Hydroxyproline is not present in significant amounts in tissue other than newly created scar and is thus useful as an indicator of collagen production.

Once the polypeptide chain is complete, it passes or is extruded extracellularly and aggregates on the cell membrane with other chains. The primary structure of the peptide chains varies in different types of connective tissue and probably accounts for different structural requirements. Three compatible chains then form covalent cross-links, and a triple-stranded right-handed helix known as tropocollagen results. In addition to collagen, fibroblasts also synthesize ground substance, consisting chiefly of mucopolysaccharides, during the second phase of wound healing. At least seven distinct mucopolysaccharides are manufactured: chondroitin, chondroitin-4-sulfate, chondroitin-6-sulfate, dermatin sulfate, heparin sulfate, keratin sulfate and hyaluronic acid. Mucopolysaccharides are complex organic molecules with repeating basic units of hexosamine, uronic acid, galactose, and 6-sulfoglucosamine. Specific mucopolysaccharides are present in high concentrations in certain tissues, and it is believed that they are responsible for the characteristics of the collagen in that particular tissue. It is thought that they determine collagen fibril size and functional capacity and participate in cross-linking reactions. For example, large amounts of chondroitin sulfate are found in the large collagen fibers of tendons, while the cornea, with its finer collagen fiber content, has a high concentration of keratin sulfate. After injury and repair of a tissue the concentrations of tissue-specific mucopolysaccharides in that tissue are lower than normal and in some instances not present at all.

MATURATION PHASE

The third phase of connective tissue repair usually commences between the second and fourth week after injury. The most important characteristic of this phase is the maturation of the newly synthesized collagen, resulting in increased tensile and breaking strength of the wound. In addition, macrophages and fibroblasts disappear and capillaries become less numerous. This maturation process continues over the next 5 to 6 months; however, the strength of the wound never reaches prewounding levels. Healed fascia has approximately 80 per cent of the breaking strength of uninjured fascia.

Maturation of collagen is due in large part to intra- and intermolecular cross-linking of the collagen. This occurs by the formation of hydrostatic, electrovalent and covalent bonds and of mucopolysaccharide complexes. It is also due to mechanical stresses which act on the wound and aid in altering the architecture of the molecule. Electron microscopy of the nascent collagen reveals it to be an amorphous mass of fibrils. As maturation occurs, collagen becomes organized into large, regular fibers the appearance of which more closely resembles normal, unwounded collagen.

During the early part of the third phase of connective tissue repair, collagen production remains elevated yet the collagen content of the wound decreases. This seemingly paradoxical situation was clarified in 1962 with the discovery of a compound capable of degrading collagen and thus named collagenase. In the healing wound, collagenase activity resides primarily in the newly proliferated epithelium and granulation tissue, but also to some degree in the mesenchyme. Experimental studies suggest that the epithelium is somehow responsible for inducing collagenolytic activity in the mesenchyme.

It has been postulated that hyaluronidase and/or other glycolytics are necessary to break the mucopolysaccharide collagen bond before collagenases can degrade the collagen. The altered molecule is then susceptible to the activity of a collagenase which splits the collagen into two fragments. One fragment contains three fourths of the molecule and the other one fourth. Lacking normal integrity, the collagen fragments are solubilized and denatured by heat into randomly coiled gelatin polypeptides which are then phagocytized.

Wound Contraction

The third major component of wound healing is a process known as contraction. It is not to be confused with contracture, an undesirable result of contraction which occurs across tissues the dimensions of which alter with motion. Wound contraction in certain areas of the body, such as the back, abdomen and fingertip, can be a highly desirable adjunct to wound healing. Most investigators in the field of wound healing agree that contraction is an active process which depends upon the integrity of viable fibroblasts. Gabbiani and associates[9] have demonstrated that wound fibroblasts under the electron microscope resemble smooth muscle cells. They have thus renamed these cells myofibroblasts. Granulation tissue from healing wounds is contractile and this property can be inhibited by smooth muscle antagonists, a fact which lends credence to their hypothesis. The myofibroblast has also been identified in the contracted bands of Dupuytren's fasciitis and in contracted intrinsic muscles damaged by ischemia.

Contraction can also be inhibited if granulation tissue is prevented from forming. Corticosteroids and irradiation both inhibit the formation of granulation tissue and therefore contraction. The process can be inhibited by skin grafts, but does not stop immediately as suggested by some authors. If this were the case, skin grafts placed on a granulating bed would remain smooth and unwrinkled, which they unfortunately do not. Furthermore, the skin graft itself, in all probability, carries to the wound new fibroblasts which undoubtedly partake in the contracting process.

Factors Affecting Wound Healing

Although there are still a great many unanswered basic questions in wound healing, our attention as clinicians should be directed toward presently controllable factors which can either adversely or favorably affect the process. Much of the voluminous surgical literature on this subject lacks scientific merit and is unconvincing to the critical reader. Anecdotal reports of powders or liquids sprinkled into, pastes smeared on, and various other physical and chemical manipulations of the wound in subjective uncontrolled clinical settings do little to increase our knowledge. There are, however, well-documented local systemic and environmental factors which do affect wound healing.

There is little doubt that excess debris, foreign bodies, and necrotic tissue present in a wound can adversely affect wound healing by prolonging the first phase of wound repair. Surgical debridement should be performed to aid this natural cleansing process. Reliance on chemical antibacterial agents to cleanse wounds of contaminated debris and microscopic organisms is not desirable. Branemark, in an excellent study,[2] has demonstrated that most of these agents are in fact toxic to cells and result in even more debris which must be removed in the inflammatory phase of repair. Irrigation of the wound with sterile saline is safer and probably just as effective in reducing bacterial contaminants as the more toxic antibacterial agents.

Exogenous nutritional factors are of great importance to the successful outcome of wound healing. Plasma protein levels do not correlate well with healing, and mild to moderate hypoproteinemia seems to have little effect on the process. Severe protein depletion, as occurs in an acute loss of 20 per cent or more of the body weight, and marked chronic protein depletion result in decreased fibroplasia and retard healing. Amino acids are the vital building blocks of collagen production. Animal investigations suggest that a single amino acid, methionine, is lacking in protein-depleted states and its replacement will correct the defect. Methionine is a sulfur-containing essential amino acid which may provide bonding sites during the cross-linking of collagen. It is also converted to cysteine, which is important for Type III and Type IV collagen production.

The earliest known nutritional disturbance of wound healing was the discovery that lack of vitamin C results in scurvy and poor wound healing. Scurvy not only retards healing of new wounds but can also cause disruption of older wounds. Subsequent studies demonstrated that lack of vitamin C prevents the hydroxylation of proline and subsequent formation of collagen, while degradation of collagen continues. Disruption of old wounds in scurvy is caused by the continuing collagen metabolism which exists in a wound even after it appears to be clinically healed. Vitamin C is not stored or manufactured by the human body; thus it is sound surgical practice to give postoperative patients supplemental vitamin C. The deleterious effects of excessive ascorbic acid administration have not been substantiated.

In experimental animals, vitamin A has been shown to be of importance in epithelial repair. Studies in humans suggest a similiar function. It has been postulated that vitamin A antagonizes the adverse effects on the wound of endogenous or exogenous corticosteroids and thus may also exert an effect on the wound other than its effect on epithelial regeneration.

Zinc levels below 100 mg/ml have been associated with poor healing. The reason for this is unknown, but zinc-deficient wounds develop atrophic granulation tissue. Administration of 220 mg of zinc sulfate per day adequately replaces the missing element. Contrary to earlier reports, supplemental zinc administered locally or systemically in a patient without demonstrable deficiency does not accelerate wound healing.

The local metabolic state of a wound is comparable to the effect of shock at the cellular level. There is no doubt that injury produces ischemia, which then results in diminished Po_2 levels, increased Pco_2 levels and an acidotic milieu. Cleanly incised surgical wounds heal well in spite of this environment. Infected wounds and chronic wounds where tissue Po_2 levels are probably even lower may fail to heal optimally because of acidosis. Increased delivery of oxygen to the local wound by increasing arterial Po_2 is said to be helpful in furthering the healing process. Continuous oxygen delivery by mask or nasal prongs in concentrations of 8 to 10 liters per minute increases arterial and tissue Po_2. These methods increase the local wound Po_2 without the potential dangers inherent in the use of hyperbaric oxygen.

Anemia has been incriminated as a major factor in retardation of wound healing. Experimental evidence suggests that this is untrue unless the hematocrit levels are in the range of 15 per cent or less. Clinically, the patient with chronic renal failure is usually quite anemic and yet his wounds heal following renal transplantation. Most of the early reports which claimed that anemia retarded healing did not recognize that their experimental models were also hypovolemic. Normovolemic animals that are anemic heal wounds normally. Subsequent studies have demonstrated that hypovolemia results in reduced arterial Po_2 and, as a consequence, tissue Po_2. Correction of the hypovolemia alone increases arterial and tissue Po_2 and normal wound healing providing the anemia is not too severe (hematocrit $<$ 15 per cent).

Temperature is another environmental factor which may affect healing. In experimental animals wounds heal better if the animals are kept in a controlled temperature of 30 to 32° C. Cold has an adverse affect on wound healing, perhaps as a result of its causing vasoconstriction and/or sludging of the blood. Denervation and the subsequent vasodilatation which develop abolish the adverse effects of cold. A positive interrelated effect of temperature and blood supply can be inferred from the fact that wounds of the head and neck region, with their increased blood supply and warmth, heal faster than those of the extremities or trunk.

Chronic corticosteroid administration adversely affects wound healing. It has been suggested that endogenous steroid released following severe trauma may also have this effect. Corticosteroids reduce inflammation and fibroplasia with a consequent decrease in collagen and mucopolysaccharide production if given during the first 3 days after wounding, but not thereafter. On the other hand, they will impair contraction if given any time after a wound has been created. Corticosteroids may also activate collagenase systems or possess inherent collagenolytic properties, as suggested by their effects on keloids.

Excessive Wound Healing

In addition to problems of inadequate and delayed wound healing, physicians and surgeons are forced to deal with the end-results of excessive wound healing. The most common example of this type of healing is a hypertrophic or keloid scar of the skin. While a great deal of effort has been expended to differentiate the two on the basis of histopathology, the distinction is best made in clinical and chemical terms. Clinically, keloids are immature scars which extend beyond the borders of the original wound and do not decrease in size over prolonged periods of time. Hypertrophic scars are usually confined to the original wound and decrease somewhat in extent as they mature over the course of several months to one year. Recent evidence suggests that both keloids and hypertrophic scars have an increased amount of metabolic and biochemical activity. Ketcham et al.[15] have shown that hydroxyproline formation and collagenase activity in both of these scars is much greater than in normal scars. Metabolic activity within the keloid is much greater than in hypertrophic scar. It would appear, then, that in keloids and hypertrophic scars collagen production and degradation are increased compared to normal scars. Since the end-result of this is an excess of scar, it can be inferred that the net effect is an increase in wound collagen. The collagen in these scars is more soluble and disorganized than that in normal scar.

Current therapy of keloids and hypertrophic scars is based on the effect of corticosteroids on collagen production and degradation, as outlined earlier. Intralesional injections of steroid in the proper dosage decrease collagen production and in all likelihood increase its degradation, possibly by activation of collagenase. A helpful adjunct in the treatment of keloids and hypertrophic scars has been the use of direct pressure against the scar by elastic stockings and sponge rubber pads for prolonged periods of time. Presumably this helps mechanically to align the collagen into a more normal pattern.

While keloids and hypertrophic scars are pathological states characterized by excessive scar formation, they represent relatively minor problems for which an acceptable solution is available. On the other hand, excessive scar formation in deep tissues, such as stenosis of a vessel following its repair or adherence of a tendon to its surroundings following repair, are more serious problems for which no good solution is currently available.

Technical Causes of Excessive Scar

Prior to discussing theoretical possiblities of scar control, a review of technical factors which cause excessive scar production and are currently controllable by the surgeon is in order. An appropriate example to utilize for this discussion is a traumatic wound of the hand involving skin, subcutaneous tissue, fascia and tendon. Immediately after injury protein-rich fluid enters the wound milieu, as in any wound. If the hand is allowed to rest in a dependent position or in an ill-fitting sling with the elbow acutely flexed, a much greater amount of protein-rich edema fluid enters the hand. The edema plus the pain from the original injury cause the patient to hold his hand immobile and in a non-functional position of comfort. The wrist is frequently flexed, the metacarpophalangeal joint slightly hyperextended, and the proximal and distal interphalangeal joints also flexed. The ligaments about these joints contract and shorten. The development of flexion deformities is promoted by the position of comfort. Bacterial infection is a distinct possibility in this situation because of the relative ischemia already present, the pabulum created by proteinaceous fluid, and the introduction of foreign bodies and bacteria at the time of the original injury. If an infection supervenes, even more edema will develop. The subsequent wound healing will inevitably involve not only the primary wound but the other collagen-containing structures in the hand—tendons, ligaments and fascia. If allowed to remain immobile in a non-functional position, deposition of collagen will cement the formerly mobile connective tissue of the hand into a fixed non-functional attitude (Fig. 30-1).

The hand surgeon should vigorously attempt to control the development of edema by resting the injured hand in a position above the level of the heart. Judicious surgical debridement and cleansing are helpful adjuncts to the natural debriding process which occurs in the inflammatory phase of wound healing. Gentle, atraumatic handling of tissue in wound repair is essential. The use of splints to maintain proper positioning and rest of the extremity is helpful. Early motion of uninjured mobile structures is essential to prevent their incorporation in the fibrotic process and to aid in the relief of congestion.

In our hypothetical wound, if primary tendon repair has been undertaken, it is obviously desirable for a dense rigid scar to develop between the tendon ends but just as obviously undesirable to have such a scar exist between the tendon and its environs. Although it is possible by the use of silicone cylinders to isolate a tendon from its milieu and thus prevent adhesion, to do so also prevents healing of the repaired tendon. Vascular adhesions and granulation tissue form about tendon repairs as they do other wounds. Because functional tendons must be mobile, however, these same adhesions must develop into a mesotendon-like structure in time, which will allow gliding and yet continue to supply blood to the tendons. This is certainly a remarkable phenomenon when it occurs and a frustrating disaster when it does not.

EDEMA AND PAIN
↓
DECREASED MOBILITY
↓
COLLAGEN DEPOSITION AND SCAR CONTRACTURE
↓
STIFF NON-FUNCTIONAL HAND

Figure 30-1. *Etiology of the stiff hand.*

Manipulation of Scar Formation

Can scar be manipulated to modify its undesirable characteristics? Efforts to find a safe agent for this purpose have been as elusive as the search for the Holy Grail and equally unsuccessful. The ideal agent should be selective enough to allow repair of injured tissue, yet avoid the detrimental effects of excess or improperly distributed scar. Since the primary component of scar tissue is collagen, it would seem that our investigations should focus on alterations of the chemical or physical structure of this molecule. Three theoretical possibilities for this control exist: (1) decrease in collagen synthesis, (2) increase in collagen degradation and (3) prevention of cross-linking of collagen subunits.

DECREASE IN COLLAGEN SYNTHESIS

Synthesis of collagen by fibroblasts can be controlled presently. Fibroblasts are living cells which can be destroyed by cellular toxins and irradiation, but these modalities are too non-specific and toxic for practical use. Another possibility is to diminish collagen production, inhibiting specific hydroxylase enzymes and diminishing production of hydroxyproline and hydroxylysine or producing local wound scurvy. Proline analogs such as cis-4-hydroxyproline are chemical substances which are similar to proline and can be substituted for it in the basic collagen molecule. Once this has occurred, proline is not hydroxylated and the end-result is failure of normal collagen synthesis. Non-hydroxylated collagen is not extruded extracellularly and builds up, instead, within the fibroblasts. Although the efficacy of proline analogs in non-toxic doses to reduce adhesions and scar formation in animals has been suggested by some investigators, others deny this. Obviously, further research is needed to settle the issue.

COLLAGEN DEGRADATION

In 1962, Gross and associates[11] discovered a collagenolytic substance in tadpole tails. Since then, a great number of heretofore unsuspected collagenolytic systems have been discovered in normal and pathological human tissue and in lower animals. Knowledge of how they degrade collagen is accumulating and certainly the answer is far more complex than our earlier simplistic explanation. It is not yet clear, however, if there are many collagenases or multiple forms of collagenase. Little human collagenase is available at this time for study. Whether or not exogenous collagenases will prove to be practical or specific enough to act as adjuncts to natural wound collagenases in selectively modifying undesirable scar formation while allowing normal tissue repair is unanswered at this time.

PREVENTION OF COLLAGEN CROSS-LINKING

Amino nitriles are a class of compounds derived from a variety of legumes. In animals, these compounds cause connective tissue to lose its structural support and tensile strength, resulting in aneurysms and skeletal deformities. This condition is called lathyrism and, because of it, these compounds are also known as lathyrogens. The most commonly used member of the group is B-aminopropionitrile (BAPN). Penicillamine, a degradation product of penicillin, while not an amino nitrile, does have lathyrogenic properties. As a copper chelator it has a secondary effect of blocking the deamination of lysine that is effected by copper-containing monamine oxidases.

Lathyrogens exert their greatest affect on immature newly synthesized collagen. They interfere with the formation of aldehydes by inhibiting the enzyme lysyl oxidase. Aldehydes are important for the inter- and intramolecular cross-linking reactions which must occur if the collagen is to mature, become insoluble, and thereby develop increased tensile strength. Systemic administration of BAPN thus results in the formation of weak scar containing immature soluble collagen.

Peacock,[22] using BAPN, has produced lathyrism in a few humans, after first performing extensive laboratory animal studies. These patients had undergone tendon replacement and were treated with BAPN for 10 to 21 days following the procedure. All 6 patients developed good tendon gliding, but no controls were available for comparison. Unfortunately, transient side effects developed in all patients, including periportal hepatitis in 2. At this time the use of BAPN in humans is rigidly restricted by the FDA and it is not generally available for clinical use.

Potential for Scar Control

The potential for scar control is real and the answer lies within the possibilities mentioned.

While BAPN has not yet developed into the safe non-toxic panacea for scar control, it has not yet been discarded and further research with it continues, albeit in rigidly controlled studies. Exciting new developments in collagenase chemistry are promising. Hopefully purified and specific collagenases will soon be available. Substitution of analogs for essential elements in collagen production likewise continues to be a valid possibility for scar control. For the present, the clinician who understands and follows the basic wound healing principles as elucidated will provide his patients with optimal wound care. He will also provide himself with the experience and knowledge necessary to scientifically and objectively assess the effects of various new modalities on wound healing.

References

1. Blackburn, W.R. and Cosman, B.: Histologic basis of keloid and hypertrophic scar differentiation, Clinicopathologic correlation. Arch. Pathol., 82:65, 1966.
2. Branemark, P.I., Albrektsson, B., Lindstrom, J. and Lundborg, G.: Local tissue effects of wound disinfectants. Acta Chir. Scand., 357 (Suppl):166, 1966.
3. Brown, R.G., Sharma, V.D. and Young, L.G.: Connective tissue metabolism in swine: II. Influence of energy level and ascorbate supplementation on hydroxyproline excretion. Can. J. Anin. Sci., 51:439, 1971.
4. Conway, H., Gillette, R., Smith, J. and Findley, A.: Differential diagnosis of keloids and hypertrophic scars by tissue culture technique with notes on therapy of keloids by surgical excision and Decadron. Plast. Reconstr. Surg., 25:117, 1960.
5. Daly, J.M., Steiger, E., Prockop, D.J. and Dudrick, S.J.: Inhibition of collagen synthesis by the proline analogue cis-4-hydroxyproline. J. Surg. Res., 14:551, 1973.
6. Ehrlich, H.P. and Hunt, T.K.: Effects of cortisone and Vitamin A on wound healing. Ann. Surg., 167:324, 1968.
7. Elias, S. and Chvapil, M.: Zinc and wound healing in normal and chronically ill rats. J. Surg. Res., 15:59, 1973.
8. Gabbiani, G., Hirschell, B.J., Ryan, G.B., Statkov, P.R. and Majno, G.: Granulation tissue as a contractile organ: A study of structure and function. J. Exp. Med., 135:719, 1972.
9. Gabbiani, G., Ryan, G.B. and Majno, G.: Presence of modified fibroblasts in granulation tissue and their possible role in wound contraction. Experientia, 27:549, 1971.
10. Gabbiani, G. and Majno, G.: Dupuytren's contracture: Fibroblast contraction? An ultrastructural study. Am. J. Pathol., 66:131, 1972.
11. Gross, J.: Specific degradation of the collagen molecule by tadpole collagenolytic enzyme. Proc. Natl. Acad. Surg., 55:417, 1966.
12. Harris, E., Jr., and Krane, S.: Collagenases. N. Engl. J. Med., 291:557,605,652, 1974.
13. Hunt, T.K. and Zederfeldt, B.: Nutritional and environmental aspects in wound healing. In: *Repair and Regeneration. The Scientific Basis for Surgical Practice.* (Dunphy, J.E. and Van Winkle, W., Jr., Eds.). McGraw-Hill, New York, 1969.
14. Ketchum, L.D., Smith, J., Robinson, D.W. and Masters, F.W.: Treatment of hypertrophic scars, keloids, and scar contracture by triamcinolone acetonide. Plast. Reconstr. Surg., 38:209, 1966.
15. Ketchum, L.D., Cohen, I.K. and Masters, F.W.: Hypertrophic scars and keloids. Plast. Reconstr. Surg., 53:140, 1974.
16. Kim, Z. and Rosenthal, S.: The effect of orally administered zinc sulfate on healing incised wounds. J. Surg. Research. 10:597, 1970.
17. Larson, D.L., Aliston, S., Evans, E.B., Dobrokovsky, M. and Linaris, H.A.: Techniques for decreasing scar formation and contractures in the burn patient. J. Trauma, 11:807, 1971.
18. Madden, J.W., Morton, D. Jr., and Peacock, E.E., Jr.: Contraction of experimental wounds I. Inhibiting wound contraction using a topical smooth muscle antagonist. Surgery, 76:8, 1974.
19. Madden, J.W., Carlson, E.C. and Hines, J.: Presence of modified fibroblasts in ischemic contracture of the intrinsic musculature of the hand. Surg. Gynecol. Obstet., 140:509, 1975.
20. Miller, S.H., Wood, A.M., Larson, L.G. and Edsmyr, F.: Keloids—Treatment by surgery and irradiation: A preliminary report. Unpublished observations.
21. Ninikoski, J., Hunt, T.K. and Dunphy, J.E.: Oxygen supply in healing tissue. Am. J. Surg., 123:247, 1972.
22. Peacock, E.E., Jr., and Madden, J.W.: Some studies on the effect of B-aminopropionitrile on collagen in healing wounds. Surgery, 60:7, 1966.
23. Peacock, E.E., Jr., and Van Winkle, W.V., Jr.: *Wound Repair.* W.B. Saunders, Philadelphia, 1976.
24. Thornton, P.A.: Vitamin D ascorbic acid association in bone metabolism. In: *Third European Symposium on Calcium and Tissues* (Fleisch, H., Blackwood, H.J.J. and Owen, M., Eds.). Springer Verlag, Berlin, 1966.

Index

Page numbers in *italics* indicate figures; those followed by t indicate tables.

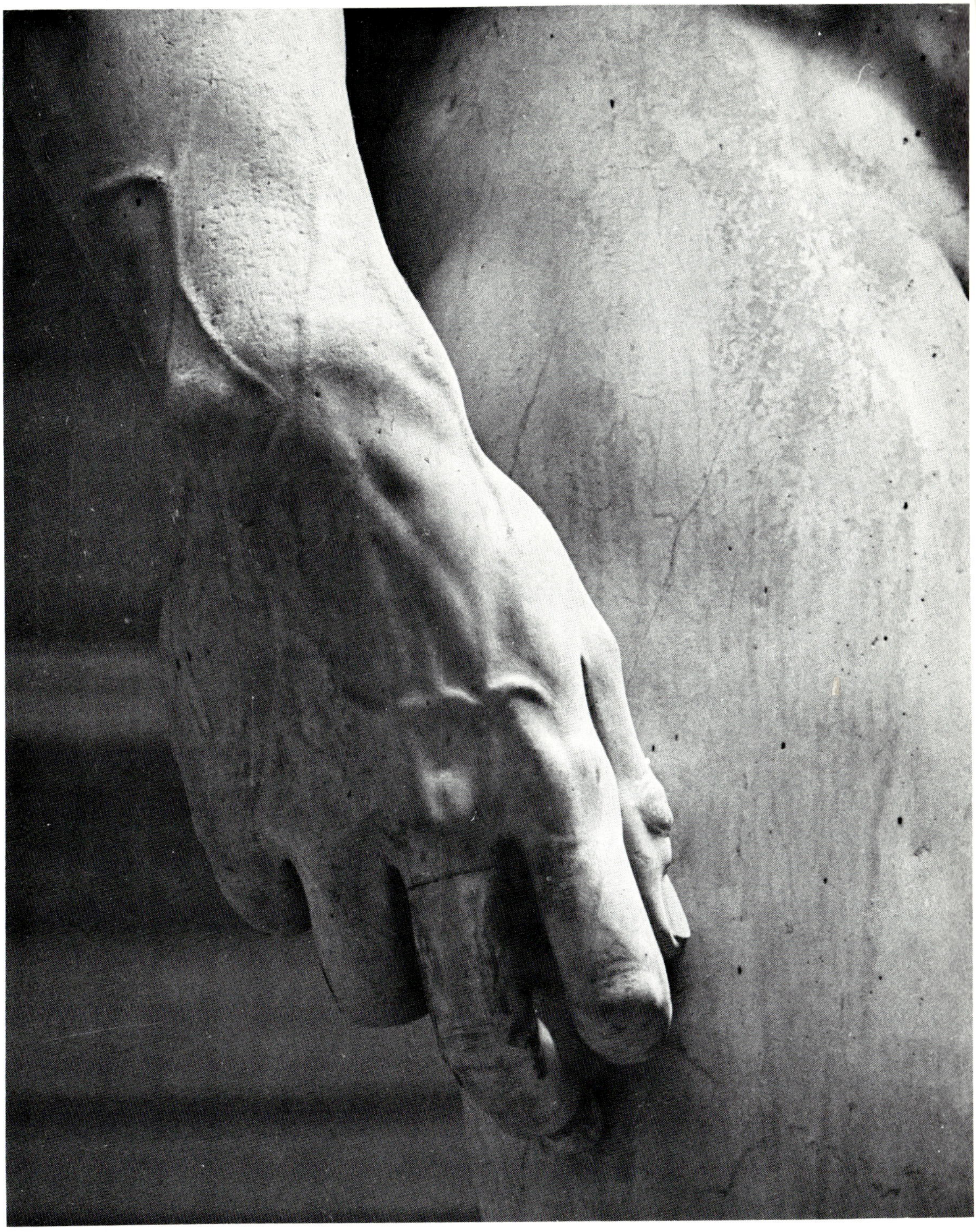

The Hand of David by Michelangelo

THE HAND

Surgical and Non-surgical Management